AF846188

Suffering and Bioethics

Suffering and Bioethics

Edited by Ronald M. Green
and
Nathan J. Palpant

OXFORD
UNIVERSITY PRESS

OXFORD
UNIVERSITY PRESS

Oxford University Press is a department of the University of Oxford. It furthers the University's objective of excellence in research, scholarship, and education by publishing worldwide.

Oxford New York
Auckland Cape Town Dar es Salaam Hong Kong Karachi
Kuala Lumpur Madrid Melbourne Mexico City Nairobi
New Delhi Shanghai Taipei Toronto

With offices in
Argentina Austria Brazil Chile Czech Republic France Greece
Guatemala Hungary Italy Japan Poland Portugal Singapore
South Korea Switzerland Thailand Turkey Ukraine Vietnam

Oxford is a registered trademark of Oxford University Press in the UK and certain other countries.

Published in the United States of America by
Oxford University Press
198 Madison Avenue, New York, NY 10016

© Oxford University Press 2014

All rights reserved. No part of this publication may be reproduced, stored in a retrieval system, or transmitted, in any form or by any means, without the prior permission in writing of Oxford University Press, or as expressly permitted by law, by license, or under terms agreed with the appropriate reproduction rights organization. Inquiries concerning reproduction outside the scope of the above should be sent to the Rights Department, Oxford University Press, at the address above.

You must not circulate this work in any other form
and you must impose this same condition on any acquirer.

Library of Congress Cataloging-in-Publication Data

Suffering and bioethics / edited by Ronald M. Green and Nathan J. Palpant.
p. ; cm.
ISBN 978–0–19–992617–6 (hardcover : alk. paper)
I. Green, Ronald Michael, editor of compilation. II. Palpant, Nathan J., 1979– editor of compilation.
[DNLM: 1. Bioethical Issues. 2. Pain. 3. Stress, Psychological. WB 60]
R724
174.2—dc23 2014005108

9 8 7 6 5 4 3 2
Printed in the United States of America
on acid-free paper

CONTENTS

PART SIX Concluding Thoughts

FOREWORD

Suffering and the Human Condition

Daniel Callahan

I can imagine nothing more fitting than to have this wonderfully rich collection on suffering open with a paper by Eric J. Cassell. Along with Leon R. Kass, Paul Ramsey, Hans Jonas, Alex Capron, and a few others, Eric was part of a group we organized at The Hastings Center in the late 1970s on death, a topic as ancient as suffering. Eric made his mark by distinguishing between pain and suffering, a distinction that everyone now takes for granted but that was not made in the early days of bioethics or medicine more generally. And what a difference it made, opening the door to the reality and complexity of suffering as a basic part of the human condition, and unavoidable in the care of the sick.

Physicians have almost always been able to relieve pain, if not wholly to abolish it, usually with opiates. Not so with the relief of suffering, often an altogether harder problem to grapple with. Why is that? My surmise is that while pain merely afflicts the body, suffering—which comes in many vexing and torturous ways—afflicts the human spirit, often forcing us to question life itself. Pain, of course, hurts and can be a misery in its own right, but if it is too deep and persistent, it shifts over to suffering, making us sorry we are even alive, a condition no opiate can effectively or more than momentarily relieve.

Partially because of my long-standing interests in cost control, technology, and the stance of medicine toward death, suffering is a thread that connects all three of those interests. Is there a duty for society to use medicine to relieve all physical and mental suffering (as a 1947 World Health Organization health study contended), and, if so, are there any economic limits that may have to be set to this venture, an idea many find abhorrent? Are there moral limits to the relief of suffering, a debate at the heart of the debate about euthanasia and physician-assisted suicide? Many dying patients suffer from an overwhelming fear of death: Is it wrong for their physicians to evade telling the truth and to inspire false hopes?

Fortunately, authors of Forewords are not required to answer their own questions, so I will not indulge myself. But here is one I will take a stab at: Just what kind of problem is suffering? The variety of ways human beings can suffer, almost uncountable, forces a confrontation with that question. Our body can make us suffer, as can our mind, our emotions, our careless, wayward desires and actions, and, of course, our fellow human beings, deliberately with war at one end of a spectrum or simply hurting our feelings at the other. Suffering in the history of love, romance, courtship, and marriage could fill a library of books, poems, and plays. The sexual revolution may be new, but the attendant emotional suffering that seems often to accompany it seems as old as human nature.

But at the core of suffering, I believe, is the puzzle about whether it is simply a problem to be solved and open to rational solutions, or a mystery to be at best endured, open to amelioration, but never to be eliminated. The Enlightenment tradition and the science that goes with it (especially in modern medicine) treat it as a problem, an effort full of hopes, possibilities, and upward progress. The much older religious traditions, and particularly the Judeo-Christian forms, see it more as a mystery, with the Old Testament story of the travails of Job and his wrestling with God telling a story as ancient as it is ever new.

I have no religious beliefs, but I am drawn to thinking about suffering as a mystery, not just a problem. I like definition number two of "mystery" in my old 1958 *American College Dictionary*: "Any affair, thing, or person that presents features or points so obscure as to arouse curiosity or speculation." It is the words "thing" and "obscure" that seem to me just right. If a "thing" is something real, then anyone who has suffered and has witnessed the suffering of others cannot doubt its reality. And if generation after generation of theologians and religious believers have tried to understand it but have been unable to achieve a consensus on the meaning of suffering, or to plumb its depths to the bottom, that suggests an enduring mystery of an obscure kind. As for the Enlightenment tradition, much younger in age, it does not seem to be doing much better.

But both traditions embrace the need to find some kind of hope in the face of suffering: the religious traditions in their belief that a good God or some spiritual force can make sense of it all in a way that only the faithful can share, and the naturalist tradition in its conviction that, with faith in reason and science, progress can be made in cutting through the obscurity. Many people these days I suspect have a foot in both camps, holding on in some fashion to their religious beliefs and the enduring mystery of suffering that it has always sought to understand—but hoping as well that reason will find ways to reduce the proclivity of humans to make war against each other and maybe, through medical research, to find a cure for cancer and Alzheimer's disease.

This collection of papers on suffering makes a unique and welcome contribution. Despite the work of Cassell and a few others, suffering is a neglected topic in bioethics, a word often invoked but rarely analyzed. That omission has occurred in great part because modern medicine is dominated by scientific methods and assumptions. Suffering is treated as an enemy to be conquered, not to be understood. Too often, moreover, some complex human realities with a long history of reflection fall outside of the methods and purview of science, in the alleged "softer," less empirical domains of religion and philosophy. Many physicians over the years have told me of their intense discomfort when patients ask them why they are suffering, what is the meaning of their suffering, and why medicine can't help them, if they must, accept and live with it. There are no good technical medical answers to questions of that kind. For many physicians, their reflex response is to call in the chaplain or social worker to handle such matters.

But why has bioethics also failed to take it on with any depth and persistence? My judgment is that bioethics in general has had a proclivity to take a procedural and policy approach to ethical problems and dilemmas, in the process bracketing questions of substance; and that is the case with suffering. One reason for the bracketing is that the substantive issues are deep and controverted, just the kind that pluralistic societies try avoid because they are often controversial and socially divisive. The meaning and place of suffering—pushed to the sidelines—makes a perfect case study in the thinness of policy and procedural tactics. I have my own favorite list of topics that have been avoided: the meaning and place of death in life and medicine, not just in advance directives; the value and scope of dignity as a way of understanding the value of human life; and the meaning and scope of progress, a core value of modern medicine, but apparently too sacred to be analyzed, much less questioned. This is not to say that nothing has been written about those problems. It is only to say that they are treated as secondary.

This book goes a long, long way to bring suffering to center stage in bioethics, to treat it in all of its substantive richness from a variety of religious, philosophical, and secular perspectives. That combination takes account of the reality of disagreement and the plurality of different approaches, but it does so by wrestling with suffering as a problem that pluralism as a value cannot wholly manage. I would hope, then, that this collection will serve as a model for bioethics, showing the centrality of substantive concepts and human realities, focusing on questions of ends and not just means.

It is not just that clinical, bedside ethics needs this kind of analysis, to help doctors and other health care workers understand the suffering of patients and their own difficulties in dealing with it, but that medicine understood more broadly as a scientific enterprise needs this corrective as well. As modern medicine moves more and more into the realm of chronic illness, where costs are high and suffering is often technologically drawn out, the topic cannot be avoided. Chronic diseases that cannot be cured, and whose only final outcome is death, are now becoming the heartland of medicine, not the whole story by any means, but a reality that cannot be evaded.

LIST OF CONTRIBUTORS

Joseph A. Amato, PhD, is Professor of History and Dean of Rural and Regional History, Southwest State, Marshall, MN. A prolific writer, Amato has written essays on suffering and values, death and dying, aging, heart surgery, and ethics. In addition to cultural histories (*Dust: A History of the Small and Invisible*, 2000, which won the *Los Angeles Times* Best Nonfiction of 2000, and *On Foot: A Cultural History of Walking*, 2004), he most recently wrote *Surfaces: A History* (2013).

Roberto Andorno, LLM, SJD, is Research Fellow at the School of Law of the University of Zurich, Switzerland. Between 1998 and 2005, he served as a member of the UNESCO International Bioethics Committee. He has published extensively on issues at the interface of bioethics and human rights, including *Bioética y Dignidad de la Persona* (Madrid: Tecnos, 2012) and *Principles of International Biolaw* (Brussels: Bruylant, 2013).

Cristiana Baffone received her MA in Philosophy from the University of Bologna (Italy), did a Diploma in Bioethics at the Centro de Investigación Social Avanzada (Mexico), and is currently a Master's student in Health Sciences at the University of Lucerne, Switzerland. She is board member of the review of Philosophy, *Diogene Magazine* (Italy). In 2011, the Dean of the Bologna University awarded her a prize as one of the best students of the University.

Jane C. Ballantyne, MD, FRCA, is Professor of Anesthesiology and Pain Medicine, University of Washington, Seattle. She is a pain management specialist, involved in the development of innovative pain management tools using rapid learning technology. Professor Ballantyne is recipient of the Alan Sharp Research Award, Oxford University, and the Will Solimene Award for excellence in medical communication given by the American Medical Writers Association.

Roberta M. Berry, JD, PhD, is Associate Professor of Public Policy at Georgia Institute of Technology and Professor of Science and Technology Law, Policy, and Ethics at Georgia State University College of Law. Dr. Berry's research focuses on bioethics, health law and policy, and the legal, ethical, and policy implications of bioscience and biotechnology research and innovation. Her publications include *The Ethics of Genetic Engineering* (Routledge, Annals of Bioethics, 2007).

She has served as principal investigator for a National Science Foundation grant on ethics education, and co-principal investigator for a National Institutes of Health grant on translational science and research ethics.

Lisa Sowle Cahill, PhD, is the J. Donald Monan Professor of Theology, Boston College. She is the author or editor of fifteen books, and more than 200 scholarly articles and chapters, in theological ethics, bioethics, feminist ethics, and the ethics of war and peace. She is a member of the American Academy of Arts and Sciences, and a past President of the Society of Christian Ethics and the Catholic Theological Society of America.

Daniel Callahan was a cofounder of The Hastings Center and is now its President Emeritus. The author or editor of 41 books, his research and writing have covered a wide range of issues, from the beginning until the end of life. In recent years, he has focused his attention on ethics and health policy.

Eric J. Cassell, MD, is a member of the Institute of Medicine of the National Academy of Sciences and a Master of the American College of Physicians. He was a member from 1997 to 2001 of the President's National Bioethics Advisory Commission. Cassell has written extensively about moral problems in medicine, the care of the dying, and the nature of suffering. He is the author of *The Healer's Art, The Place of the Humanities in Medicine, Changing Values in Medicine,* two volumes on doctor– patient communication entitled *Talking with Patients, Doctoring: The Nature of Primary Care Medicine,* and *The Nature of Suffering,* now in its second edition. His most recent book is *The Nature of Healing: The Modern Practice of Medicine*.

Mark J. Cherry, PhD, is the Dr. Patricia A. Hayes Professor in Applied Ethics and Professor of Philosophy, St. Edward's University, Austin, Texas. He is author of *Kidney for Sale by Owner: Human Organs, Transplantation and the Market* (Georgetown University Press) as well as numerous articles, book chapters, and other publications. He is Editor of *The Journal of Medicine and Philosophy* (Oxford University Press), Associate Senior Editor of *Christian Bioethics* (Oxford University Press), and Editor-in-Chief of *HealthCare Ethics Forum* (Springer).

Jean Decety (PhD in Neurobiology) is Irving B. Harris Professor of Psychology and Psychiatry at the University of Chicago. He is a leading scholar on the social neuroscience of empathy, morality, and prosocial behavior, as well as other topics related to the neurobiological underpinnings of social cognition. His work has led to new understandings of empathy, affective processes, and moral decision making in typically developing individuals as well as psychopaths. His research uses neuroimaging techniques (functional MRI and high-density EEG) and genetics to examine how biological and social factors interact in contributing to empathy and the motivation to care for the well-being of others. Dr. Decety is the President of the Society for Social Neuroscience. He recently edited the *Oxford Handbook of Social Neuroscience* (2011) and *Empathy from Bench to Bedside* (2012).

David DeGrazia, PhD, is Professor of Philosophy at George Washington University and Senior Research Fellow in the Department of Bioethics, National Institutes of Health. His books include *Taking Animals Seriously* (Cambridge University Press, 1996), *Human Identity and Bioethics* (Cambridge University Press, 2005), and *Creation Ethics: Reproduction, Genetics, and Quality of Life* (Oxford University Press, 2012). DeGrazia's articles have appeared in such journals as *Philosophy and Public Affairs, The Hastings Center Report, Bioethics*, and *The Philosophical Forum*.

H. Tristram Engelhardt Jr., MD, PhD, is Professor in the Department of Philosophy, Rice University, and Professor Emeritus in the Department of Medicine and in the Department of Community Medicine, Baylor College of Medicine. Dr. Engelhardt is senior editor of the *Journal of Medicine and Philosophy, Christian Bioethics*, the Philosophy and Medicine book series with more than one hundred ten volumes in print, and the book series Philosophical Studies in Contemporary Culture. He has authored more than three hundred eighty articles and chapters of books. His books include *Bioethics and Secular Humanism: The Search for a Common Morality* (Philadelphia: Trinity Press International, 1991), and the second, thoroughly revised edition of *The Foundations of Bioethics* (New York: Oxford University Press, 1996). His most recent book is *The Foundations of Christian Bioethics* (Salem, MA: Scrivener Publishing, 2000). Recent edited volumes include *Global Bioethics: The Collapse of Consensus* (Scrivener, 2006), *The Philosophy of Medicine Reborn* (Notre Dame, 2008), *Innovation and the Pharmaceutical Industry* (Scrivener, 2008), and *Bioethics Critically Reconsidered* (Dordrecht: Springer, 2012).

Ronald M. Green, PhD, is The Eunice and Julian Cohen Professor for the Study of Ethics and Human Values in the Department of Religion, Dartmouth College, Hanover, New Hampshire. He is the author of nine books, including *The Human Embryo Research Debates: Bioethics in the Vortex of Controversy* (Oxford University Press, 2001) and *Babies by Design: The Ethics of Genetic Choice* (Yale University Press, 2007), and more than 160 articles in theoretical, applied, and professional ethics, many with a special focus on bioethics. In 2005, Professor Green was named a Guggenheim Fellow.

Daniel B. Hinshaw, MD, is professor of surgery at the University of Michigan, consultant in palliative medicine in the University of Michigan Geriatrics Center and VA Ann Arbor Health Care System, Ann Arbor, Michigan, and visiting professor of palliative care at St. Vladimir's Orthodox Theological Seminary in Yonkers, New York. Dr. Hinshaw's research interests have ranged from the basic mechanisms of cell injury and death to complementary therapies and spirituality in palliative care. He is the author of more than eighty-five scientific articles and chapters. SVS Press published his first book, *Suffering and the Nature of Healing*, in August 2013.

Barry Hoffmaster, MA (Public Affairs) and PhD (Philosophy), is Professor in the Department of Philosophy at the University of Western Ontario. He teaches and works in bioethics and philosophy of law, and he currently is collaborating with Cliff Hooker on a project called "Re-Reasoning Ethics," which recognizes that judgment pervades bioethics and our lives and provides an account of how judgment can be rational. He is an elected Fellow of The Hastings Center and a past President of the Canadian Bioethics Society.

Catherine Q. Howe, MD, PhD, is Assistant Professor at the University of Washington, Department of Psychiatry and Behavioral Sciences. Dr. Howe does outpatient consultation-liaison psychiatry in the areas of chronic pain and psycho-oncology.

Peter D. Jacobson, JD, MPH, is Professor of Health Law and Policy, and Director, Center for Law, Ethics, and Health, at the University of Michigan School of Public Health. Jacobson's research focuses on the role of the courts in shaping health and public health policy. Jacobson is Associate Editor for Health Law and Public Health at the *Journal of Health Politics, Policy and Law*, and recently served as President of the Public Health Law Association.

Daniel Krashin, MD, is Acting Assistant Professor in the Departments of Psychiatry and Pain and Anesthesia at the University of Washington. He has done research and published in the fields of pharmacological and behavioral treatments of pain, HIV treatment, somatic treatments of psychiatric illness, and the history of medicine.

Paul Lauritzen, PhD, is Professor of Religious Ethics at John Carroll University. He is the author of five books, most recently, *The Ethics of Interrogation: Professional Responsibility in an Age of Terror*. He has held the Paul E. McKeever Chair in Moral Theology at St. John's University and the Brady Distinguished Visiting Faculty Chair at Northwestern University.

Karen Lebacqz, PhD, is the Robert Gordon Sproul Professor of Theological Ethics, emerita, at Pacific School of Religion in the Graduate Theological Union, Berkeley. Author or coauthor of some eight books and dozens of articles, her specialties include bioethics, theories of justice, feminist ethics, and professional ethics. She is a former member of the National Commission for the Protection of Human Subjects of Biomedical and Behavioral Research and has served as Bioethicist in Residence at Yale University.

Mary Anderlik Majumder, JD, PhD, is an associate professor of medicine with the Center for Medical Ethics and Health Policy at Baylor College of Medicine,

Houston, Texas, and Co-Director of The Methodist Hospital System Biomedical Ethics Program. Professor Majumder's research interests include ethics consultation; ethical and policy questions related to problems of cost, quality, and access in health care; the ethical and social implications of new technologies; and the intersection of religion and spirituality and biomedical ethics.

Gordon D. Marino is Professor of Philosophy and Director of the Hong Kierkegaard Library at St. Olaf College. He has been a lecturer in bioethics at the University of Florida Medical School, is Editor of *Ethics: The Essential Writings* (Modern Library Classics), and, in 2003, was the recipient of the Richard J. Davis award for writing on ethics and the law. In addition to his scholarly work on Kierkegaard, Marino's writings have appeared in the *New York Times, Atlantic Monthly, Newsweek, Wall Street Journal*, and other periodicals.

Susan E. Marino, PhD, is Assistant Professor Experimental and Clinical Pharmacology and Director of the Center for Clinical and Cognitive Neuropharmacology at the University of Minnesota. With undergraduate training in philosophy and psychology, and a PhD from the University of Pennsylvania in behavioral neuroscience, Dr. Marino has published widely in academic journals and has received major National Institutes of Health funding for her interdisciplinary approach to the study of drug effects on neurocognition.

Natalia Murinova, MD, MHA, is Clinical Professor of Neurology and Co-Director of the Headache Clinic at the University of Washington. She has done research and published in the fields of headache medicine, behavioral pain management, telemedicine, and bioethics.

Nathan J. Palpant, PhD, is Acting Instructor in the Department of Pathology at the University of Washington, Institute for Stem Cell and Regenerative Medicine. His scientific work focuses on developmental fate choices and therapeutic applications of lateral plate mesoderm derivatives. Dr. Palpant's work in bioethics has focused on the translational implications of nuclease-mediated genetic engineering and human embryonic stem cells. He is coeditor of *Human Dignity and Bioethics: From Worldviews to the Public Square* (Routledge, Annals of Bioethics, 2013).

Abdulaziz Sachedina, PhD, is Professor and IIIT Chair in Islamic Studies at George Mason University in Fairfax, Virginia. Dr. Sachedina, who has studied in India, Iraq, Iran, and Canada, obtained his PhD from the University of Toronto. He has been conducting research and writing in the field of Islamic Law, Ethics, and Theology (Sunni and Shiite) for more than two decades. In the past ten years, he has concentrated on social and political ethics, including Interfaith and Intrafaith Relations, Islamic Biomedical Ethics, and Islam and Human Rights. Dr. Sachedina's publications include *The Islamic Roots of Democratic Pluralism* (Oxford University Press, 2002), *Islamic*

Biomedical Ethics: Theory and Application (Oxford University Press, February 2009), and *Islam and the Challenge of Human Rights* (Oxford University Press, September 2009), in addition to numerous articles in academic journals.

Jens Schlieter, PhD, is Professor for Theory of Religion at the Institute for Science of Religion and Director of the Center for Global Studies, University of Berne, Switzerland. His work comprises contributions on methodological and theoretical questions concerning the study of religion, on Buddhist ethics and bioethics, and on comparative philosophy.

Margaret Somerville, AuA (pharm), DCL, is Samuel Gale Professor of Law, Professor in the Faculty of Medicine, and Founding Director of the Centre for Medicine, Ethics and Law at McGill University, Montreal. She has an extensive national and international publishing and speaking record and is a frequent commentator on social-ethical-legal issues in all forms of media. She delivered the nationally broadcast CBC 2006 Massey Lectures, published as the book, *The Ethical Imagination: Journeys of the Human Spirit* (Anansi, 2006). Professor Somerville has received many honors and awards including the Order of Australia and eight honorary doctorates and is a Fellow of the Royal Society of Canada. In 2003, she was chosen by an international jury as the first recipient of the UNESCO Avicenna Prize for Ethics in Science.

Marisa P. Weisel, MPH, is a Research Associate at the University of Michigan School of Public Health in the Department of Health Management and Policy and in the Department of Health Behavior and Health Education. Her work is in the field of public health advocacy, and her research focuses on public health policy and regulation. Ms. Weisel also studies implementation of the Affordable Care Act at Federally Qualified Health Centers.

Laurie Zoloth, PhD, a Charles Deering McCormick Professor of Teaching Excellence, is Founding Director of the Brady Program in Ethics and Civic Life at Weinberg College of Arts and Sciences at Northwestern University, where she also teaches in the Medical Humanities and Bioethics Program and in the Jewish Studies program and is Professor of Religious Studies. She has served as President of the American Society for Bioethics and Humanities and the American Academy of Religion. Her book, *Health Care and The Ethics of Encounter*, on justice, health policy, and the ethics of community, was published in 1999. She is also coeditor of four books, *Notes from a Narrow Ridge: Religion and Bioethics*, with Dena Davis; *Margin of Error: The Ethics of Mistakes in Medicine*, with Susan Rubin; *The Human Embryonic Stem Cell Debate: Ethics, Religion and Policy*, with Karen LeBacqz and Suzanne Holland; and *Oncofertility: Ethical, Legal, Social and Medical Perspectives,* published in 2010, with Teresa Woodruff, Lisa Campo-Edelstein, and Sarah Rodriquez.

Suffering and Bioethics: An Introduction to the Volume

Ronald M. Green and Nathan J. Palpant

Beaune, France, has at its center the beautifully restored Hôtel-Dieu, a hospice established in 1443 by a local noble family as a hospital for the poor and the needy. Comfortable beds line the hospice's walls. A dedicated core of nursing nuns worked long hours to comfort those for whom death was usually imminent. Although many other Hôtel-Dieus across France and Europe later evolved into modern hospital centers, the hospice of Beaune reveals the original impulse behind much of Western medicine. Disease could only rarely be cured, and death could not easily be put off. The immediate goal was the relief of suffering through merciful acts and the presence of caregivers who cared.

Despite its precedence in medicine, attention to the relief of patients' suffering has often taken a back seat in modern biomedical research and treatment. To suffering's many forms—epidemics, premature death, painful disease conditions, and prolonged dying—there seemed one obvious response today: increase research on disease and its causes, and translate this research as soon as possible into effective clinical therapies.

Modern bioethics, too, has been slow to come to terms with suffering. As Barry Hoffmaster observes in this volume, "Suffering is largely foreign territory for bioethics, medically and morally."[1] In the world of bioethics, attention to ethical quandaries or the philosophical analysis of hard medical choices has sometimes displaced attention to patients' experience and its implications for the training and conduct of researchers and clinicians. This is not to say that bioethics is uninformed by the reality and weight of suffering. In fact, modern bioethics was born in engagement with the question of whether there are limits to the biomedical eradication of suffering, a question raised by the cruel experiments of the Nazi era. Although some Nazi researchers and doctors were motivated by little more than sadism and professional ambition, their cruel and inhuman research was often justified in terms of the relief of suffering. "A few would have to suffer so that the many, the Volk, could forever be cleansed of ancient maladies." Faced with such reasoning, the Nuremberg code and other charter documents of biomedical ethics introduced other values to offset any single-minded attention to minimizing suffering.

Foremost among these was the insistence on autonomy and free, informed consent to research and treatments. Subsequent developments have widened and deepened the range of values competing with suffering in the bioethical program and have revealed new conflicts. For example, does the relief of suffering now justify the subordination of patient autonomy, as some advocates of involuntary or nonvoluntary euthanasia argue? Does autonomy itself became a source of suffering, as when patients reject treatments or palliative measures that their physicians and caregivers deem advisable?

Recent literature reveals an increase in the number of conflicting inclinations when it comes to the obligation for modern medicine to alleviate suffering as a goal *in itself*. In response to new medical possibilities in the areas of genetic manipulation, nanotechnology, and pharmacology, transhumanist ideologies have pushed for the advancement of science at all fronts, believing that "human dignity" requires transcending the "limitations" of our current body and mind. Some transhumanist scholars hold a negative utilitarian ethic, advocating that the strongest ethical mandate is the abolition of suffering among sentient beings. In contrast, other scholars, some of whom have drawn on religious perspectives, have asked whether the "relief of man's estate" should be the archetypal goal of medicine and science. These thinkers suggest that the use of science and technology in the alleviation of suffering can, in some cases, diminish our understanding of "human dignity" and what it means to be human. During the first decade of this century, these issues marked the work of the President's Council on Bioethics and stirred debate between the Council and its critics. Today, we are a long way from the hospice of Beaune, where the meaning of suffering was clear and widely understood and where the extent of the obligation to relieve suffering was straightforward.

Understanding the role of suffering in moral decision making is a more complicated matter than ever, requiring rigorous academic attention at multiple levels. The aim of this book is to undertake a new foray into this "foreign territory." It is organized to examine suffering in depth, in its biological, psychological, and clinical dimensions, and in many of the ways its concept and reality influence bioethical decision making.

Part One: The Nature, Meaning, and Experience of Suffering

The first section of the volume begins with an essay, "Suffering and Human Dignity," by Eric J. Cassell that takes us back to his landmark 1991 book, *The Nature of Suffering and the Goals of Medicine*. Once again, Cassell affirms that suffering involves the disruption or destruction of a person's intactness or integrity, but he broadens this to place suffering in the context of threats to the patient's dignity. It would seem that new emphases on patient-centered care and personal medicine would intensify medicine's focus on patient suffering and dignity, but Cassell sees just the opposite occurring. Using a series of cases to illustrate his point, Cassell maintains that the growth of scientific medicine and a focus on objective data have reduced physicians' and other caregivers' attention to the patient before them and their ability to perceive this patient's suffering.

Following this, in "Understanding Suffering," Barry Hoffmaster reinforces Cassell's theme of medicine's neglect of suffering and extends it to the field of bioethics itself. Orthodox bioethics, Hoffmaster asserts, is impervious to suffering because it is "bedazzled by theory that subverts the richness of human experience." Hoffmaster believes that suffering results from profound loss that impairs a life. It becomes intolerable if the values lost cannot be redeemed by other values found in and through the experience of suffering. Using the cases of the biblical Job and the contemporary story of Dax Cowart, whose own encounter with suffering remains foundational for modern bioethics, Hoffmaster illustrates the potentially transformative role that suffering can play in an individual's life, a role that medical care and bioethics must not ignore. An emphasis on patient autonomy alone, as is the case in so many contemporary bioethical discussions, may actually harm a patient. The real value of autonomy, Hoffmaster maintains, lies not in simply being able to choose, but rather in being able to choose the good and avoid the bad. Suffering can play a role in informing that deeper value choice.

Susan and Gordon Marino's essay, "Paying Homage to the Silence of Suffering," continues this attention to the experiential dimensions of suffering and picks up the theme of the meaning of suffering for bioethics' cherished value, autonomy: "... severe, prolonged agony of the sort that disease and frequently the treatment of disease deliver incinerates our ability to communicate and, in the same stroke, robs us of a degree of agency."[2] The sheer incommunicability of severe suffering impedes caregivers' ability to assess the patient's condition and make reasoned treatment decisions. It can do the same thing to patients themselves, leading to the extreme of foregoing needed treatments or palliative alternatives. Drawing on Elaine Scarry's observation, the Marinos observe that suffering is often torture without a torturer.

Joseph A. Amato's "Suffering, and the Promise of a World without Pain" returns us to Hoffmaster's observation of the dual nature of suffering: its threat to values and its ability to affirm value. "Is suffering an intrusion or a gift? Is it of deep tragedy and an exchange with destiny and the gods?" Amato sketches a narrative history of Western culture, from its Greco-Roman roots, through the biblical traditions, and into post-Enlightenment civilization. Throughout this history, suffering has been seen not just as something to be avoided or minimized but also as something that creates, identifies, and affirms a civilization's deepest values. In this culture-creating role, self-inflicted suffering in the form of sacrifice has often been used "to secure rebirth; solidify and purify social orders of wrongs, crimes, and sins; and renew broken human and divine relations."[3] Amato acknowledges the power of the post-Enlightenment quest to reduce suffering through medical, scientific, and technological means, but he asks whether this may not be accomplished through the infliction of new and potent forms of suffering. "Medical dialogues," he concludes, "must walk the edge of identifying the suffering and pains to be negated and defeated and those to be acknowledged and left to exist and even embraced and reverenced."[4]

Part Two: Suffering in Biology

This section of the volume discusses the nature of suffering in the biology of sentient beings. It addresses fundamental questions of what kinds of species can suffer, how suffering manifests biologically, how suffering and pain differ, and how our understanding of the biology of pain has shaped our treatment of suffering and pain in clinical medicine.

We start with Jean Decety's "Social Neuroscience Meets Philosophy: Suffering, Empathy, and Moral Cognition," which draws on the findings of neuroscience and functional imaging technologies to develop our understanding of the links between sensitivity to suffering and the capacity for moral judgment. Decety observes that the long history of mammalian evolution, especially the role of parental care in these species, has shaped our brains to recognize and respond with care to signs of the suffering of others. These abilities also seem to be morally significant, with the perception of others' physical and social distress proving central to caregiving motivation and prosocial behaviors. Highlighting these points, Decety closes with an examination of the ways in which newer studies of psychopathy illustrate how lack of sensitivity to others' suffering contributes to a callous disregard for the welfare of others and amoral conduct.

Following this, "Biology of Suffering" by Daniel Krashin, Natalia Murinova, Catherine Q. Howe, and Jane C. Ballentyne moves us from the lived experience of suffering into an exploration of its underlying physiological and biological causes. Suffering must be distinguished from pain because not all pain causes significant suffering, and people can experience suffering from many causes. Both pain and suffering result from a complex interaction between sensors in the body and the brain, where these somatic signals are analyzed and understood. Psychiatric illnesses like major depression and post-traumatic stress disorder are equally complex, involving subtle changes in brain chemistry and systems that enable the body to manage stress, some of which are shaped by genetic inheritance. Psychiatric suffering also has a social aspect, with lack of social support having a direct effect on mental health. In severe suffering, all these factors work together. The authors observe that recent studies using functional imaging have revealed that the pain of social exclusion is felt in much the same way, using many of the same brain systems, as the pain of physical injury. Current biological research thus supports many of the insights offered by experiential accounts of suffering.

David DeGrazia's chapter utilizes insights derived from biology and neuroscience to address questions laden with ethical import: "What Is Suffering and

What Sorts of Beings Can Suffer?" The essay opens with a conceptual investigation of suffering and distinguishes broad and narrow conceptions. Suffering in the broad sense covers any experience that registers negatively for the subject just on account of how it feels. Suffering in the narrow sense is defined as a highly unpleasant emotional experience associated with significant pain or distress. In view of these definitions, DeGrazia then asks, what sort of beings can suffer? Dismissing as unreasonable theoretical positions that deny that animals are capable of consciousness, DeGrazia argues that there is a strong empirical case for the proposition that many animals, and not only mammals, are capable of suffering in both the broad and narrow senses of the term. The chapter concludes with a discussion of the implications of these arguments for bioethics, especially for the use of animals in biomedical research.

Part Three: Suffering in Policy and Law

This part examines the interactions between the experience of suffering and developments in the regulatory and legal arenas, with suffering often being a spur to reform but, sometimes as well, the consequence of specific legal or regulatory innovations. In the first essay in this part, Daniel B. Hinshaw, Peter D. Jacobson, and Marisa P. Weisel examine how "Individual and Social Callousness toward Human Suffering," notably in egregious research ethics violations like the Tuskegee syphilis experiment, have spurred the development of the vital research protections put in place in the United States following the Belmont Report. How can we explain the callousness to suffering, both here and abroad, that necessitated these reforms? The authors present various rationalizations that were used to justify this unconscionable research: "we had no choice; it was for their benefit; others created the problem; and scientific progress justified the behavior." Paradoxically, therefore, the relief of suffering was used to justify the deliberate imposition of suffering by physicians and researchers. Although Hinshaw, Jacobson, and Weisel applaud the regulatory structure that has grown out of these tragedies, they also argue that new cultural shifts, particularly in the area of palliative care, will be necessary for medical researchers, physicians, and caregivers to make the easing of suffering their highest priority.

In "Human Rights and the Moral Obligation to Alleviate Suffering," Roberto Andorno and Cristiana Baffone examine the human rights enterprise that has progressed since the Second World War as a social response to suffering. Their overall argument is that human rights norms are primarily focused on preventing the worst forms of human suffering. They observe that human rights theory traditionally paid little attention to the problem of suffering as such, which was usually regarded just as the implicit psychological underpinning of human rights concerns, but not as a legally relevant concept in itself. Only in the past few decades has greater awareness developed about the need to take pain and suffering more seriously and explicitly into account in the implementation of every human rights policy, including policies related to such issues as the involvement of physicians in harsh interrogation practices and the human right to medical care. Suffering, they contend, is the true parameter that determines the degree of urgency in the identification and implementation of human rights.

How should the law deal with suffering and how does it do so in relation to bioethical issues? This is the question posed by the Canadian ethicist and legal scholar Margaret Somerville in her essay, "Exploring Interactions between Pain, Suffering, and the Law." Somerville begins by discussing the 2010 extralegal development of the Declaration of Montreal. In establishing the principle that failure to provide fully adequate pain management is a breach of a person-in-pain's human rights, this Declaration highlights the positive role that attention to pain and suffering must have in a legal and ethical context. She develops the negative side, however, in an intensive engagement with the Carter case, a recent Canadian decision in which the words "suffer" and "suffering" appear 212 times. In Somerville's view, this case illustrates a perilous judicial tendency to equate suffering with the loss of dignity, and the loss of dignity with a loss of autonomy and self-determination. The consequence is that the relief of suffering comes to trump all other bioethical values, and thus the road to various forms of medical killing, including involuntary euthanasia, is paved. Such analysis, Somerville believes, ignores less tangible values than suffering, such as respect for human life. The risk in such privileging of the relief of suffering, she says, is a degradation of the "metaphysical ecosystem" of values and trust on which a humane bioethics and humane society depend.

Part Four: Religious Perspectives on Suffering and Medicine

Theologians and religious thinkers played an active role in the birth of modern bioethics. Their insights are crucial for the understanding of the relationship between suffering and the value of medicine and medical care. This part explores this relationship across a variety of religious traditions, beginning with Lisa Sowle Cahill's "Suffering: A Catholic Theological-Ethical View," which traces a deep tension or ambiguity in the body of relevant Catholic teachings. Although caregivers are urged to relieve suffering, Cahill notes that various teaching documents encourage patients to find meaning in suffering by identifying with Christ's suffering on the Cross. She believes this encouragement gives suffering a "redemptive meaning" and is theologically problematic for several reasons. It seems to make the suffering of human beings (Christ or others) desirable and pleasing to God. It reinforces the discredited theological idea that the whole point of Jesus' life was to suffer and die, rather than to proclaim the kingdom of God as a realm of compassion, love, and mercy. And it militates against the ability of Christian caregivers to offer holistic, humane care and companionship, within an assurance of God's love, as the best way to a meaningful life. Cahill believes that emergent emphasis on the alleviation of suffering through the provision of holistic care, along with a continuing distinction between intentional killing and allowing to die, provides the best expression of Catholic bioethics today.

H. Tristram Engelhardt's "The Orthodox Christian View of Suffering" also exposes a tension between religious efforts to provide "answers" to the problem of suffering that explain its presence in the world and the need to value and justify the relief of suffering through medical care and medical interventions. Because the Orthodox Christian appreciation of life, death, and suffering turns on the pursuit of salvation, says Engelhardt, its account is more homiletic than scholastic in tone compared with Western Christian, especially Roman Catholic, accounts. In Orthodoxy, he says, suffering does not discharge any temporal punishment due to sin, and it does not play a role in an economy of salvation, as has sometimes been true in Roman Catholicism. This means that suffering for Orthodox Christianity has no intrinsic value and is in fact disvalued, all things being equal. Suffering can gain positive value only insofar as it aids in leading to salvation through breaking our pride or serving as an occasion for repentance. Medicine is a gift of God, and its use is affirmed as long as a particular intervention is not a stumbling block to our spiritual lives. Like Catholicism, however, Orthodox teachings absolutely prohibit euthanasia and abortion

Karen Lebacqz's essay, "Redemptive Suffering Redeemed: A Protestant View of Suffering," directly challenges those traditions in religious ethics that see suffering as redemptive or that otherwise bestow intrinsic value on suffering in ways that limit medical efforts to reduce or alleviate it. According to Lebacqz, neither classical nor contemporary Protestants find the natural suffering that can accompany disease to be redemptive. Rather, the only suffering that is redemptive is that which is undertaken in the struggle for justice and human dignity. Drawing especially on the work of Martin Luther King Jr. and of Sharon Thornton, she argues that the category of redemptive suffering should be limited to suffering voluntarily undertaken in the face of a struggle to overcome oppression and to work for human rights and dignity. Because suffering itself is not redemptive, Protestants in the field of bioethics have a mandate to remove or reduce suffering to the extent possible, to stand in solidarity with those who suffer, to investigate and work to obviate social and political causes of suffering, and to avoid the temptation to deliberately choose suffering as a way of imitating Christ.

Laurie Zoloth's "Suffering: Reflections from the Jewish Tradition," addresses how the textual tradition of Jewish thought regards the problem of human suffering in theological and moral terms. The essay looks at the historical view of suffering, finally showing how one rabbinic text structures a response of "reversibility" between healer and patient. It ends with some suggestions for how an appreciation of the different voice that Judaism brings to ethics, in such matters as stem cell research and end-of-life care, may largely be because of its different (and largely negative) evaluation of suffering.

Of the Abrahamic traditions, Islam has sometimes displayed the greatest amount of tension between appreciations of the spiritual value suffering and the religious mandate to avoid and reduce suffering through medical care. In his "Human Suffering through Illness in the Context of Islamic Bioethics," Abdulaziz Sachedina traces the presence of both these motifs. On the one hand, he says, the Islamic approach to illness inculcates faith in God's goodness and an acceptance of suffering as part of the overall divine plan for humanity's spiritual and moral development. On the other, Islam has usually actively encouraged recourse to medical care and the development of medical institutions. The Qur'anic basis for the latter is a tradition that has the Prophet saying, "O servants of God, seek the cure, because God did not create a disease without creating its cure, except for one disease . . . senility."[5]

Jens Schlieter's "Endure, Adapt, or Overcome? The Concept of 'Suffering' in Buddhist Bioethics," follows with a comprehensive assessment of the implications of Buddhist teachings for the relationship between suffering and biomedicine. Of all the religious traditions examined here, Buddhism probably has the most penetrating analyses of suffering, tracing it not simply to present physiological or emotional states but also to a fundamental philosophical misunderstanding: the failure to realize that existence itself is suffering. Buddhist texts thus stress the central place pain and suffering have in the mental life of human beings, but, according to Schlieter, they nevertheless preserve a positive and optimistic commitment to combatting suffering on all levels: medical, psychological, and philosophical. What are the bioethical implications of this? Schlieter traces differing Buddhist views on the active relief of suffering at the end of life, whether through palliative care or suicide and euthanasia. Some thinkers, he observes, see karmic value in the improved state of mind and tranquility these measures might induce, whereas others see these measures as seeking to avoid the reality of suffering and even provoking greater suffering through their future karmic consequences. Schlieter explores similar tensions with respect to biomedical enhancement technologies, and he traces the complexity resulting from the relative priority given in different Buddhist teachings to intentions or deeds in the treatment of nascent human life.

This part closes with Mark J. Cherry's "Human Suffering and the Limits of Secular Bioethics," a broad and sharp indictment of much contemporary bioethical discourse. Cherry argues that to honestly face the challenges of human suffering in an age of life-sustaining therapy, one must first come to terms with human finitude, when confronted with the collapse of human abilities, suffering, and death. To provide a definitive response to such existential concerns, however, Cherry insists, requires a canonical morality, a binding moral standpoint from which to know truly the nature of the right, the good, and the virtuous. But secular bioethics today possesses no such definitive moral foundation, and secular reason cannot secure a single authoritative account of the characteristics of the appropriately flourishing human life. Instead, such matters are left to individual, potentially idiosyncratic, choice. As a result, Cherry concludes, all bioethical thinking today is set fully within the specific interests of particular persons, with secular bioethics routinely sanctioning unhampered access to nearly any medical means to satisfy individual life- and death-style choices.

Part Five: Suffering in the Ethics of Contemporary Medicine and Biotechnology

The extent of our obligation to relieve suffering has become a matter of debate in the development of new biomedical approaches and technologies. This part asks whether, with any given technology, there are morally required boundaries or extensions to our obligation to alleviate human suffering. Although it is not clear whether Paul Lauritzen would agree with Cherry's broad indictment of modern bioethics at the end of the previous section, in "Reproductive Technology in Suffering's Shadow" he offers a critical assessment of the medical enterprise as representing a limitless and morally questionable assault on suffering. Lauritzen highlights two serious dangers when infertility is approached largely as a matter of patient suffering: the medicalization of suffering and suffering's trivialization. What Lauritzen calls the "shadow side of medicalization" appears when we ask whether every case of involuntary childlessness is one that merits a medical response. Should the only check on what reproductive medicine provides be the desire of a patient who is suffering? When the answer to these questions is "yes," patients come to be seen as consumers, and medicine is treated as simply another marketplace commodity. It then becomes extremely difficult to evaluate and prioritize the sort of suffering that should have a moral claim on us. For example, in the effort to alleviate infertility, reproductive medicine has contributed to a major increase in the birth of twins and triplets and has precipitated the many medical and developmental problems associated with these multiple-gestation pregnancies. When patient suffering alone functions as a kind of currency in the commoditized world of medicine, says Lauritzen, then unqualified attention to suffering begets even newer and more threatening forms of suffering.

The two essays that conclude Part Five wrestle in different ways with the new philosophical, ethical, and medical questions raised by accelerating advances in genetics and their applications to both therapeutic and reproductive decision making (a biomedical region that some have labeled *reprogenetics*). Roberta M. Berry's "Genomic Information and Suffering in the Genomic Era" explores the implications of the fact that the generation of genomic information is often, at best, only a "halfway house" to the generation of cures and thus a source of unintended negative consequences. One problem is that genomic research can identify gene sequences associated with a disorder well before treatments are developed for the disorder. Another problem is that test results are often not definitive but only probabilistic. Genetic testing, therefore, sometimes unnecessarily exposes patients (and their blood relatives) to a host of harms, ranging from employment and insurance discrimination to personal stigmatization. At its worst, as in the case of Huntington's disease, testing becomes a new source of suffering in revealing dreaded but unpreventable health futures. Berry observes that a "simple account" sees the actors in this story—the scientists and technologists, public agencies that support their efforts, commercial entities that translate their efforts into deliverables, health care providers who deliver relief, and policy makers who guide the enterprise—as allied in the pursuit of knowledge for the relief of human suffering. While not denying the truth of this simple account, she points to a "more complex account" that involves such matters as the financial (and patent-driven) motivations of researchers and the companies that finance them. This complex account throws open to question—but may not invalidate—how much the relief of suffering results from genomic research.

Mary Anderlik Majumder's essay, "Preimplantation Genetic Diagnosis and the Prevention of Suffering" picks up where Berry leaves off, focusing on the procreational and reproductive implications of genomic interventions. As Majumder observes, this is an area marked by bioethical controversies, some of which revolve around the issue of suffering. Like euthanasia, preimplantation genetic diagnosis is regarded by some as problematic because it prevents suffering by eliminating the potential sufferer. The complex balancing of suffering and parental autonomy raises a further series of questions in this area. A memoir of parents of a child with osteogenesis imperfecta, a disorder that renders the child highly susceptible to broken bones, raises the question of how we balance suffering for a child and its parents against the positive aspects of the child's life and the joys of parenting. As Majumder says, this is a realm of experience in which we witness the "intertwined nature of suffering and joy." Similar questions are raised by the deliberate selection of a child with a disability, as when parents request medical assistance in having a deaf or short-statured child. Majumder closes with a look at the policy implications of these bioethical quandaries and offers a caution against premature legal prohibitions.

Part Six: Concluding Thoughts

This part offers the coeditors of this volume an opportunity to take stock of what has been accomplished and to indicate how they have been informed by all the discussions. The two do not always agree, and their disagreements rehearse many of the tensions that are evidenced throughout the essays in this book.

In "Suffering and Ethics in an Age of Empowerment," Nathan J. Palpant begins by supporting the shared view that suffering is intrinsically evil and its alleviation ought to be a high moral priority. However, because the alleviation of suffering is inherently only a prima facie duty, the core of his reflection centers on trying to understanding the limits to our obligation to alleviate suffering. He asserts that it is the misunderstanding of the limits to our obligation to alleviate suffering that can open us to callousness toward human suffering and undermine our sensitivity to discern those manifestations of suffering that absolutely and morally demand our intervention. He points out that our ethics about suffering are informed by two related matters. In the first place, we cannot know how to alleviate suffering unless we know the good we seek in its remediation. Second, the good we seek is integrally tied to the powers we choose to employ. It is the relationship between the goods we prioritize and the powers we use that markedly influences our ethical priorities about how to approach human suffering. Using psychotropic drugs as an example, Palpant addresses our proclivity to evaluate suffering in light of powers we are capable of, which puts at risk our sensitivity to the meaning of suffering in the human experience. In closing, Palpant outlines two ways that disorient our priorities about suffering in the human experience. First, there is significant moral risk around decisions made from the desire for circumstantial well-being in which suffering without malady is the currency of justification for intervention. Second, the powers we acquire in medicine and technology often define the goods we seek, and we ought instead to use the powers we are capable of to protect the goods we value and bring meaning to the human experience.

Ronald Green's "The Evil of Suffering" begins with the assertion that suffering is intrinsically bad. It is something we all seek to avoid and that, as Jamie Mayerfeld has insisted, we have a prima facie duty to relieve for others. This is true not just for human suffering but, as David DeGrazia argues, also for the suffering of animals, an observation of great importance for biomedical research. Green does not deny that there are limits to our obligation to prevent or relieve suffering, including deontological limits indicated by duties not to kill, lie, cheat, or steal. But he believes that all these countervailing reasons and obligations are traceable back to our desire to avoid suffering and our moral obligation to prevent or relieve it. The currency of all such calculations of limits and constraints is suffering itself. Green here takes issue with Mark J. Cherry's assertion that "to make unequivocal moral judgments in response to suffering requires a canonical morality, a binding moral standpoint from which to know truly the nature of the right, the good, and the virtuous."[6] The avoidance of suffering, Green replies, does not depend on any comprehensive ethical or metaphysical position. Rather, it is a negative primary good, an undeniable component of any moral view. This insight, Green affirms, grounds the prestige of medicine as a profession and justifies those reasonable limits to the relief of suffering that are currently argued for in relation to such areas as end-of-life care or reproductive decision making. After applauding the progress in theological insight among the essays in this volume dealing with religion, medicine, and suffering, Green concludes by critically engaging Paul Lauritzen's treatment of medicalization and commoditization in infertility medicine. Against Lauritzen, Green argues that there are no clear limits to what physicians can do in response to patient requests to relieve suffering. Distinctions such as "treatment versus enhancement" or "physiologically indicated versus merely desired" will not do, he says. What is involved, instead, is a multifactorial judgment about which policy best serves all of our interests and is most likely to reduce suffering.

This volume brings together a wide spectrum of approaches to discuss the nature of suffering in the human experience and the implications for bioethics. Its contents present in-depth engagement with the moral gravity we face in our obligations to alleviate suffering, including what happens when we don't take this seriously, and wrestles with the challenging questions we face when we encounter or try to define the boundaries around our obligation to alleviate suffering. We hope that the contents will inform the field of bioethics in policy making and practice by bringing to the fore a long missing conceptualization of suffering in bioethical decision making. Having surveyed the essays outlined in this volume, we now turn our attention to the contributions.

Notes

1. *Suffering and Bioethics*, Chapter 2, p. 45.
2. *Suffering and Bioethics*, Chapter 3, p. 54.
3. *Suffering and Bioethics*, Chapter 4, p. 66.
4. *Suffering and Bioethics*, Chapter 4, p. 82.
5. *Suffering and Bioethics*, Chapter 15, p. 305.
6. *Suffering and Bioethics*, Chapter 17, p. 338.

PART ONE

The Nature, Meaning, and Experience of Suffering

1

Suffering and Human Dignity

Eric J. Cassell

Suffering is the severe distress that attends or follows injury. The first lesson of suffering is that bodies do not suffer, persons suffer. The injuries from which suffering follows can occur in any part of the person, from a body part to the social being to spirituality, if those injuries are of such severity or extent that the person is no longer intact. Suffering, it follows, is always personal. Because all persons are different from one another in every respect, suffering is also individual. Suffering always involves self-conflict because persons are not "of a piece." The source of suffering is usually seen as outside the sufferer—the cause of the pain or the pain itself, or the circumstance or fate. The clue lies in the fact that meaning enters into suffering. The threat to the person's intactness lies in the meaning of the pain or injury, and persons are seldom of one mind about the meaning of things. The self-conflict within a righteous Job is an example: every fiber of Job's being knows that God is just, and yet his God who "sees my ways and counts my every step" (31:4) is causing him to suffer the punishment of the wicked when he is not wicked. This conflict within himself is far worse than the many harms inflicted on him. There may be conflict between the self and body or between the social self and private self. All suffering involves loss of or profound change in purpose. Purpose pervades every moment and every part of being leading to central purpose—the being of oneself. In the sufferer, purpose is diverted to the suffering or its source. Finally, suffering is always lonely because it is misunderstood owing to the sufferer's withdrawal from others and from the social world.

When suffering starts, it is the suffering that is the primary distress. It is no longer simply pain; it is suffering. It is not helplessness; it is suffering. It is no longer the abuse; it is suffering. It is not grief; it is suffering. Suffering is suffering is suffering and not another thing. I emphasize this because, in medicine, the injury to the person that initiates suffering—for example, pain, fear of suffocation, or abuse in treatment—tends to be seen as the primary problem rather than the suffering that has supervened. In fact, the pain (say), or dyspnea, or object of fear may be relieved, but the suffering continues. Suffering may be acute and short lived, it may become long lasting and be the person's state of being, and it may be severe or mild. Disruptions of personal intactness or the integrity of a person probably occur in everyone from time to time to some extent or another. They may be mild or (to the person) insignificant and easily dismissed. One way to understand this is to use the integrity of the skin as an example. The skin is a vital barrier against intrusions of the environment, which if lost to a significant degree, as in a serious burn, results in death or severe illness. Small lacerations, on the other hand, or burns, wounds, punctures, tears, bruises, and the like commonly disrupt the barrier function of the skin but usually do not threaten the person; they quickly heal or are easily treated. One problem with this comparison is that the skin is a physical object, whereas the person is not an object except in a physical sense.

Difficulty of Defining Human Dignity

Dignity, human dignity, is a quality of all persons whose injury or destruction may lead to suffering. It is usual to define important terms, but that is a problem with human dignity. Human dignity is seen by the Catholic Church as present because humans are said to be created in the image of God. For others, human dignity is an inalienable right from which follow other rights. Acting against such rights makes the person an object, and the German Constitutional Court ruled that forbidden. (The Germans know well where that forbidden act leads.) Most consider that human dignity, or the dignity of an individual human, derives from all the ideas wrapped up in terms like *self-respect* and *self-worth* or *worthiness*. The feeling of empowerment is another extension of these ideas of an individual's dignity. The history of the term and its earlier application to nobility tells us that common people were not originally considered to have dignity—that dignity came from the outside or was bestowed. It fits the history of humankind, particularly in the Western democracies, to see dignity as a more recent bestowal arising from truths that "we hold to be self-evident." That seems fitting particularly because the wide acceptance of subjectivity itself only came into being at about the same time as the American Declaration of Independence. Definitions of terms are particularly endorsed—even vital—in medicine and medical science, and although one can understand the need for standardized terminology, this requirement has made the human biology described by medical science particularly essentialist. The remainder of biology moved on quite a while ago and is now appropriately described as evolutionary biology that understands the invariance of *individual variation*—individual variation in all living things, in disease states, and in human structure and physiology. It would appear that there is individual variation in the meaning of human dignity. As a consequence of this, I do not believe a definition of dignity is possible, as in, "he is dignified," or "she kept her dignity," or "I have my dignity if nothing else." I had for many years a patient who spent his life in menial tasks that others would not do. He had a number of children who, because of legal difficulties, moral problems, numerous illnesses, or substance abuse, all died. He became increasingly proud and dignified because he had outlived them all.

When we leave bishops and even presidents who are dignities by office, it might be difficult to find out precisely what a person means when speaking about dignity or even self-respect or self-worth. I know that the words have meant different things to me at different times in my life. Dignity like suffering is ineluctably subjective. Subjectivity and that which is subjective are a problem for medicine. The experience of suffering is subjective and cannot be made objective. This is true even though persons who are suffering will begin to appear and act differently than others, with these changes becoming apparent to knowledgeable observers. The longer suffering goes on, the more apparent it becomes. The longer it lasts, the greater are the changes that suffering persons experience of themselves. Understanding subjectivity becomes necessary to understanding suffering.

Suffering Is Important to Bioethics

These characteristics of suffering and its causes are important to clinicians, but they are also important to bioethicists. At its heart, bioethics is concerned with persons because ethics itself has most often to do with the relations of persons to others separately or joined to others or to those things that have an effect on persons. Bioethicists have too often acted as though persons are constants, and they have been concerned primarily with (say) the rights and wrongs of actions or events in themselves rather than the particular effects of these on individual persons. Respect for persons and autonomy is of cardinal importance, but do those words translate into the same actions in relation to everyone? Allowing that sufficient cognitive capacity is present, does autonomy really mean precisely the same thing for the very sick as for the healthy person?

Case Examples

Frequently in medicine it takes actual cases—examples of sick persons—to clarify a problem. Here are three cases written as personalized anecdotes about patients who said they had suffered and who lost dignity. These cases allow us to go further into the nature of persons, human dignity, and the relation of suffering to dignity.

> What if you have been tolerating pain for hours and hours and days and it never stops? Now you're in the emergency department. You are so exhausted because the pain has kept you from sleeping. You've tried so hard not to cry and call out to every passing doctor and nurse. And they don't stop anyway because they are too busy for you. When they do stop, it's because they want

something, a signature or something. It goes on and on and on. Finally you have no stamina, no strength left anymore—and no control. And you just start to whimper, and you don't even hear yourself anymore because there is no "yourself" anymore, just pain.

What if you have always been proud of your appearance and now everybody always told you how beautiful you are? And forever proud of the way you look, really proud, and very careful about dressing? Then lately you start having diarrhea—all the time, constantly. For days on end. And they won't give you anything to stop it because—you're not sure why. And when you finally come into the hospital, the nurse undresses you standing up, and there is shit running down your legs and on your clothes and everywhere. And everybody just goes in and out of the room.

What if you've always been a good patient and tried to do everything they asked you to do? Because you've always been good and did the right thing even as a kid. And everybody always said you were special—even strangers. And you came into the emergency room because this time you're really sick. And you've been lying on a gurney for eleven hours waiting for a bed. And you're not sure what's happening. You're so thirsty and cold, for hours, but nobody helps. When people do stop, they tell you how busy everybody is and to just be patient. When you try to find out what's happening, nobody listens. And some are just mean and short. And you're so cold.

Our View of These Cases Depends on Who We Are at This Time

As we read these cases, we can understand that these patients suffered, even have ideas about why, and perhaps have thoughts about what to do for them. Thoughts also about what should be done about the environment in which these cases occurred. I believe, however, that no matter how much understanding and even compassion we have, what we see and how we understand it in each case may be restricted because of the world in which we now live in the United States and in the several decades that came before. Further, I believe the changes in the way we see and understand persons and, in fact, changes in the actual nature of people in the United States are almost invisible despite their impact on our ideas about ourselves and about what persons are and what they can do. The changes I will describe came about because of social influences—the social context—that have also had an important effect on medicine and bioethics. To demonstrate what I mean, a brief excursion is necessary into the history of the past sixty years in the United States, particularly the history of medicine and medical science. Many of the things I am going to mention took place over a considerable number of years. It always takes appreciable time for social change to manifest itself. As with all important changes, many factors can be at play simultaneously.

Emerging from World War II

The United States and most of the world came out of the awfulness of the Second World War with a powerful embrace of freedom, personal liberty, and individuality. This was demonstrated after an initial quiet decade in the United States by the growing force of the civil rights movement and the women's movement. As part of these social changes, previously marginalized groups became full-fledged persons. Patients also became persons and were granted agency. In the 1950s came the Beat generation, Hippie movement (in the 1960s), and the "flower children," emphasizing a revolt against what was believed by these groups to be a hierarchical and stultifying society. Birth control pills introduced in 1960 helped along the already burgeoning growth in sexual freedom—an important step in the change of the status of persons. In this atmosphere, not surprisingly, in the 1960s came the birth of bioethics and its dedication to the protection of persons and personal freedom. During this same period, the country became more affluent, generally better educated, and healthier. Gaining a college education became available to many more than previously and was less restricted by class. This was largely an effect of the GI Bill but also occurred because returning veterans were more mature and had earned enlarged expectations.

What Persons Were Like

During this same period, persons in general were increasingly *understood* as deeper, more complex, and many layered, with subjectivity and emotion counting for more. What one could see of a person or what they said or did were considered just the surface; it was accepted that there were many aspects of the person below the surface. These ideas, which became widely accepted, emerged initially because of the influence of psychoanalysis and other new psychologies. Seeing the psychology of persons in this rich and elaborate manner and the labyrinthine workings of the unconscious mind had been gestating since the beginning of the twentieth century. Much illness was attributed to psychological and unconscious sources in the individual. Freud, Jung, Horney, Erikson, Alexander, Melanie Klein, and many other psychoanalytic pioneers were well known names in the 1960s and 1970s. Psychoanalysis and psychotherapy were commonplace at this time, especially in New York and Los Angeles, but also were widely thought about. Many departments of psychiatry in medical schools were psychoanalytically oriented. (Academic psychology, which tried to become a laboratory science in emulation of the hard sciences, contributed little during these years.) Overall, the result of all these forces were persons politically enhanced, better educated, more complex, and personally more interesting.

Doctors in the United States came out of World War II with increased stature and more authority. It does not go too far to say that they were often trusted and revered as representing a sacred vocation from the beginning of the twentieth century as medicine itself grew in stature with the development of the famous medical schools and clinics—Johns Hopkins, University of Pennsylvania, Harvard, Yale, the Mayo Clinic, and others. Through the 1950s,1960s, and early 1970s, doctors themselves, not just their science, were at their peak.

The Start of the Hegemony of Science

Science in medicine is a crucial *social* force because of the enormous growth of medical science and scientific influence since the 1950s. This was marked in medicine by the huge increase in budgets of the National Institutes of Health and the medical science establishment. From the beginning of the twentieth century, there had been moves toward full-time science-oriented faculties in medical institutions. After World War II, however, it became the accepted reality: medical schools and teaching hospitals had full-time scientifically oriented faculty. The days of the special influence of experienced clinicians were numbered (and are now over). The change in the faculty and staff was underlined by two other trends: the rise of medical specialties and later the increasing importance of medical technology. It became accepted belief that it was medical science and science-born technologies that made the diagnosis and that made patients better. The scientific knowledge was what counted. Who the doctor was that conveyed that knowledge did not matter; it was the knowledge that did the work. (I was told this at New York University School of Medicine when I graduated in 1954.) The ideal doctor became the doctor-scientist, the research doctor. The wise, knowledgeable, and trusted clinician who took care of sick patients began to lose status and disappear. One of the best of these clinicians and an excellent teacher at The New York Hospital in the early 1970s looked forward to his retirement from practice when he would start teaching full-time. Within two years, he left, a crushed man. The medical students had made it clear that they were no longer interested in what he had to teach.

The Central Tenets of Science that Spread throughout the Culture

The ideas and ideals of science became universal in medicine and then spread out to the entire culture, where they are present in great strength and wider influence. These ideas include the belief that only objective data have validity. In medicine, *objective* generally means "measurable." Only objective evidence counts in understanding the sick, sickness, and everything else. Subjective information and subjectivity itself are always suspect. Information or knowledge gained from narratives about a particular patient or episode is "anecdotal medicine" and as such is believed to be of almost no value (even though anecdotes are frequently used in support of actions). Scientific thought is linear. Linear thinking is a process of logical thought following a known step-by-step progression. The response to a step must be elicited and carefully defined before the next step is started. That step must be defined and explicated before the next step, and so on. Where there are leaps of thought, even when great creativity is involved (e.g., the idea of the double helix as the form of DNA), before the idea can be accepted, the careful stepwise process of defining, clarifying through logical reasoning, and empirical testing must be undertaken. All scientific findings are open to confirmation or denial through replication of the original proof. Then, the scientific results should return to operation in the original field of experience where the questions arose.

There are situations that do not fit these ideals. For example, students learning clinical psychology know that there are things they learn about their patients that are difficult or impossible to quantify. That does not change their thinking; they know they must keep looking for evidence and that finding evidence on which to base their actions is crucial. They remain true to the scientific ideals they were taught even when they cannot, on occasion, meet the goal.

The Scientific Ideal Takes over Clinical Medicine

In 1967, Alvan Feinstein published the book, *Clinical Judgment,* which showed how mathematical concepts and mathematical precision could be brought to clinical medicine. Feinstein, importantly, was primarily interested in the care of the individual patient, and he never lost that focus. The field of clinical epidemiology that grew out of Feinstein's work, however, lost his concern with the individual. Instead, while applying mathematical methods of epidemiology to the care of patients, it increasingly emphasized mathematical methods derived from populations. These primarily statistical methods refined the precision of diagnostic and therapeutic evidence. They were always focused on disease and its objective physical manifestations. This major and increasingly important trend culminated in the movement called *evidence-based medicine* (EBM). "EBM is the use of mathematical estimates of the risk of benefit and harm, derived from high-quality research on population samples, to inform clinical decision-making in the diagnosis, investigation or management of individual patients"[1] EBM has taken over medicine. Those aspects of sickness and the sick person that cannot be numerically measured are put aside. EBM has spread to allied health fields like dentistry, nursing, and psychology, and even further out into education and educational theory. The physicians and their independent judgment earned through training and experience have been actively put in doubt. In their place have been put algorithms and guidelines developed to instruct almost all the actions of physicians.

There are problems with this, the biggest being that for science to be preeminent, medicine had to be defined as the treatment of disease and the fact of the patient, and the relationship between doctor and patient had to be demoted to somewhat romantic old-fashioned notions—the art of medicine. Disease had to be reduced to problems that could be explored in the laboratory under controlled conditions. Treatment had to be explored meeting the stringent requirement of EBM. All these conditions moved medical science further away from clinical medicine—as well as distant from the ideals of science. Science starts from "the radically untidy, ill adjusted character of the fields of actual experience. To grasp this fundamental truth is the first step in wisdom when constructing a philosophy of science."[2]

The Role and Training of Physicians Have Changed

As a result of clinical epidemiology and EBM (and similar trends), physicians are expected to make patient care choices and assist patients in making choices based on validated clinical methods. The physician is subservient to the methods, guidelines, and algorithms. This is true even in the training of medical students. The great advance in the training of physicians, bedside teaching with "the patient as text," introduced by Sir William Osler at the end of the nineteenth century and now present throughout Western medicine until a few years ago has virtually disappeared. The students, by their choice, are now taught in front of the computer where test results, x-rays, magnetic resonance images, and other images can be displayed. It is "the numbers" that count, along with the many forms of diagnostic images and tests. Many studies have documented the diminished ability of contemporary students and recent graduates to take patient histories and do physical examinations—the basis of the clinical method. The emphasis on health care costs and on the organization of medical services based primarily on cost has been an added depersonalizing force. Both patients, whose "numbers" and tests are considered most important, and physicians, who are less valued than "the method," are diminished by these changes.

Reductionism Always Wins

Throughout our society—modern society in general—medical science and its methods, values, and reductionist focus have become a dominant force. Reductionism—reducing problems to their parts and focusing on the parts rather than the whole—always seems to win. It will be that way as long as we remain within the scientific worldview. Reductionism only loses when whole persons are considered as the complex functioning beings that they are, with their life's goals and purposes being the major focus. This is not medicine's primary concern. In professions other than medicine, it has also become the "method" that is important. Even in the early grades, teachers are expected to follow the validated method. Then, they see their students not as themselves but as subjects of the method. The interaction of teacher with student and thus the importance of the teacher as a person and the relationship of teacher to student become subservient to scientifically proven methods.

Devaluation of Physicians

The general result is a depreciation of individuals. When expertise is derogated—it is not the person that counts, it is the facts—it is the expert *person* who is devalued. As I noted earlier, it is not the physician who diagnoses and treats the patient, it is the scientific knowledge. It follows that whoever has the knowledge can do as well as the expert. This pervades society and can be found at all levels and in all areas of life. It seems at first as if it is just authority in general that is being discounted, but that is a result, not an initiator, of the problem. This would seem not to be the case because of the increasing concern over the past several decades that medicine be patient centered. Now, every hospital medical center and medical school declares that it is centered on the patient. The term *patient centered* came to denote a focus on patients' wants, needs, desires, concerns, and preferences and a demand that patients have the education and support needed to make decisions and participate in their own care. Physicians have frequently moved to an advise-and-consent function, whereby the patient is asked to make the decisions. The care in these hospitals and medical institutions remains, not less than before, steadily focused on disease and its bodily manifestations. It could not be otherwise because of the increased influence of the methods, values, and inevitable reductionist focus of science. (For example, genomic medicine, which aims to find the origins of the disease in the genome of the individual, has come to be known by its experts as "personalized medicine.")

Debasement of Persons in General

The depth and complexity of persons that was arising and valued by the 1950s has begun to disappear. What happened to the unconscious and the rich psychological life that was widely discussed and even celebrated in mid-twentieth century? The unconscious and all the associated ideas, including the importance of psychogenic factors in illness, have disappeared. Depth psychotherapy (and depth psychic growth) have gone away and have been replaced by a generalized psychological method—cognitive and behavioral therapy. (One size fits all.) Departments of psychiatry and psychiatrists focus on biological factors in psychological illness and on psychotropic medications. When persons and their complexity are debased, so, too, are their relationships. Personal relationships—from friendship to love, family relationships, and certainly professional relationships, including doctor and patient, teacher and student, and expert and neophyte—and their depth, intensity, and complexity are lessened. (There are, of course, individual exceptions.).

What Do We See When We See a Person?

The issues I have raised in this major digression are central to the question this chapter addresses: suffering and human dignity, both of which are, at heart, problems of subjectivity and the subjective life. What do we see when we see a person? There is, of course, the visual image, just as we see the visual image when we see a tree: we see an interpretation of the browns and greens, of the straight and wrinkly surfaces; we see a meaning. It is impossible not to see the meaning of the conglomerate that is the percept because, as the neuroscientists have shown, meaning is not something applied after the original percept is received; rather, it is part of the process of vision. For example, even though it is possible to restore some persons' sound reception with hearing aids, they still cannot "hear" because they have lost the cognitive ability to apply meanings to the sounds. In the same way, when we see a person, because of our interest in seeing this particular person, ideas come to mind of other patients or situations in the past or other circumstances that lead to thinking about differences or similarities. Others are also brought to mind and may or may not enter consciousness because of similarities or because the topic of thought about this primary person applies to others. If the person is a patient, that person's illness or symptoms remind us of others. We also are put in mind of others who are similar or contrasting in one or more respects. We know this complexity must be true because we draw conclusions, and these almost invariable involve other instances that lend support to our thoughts.

The Woman with Diarrhea

Look at her, if you can bear it (one is afraid of embarrassing her), a beautiful naked middle-aged woman standing straight up, with an agonized look on her face, her dirty clothes at her feet, and her inner thighs and legs stained with feces as the nurse cleans her with a basin and washcloth. Is the agonized look hers, or have we made it so because that is how we would be in her place? Is such a complicated image ever of just a naked woman standing with feces-stained legs, or is the image inevitably also a reminder of the past? A little boy has brought his parents and two grandparents from the living room and has them sit in a circle of chairs in his room as he then sits on the potty, the focus of their attention, and has an intentional bowel movement. Toilet trained! Or a soiled little girl is running on the street toward her house, crying, "I didn't mean to Mommy, I didn't mean to!" Look at the attendant and nurse's aide who just walked in to do things in the room, despite her nakedness. Have they no feelings? If this is not wretchedness, what is? Perhaps we have got it wrong, and she is the image of dignity and pride at being able to rise above the terribleness and be, as always, her beautiful self. We have admiration knowing that we would not be able to convey such dignity. This is improbable for her, also knowing what we know of persons.

Seeing her brings to mind other naked women. Physicians see her mons pubis and scant pubic hair common at this age but also probably affected by alcoholism. Most people who look at a naked person do not register the details of the genitalia probably because of their own modesty. We also think how awfully unfair this situation is and that reminds us of other scenes of sickness that are also unfair. The idea of dignity and indignity come to mind, and of suffering. Is she suffering? This parade of thoughts occupies less time than reading the 340 or so words. She remains in our thoughts after we leave her. The diarrhea is a result of her alcoholism. Again, we can believe she is suffering and that her suffering is a result of the loss of dignity because of the awful situation, compounded by her shame at not being able to end her continual overuse of alcohol. Dignity is an aspect of the person that arises related to other persons or the group. Were there no others, was there no world looking on, were there no expectations of the group, was there no family, was there no past or predicated future self to judge the present, there would be, perhaps, no deep rupture or breach in the intactness of the present self that is the basis of the indignity and thus the suffering.

Is the embarrassment at looking at her a part of the visual object that is she? All these other meanings and memories—are they her? Yes to both questions. If you believe that if you saw another similar (but not the same) woman, you would have all the same thoughts, you do not understand what it means to confront the complex percept that is a person. All these thoughts—similar images of the past, reminders of other scenes, memories like the little boy and the little girl—belong to the knowing of this woman. They might all or in part (plus other things) be part of another similar visual object asking to be known. How many precisely similar experiences will you have? Precisely and exactly the same? None, because the person will be different—the day, time of day, nurses, hospital room, and so on. Do we, perceiving her standing there, know what the experience means to her rather than to us? We cannot because an experience is a many layered thing, and everything that contributes to its meaning may not be consciously known to the subject or to the onlooking clinician. Do the other layers contribute to (say) her losing her dignity? They may or they may not. Suppose her father was an alcoholic who died of the disorder. Or her mother had ulcerative colitis, and she, as a child, saw her mother in similar situations because of the bowel disease. Perhaps the diarrhea is not the problem, but only the feces, the mess, or the smell? It matters not because, in any case, she has constructed herself as an adult around or over these damaged places, these faults in her life. The experience would then start the suffering because it breaks through to those aspects of herself that she had covered up.

We cannot even pretend that thought about this woman is linear in the sense that science engages in linear thought. On the other hand, to see her in all this complexity is to see *this particular individual.* The clinician with long experience sees her knowing that the intricacy and tangle of memories and meanings marks humankind. To deny complexity to the person in the percept is to deny humanness.

The experienced clinician seeks those aspects of the woman needed for her care. To make her a simple female patient with diarrhea is to focus on diarrhea and deny her personhood.

The Whimpering Woman in Pain

This pitiable woman, that inimitable sound—uhh, uhh, uhh, uhh. The sound is awful to hear. Even worse because when she is asked to stop, she does not know she is making any sound. The head nurse tells you how annoying she is; she has been groaning for hours. Has she gotten pain medication? "Some morphine a few hours ago, and it is too soon to give her more. Besides, she is soon going to a bed upstairs, and the doctor did not want to force the hand of the admitting intern." In fact, however, no one is paying much attention to her because she is just on the gurney waiting for a bed upstairs. She is not a person, she is an annoyance—and probably no one is actively aware of how long she has been on the gurney. If you want to know more about her, her chart is stuck under the pillow on the gurney. She is in pain because of widespread metastatic cancer for which she has been treated unsuccessfully. That aspect of her for which one might think she would get sympathy or compassion is put aside by her irritating quality. People have sympathy or compassion for someone obviously sick lying on the gurney, but because she is both sick and in pain and has become depersonalized, it takes training and experience to reach out to her and know that she needs intensive pain relief to become a person again. Doing that requires recognizing her as a person, commenting on her awful state, asking her what she would like done first while the opioid takes time to act. Actually, her medication should be given intravenously so that pain relief is achieved while talking to *her.* Dignity belongs to persons; when personhood is absent, dignity is also absent. Her present state is a state of profound suffering. Did the loss of her personhood remove her dignity, or did her suffering lead to the loss? It matters not which is put first.

She brings to mind a 65-year-old patient with recurrent urinary tract symptoms who was seen in the clinic by a fourth-year medical student. The student responded correctly and quickly to the urinary problem, but there was still almost twenty-five minutes left for the visit. The student seemed caring, and the patient began telling him about her recent spine surgery. The medical student appeared to be interested in her, and she continued speaking. This operation, she said, reminded her of a spinal operation when she was considerably younger. Then she related an awful story of continuing spousal abuse and then abandonment while she had three young children to care for without money, adequate housing, or help from anyone. Her parents both died while the abuse was going on, and shortly after that, her brother and her sister were killed in an automobile crash. That latter part of the story was delivered through tears while the student asked many unnecessary brief questions about other body systems. Then, as his time with her (by the clock) came to an end, he said in a few words that she had the classic symptoms of depression but there were good medications for this, and he wrote out a prescription and ended the visit without another word. This depersonalizing indignity is known because the student was observed throughout the interaction by his family practice teacher on the other side of a one-way vision window.

The Woman Who Has Always Been Good

This woman's suffering started while she was still lying on the gurney. She was sure that she had been intentionally abused. The "unfair abuse" was the initiating cause of her suffering. (What patients perceive to be intentional abuse of this type is a common cause of suffering.) Very long waits for an in-patient bed have become common all over the United States for patients admitted to the hospital from emergency departments. (In the United States, a few years ago, the average waiting time was eleven hours.) She actively tried to be a very good patient doing eagerly what she was told to do. Her enthusiasm for the staff was odd from their point of view; several of the nurses and the doctors commented that she seemed strange. She was obviously ill, but when some contents of her bedpan spilled on the floor, she climbed off the gurney to clean it up. Then she had to be helped back to the stretcher, and the nurse was annoyed, not grateful. After that, the patient tried even harder to do what the doctor wanted even before being asked. Between the depth of her sickness and this "kindergarten behavior" (the nurse's description), the staff was glad to finish with her and get her out into the corridor on her gurney to wait for her bed. She had sent her husband home telling him how well things were being done. In his absence and out in the corridor, one of a number of patients waiting there on their gurneys, she had no one standing by to get water or help her to the toilet. After the enthusiastic and helpful self that she had demonstrated to the staff, she could only think that someone must be intentionally keeping her in the cold corridor. As the hours went by, her resentment and then anger increased, using up even further her small reserve of strength.

Alfred Schwartz was similar to her, I remembered. He had a high fever and a urinary tract infection and some bloody urine spilled from his urinal. We found him lying on the floor. He had tried to clean it up and then could not get back on his bed. He was so embarrassed and said again and again that he did not want to be a bother. There were also others who behaved like that. Acting as if this was a personal problem like a similar mess at home. The staff was going through their duties, and to them, their patients were just patients. A mess was just a mess; it was not anything personal. A mess was not anything out of the ordinary, and there were procedures and clean-up people in place just to handle such things. If something like that happened, or some other incident occurred that was really different or difficult, then the doctors and nurses would have to think their way through or around the problem. If that happened, their minds would actually register the patient and the circumstances, and they would begin to have actual awareness of other possibilities, openly thinking about the specific patient and the problem. Reflecting on that, I could see the difference between how physicians and other medical staff assessed persons who were patients and persons who were not patients, how differently the two groups in our lives—patients and simply persons—registered cognitively.

Immediate Lessons from These Examples about Dignity and Subjectivity

These three women suffered, and loss of dignity contributed differently in the genesis of their suffering. In the beautiful woman being cleaned up from soiling herself, shame was involved. She might be ashamed because of what actually happened, ashamed because she had soiled herself apart from the indignity of being cleaned up in full view (the memories of the two children helps here), and ashamed because uncontrolled alcoholism was part of the problem. The whimpering woman had been stripped of her personhood by the overwhelming pain, and then, projecting nothingness, she was treated as nothing by the staff. The behavior of the staff was partly a response to her state and partly a cause of it. Her situation demonstrates how the behavior of others is a determinant of our state of being. The woman who was always good finds that the response of others—doctors, nurse, and other staff in this instance—is distinctly different in this situation from the response of others when she is in a personal or family situation. She cannot understand this, and so she responds as if she had been abused. If it happened at home, it would be abuse, but in the emergency department, it was simply "impersonal." The first lesson is that dignity is a subjective state that can be an attribute of the person or assigned to the person by others, but it always reflects the fact that persons live in a world of others. Intersubjectivity is continuous and a constant. The way in which patients are treated by physicians and other members of the medical staff contributes to the presence or absence of dignity in the person's own eyes and in the perspectives of others.

How Physicians See the Person of the Patient

In each instance, the person of the patient as seen by the medical staff was simplistic and one-dimensional, as contrasted to the view of the person that emerged from the material and memories evoked by reflection about each particular patient. This was most completely demonstrated and discussed for the patient soiled by feces but was true of all. To think of patients in this simplistic manner denies their humanness and is more the way an object of science is considered. The history of the past fifty years during which science and the scientific worldview have dominated medicine suggests one reason that persons are seen in this unilayered manner. The richness and complexity of persons that were emerging in the 1950s and 1960s should have led to continued growth of a multidimensional view of persons so that, by this time, psychological, personal, political, social, and spiritual aspects of the person would be part of the medical perspective each time a physician considered a patient. Sometimes, this would be a miniscule part, but at other times, where appropriate, it would be a much larger aspect by contemporary physicians of the fulsome nature and depth of patients. That direction of study and thought died a premature death. The debasement of persons, resulting like a side effect from the contemporary culture of science, seems to have been responsible. Let me say this again in a different way. Considering how widespread dynamic and in-depth ideas about person were and how they permeated departments of psychiatry, ideas about personhood would have been expected to continue to evolve.

The famous article in 1977 by George Engel about the "biopsychosocial" nature of persons should have led to an expansion and development of the idea and its use in practice, but that did not happen.[3] Engel's paper was and is frequently cited, but it did not lead to continuing new research or intellectual development. That was not the direction taken by clinical medicine, science, or even psychiatry. Let me illustrate from another field. Suppose, as impossible as the idea is, that knowledge of the human genome had suffered a similar fate. In the past fifty years, genetic analysis of microorganisms, important molecules like insulin, and other organisms or parts of organisms have step by step been accomplished with concomitant technological advances leading to the sequencing of the complete human genome in this century. If, for ideological reasons, the genome had been declared off limits in the 1970s (a laughable idea), science would have stopped genetic knowledge at simian virus 40!

The View of the World of Dailiness Rules Everyday Thinking

In "The Phenomenology of Spirit," by Georg Wilhelm Hegel, spirit is the total real being of the world divided on the one hand into the hard reality of universally shared culture and on the other hand into a universal reality of faith and truly appreciated knowing. It is a difficult concept, but the basic insight is that we are all separate beings but are all inseparable from spirit, which is the spirit of the larger community. For Hegel, spirit (as the sum of us and our knowledge and as our nurturer and source of growth) itself gradually learns and evolves *pari passu* as cultures and individuals also slowly evolve spiritually and in terms of what can be known and accepted in the world. It is not important to criticize or defend Hegel (who did pretty well on his own), but it does help us understand phenomena like the growth and overwhelming dominance of medical science in the twentieth and early twenty-first centuries in the Western world. After this has happened, ideas foreign to science or not acceptable to medical science like subjectivity in its fullest sense will fall by the wayside, not to return until the worldview changes.

Fundamentally, the Worldview of Medical Science Has Failed the Sick

The idea that it is medical science itself—its knowledge and ideas—that treats the patient has failed. Actually, the idea that medical science treats the disease and that the patient is subservient to the disease is problematic. The difficulty with that formulation, which can neither be proved nor disproved, is that it is the patient that is most important, not the disease, and that it requires a person to understand and treat a person. This is illustrated by the problem of human dignity. The simple question is whether a seriously ill patient who is suffering because of the injury to intactness resulting from the loss of dignity will have the same chance of treatment success as the person whose dignity is intact and is not suffering. The question cannot be answered by medical science because the answer would involve a treatment trial that would compare enough patients suffering and without residual human dignity with patients who have the exact same affliction but whose dignity is intact and who are not suffering. Let us put aside the problems raised by scientifically defining dignity or its absence.

In the absence of an understanding of subjectivity and the knowledge of persons for which it is essential, neither human dignity nor suffering can be fully comprehended as concepts and in their actual presence in sick persons. Objectivity in the absence of subjectivity renders persons one-dimensional and robs medicine of the compassion and human relationships that define it in history and in the care of an individual sick person.

Notes

1. D. L. Sackett, W. Rosenberg, J. Gray J et al., "What is EBM (Evidence Based Medicine)?" *British Medical Journal* 312 (1996): 71–72.

2. Alfred North Whitehead, *The Organization of Thought: Educational and Scientific.* (London: Williams and Norgate, 1917), 110.

3. George L. Engel, "The Need for a New Medical Model: A Challenge for Biomedicine," *Science* 196 (1977): 129–136.

2

Understanding Suffering

Barry Hoffmaster

> We cannot know why the world suffers. But we can know how the world decides that suffering shall come to some persons and not to others. While the world permits sufferers to be chosen, something beyond their agony is earned, something even beyond the satisfaction of the world's needs and desires. For it is in the choosing that enduring societies preserve or destroy those values that suffering and necessity expose. In this way societies are defined, for it is by the values that are foregone no less than by those that are preserved at tremendous cost that we know a society's character.
>
> Guido Calabresi and Philip Bobbitt, *Tragic Choices*[1]

We know that human beings suffer because of their inherent biological finitude and fallibility, but we do not know why human beings are constitutionally vulnerable to suffering, and we do not know why some human beings are innately more vulnerable than others. Many things can go wrong in the conception, gestation, and birth of a child, for instance, and given that, it is miraculous that more things do not go wrong more often. Nevertheless, when something does go wrong, it seems capriciously unfair to those who are harmed and suffer. Why are the probabilities as they are, and why do the probabilities play out as they do? Despite the often desperate quests for answers to these tormenting questions, they remain inexplicable.

We do know, however, why some human beings are more socially vulnerable to suffering than others. Societies make policies and refrain from making policies based upon their priorities, and those choices, whether explicit or implicit, can impair well-being and create or prolong suffering. Examples abound: teenage women who are pregnant do not get adequate prenatal care and nutrition; disengaged, disillusioned youth become addicted to drugs; unemployment insurance runs out. The choices a society makes about suffering expose the values of that society. They are the collective values that prompt responses to some kinds of suffering and perpetuate neglect of other kinds of suffering; that determine how scarce resources will be allocated to mitigate the suffering deemed compelling; and that either reveal or conceal the ways in which these social decisions are made.

We also know how human beings suffer because we suffer. Extrapolating from our own experiences and what we know about the world, we can observe when others are suffering, and we can comprehend the source of their suffering and the intensity of their suffering. We can empathize with them because we know the sorrows that cause suffering and how suffering feels. To understand the suffering we share is to understand what suffering means for us, and to understand what suffering means for us is to understand the values our suffering exposes. For individuals who are suffering, those values are the personal values that give life purpose and vitality but have been denied or lost, whether temporarily, as in the case of fighting a war, being taken as a hostage, or being imprisoned, or irretrievably, as at the end of life with the inevitable breakdown of body and mind.

The meager attention that suffering receives in bioethics exposes both the defining values of its theoretical orientation and the controlling values of the health care settings within which it is practiced. The values of the academic discipline of bioethics are the values that identify what issues are amenable to and worthy of scholarly attention and that subject those issues to prescribed scholarly methods, the result of which is that prosaic, merely subjective matters of suffering are relegated to the margins of bioethics. The values of the practice of bioethics are the encompassing operational values of the health care institutions that employ bioethicists. Particularly in dire economic circumstances, the paramount organizational values are efficiency and productivity, which in the delivery of health care mandate timely treatment of patients and speedy resolutions of problems, including moral problems. To acknowledge suffering as a problem that deserves attention, even if bioethicists were competent to address suffering, would be to legitimize slowness, delay, and inefficiency.

The goals of this chapter are to provide a coherent depiction and appreciation of the human experience of suffering and to explain why suffering is not prominent in bioethics. The complexity, diversity, and force of suffering cannot be reduced to the abstract terms of a neat, exhaustive definition or theory. Moreover, we ultimately would use our familiarity with the experience of suffering to test the adequacy of any putative definition or theoretical account of suffering. Because suffering needs to be comprehended through the experience of suffering, this chapter uses examples and illustrations to elucidate the nature of suffering and responses to suffering.

The orientation of the chapter is borrowed from the epigraph. Suffering results from profound loss that impairs a life. Loss is profound when it forecloses the satisfaction of values that define and drive a life. When lost values can be redeemed by other values that give life integrity and vitality, suffering can be accepted and could be ennobling. When lost values cannot be redeemed by other values, suffering can be intolerable and might be ended by ending the life of the person who is suffering. Suffering is understood through the values that suffering exposes and the values that are endorsed and suppressed in responses to suffering.

Features of Suffering

The experience of suffering is deeply personal and highly contextual. Suffering has been simultaneously described as "common to us all," yet "radically personal," so much so that "the felt reality of suffering is in an important sense ineffable, un-sharable."[2] Care must be taken to avoid expanding a truth about feelings into a gratuitous philosophical solipsism about suffering—that we each live in our own unknowable world of suffering. In what "important sense" is that felt reality ineffable and not shareable? One person's "felt reality" is indeed not shareable because we cannot share, that is, experience, somebody else's feelings. We cannot feel what others feel. That claim is true in virtue of the meaning of "felt reality." But what follows from it? Not that suffering is ineffable, in the sense of being too overwhelming to be expressed or described in words or to be too awesome or sacred to be spoken. And not that somebody else's suffering or suffering itself is opaque to us. The same point applies to Eric Cassell's description of suffering as "ultimately a personal matter—something whose presence and extent can only be known to the sufferer."[3] How is the qualification, "ultimately," to be understood, and what exactly is that "something" that only the sufferer can know (with certainty?)? Reducing suffering to its "felt reality" decocts suffering to the powerful feelings and emotions that are the phenomenological essence of suffering, but those personal feelings and emotions are products of the biological and social components of suffering that are "common to us all."

We can recognize when others are suffering, and we can discern elements of suffering and sources of suffering. We learn to do that collectively because suffering—not the felt reality of suffering—is collective. When we suffer, how we suffer, and why we suffer are determinants of our collective experience and understanding of suffering. A child can begin to learn what suffering is by, for example, watching his grandmother mourn the accidental death of her youngest son, his favorite uncle. Over time he will experience his own losses and the emotions attached to losses such as the death of a devoted pet, rejection by a long-time girlfriend, and being fired from a prized job, and he will observe the losses of others and their reactions to their losses. He will console and be consoled. He will come to know, with others and from others, what suffering is. He will not know with certainty because there is no certainty in life, and in fact the unpredictability of suffering is the best teacher of the contingency of life. He never will know the "felt reality" of another person's suffering, but, given the collective nature of suffering, his experience, and his capacity to make inferences, he will be able to recognize that suffering and empathize with it. There is much more to suffering than the private, idiosyncratic "felt reality" of suffering. Suffering is not just "radically personal." Indeed, it is the commonality of suffering that ultimately makes our radically personal felt reality feel the way it does, and it is that commonality that we evince in our own suffering and recognize in the suffering of others.

Understanding what something is often begins with understanding what it is not. Suffering is not pain, not the localized bodily sensation of hurting caused by physical injury, disease, disorder, malformation, or degeneration. Suffering is mental, emotional, and spiritual, and it manifests grief, despair, and sorrow. Suffering can result from disabling pain, but it is qualitatively different. The enervation, incapacitation, anxiety, worrying, withdrawal, and other forms of distress that accompany pain are distinct from the pain. They are not the throbbing of a migraine or the aching of a back or the burning of childbirth. They are the despair of a person. And whereas pain scales crudely quantify the magnitude of pain, there is no comparable quantification of suffering. Assessing the severity of suffering is elusive because it depends on the disparate features of our lives that we value, such as the ease, convenience, and importance of doing things for ourselves, comfort at being touched, warmth from the affection of our children, and the fun we have with friends. Different persons value different, idiosyncratic, incommensurable combinations of the fundamental elements of life and the manifold joys of life. We understand that being deprived of the opportunities and rewards of life causes suffering, and we can judge whether the apparent intensity of suffering is commensurate to the magnitude of a loss. But we cannot quantify, however crudely, the depth of the suffering that attends a particular life.

Suffering comes in myriad forms and in myriad ways. Its presence can be illustrated by its manifestation in three different kinds of lives. The first is a constrained life, a life that has few, if any, prospects beyond mere existence and might hold suffering. That is the life of a person born with extensive, severe physical and mental handicaps who responds to little, if any, sensory stimulation, shows signs of being in discomfort and pain, and is restricted to a bed or a wheelchair. We readily assume that such a person is suffering, either as a consequence of pain or independently of pain, or both, but that assumption is a projection of the kind of life we have onto the kind of life we see, which we have difficulty imagining and comprehending. Persons who are less physically handicapped but severely mentally handicapped can engage in serious self-abuse, for example, banging their head against the corner of a table, and have to be controlled with drugs or physical restraints and protected with helmets. Might the pain they seek be a way of escaping suffering they find intolerable? Persons with less severe physical and mental handicaps can become aggressive to others who have what they do not have and never will be able to achieve. Might causing others to suffer allay their own suffering by evening the score and giving them company? Perhaps. We do not know whether they suffer and, if so, how they suffer.

A constrained life need not contain physical handicaps, or pain, or suffering, however. When I started out in bioethics, I spent time in a diagnostic, assessment, and treatment facility for children with serious mental and physical handicaps. I met the cutest little boy I have ever seen there, and for months every time I went into his building, I would go straight to the play room, pick him up, and carry him around in my arms. I never saw him smile, and I never received any acknowledgment whatsoever of my existence from him. I have no reason to believe that he was suffering. Attributing suffering to him would have to be based on what he knew was happening and what he realized he had lost, but he did not have the mental capacity to understand his situation. His parents undoubtedly suffered, though.

The second kind of life is a compromised life, a life that is missing some of the important opportunities and goods that make living rewarding and enjoyable or that has some serious impediments, disadvantages, or troubles that impair or remove much of the satisfaction of living. An example is a teenager who is struggling with and succumbing to the array of challenges to maturing and becoming a confident, proud adult and resorts to cutting herself, probably to gain attention but also, in some way, to relieve her suffering. Unlike children, teenagers have formed at least a protean sense of what they value and what it is to have a good life, and they can fear that they do not have the capacity to have a good life now or in the future because of problems with peers, family, or school, say. They have lost a nascent good life, temporarily, one hopes, and with that they have lost hope for a good future life. Their despair, at a pivotal time when lives are unfolding and being shaped and hopes and dreams are fervently proliferating, is a sign and a source of their suffering. Cutting could be a way of coping with their amorphous, confusing, intangible suffering by converting it to pain, which they understand. They can see the wound and the bleeding, and they know that wounds heal in a limited, predictable time. Cutting might enable them to make some sense of their suffering and give them the feeling that they can constrain and have some control over their suffering. Persons addicted to alcohol or drugs have similarly compromised lives that are a source of their suffering.

The third kind of life is a life that has vanished or has become evanescent.[4] A life that had its inevitable setbacks, disappointments, and failures but overall has been productive, rewarding, and enjoyable can unexpectedly be closed by accident or disease or can be fading because of disease or aging. Values that inspired aspirations and ambitions, formed and developed relationships, built confidence and integrity, and instilled pride are gone. Those values created, sustained, and invigorated a life but now have been replaced by values that are imposed, alien, and unpalatable.

A drastic example conveys the suffering that accompanies the sudden, irretrievable loss of a flourishing life. Jean-Dominique Bauby, 44 years old, was married and the father of two children and the editor-in-chief of *Elle*, a famous fashion magazine in Paris, when he suffered a massive stroke. He describes the result:

> ...Improved resuscitation techniques have now prolonged and refined the agony. You survive, but you survive with what is so aptly known as "locked-in-syndrome." Paralysed from head to toe, the patient is imprisoned inside his own body, his mind intact, but unable to speak or move. In my case, blinking my left eyelid is my only means of communication.[5]

Bauby was able to dictate a book about his experience by blinking his eyelid to identify letters of the alphabet. He describes his life as "forced solitude" and "taking up residence in my cocoon." His life before the stroke was replete with the perquisites and pleasures of wealth and power, but he misses one pleasure in particular:

> ...My communication system disqualifies repartee: the keenest rapier grows dull and falls flat when it takes several minutes to thrust it home. By the time you strike, even you no longer understand what had seemed so witty before you started to dictate it, letter by letter. So the rule is to avoid impulsive sallies. It deprives conversation of its sparkle, all those gems you bat back and forth like a ball—and I count this forced lack of humour one of the great drawbacks of my condition.[6]

That loss, albeit a "great drawback," is not, in itself, a source of suffering but a source of sadness and regret. Someone who has long loved to play tennis might have to give it up because of injury or aging, and although that would be a great disappointment and loss of much pleasure, it would not be a source of suffering. Suffering is more general and more diffuse and not linked to what Cassell calls "the loss of a piece of oneself."[7]

This is suffering:

> Sunday. I dread Sunday, for if I am unlucky enough to have no visitors there will be nothing at all to break the dreary passage of the hours. No physiotherapist, no speech pathologist, no shrink. Sunday is crossing the desert, its only oasis a sponge bath even more perfunctory than usual....The bath I am given bears more resemblance to drawing and quartering than to hydrotherapy. A triple dose of the finest deodorant fails to mask the reality: I stink.[8]

Loneliness, boredom, objectification, disgust. And this:

> For half an hour the alarm on the machine regulating my feeding tube has been beeping out into the void. I cannot imagine anything so inane or nerve-racking as this piercing beep beep beep pecking away at my brain. To make matters worse, my sweat has unglued the tape that keeps my right eyelid closed, and the stuck-together lashes are tickling my pupil unbearably. To crown it all, the end of my urinary catheter has become detached and I am drenched.[9]

Distress, embarrassment, impotence, humiliation. And this devastatingly poignant time with his son:

> ...We...play hangman, the national pre-teen sport. I guess a letter, then another, then stumble on the third. My heart is not in the game. Grief surges over me. His face not two feet from mine, my son Théophile sits patiently waiting—and I, his father, have lost the simple right to ruffle his bristly hair, clasp his downy neck, hug his small lithe warm body tight against me. There are no words to express it. My condition is monstrous, iniquitous, revolting, horrible.

> Suddenly I can take no more. Tears well and my throat emits a hoarse rattle that startles Théophile. Don't be scared, little man. I love you. Still engrossed in the game, he moves in for the kill. Two more letters: he has won, and I have lost. On a corner of the page he completes his drawing of the gallows, the rope and the condemned man.[10]

Pathos. No words to express the felt reality but words to express the suffering. The feelings and emotions are displayed by the body, but the unendurable losses are suffered by the person. Before his family leaves, his children go for a run on the beach while his wife stays with him: "... Sylvie and I remain alone and silent, her hand squeezing my inert fingers. Behind dark glasses that reflect a flawless sky, she softly weeps over our shattered lives."[11]

Suffering is the realized loss of the values that give a life integrity and make life meaningful and enjoyable, loss that is profound in the sense of being intensely felt and in the sense of being thoroughgoing. The loss in a constrained life is thoroughgoing but might not be felt, let alone intensely felt. The loss in a compromised life and the loss of a once-flourishing life are both thoroughgoing and intensely felt. Suffering can be compounded when loss is not just profound, but senseless—loss without reason, without explanation, without meaning. Not all suffering is senseless. A divorced father distraught about being estranged from his children, for example, might come to comprehend and bemoan the behavior that caused those rifts and concede the responsibility he bears for his suffering. But much suffering is senseless. A person whose life has been devastated by a catastrophic stroke or a parent whose life has been emptied by the death of a child searches for answers to imponderable questions: "Why me?" "Why now?" "How can I go on with my life?" "Who am I now?" The sheer arbitrariness of the occurrence and timing of a loss can itself be devastating.

Responses to Suffering

Much suffering is accepted and endured. People with strong religious commitments can believe that suffering is necessary to obtain peace and grace in an eternal afterlife. Others suffer for an array of reasons, such as resignation to the vicissitudes of life and deference to the desires of families. Acceptance is an attempt to deprive suffering of its uselessness by making it a means to some good. Silence is a natural accompaniment to acceptance because it "allows sufferers not to speak of something that is painful and does not trivialize their suffering with all-too-easy words of understanding."[12] Silence poses a danger, however. I once heard Dan Gottlieb, a psychologist in Philadelphia, say in a public talk that the more we suffer, the more we become self-absorbed, and the more we become self-absorbed, the more we suffer. By deepening that self-absorption, silence could reinforce that vicious circle.

The goal of responses to intractable suffering is, as Arthur Frank puts it, to make suffering livable.[13] What he calls his "unoriginal premise" is that "suffering is intensified when people feel alone."[14] And withdrawal, loneliness, isolation, perhaps even claustrophobia can make people feel crazy. Frank explains that "one of the most frequent and most poignant comments that ill people have made to me about my own memoir of illness is that reading it made them feel less crazy."[15] Craziness starts in isolation and fosters isolation, and isolation magnifies suffering. Frank believes that recognizing the dramatic in suffering and sharing dramas of suffering with others can make suffering livable. Because drama is communal, "to render suffering dramatic can help to *communalize* it," and communalizing suffering can prevent craziness from becoming destructive and all consuming.[16]

The communality of companionship can interrupt isolation and diminish loneliness, as when a nurse in a long-term-care facility eats her lunch and shares stories with a resident whose children are distant and visit infrequently. And companionship can be an important source of comfort, consolation, and compassion. Modifying circumstances also can mitigate suffering. Reassurance can allay anxiety, for example, by regularly reminding a patient that the doctor will talk to her soon about changing her medications. Other strategies for lessening suffering are engaging and distracting, by, for instance, organizing social events such as card games and having a television on constantly in a nursing home. Mitigation can provide solace, but it is sporadic, and its effects are transient. The most formidable obstacle to mitigation is a shortage of resources, human and material.

Two more drastic responses to extreme, refractory suffering are transformation of the person who is suffering and ending the life of the person who is suffering. Bioethics and the Bible provide dramatic examples of transformation. The bioethics example is Donald Cowart, an active young man who was terribly burned in an accident and who endured horrific pain and suffering that drove him to request that his life be ended.[17] The Biblical example is Job, who had everything but his life taken by Satan. Donald Cowart dealt with his suffering, William May explains, by becoming a new person.[18] Job dealt with his suffering, Herbert Fingarette explains, by transcending the person he was.[19]

May understands that Donald Cowart's tragedy lies beyond the conventional invocations of autonomy and quality of life because it poses a fundamental existential plight:

> The patient... resembles... the agonist in Greek tragedy or the stricken religious figure cut off from the safeties of family and city. I cite these analogies not in order to flatter the patient, but simply in order to locate him. He bears the mark of the uncanny, the German term for which is the *Unheimlich*, literally, the one "not at home," the alien, the one driven out beyond the precincts of hearth and city gates, where no one in his right mind would want to venture, and who therefore sends a shudder through the rest of the community.[20]

Donald Cowart built a successful, rewarding life that he never will reclaim. Most people have only one life to live, but Donald Cowart has the choice to live another life. He realizes that if he is to live, he must forge a new life defined by values fundamentally different from the values of his old life. As May so trenchantly puts it, "his life must reconstruct from the grave up."[21] His choice implicates the values that would shape and give worth to the kind of life he could have, and, more profoundly, it exposes values about not just the preciousness and sanctity of life but also the dignity of life, as May recognizes:

> Should he choose to live, he cannot choose simply to take up his old life. He must become a new man. Don Cowart becomes Dax. . . . To travel into that darkness requires an interior transformation, it requires ethics at the deepest level, not trivial problem-solving, but the reordering of one's identity from the ground up. The community can and must assist in countless ways. But without consent to transformation the patient cannot move from saying "please let me die" to "I am glad to be alive." That heroic movement does not vindicate his doctors, because the deeper decision must be his, and only as it is his do we see in him not simply a patient encased and obscured by the surgeon's art but the uncanny radiance of a man.[22]

Donald Cowart's suffering also reveals the values of the community. They are the values of attending to the vulnerable—caring, compassion, community; empathy, sympathy, kindness; patience, understanding, help. And admiration of Donald Cowart's courage and awe at his resoluteness.

It is tempting, perhaps irresistibly so, for bioethics to wrap all of that up in autonomy, and then the answer is easy.[23] Everybody I know who has seen the tape of the psychiatric interview with Donald Cowart—and I have been showing it to students for years—has no doubt that he is competent. If autonomy is a matter of respecting the decisions of competent persons, Donald Cowart should be allowed to die. The obstacles to that outcome at the time of his hospitalization decades ago were fear of legal culpability and uncertainty about how to bring about his death without inflicting even greater pain and suffering. That approach manifests the narrowness and superficiality of quandary ethics.[24] The values that Donald Cowart's suffering expose reveal that "the deeper decision must be his" not because nobody is morally entitled to decide on his behalf but because nobody could possibly decide on his behalf.[25] The complex concatenation of values that makes life valuable and worth living is too diverse, too grand, and too idiosyncratic. "Ethics at the deepest level," as May puts it, is a matter of appreciating the momentousness of what is at stake and finding a way of struggling with that momentousness. The loss of Donald Cowart will not disappear, and Dax will suffer that loss throughout his life. His suffering is unimaginable, and only a commitment to life and a transformation—a reconstruction of who he is—could make his suffering bearable.

The suffering of Job is just as unimaginable because it is so complete. When Satan challenges the purity and sincerity of Job's scrupulous obedience to God,

God allows Satan to take away everything from Job except his life. His seven sons and three daughters are killed when the house in which they are eating is blown down; his livestock are stolen and his servants murdered; his relatives and friends desert him; he becomes diseased and pustulous. There is no more exhaustive depiction of loss than the contrast between Job's life before and after Satan's depredations. Job suffers from the totality of his losses, but he also suffers, perhaps even more, because he does not know why he is suffering. God says to Satan: "Hast thou considered my servant Job, that *there is* none like him in the earth, a perfect and an upright man, one that feareth God, and escheweth evil? and still he holdeth fast his integrity, although thou movedst me against him, to destroy him without cause."[26] Job's suffering is more than senseless—it is incomprehensible. Job is bewildered because his suffering violates the orthodox understanding of God as lawgiver. God makes the law and enforces the law by rewarding those who obey and punishing those who disobey. Job knows that he has been unfailingly obedient, and Job knows that God knows that he has been unfailingly obedient. Why, then, has he been punished? Job believes he deserves an answer, and he seeks that answer from God.

The Book of Job reveals that Job cannot come to understand his suffering from an interlocution with God. Suffering cannot be understood by reason, by the kind of questioning and argumentation that Job envisages in a hearing before God. An understanding of suffering, Fingarette explains, can be grasped only through experience:

> The wisdom taught by suffering is the wisdom learned in living, not in books; it is the experience of the finitude and fallibility of the personal will, and also, in the perspective of human mortality, of its ultimate impotence and defeat. The message of suffering is thus implicit in suffering itself; it is not a lesson only contingently associated with and conveyed through suffering. The experience gives wisdom when we see the fact for what it is, when we experience the humbled will and see at last the will as humble, inherently finite, and fallible, and when we accept this truth in our very bones and not merely in theory.[27]

We know that suffering exists, but that knowledge remains abstract and aloof as long as it is about the suffering of others.

That suffering will come to us because we, too, are finite and fallible is the message delivered to Job by Elihu and a whirlwind and expressed through poetry and music:

> Elihu does not explain all this, but he announces it. God's message comes in suffering; an appreciation of the message comes only when we despair of our own powers, thus accepting the inevitability of the humbled human will and accepting suffering as intrinsic to our mortal existence. The implication of the message is that salvation and reconciliation with creation can not be accomplished by depending fundamentally on our own personal will. There must be a *goel* or an intercession from outside. No *goel* can save us, however, until

> we have learned the essential wisdom that consists in abandoning hope in our personal power to make things as we will them to be.[28]

The wisdom of the Book of Job is that our agency in life and our control over life are limited, but those limitations do not threaten our dignity or our integrity:

> The point is that Job does achieve humility; the self-assertive "I" has dissolved. But this humility is the very opposite of humiliation. Humiliation presupposes an "I" which exists and is assertive even in its impotence, an "I" that is coerced and self-denigrating. This suffering is what we ordinarily recognize as suffering: it is misery. But authentic humility reflects neither impotence nor self-deprecation; it is as if the self-assertive "I" had been a cloud over the soul that has dissipated.... Authentic humility is never associated with being put down, but on the contrary it is an aspect of the transcendent elevation of consciousness.[29]

To ignore the suffering of others is egoistic, callous, selfish; to ignore the possibility of one's own suffering is denial, conceit, pride. When suffering comes, the response to its humiliation of the assertive, independent self—to incapacity, debilitation, dependency, embarrassment, and shame—can only be transcendence of that self. What remains is the "uncanny radiance" of a human being that May sees in Dax, a self that has been humbled but not humiliated.

The responses of Dax and Job to overwhelming suffering are extreme. Donald Cowart's conversion to Dax and Job's acceptance of humility expose the profound values that severe suffering implicates. The fortitude, courage, and will of Dax will be admired but seldom emulated. In a society that exalts appearance, beauty, and perfection, and where much time and money is spent to hide or correct minor physical imperfections and signs of aging, deciding to endure enormous pain for a disabled, disfigured body that will make life agonizing and exhausting and will disconcert and distress others—to become *unheimlich*—seems folly. The humility of Job will be esteemed but seldom emulated. Humility is a scarce virtue in a society enthralled by the assertion and promotion of self and devoted to the independence and control enshrined in autonomy.[30] The Book of Job will continue to be regarded as a great sacred text and literary masterpiece, but its wisdom of suffering will, if understood, be ignored.

The compelling transformations of Dax and Job are, nevertheless, emblematic of the most profound value that suffering reveals—human dignity. Traditional accounts of dignity locate it in the uniqueness of human beings. From a theological perspective, human beings are creations of God; from a secular perspective, human beings possess reason. Those are generic, impersonal attributions of dignity. Suffering provides a personal, humane perspective on dignity. Throughout their suffering—through helplessness and humiliation—Dax and Job retain and display their dignity. They refuse to be diminished or demeaned by their unrelenting suffering. The transcendence of suffering is the transcendence of our finitude and fallibility, and that transcendence is both a demonstration and an affirmation of our dignity. The dignity of Dax and Job is not the dignity of personhood, but the dignity of persons. Although Dax and Job are exceptional examples, the dignity of suffering is an ordinary and common phenomenon. Children dying from leukemia, for example, transcend their fears and their sadness in their concern for their parents,[31] and persons with progressive dementia transcend their plight in their flickering, sporadic reversions to and reaffirmations of their disappearing lives.

The loss of dignity through degradation and humiliation is the consummate form of human suffering. Slavery, of course, is the consummate example of that suffering. The debilitation of serious disease and illness and the decrepitude of aging bring losses that impose multiple incapacities and sweeping dependency. The resulting helplessness and humiliation can threaten the dignity of a life and thereby create overwhelming suffering.

An emerging response to such great suffering is to end the suffering by ending the lives of those who are suffering, and that alternative is where suffering most directly engages bioethics. Because severe pain can generally be controlled, the primary reason for ending a life is unceasing, intolerable suffering. In the Netherlands, intentionally ending a life remains a criminal offence in principle, but doctors who perform euthanasia are exempt from criminal liability if the patient has a medically classifiable illness, the patient is experiencing unbearable suffering with no prospect of improvement, and the legally prescribed criteria for due care are satisfied.[32] An ethical analysis by Theo Boer of 1,200 reports submitted to one of the five Regional Review Committees on Euthanasia in the Netherlands from 2005 to 2009 displays the values that motivate requests for euthanasia.[33] Patients cite an array of reasons for their unbearable suffering: "Pain is mentioned in 43 percent of the cases, nausea in 41 percent, dependence on others for daily care in 48 percent, loss of autonomy in a wider sense in 18 percent, dyspnea in 29 percent, extreme fatigue in 22 percent, anxiety in 22 percent of the cases, a loss of body functions (incontinence, a loss of speech) in 11 percent, and meaninglessness (including loneliness) in 11 percent of the cases." (55) Details in the reports submitted by patients and doctors elucidate the losses and the suffering behind those numbers:

> "Her sister vividly explains her predicament. There is nothing left she can do: she can't even wipe the tears from her own eyes." (55)
>
> The doctor of a patient with metastases in the bones writes: "Last week he broke two ribs when he was assisted in going to the bathroom. The next day he sneezed and broke another rib. Now he won't let anyone touch him, not even his own wife." (55)
>
> A woman with severely disfiguring facial cancer who has small children explains that "she wants euthanasia before her children start avoiding her and no longer show affection to her." (56)

Three primary reasons are given for the existence of unbearable suffering: dependence, humiliation, and a life that is meaninglessness or is not a good life.

Dependency can cause enmity and resentment, but it also can be a source of great suffering, particularly when it is comprehensive and when it occurs in societies with a worldview that promotes and rewards individualism, freedom, self-sufficiency, and control.[34] Dependency is especially despairing when it involves the daily needs of life because patients can feel that they no longer are full human beings but mere objects of care and pity. (54) In explaining what makes her suffering unbearable, a woman replies: "It is having to ask others for help. 'Asking, asking, asking, I can't and I won't!'" (60) Some people regard admission to a nursing home as a confirmation of dependency and an imposition of its correlative unbearable suffering. That view, in fact, is so pervasive that it has been incorporated into advance directives: "If my condition would justify admittance to a nursing home, it is my wish to have my life terminated." (55)

Humiliation caused by insensitive and inadequate care can prompt patients to request euthanasia, as a doctor describes:

> Patient never thought about giving up because she found her life worth living, despite everything. But that changed during her last hospitalization. For the duration of her six day stay she received not half of the help she needed. One afternoon she was stripped to the waist so she asked a nurse to help her arrange her pyjamas. The nurse refused. On the afternoon of her departure there was no one to help her. There was no wheelchair and she and her husband had to arrange their own taxi. At that moment something snapped. These six days were so dehumanizing that she blew a fuse. Her husband affirms this. "On top of her physical condition," he affirms, "his wife's suffering was caused by the humiliation she underwent in the hospital." (62)

Pride likewise can motivate a request for euthanasia. A doctor writes: "This proud lady rejects being admitted to a nursing home. For her this equals unbearable suffering." (60) An elderly man explains, "My bare bottom washed by a young girl, never!" (60)

Patients who feel that their life has become meaningless or no longer is a good life also can request euthanasia, as several doctors report:

> The pain and nausea are under control, but the real problem is that we haven't succeeded in finding a meaningful activity during his last weeks. He bluntly refuses every suggestion we make. (56)
>
> Patient has a tan and gives a vital impression. What really causes her suffering is that she can no longer make any essential contribution to the lives of others. (56)
>
> She has been a nurse all her life, but having others take care of *her* is the last thing she would accept. An important part of her self-esteem has always consisted in taking care of others. Now that she can no longer care, her life lacks meaning. (55; emphasis in original)
>
> All this respectable and once active lady can do is sit at the window and chase away the crows with her cane. (56)

> Patient is known to be a true *bon vivant*. Being bed-ridden is not compatible with his conception of a good life. (57)

Patients explain:

> It's like floating in space, there is no goal, no fixed points, just uncertainty and lack of meaning. (56)
>
> I am bored all day. The only thing I notice are cars parking in and out. Lying in bed and staring at the ceiling all day makes no sense. (56)
>
> Tinkering with embroideries in some room, singing songs to keep up our spirits, I don't want all that. (60)

These people are distressed because they realize how much they have lost and what they never will have again, and they find their suffering unbearable.[35]

Suffering also can be caused and exacerbated by institutional settings in which care is unavailable or poor. Many people fear being placed in a nursing home, and their fear might not be misplaced: "The bad reputation of nursing homes, which is one of the reasons for qualifying a future transfer into such an institution as unbearable suffering, at least in part goes back to real problems: shortage of staff, insufficient hygiene, lack of privacy, a socially untrained staff." (61) Care provided in a hospital, a doctor relates, also can create suffering:

> One patient in a hospital indicates that one of the motives for his euthanasia request is the fact that he never sleeps through the night. "Staying in a four-bed room, I am constantly being woken up by noises." "The institution he is in has a serious shortage of staff. Apart from the pain and the distress, he tells me he has lain in his own excrements a couple of times now, and he does not want that to happen again." "The severe suffering of this man is intensified by the impersonal setting of his care institution." (62)

Suffering cannot be disengaged from the settings and circumstances in which it arises and in which it is experienced.

These accounts of the nature and sources of suffering, combined with the various responses to suffering, raise challenges for how bioethics should be conceived and conducted. What could bioethics do about suffering?

Suffering and Bioethics

Before Fingarette begins his discussion of Elihu's appearance to Job, he cannot resist digressing to tell a story:

> . . . Most of the newly deceased, as they arrive at the pearly gates, are greeted by the attending angel and directed to a broad avenue that will lead them to the Divine Presence; but on the occasional arrival of a professor of philosophy or theology, the angel obligingly points out, instead, a different path leading to an auditorium where there is a lecture on God.[36]

And he cites an analysis by Jack Kahn, a psychiatrist, who in his book, *Job's Illness: Loss, Grief, and Integration*, undertakes "to draw conclusions about . . . [Job's] experiences using the kind of reasoning which would be available to a clinician. . . ."[37] Fingarette notes that many readers complain about "the shift from argument as a mode of teaching to direct revelation through poetry" and the whirlwind passages that Elihu brings, and he identifies the source of this dissatisfaction: "Instead of listening to the music of song and poem and opening the self to what the poet does—in short, instead of suffering—such a reader insists on continuing to act or to impose on the text the old categories and modes of inquiry."[38]

Suffering is largely foreign territory for bioethics, medically and morally.[39] Suffering is not a disease or an illness, but a phenomenon of the human condition—our finitude and fallibility—that attends serious disease and illness as well as other devastating misfortunes. Suffering remains peripheral to the mainstream bioethics that is grounded in analytic moral philosophy, which has little interest in the human condition.[40] Had bioethics not been transferred from theologians shortly after its inception, suffering might occupy a more prominent place in bioethics today.[41] Now, however, not only the kind of revelation Fingarette describes but also suffering itself are rebuffed for being subjective and nonrational, if not irrational, according to the prevailing canons of philosophical respectability and objectivity. There is a steep price to be paid for that vaunted objectivity, however, because it dissolves the humanity of morality in its presumptive universalizability.

Yet a number of prominent bioethicists recently had a sobering "direct revelation" about the objectivity of bioethics from being diagnosed or having a member of their family diagnosed with cancer.[42] That whirlwind shifted their focus from the professional to the personal—the subjective. They discovered that receiving the diagnosis was overwhelming; they experienced regression and felt dependent; they had to make decisions in the face of uncertainty and complexity; and they made decisions that they subsequently realized were not good. They came to appreciate the diversity of the illness experience, both across and within individuals. They experienced distress, grief, and despair; they lost control; and they discovered how limited their autonomy was. They had difficulty figuring out which treatment options were most compatible with their values and goals, and they were torn between quantity of life and quality of life: "In the end, quantity of life usually took priority. We were a little surprised at the burdens we were willing to accept in exchange for a better chance of survival. We now know why so many patients desire those expensive cancer drugs that rarely extend life more than a few months."[43]

These bioethicists naturally related their personal experiences to their professional roles. Leon Kass asked the group, "Without a good understanding of what it is like to be overwhelmed by the experience of illness—one's own or that of a loved one—how can the doctor or ethicist appreciate the human situation the doctor must address?"[44] Throughout their experiences, the bioethicists were patients or caregivers, but they also were ethicists observing and assessing what was transpiring with professional interest and detachment. They were ethnographers (some professional and some amateur) doing research in the field.[45]

What should be made of their findings? The group understood that their personal experiences could, and likely would, be readily dismissed by colleagues because they are not relevant to "real" bioethics. Yet what they learned is "about the distance between medical ethics in books and classrooms and medical ethics on the ground," in particular, that "fear, guilt, isolation, fatigue, and despair populate the world of serious illness."[46] They learned that people dealing with serious illness are concerned about dignity, mortality, and grief and that a bioethics that ignores their suffering and their values is decidedly limited.

The unpredictability of suffering also shows that the respect for autonomy that dominates analytic moral philosophy and bioethics is decidedly limited. Fingarette acknowledges the sobering message that the Book of Job delivers for autonomy:

> This teaching may seem to be grim and despairing. But it is only grim to one who has placed all hope, consciously or unconsciously, in a happiness that relies on the fulfillment of the personal will, and, more specifically, the hope that we can impose our will on existence because our existence is essentially lawlike and because we can manipulate existence through knowledge of its laws. Loss of such hope is "despair" in the literal meaning of that word, without hope; it has this meaning only in regard to the deceptive hope of imposing one's will on life. To surrender that hope, is by no means to surrender all hope.... That concept is the truth that the *Book of Job* teaches.[47]

The currently burgeoning industries of academic and popular writing on happiness affirm the preeminent goal of our society—the pursuit of "happiness that relies on the fulfillment of the personal will." Moral philosophy and the bioethics derived from it embrace the means of attaining that goal—the exercise of autonomy, which embodies and promotes "the hope that we can impose our will on existence." One needs only to look at John Rawls' monumental work, *A Theory of Justice*, for a declaration of the centrality of planning a life to moral philosophy.[48] For Rawls people have to have plans of life, and a rational plan of life determines the good of a person. Rawls explains that he is simply adapting Josiah Royce's proposal that "a person may be regarded as a human life lived according to a plan."[49]

That view of persons and the good of persons exhibits an overweening confidence in the transparency and benignity of the world and in the capacities of human beings to predict events and anticipate the vagaries of life. Writing after he was widowed, Renato Rosaldo relates an anecdote about a man, widowed by his wife's unexpected death, who put a sign on his refrigerator that said, "Life is what happens to you while you're making other plans."[50] Rosaldo offers a more realistic depiction of life and its contingencies:

> ...In everyday life the wise guide themselves as often by waiting to see what happens as by using rules, plans, and expectations. When in doubt, people find out about their worlds by living with ambiguity, uncertainty, or a simple lack of knowledge until the day, if and when it arrives, that their life experiences

> clarify matters. One can, in other words, learn by doing Human beings often do muddle through, improvise, and make things up as they go along.[51]

That account of ordinary life captures the wisdom of ordinary people but unintentionally and unwarrantedly demeans it by characterizing it as just muddling through. People, including children, indeed learn from their experience and by doing, and they develop skilled judgment in that process. They do all that because they are rational, not in the sense of the formal reason that makes logic and mathematics rational, but in the sense of a more expansive, process-based nonformal reason that can vindicate the rationality of judgment.[52] They make judgments about when to plan and use rules and when to wait and see, when they need help, when they need more information, when they must improvise, when matters become sufficiently clear, and endless other issues in their lives. Their judgments are rational not because they can be derived from principles but because of the process of deliberation from which they emanate and the tools they use in that process: observation to learn about the world and from the experiences of others; creativity to develop options and ways of testing those options and to improvise; formal and informal reasoning to understand the implications and consequences of alternatives; and comprehensive critical assessment to determine how they can improve their deliberation, when they have deliberated enough or waited enough, and which option is preferable. With that broader conception of nonformal reason, bioethics would not have to consign suffering to the merely subjective. Nor could the personal revelations and insights of those serendipitous bioethicist ethnographers be dismissed because they do not belong to "real" bioethics. Rather, their experiences would be recognized as the real "real" bioethics. Cassell observes that "since antiquity there has been a prejudice in favor of reason and against experiential knowledge,"[53] but that inveterate dichotomy and the ensuing prejudice exist only if reason is reduced to and equated with formal reason. The rationality of real human beings extends well beyond the narrow confines of the formal reason that dominates the academy and, in turn, bioethics.

Yet the sway of autonomy remains undiminished and, if anything, is expanding. The exercise of autonomy can itself produce unbearable suffering by, for example, refusing palliative care, admission to a nursing home, or supportive care, and the resulting unbearable suffering then can be invoked to request euthanasia.[54] A doctor in the Netherlands reports: "Palliative care could be better, but the patient rejects the alternatives. Euthanasia is all she wants." (60) Another doctor says of a 50-year-old man handicapped after a motorcycle accident: "He deserves better care than he gets, but refuses. Getting washed and dressed takes hours. The severity of his suffering is related to a total lack of a social network." (60) In such circumstances, Boer reports, physicians "nevertheless—albeit hesitantly—grant the patient's request." (60) Physicians and patients have different understandings of euthanasia: "Physicians continue to see euthanasia as a last resort; patients increasingly regard it in terms of a right." (54)

Appeals to autonomy will continue to exert inexorable pressure to expand that right. A euthanasia advocacy group, Right to Die–NL, in the Netherlands now is promoting legislation that would make euthanasia available to any person over the age of 70 years, regardless of whether they have a terminal illness.[55] Dr. Petra de Jong, a Dutch pulmonologist who has helped people to die since 1989, says, "We think old people can suffer from life."[56] The next development in the Netherlands, not surprisingly given the kinds of requests for euthanasia that already are approved, could be purely autonomy-based euthanasia for veterans of life. Dr. Paul Root Wolpe, Director of the Center for Ethics at Emory University, is "generally supportive" of "people's right to choose their own death," but he is concerned about the enforcement of such a policy: "When you switch from purely physiological criteria to a set of psychological criteria, you are opening the door to abuse and error."[57] That concern already exists with respect to the requirement that suffering be unbearable, where it does not seem to substantially constrain the approval of requests for euthanasia.

How impervious bioethics is to suffering exposes not just the substantive but also the constitutive values of orthodox bioethics. Arthur Kleinman warns those in the humanities of the danger that "all the interest we have in theory subverts what the human experience is about."[58] The theoretical underpinnings and methods of bioethics are drawn from academic disciplines committed to and bedazzled by theory that subverts the richness of human experience. The orientation of bioethics to health care remains largely medical, with nursing and its dedication to caring decidedly subordinate and physical therapy, occupational therapy, speech therapy, and social work absent. Just as there is much to be learned about the character of persons and societies from how they respond to suffering, there is much to be learned about the character of bioethics from its shallow response to suffering: avoid it or end it.

Conclusion

This chapter is about how to understand the suffering—"the heartaches and the thousand natural shocks that flesh is heir to"—imposed by the rampant contingencies of life and the ways in which people and bioethics respond to suffering. Suffering is, however, more complex, more commodious, and more nuanced than this limited analysis conveys. The choices that individuals make about suffering reveal their values; the choices that bioethics makes about suffering reveal its values; and the choices that societies make about suffering reveal their values. Each domain provides a partial, independent, discrete perspective on suffering. Suffering needs to be understood holistically, as the manifestation of a complex, dynamic system that encompasses individuals, institutions, governments, bioethics, and society and within which the values of each component interact, conflict, mutate, and coalesce. Suffering and its place in that system then can be better comprehended and addressed more productively. Moreover, choices have to be made not just about how to respond to suffering that is imposed but also about what, if anything, should be done with respect to suffering that can be foreseen. Perhaps the most compelling case for the legalization of assisted suicide is the enormous suffering that persons with amyotrophic lateral sclerosis, or Lou Gehrig's disease, have to endure. That issue exposes a panoply of values beyond the values of personal suffering, some of which, such as the sanctity of human life and the worthiness of the lives of handicapped persons that might be endangered, mitigate against changing the law to relieve great suffering. The moral issues of suffering go beyond alleviating suffering to considering the good that might come from suffering and from tolerating suffering and the values that might override the alleviation of suffering.

Suffering eludes the limitations of current bioethics. The constitutive morality of orthodox bioethics is a moral theory comprising four canonical principles. The principle of nonmalificence—do no harm, in medicine—is the most stringent, and it prohibits imposing suffering, through torture or in other ways, but disease, accidents, and aging do not obey principles. Of the quadruplet, the principle of beneficence—doing good—is the weakling. Philosophers struggle to justify a general duty of beneficence, regarding it as virtue or charity instead, so an obligation to help a specific person generally is grounded in and defined by a relationship to that person, such as being a spouse, a child, a friend, or a health care provider. The abstruse principle of justice is no match for the captivations of politics and ideologies. For suffering, that leaves, by default if not by design, the pinnacle principle of respect for autonomy. Unfortunately, the value of autonomy is reduced to the ritual exercise of protecting the freedom to choose, thereby avoiding substantive assessments of the goods that freedom to choose should be used to select and the bads that freedom to choose should be used to reject. To be able to say more than, "It's your choice," to a person who is suffering, bioethics needs to learn from the experience of suffering and to incorporate that learning into what it means to do bioethics.

The theoretical foundations of bioethics do not provide a moral mandate for the amelioration of suffering or the acceptance of suffering simply an escape from suffering lodged in an ethos of individualism. Kleinman's warning that a preoccupation with theory subverts an understanding of experience, let alone an appreciation of experience, explains why. Suffering does not matter for bioethics twice over: the moral theory of bioethics applies only tangentially to suffering, and bioethics proceeds from that theory, not from experience.

The practical obstacles to suffering becoming an important, integral dimension of bioethics are equally formidable. The academic institutions and programs within which bioethics is taught and research is conducted propagate the moral theory that establishes the intellectual credibility of bioethics, and the acute care institutions in which bioethicists typically work relegate the relief of suffering to ancillary services such as home care, long-term care, nursing homes, and volunteer programs. With resources becoming progressively more scarce everywhere in society, suffering will assuredly not become a higher priority, even for those who most deserve it, such as soldiers who served their country.

This analysis is pessimistic but realistic. Understanding emerges from experience, as those bioethicist ethnographers discovered. Before any challenge, however large, can be met, it must be understood. Bioethics will understand suffering only if and when it comes to appreciate the experience of suffering.

Acknowledgments

I thank Arthur Frank, G. Toni Swart, Daniel Callahan, and Sidney Callahan for their insightful criticisms of and suggestions for improving a draft of this chapter and the staff of the Hastings Center for their helpful assessments of it. I am grateful to Nathan Palpant and Ronald Green for the invitation to write this chapter and indebted to them for the guidance and the acute critical and editorial recommendations they gave me throughout the preparation of the chapter.

Notes

1. Guido Calabresi and Philip Bobbitt, *Tragic Choices* (New York: W. W. Norton, 1978), 17.
2. "Illness and Suffering," *Hedgehog Review* 8, no. 3 (2006): 5.
3. Eric J. Cassell, *The Nature of Suffering and the Goals of Medicine*, 2nd ed. (New York: Oxford University Press, 2004), 33.
4. With Cassell's definition of suffering, the anticipation of loss also can cause suffering: "Most generally, suffering can be defined as the state of severe distress associated with events that threaten the intactness of person." Ibid., 32.
5. Jean-Dominique Bauby, *The Diving-Bell & the Butterfly* (London: Fourth Estate, 1997), 12. Translated by Jeremy Leggatt from *Le Scaphandre et le Papillon* (Paris: Robert Laffont, 1997).
6. Ibid., 78–79.
7. Cassell, supra note 3, 42.
8. Bauby, supra note 5, 107–108.
9. Ibid., 65.
10. Ibid., 79.
11. Ibid., 82.
12. Supra note 2.
13. Arthur W. Frank, "Telling the Dramas of Suffering," *Hedgehog Review* 8, no. 3 (2006): 9.
14. Ibid.
15. Ibid.
16. Ibid. (emphasis in original).
17. For the initial presentation of Donald Cowart's tragic plight, see Robert B. White and H. Tristram Engelhardt Jr., "A Demand to Die," *Hastings Center Report* 5, no. 3 (1975): 9–10, 47.
18. William F. May, *The Patient's Ordeal* (Bloomington, IN: Indiana University Press, 1991), ch. 1.

19. Herbert Fingarette, "The Meaning of Law in the Book of Job," *Hastings Law Journal* 29 (1978): 1581–1617.

20. May, supra note 18, 35.

21. Ibid., 33.

22. Ibid., 35.

23. That is Engelhardt's moral orientation: "... Individuals, when able, must be allowed to decide their own destiny, even that of death.... When the patient who is able to give free consent does not, the moral issue is over. A society that will allow persons to climb dangerous mountains or do daredevil stunts with cars has no consistent grounds for paternalistic intervention here.... Competent adults should be allowed to make tragic decisions, if nowhere else, at least concerning what quality of life justifies the pain and suffering of continued living. It is not medicine's responsibility to prevent tragedies by denying freedom, for that would be the greater tragedy." Engelhardt recognizes that it is a "uniquely intimate choice concerning the quality of life: the amount of pain which is worth suffering for a goal" but says nothing about the nature of that goal. White and Engelhardt, supra note 17, 10, 47.

24. For a criticism of quandary ethics, see Edmund Pincoffs, "Quandary Ethics," *Mind* 80 (1971): 552–571.

25. The decision-making process that best fits Donald Cowart's situation involves the creation and evaluation of imaginative scenarios of what his new life after he left the hospital would be like. For an account of the rationality of that kind of deliberation, as used by women making decisions about whether to try to become pregnant after receiving genetic counseling, see Barry Hoffmaster and Cliff Hooker, "How Experience Confronts Ethics," *Bioethics* 23 (2009): 214–225.

26. The Book of Job, *Holy Bible*, King James Version, 2:3 (emphasis in original).

27. Fingarette, supra note 19, 1605.

28. Ibid.

29. Ibid., 1612.

30. There is at least one philosophical companion to this theological view, albeit not from analytic philosophy. Card says: "For Schopenhauer, salvation comes with a quieting of the will, the stoicism of ceasing to value what inevitably brings suffering. His solution is an escape after all, not from suffering or harm but from experiencing it as intolerable, an ingenious escape through a revaluation of suffering. For Schopenhauer, salvation lies not only beyond ethics but beyond the phenomenal world." Claudia Card, *The Atrocity Paradigm* (New York: Oxford University Press, 2002), 168.

31. See, in particular, the description of how children who know they are dying create and sustain the practice of mutual pretense in Myra Bluebond-Langner, *The Private Worlds of Dying Children* (Princeton, NJ: Princeton University Press, 1978).

32. Information about the practice of euthanasia in the Netherlands is available at http://www.government.nl/issues/euthanasia. Accessed March 3, 2014.

33. Theo A. Boer, "Euthanasia in a Welfare State: Experiences from the Review Procedure in the Netherlands," *Philosophy Study* 2, no. 1 (2012): 51–63. Page references are given in the text.

34. For discerning, instructive constructions of the two worldviews that generate different approaches to disclosing the diagnosis of a terminal illness in the United States and Italy, see Deborah R. Gordon and Eugenio Paci, "Disclosure Practices and Cultural

Narratives: Understanding Concealment and Silence around Cancer in Tuscany, Italy," *Social Science and Medicine* 44 (1997): 1433–1452.

35. For a discussion of a person's loss of the sole source of meaning in life, or the integrity of a life, that led to death from a dose of lethal drugs provided by a psychiatrist, see Henri Wijsbek, "'To Thine Own Self Be True': On the Loss of Integrity as a Kind of Suffering," *Bioethics* 26 (2012): 1–7.

36. Fingarette, supra note 19, 1608.

37. Jack H. Kahn, *Job's Illness: Loss, Grief, and Integration* (New York: Pergamon, 1975), 24.

38. Fingarette, supra note 19, 1608.

39. For notable exceptions, see Cassell, *The Nature of Suffering and the Goals of Medicine*, supra note 3; Arthur W. Frank, *At the Will of the Body* (Boston: Houghton Mifflin, 1991; reprinted 2002) and *The Wounded Storyteller* (Chicago: University of Chicago Press, 1995); and Daniel Callahan, *The Troubled Dream of Life* (Washington, DC: Georgetown University Press, 2000). For philosophical examinations of suffering, see Jamie Mayerfeld, *Suffering and Moral Responsibility* (New York: Oxford University Press, 1999); Erich H. Loewy, *Suffering and the Beneficent Community* (Albany, NY: State University of New York Press, 1991); Joseph A. Amato, *Victims and Values: A History and A Theory of Suffering* (NewYork: Praeger, 1990); and John Portmann, *When Bad Things Happen to Other People* (New York: Routledge, 2000).

40. The entry for "Suffering" in the index of the fifth edition of the canonical bioethics text, *Principles of Biomedical Ethics*, contains 52 references, most of which are to one page and all of which are to no more than occurrences of words such as "suffering" or phrases such as "suffered from." One example is the decision in World War II to give the scarce resource of penicillin to soldiers "suffering from venereal disease" instead of soldiers "suffering from battle wounds." (270) The entry for "Suffering" says, "*See also* Pain," and the entry for "Pain" says, "*See also* Suffering." Tom L. Beauchamp and James F. Childress, *Principles of Biomedical Ethics*, 5th ed. (New York: Oxford University Press, 2001), 452.

41. For a theological view of suffering, see Sidney Callahan, *Created for Joy* (New York: Crossroad, 2007).

42. Rebecca Dresser, "Bioethics and Cancer: When the Professional Becomes Personal," *Hastings Center Report* 41, no. 6 (2011): 14–18.

43. Ibid., 15.

44. Ibid., 17.

45. For a call for qualitative social science research in bioethics, seeBarry Hoffmaster, "Can Ethnography Save the Life of Medical Ethics?" *Social Science and Medicine* 35 (1992): 1421–1431.

46. Ibid., 18.

47. Fingarette, supra note 19, 1606.

48. John Rawls, *A Theory of Justice* (Cambridge, MA: Harvard University Press, 1971), 408.

49. Ibid.

50. Renato Rosaldo, "While Making Other Plans," *Southern California Law Review* 58 (1985): 19.

51. Ibid., 20.

52. For an introduction to nonformal reason in the context of health care, see Barry Hoffmaster and Cliff Hooker, supra note 25. For an illustration of how children with

leukemia used nonformal reason to discover their diagnosis and that they were dying that is based on the work of Bluebond-Langner, supra note 31, see Larry Hoffmaster, "The Rationality and Morality of Dying Children," *Hastings Center Report* 41, no. 6 (2011): 30–42. For an extended presentation and defense of nonformal reason, see C. A. Hooker, "Rationality as Effective Organisation of Interaction: Towards a New Naturalist Foundation for Rationality," *Axiomathes* 21 (2010): 99–172.

53. Cassell, supra note 3, ix.

54. The exercise of autonomy can, of course, reduce suffering, notably when it relieves the trepidation of patients about having unwanted surgery or investigations. But autonomy must be understood carefully and used judiciously because it also can, wittingly or unwittingly, produce suffering. In addition, the unanticipated consequences of respect for autonomy in health care settings need to be appreciated. Mol, for example, argues that institutionalizing autonomy gives health care workers the alibi that whatever happens is the patient's "choice." See Annemarie Mol, *The Logic of Care* (New York: Routledge, 2008). I thank Arthur Frank for this clarification and amplification.

55. David Jolly, "Push for the Right to Die Grows in the Netherlands," *New York Times*, April 2, 2012. Available at http://www.nytimes.com/2012/04/03/health/push-for-the-right-to-die-grows-in-the-netherlands.html?pagewanted=all.&_r=0. Accessed March 3, 2014.

56. Ibid.

57. Ibid.

58. Jennifer L. Geddes, "A Conversation with Arthur Kleinman," *Hedgehog Review* 8, no. 3 (2006): 85.

3

Paying Homage to the Silence of Suffering

Gordon D. Marino and Susan E. Marino*

In her classic *The Body in Pain,*[1] Elaine Scarry makes a painstaking study of the effects of torture on discourse. Scarry argues that waterboarding and other procedures from the horror shop of human inventions leave a person bereft of speech and in the cell of their own dark, private world.

In this short essay, we suggest that torture is not required in order to bring us to the sad extremes of tormenting silence etched in Edvard Munch's "The Scream." Some researchers distinguish between pain and suffering. However, no matter what the terms, whether it be by torture or tortuous illness, severe, prolonged agony of the sort that disease and frequently the treatment of disease deliver incinerates our ability to communicate and, in the same stroke, robs us of a degree of agency.

As Pascal sighed, the fifth act is bloody. It was bloody in his time, and it remains bloody today. Before the curtain crashes down, there is a good chance that we will suffer from some debilitating illness and be dragged through the klieg lit surgery theaters of modern heroic medicine, which of course can be downright medieval in the suffering it inadvertently inflicts. Once again, the throes of disease and severe injury are not far removed from the pincers and thumbscrews. After all, it is no mistake that people caught in the maws of illness invariably moan, "This is sheer torture." Yes, torture without a torturer—but all-consuming affliction just the same.

You do not have to be a Utilitarian to acknowledge the fact that much of life is concerned with negotiating pleasure and pain. The philosophers, the lovers of wisdom, have long understood that the content of our character will in part be decided by the way we negotiate this almighty duo. Pleasure, of course, has been a frequent object of contemplation for members of the Socrates guild; however, that same august group has frequently turned a cold shoulder to the experience that in time will not forget to remember us. We need to think about the meaning of pain.

---

* This jointly authored essay is written in the first person to avoid confusion that might stem from the discussion of personal experiences.

After all, everyone with moral aspirations has some degree of focus on how we can best diminish the suffering of our fellow human beings.

Following pages of vivid descriptions of the experience of torture victims, Scarry surmises that one dimension of pain "is its ability to destroy language, the power of verbal objectification, a major source of our self-extension, a vehicle through which the pain could be lifted out into the world and eliminated."[2] It is a canonical presupposition of all psychotherapy that beginning to talk about something is the first step to mastering that painful something. By expressing ourselves we "get it out," separate ourselves from an experience that seems to have absorbed our identity. By articulating what we feel we gain a measure of distance and perhaps control over our feelings. But when we are under the siege of severe suffering, we can only scream or, perhaps, what amounts to the same, grit our teeth, close our eyes, and lapse into stony silence. The most common word used to describe pain at its white-hot pitch is "indescribable." It takes a poet to capture love, and it takes an Emily Dickinson to fill in the blank that Dickinson takes pain to be.

In her poem, "The Mystery of Pain,"[3] she writes:

Pain—has an Element of Blank—
It cannot recollect
When it begun—or if there were
A time when it was not –
It has no Future—but itself –
Its infinite contain
Its past—enlightened to perceive
New Periods—of Pain.

Pain consumes the consciousness of the individual in which it has taken up a home.

Again speaking of the unspeakable, Virginia Wolfe sighs, "English, which can express the thoughts of Hamlet and the tragedy of Lear, has no words for the shiver or the headache.... The merest school girl when she falls in love has Shakespeare or Keats to speak her mind for her, but let a sufferer try to describe a pain in his head to a doctor and language at once runs dry."[4]

When I complain to an acquaintance that I have a headache, she can tether my statement to a personal experience. She can imagine that what I am feeling is akin to what she has felt when her head was throbbing. But what happens when we endure a degree or quality of agony that is not common experience? G. D. Schott observes:

> The pain of angina will be difficult to express to anyone who has not experienced myocardial ischemia.... Few will have experienced, or could even envisage prolonged sensory and affective consequences associated with pain that follows spinal cord injury, stroke, or shingles.... For these sufferers, communication of such alien experience becomes particularly difficult....[5]

Suffering reaches its pitch when there is no hope of release from it—when it does not, as with childbirth, promise to lead to a positive outcome. At these times, it would never do to suggest, "multiply a migraine one hundred times and you will have some inkling of what I am feeling."

Consider a terminally ill mother who has endured surgery, chemotherapy, and radiation. When taken to the edge, these treatments sear her and rob her of control over her bodily functions and of our sense of dignity. In addition to the physical pangs, there is the psychological ordeal. Her 4- and 6-year-old children come to the hospital. They sit on her bed, nestle up close. The mother can feel their palpable, urgent need for reassurance, for things to be all right again. But what can she tell them? Banging around behind her eyes is the stabbing certainty that she is not going to survive to see her children grow up. It is not hard to imagine that this woman might legitimately feel that she is hanging on a cross that no one, save perhaps a fellow cancer patient, could begin to fathom.

Kierkegaard once wrote, "All human speech ... about the spiritual is essentially metaphorical speech."[6] The same holds for severe suffering. We can only talk about pain in figurative terms, and to continue with that figurative language, five-alarm pain drives us into ourselves, cuts us off from the world. Drawing from his own experience engulfed in the flames of an agonizing and life-threatening illness, Dr. David Biro[7] recalls,

> When I was in the hospital, although I was surrounded by the people I loved most—my wife, parents, sisters—I felt completely detached. The only thing in the world that mattered was what was happening inside my body—the disease in my bone marrow, its response to chemotherapy and radiation, *my* response to chemotherapy and radiation."[8]

"I felt," Biro continues, "like the French journalist Jean-Dominique Bauby. After a stroke left him completely paralyzed, he imagined himself imprisoned in an old-fashioned diving bell suspended in the ocean depths, sinking farther and farther away from his family and friends."[9] It is worth noting that Biro and Bauby were only able to describe their experiences when they were in the rearview mirror. Pointing again to that amorphous colossus, Biro[10] quotes Arendt, "... the most intense feeling we know of, to the point of blotting out other experiences, namely, the experience of great pain, is at the same time the most private and least communicable of all."[11]

The philosopher-poet of suffering E. M. Cioran wrote, "all genuine suffering is long-lasting—though purifying in its first phases, unhinges the reason, dulls the senses, and finally destroys." Cioran continues, "To have the monopoly of suffering is to live suspended above the abyss. All suffering is an abyss."[12] And in the abyss, mental activity, which is always, or rather, almost always intentional, ceases to point beyond itself. Anger, joy, and other feelings are about something, they point to something outside the self, they link us to the world. But not pain. To heed Scarry's analysis, pain obliterates "the content of consciousness. Pain annihilates not only the objects of complex thought and emotion but also the objects of the most elemental acts of perception."[13] Once in its firm clutches, the afflicted can only think of escaping affliction.

Pain takes the words to describe pain right out of our mouths. But it is not just a matter of the boulder of pain being a hard one for language to lift. The earnest student of suffering must be honest enough to pay homage to the powerful resistance we face in ourselves to listening to pain. It is agonizing to be with someone under the whip when you are impotent to assuage their suffering. I have sat at the bedside of a beloved friend, one who was nearing the falls. Wriggling on the hook of severe nerve pain, there was almost nothing he could do but moan. Over and over, he howled, "Oy vey... oy vey... oy vey." Now and again, between groans he would beseech me to hand him the bottle of pills that could end his life and the torture.

He knew and I knew that this was the end; that he was not going to get out of this one alive. There was a part of me that feared that the cold flames of constant pain that were licking at him might consume all his good memories and feelings. He was the kind of man who took the task of being a loving person quite seriously, and the thought dripped in me—this pain is going to drive him into himself and render him indifferent to everything about himself and his world that he cherishes. It will, I feared, rewrite his memory of life. I thought seriously about helping him through the escape hatch in the bottle, but rightly or wrongly, I ended up just going back and forth between putting my hand on his back and my head in my hands. It was such an infinitely sad and hopeless place. Maybe my friend was actually succeeding in communicating his pain, but either way, I could not wait to find some good excuse to leave that bedside.

The inability to soothe is not the only obstacle to being able to hear pain. Real-life witness can serve to unpleasantly remind us of what is probably around the bend for us personally. And the morphine drips and ice chips of the fifth act are things that people clad in "Life is Good" tee shirts are not eager to appropriate. Not only is pain difficult to translate into language, but also we are averse to understanding it because we fear the night that it will knock at our door. Apparently, the unwillingness to listen to pain holds for physicians as well as laypersons. Dr. Biro reports that time and again, studies show that physicians underestimate and are perhaps even skeptical about the pain of their patients. Scarry offers this rather scary assessment:

> [M]any people's experience of the medical community would bear out... the conclusion that physicians do not trust (hence, hear) the human voice, that they in effect perceive the voice of the patient as an "unreliable narrator" of bodily events, a voice which must be bypassed as quickly as possible so that they can get around and behind it to the physical events themselves.... Medical contexts, like all other contexts of human experience, provide instances of the alarming phenomenon noted earlier: to have great pain is to have certainty; to hear that another person has pain is to have doubt.[14]

And as Scarry underscores, "The doubt of others . . . amplifies the suffering of those already in pain."[15]

Implications for Biomedical Ethics

What, then, follows from the phenomenological understanding of the strangling impact of prolonged pain? One point can be fixed: those in the healing arts need to cultivate a humble awareness of the fact that there are special obstacles to being able to take the coordinates of suffering. Those who find themselves behind the lectern in medical school biomedical ethics classes should devote serious effort to reminding future physicians, some of whom might be brimming with confidence in their intellectual and empathic abilities, that the experience of pain varies enormously from individual to individual and that intense suffering of both the psychological and physical ilk severely reduce and perhaps even rob us of our vocabulary for expressing pain.

The ubiquitous one-to-ten scales and lines from smiley to frowny faces cannot capture the reality of pain. It is no surprise that nurses will often put these in a patient's hand with an ironic smile, as if to say, I know that this is a long way from providing a window into your experience. After all, one person's three might be another's ten. When taken too seriously, these instruments could even prod a false conviction that we understand something we are in the dark about, and as result, they might serve to reinforce the tendency to repress the difficulties of hearing the pain of others.

At the risk of repeating, meditation on pain should make it plain that madly firing synapses can turn us into veritable objects and as such diminish our sense of agency. In times of severe affliction, most of us are in no position to think through and make rational choices. In an article addressing the ethical issue of pain control, E. I. Lisson insists:

> Pain destroys autonomy: the patient is afraid to make the slightest movement. All choices are focused on either relieving pain or preventing greater future pain, and for this, one will sell one's soul.[16]

According to L. F. Post and her coauthors,[17] autonomy "underlies decision making that gives priority to the values and wishes of the individual when they are both restricted by the rights of others." They continue, "It is only when the individual's wishes are obscure, inaccessible, or overridden by competing principles that the judgment of others is substituted."[18] Extreme suffering obscures our deepest wishes and life plans and as such should raise eyebrows about the sometimes inordinate weight given to autonomy in the medical decision-making process.

Case histories can be abused, but they can also illuminate. I had an elderly friend who was in the terminal stages of lymphoma. He was in terrible pain and desperately trying to adjust to the fact that the far edge of his life was only weeks away. A health nut who always kept himself in great condition, he was one of those people who had expected to live at least another decade or two. Then the gavel came down. He was so disappointed. He was bombarded by chemotherapy and radiation, but neither of them did anything to halt the armies of his cancer. No matter, because of his incontinence and the embarrassment it caused him, doctors started pressing him with the choice as to whether or not he wanted to have bladder surgery. Against the advice of the family and perhaps imagining that this would give him a reprieve, he elected to have the ridiculous procedure, only to perish a few days later. Yes, he consented, but because of his pain and anguish, he was in no more of a position to make a decision than a drowning swimmer going down for the last time.

When intense pain is a clarion announcing the progression of an underlying disease or disorder, how can the physician expect the patient strapped to the harrowing machine to choose rationally among treatment options?

Of course, there is nothing akin to an algorithm for adjudicating the relative weight of moral principles in the medical decision-making process.

Nevertheless, as people descend into the pit of seemingly bottomless suffering, a physician's thinking should be steered by the aim of compassion rather than narrowly focused concerns about autonomy. This change in perspective could involve the difficult decision of increasing pain medication even when patients fail to press for it. It may also require the physician to choose, without the direct consent of her patient, a therapeutic intervention for the underlying condition that she thinks is best. But at what number on the pain scale does that choice become ethical?

We have argued that the language of pain is virtually untranslatable, so how can caregivers, nurses, and physicians recognize the point at which the sufferer can no longer make autonomous decisions? As a result of the highly subjective and multidimensional nature of pain, developing valid and reliable assessment tools that accurately reflect pain intensity and suffering has been challenging, to say the least. More research into the physiology and genetics of individual pain perception will be needed before objective measures for pain are fully realized.

Until then, we must remind our clinicians that they, as healers within the Hippocratic tradition, must not turn away from, but instead learn to listen carefully to, the pain and suffering of each patient and, as the oath itself provides, "apply dietetic measures for the benefit of the sick according to [their] ability and judgment; [and to] keep [the sick] from harm and injustice."[19]

Notes

1. Elaine Scarry, *The Body in Pain: The Making and Unmaking of the World* (New York: Oxford University Press, 1985).

2. Ibid., 54

3. Emily Dickinson, *The Complete Poems of Emily Dickinson*, ed. T. H. Johnson (Boston: Little, Brown, 1955), poem 650.

4. Virginia Woolf, "On Being Ill," in *Collected Essays* (New York: Harcourt, 1967), 194.

5. G. D. Schott, "Communicating the Experience of Pain: The Role of Analogy," *Pain* 108 (2004): 209–212.

6. S. Kierkegaard, *Works of Love*, ed. and trans. Howard and Edna Hong (Princeton, NJ: Princeton University Press, 1995), 209.

7. This essay was inspired by and is deeply indebted to David Biro, *Listening to Pain* (New York: W. W. Norton, 2010).

8. Ibid., 24–25.

9. Ibid., 25

10. There is a lively philosophical debate as to whether pain, or for that matter any subjective experience, is intrinsically ineffable. In his splendid treatment of this question, David Biro (cf. *Listening to Pain*, 48–55) discusses and seems convinced by Wittgenstein's private-language argument, which holds that it cannot be the case that there are thoughts which we can express to ourselves but not to others. The present authors do not take any absolute position on the issue of the intrinsic ineffability of pain. It is enough for us to follow Scarry, Biro, Schott, and a host of others in affirming that there are special problems in communicating the experience of severe pain.

11. Hannah Arendt, *The Human Condition*, as quoted in Biro, op. cit., 23.

12. E. M. Cioran, *On the Heights of Despair*, trans. I. Zarifopol-Johnson (Chicago: University of Chicago Press, 1992), 54.

13. Scarry, op. cit., 54

14. Ibid., 6–7.

15. Ibid., 7.

16. E. L. Lisson, "Ethical Issues Related to Pain Control," *Nursing Clinics of North America* 22 (1987): 654.

17. L. F. Post, J. Blustein, E. Gordon, N. N. Dubler, "Pain: Ethics, Culture, and Informed Consent to Relief," *Journal of Law, Medicine & Ethics* 24 (1996): 351.

18. Ibid., 351.

19. L. Edelstein, *The Hippocratic Oath: Text, Translation, and Interpretation* (Baltimore, MD: The Johns Hopkins University Press, 1943).

4

Suffering, and the Promise of a World without Pain

Joseph A. Amato

Humans have increasingly endowed themselves with transformative powers. Among their principal agencies are innovative technology and science, global capitalism and industry, and centralizing nation-states and democratic and mass society. Insofar as these powers are directed by mind to human wish and design, their guiding vision is secular, progressive, and redemptive. This vision has its sources in the universalizing reason and humanism of the Enlightenment, the messianic sympathy of romanticism, and the revolutionary platforms of liberalism, socialism, democracy, and positivism and technocracy.

At the outer ken of this utopian secularism stands belief in the modification of humans and the earth as a living entity. It summons to its proof and cause indisputable beneficent revolutions in medicine, scientific research, and medical legislation against the perennial borders of birth and death. In defiance of almost all evidence of what humans and society were in traditional village and valley and what they have become in collective, centralized, and affluent society, redemptive secularism professes the extreme utopian faith that humans have not just the potential but also the ethical duty to eliminate suffering itself.[1] Such a commanding wish assumes that suffering is somehow static and a physically fixed target, that it does not in fact increase or equilibrate as corporal abundance is secured, individual choice and freedom are increased, and collective and centralized life becomes paramount in controlling and directing humanity at large. It further assumes that suffering is diagnosable and treatable as the sum of discrete pains—and its proponents must suppress or, at least, suspend the possibility that ever-artificial and invented humanity could well be equipping itself by innovation and dependency to destroy itself and life on the planet.

In the words of historian Wilfred McClay, we have arrived at or are quickly approaching the peril of acting on this dream. We take "pride in freeing ourselves from material necessity and from outdated traditions and take for granted an ever-growing knowledge of, and control over, the physical mechanism of our condition. We feel confident that there are no mysteries or constraints that our knowledge cannot master; no diseases it cannot cure, no possibilities it cannot open to us." McClay concludes, "The momentum of innovation at times seems unstoppable, answerable to neither effective political control nor to effective moral interdictions grounded in a shared metaphysics." Standing before us is "the very real possibility that our biogenetic mastery will give us the power to replace human procreation with the willful arts of manufacture, remaking our conditions by engineering human life and 'hybrid' forms of transhuman life."[2]

Against this utopian vision of the future, we assemble the entire experience of the past. We know that suffering has too large, deep, and diverse a hold on human life to be reduced to technical, therapeutic, psychological, and sociological quadrants. Even the keen philosophers and scientists do not have a periodic table of pains and sufferings. Suffering remains too much a multiplicity—an ache; a life of woe, travail, and grief; an inner affliction; and simply the condition of being vulnerable to a precarious, cruel, and fickle world. Suffering, to quote an old folk proverb, comes on horseback but departs on foot. It overwhelms body and spirit with its cruel epiphanies about our place in life with drought, flood, famine, plague, and war; it resides in the deepest basements of memory and yet in the best of our ways and the brightest of our days.

Bioethics, a new field, cannot but register the dichotomies, ambiguities, and raw contradictions between contemporary hopes and old-world truths. As much as bioethics might wish to establish the most ambitious of programs of a curative and progressive humanism, it also must realistically recognize, lest it cut its tie with all of humanity's past, that humans will always suffer in some way. Alive to contemporary practice and possibilities and traditional ways and values, bioethics vacillates before the advancing transformations of medical practices and rights and the potential of human life. A neologism in 1970, bioethics, emerging out of the intersection and collision of medicine, theology, politics, the life sciences, law, and moral philosophy, soon found itself walking the line between reality and possibility as it sought to establish values and terms for social movements, technological developments, innovative lines of experiment, the setting of legal precedents, the breaking of medical scandals, changes to the institutions of medicine, the appearance of new diseases and the return of resistant diseases, and yet entire new interventions and procedures for saving, treating, prolonging, and redesigning life.[3]

Perhaps, suffering can serve as a North Star for bioethics. It surely invites us to puzzle how we know and meet suffering. Is suffering born out of immediate perceptions, elaborated conceptions, or only long reflections and acute judgments? Is suffering singular or plural? And can it be identified as distinct types of pain? Does suffering have a value? And do humans lose their dignity if they cannot intentionally make and embrace select acts of suffering as sacrifice and dedicate them as a gift and a tribute to a person or an end?

Aside from offering implicit answers to these questions, in this essay I use cultural and intellectual history to offer a brief narrative of suffering as a differing value by commenting on its place in both classical and Judeo-Christian traditions and its development in the Middle Ages and the Reformation and in Enlightenment and romantic thought. Additionally, I hope to sketch the contradictory place of suffering in modern and especially contemporary thought and practice. Untangling this roping and rigging might clarify the premises, assumptions, and problematics of bioethical discourse as its students seek to confront new realities and potentials of human action on life, while seeking to thread their way through disparate and adversarial philosophies and irreconcilable ethical systems.

All and Ever-Present Suffering

Body, mind, life, society, politics, and values are deeply tongued with suffering. Suffering gives rise to pity, sorrow, lament, supplication, and pleasure; it occasions judgment, punishment, and war; it can be a source of forgiveness and the grounds for mercy. Analogous to reflective and absorbent light, suffering bombards skin and mind with photons of pain, ordeals, woes, and tragedies. The mind churns with pains and suffering in senses, images, and words of sickness, conflict misguided passions, violent wills, and anxiety honed by uncertainty and pent-up times. And hopes and happiness can seem frail bridges across suffering seen, experienced, and foreboding.

Suffering goes to the depths of consciousness and scores the everyday surface of experience. Suffering comes with the ever-expressive, though not necessarily truthful, human face, a person's countenance, appearance, gestures, and of course voice—or as contemporary Michael Palma writes of poet W. H. Auden:

> Through all, he honored us,
> By wearing the helplessness
> Of being one of us.[4]

We see, hear, and even smell suffering. It silences us in sorrow and steels us in action. It measures the inner depths of the wounds we touch. We know the flesh I sketch in the squalid valley below. Suffering draws us to it. It is among the first things we acknowledge and the lasting residues of our lives. There is suffering we cannot forget and suffering that departs like morning's dew. It moves on trembling lips, and yet the most calloused walls of perception and conception block it. And, we encounter the paradox that the more industrialized and civilized humans improve conditions of life, the more likely suffering, even suffering past, is cultivated, becomes incorporated in public rhetoric, is registered as an actionable complaint, and justifies activist plans and programs. (Even slaughter of twenty children—I think of the massacred innocence at Sandy Hook—precipitates a river of public responses even before a period of mourning and meditation is observed.)

Arguing about suffering, proposing means and cures, leaves a problem-solving civilization inured, even hardened, to suffering. We have been taught, and we have taught ourselves, to look away from its interrogating face. At the same time, only the hypocrite presumes to take the sufferings of others fully and purely to heart, denying a complex of ambivalent feelings, including hate for source and agency of the suffering; revulsion and superiority to suffering victims; and senses of pleasure, justice, and rectitude before the afflictions and misfortunes of others. And if we contemporaries, surely hypocrites of a time and an age, are to explore suffering in the past, we must admit that so much of our loudly lauded and touted sympathy, concern, and empathy is the tinsel of a posturing sensibility and ideological pretense that belongs to democratic rhetoric and abundant material well-being and the pretense that our sincere and natural hearts of fellow feelings are equal to the compassion of Buddha and the divine embrace of Christ.

Aware that perceptions are not conceptions, that images are not thoughts, and that contemporary sensibilities and ideologies are far truth and useful analytic propositions, we start into the past knowing that suffering constitutes vast kingdoms we cannot traverse. With immense variation, it belongs to what we see and sense and have experienced, learned, and incorporated into words and gestures, cultures, art, philosophies, and religions. Suffering forever belongs to manifestations and interpretations. It cannot be bisected sharply between body and mind, thought and imagination, description and prescription. Equally, we cannot disengage suffering from experience, memory, and the cultures in which it existed and in which we exist and through which we think. Its myriad forms belong to complexes of emotions, sensibilities, languages, and metaphors—as well as, which is especially important to bioethicists, the definitions of customs and law, the cannons of medicine, and professional codes. In more concrete terms, suffering comes with the surfaces of things: it wears the faces of flesh and life, landscapes, buildings, tools, books, and arts. It speaks with its very appearance to us—an inseparable mix of animal and human—of friend and enemy, street and battlefield, hospital, laboratory, and operating room.[5]

Such a phenomenological approach reveals suffering manifest and concealed at the very depths of spirits and minds. Cultural and intellectual histories of suffering broaden and deepen our awareness of its permanent, rich, and yet changing place in human perception, sentiment, worldviews, and representation. As contemporary citizens of the West, it helps us grasp how suffering was developed and differentiated by Greek, Jew, and Christian. It teaches how the modern centralizing state and the spreading doctrines of natural and individual rights and democracy reinterpreted and secularized suffering's multiple meanings. At the same time, we grasp how suffering, though not comprehensively, belongs to the purview of advancing science and technology, encompassing law, social, and reform agencies, and, as suggested, the revolutionary proposition that humans, as a whole species, belong to one another by covenant, potentiality, and responsibility for a shared earthly happiness.

Before Philosophy

Before any historical or anthropological discussion, certain perennial truths about the human condition and suffering's place can be offered. Suffering reaches across and through human experience. It belongs to the opposing polarities of body and spirit, normal and abnormal by which we know and value, differentiate and classify life. It stands as both source and result of the dichotomies and contradictions of experience and consciousness. To suffer or not to suffer, I analogize, is light and dark of our being. As much as suffering has it sources in our biological and evolutionary roots and the disjuncture between general nature and individual creature, it also depends on the increasingly complex history of humans as social and symbolic beings. It belongs to our deepest history, which includes the formation of a social nature, tool use, and the development of language. It is inseparable from the formation of human consciousness and is connected to one's condition as contingent: a result of necessity, risk, and even choice. It hinges on our ability to project self and group into places and times, and it shapes our faculties of memory, will, judgment, imagination, and even conjecture. At the same time, suffering leads humans out of themselves and into the world for a cure and an understanding of their suffering.

An abscessed tooth rules the behavior of a dinosaur and the mind of a wise philosopher. A king's dread, a queen's envy, and a prince's unsettling melancholy, as Shakespeare tells us, can overturn a kingdom. Neither mind nor body minister well to each other—no more than self and other have conjoined hearts and shared ends. At play in taking cognizance of suffering is not just reason but also emotion, compassion, and pity—justice and vindication, pleasure and cruelty too—and as Montaigne writes of our mixed and flawed nature, "For in the midst of compassion we feel inside ourselves some sort of malicious pleasure in seeing someone else suffer."[6] Humans identify suffering across the whole arc of approval from the elevating and ennobling to the deserved, degrading, and altogether contemptible. We take suffering's source as a bad to be alleviated and cured—a certain outcome from a form of action and justly merited punishment for vice, abuse, and stupidity; or, we judge it on a metaphysical plane, as a reality arising out of the depths of human freedom or inextricably rooted in evil.

Suffering binds us, like atoms and ions secure molecules, to chains of multiple narratives. It binds and joins us one to another inextricably by affection, loyalty, anger, resentment, and the weave of memory. And so it gives rise to endless chronicles and histories. The being called *human* anguishes at birth, grieves a lost thing, place, or state; confesses impotence; and concedes the certainty of death. And so humans enter into the kingdom of consciousness, suffering in the worlds of their own bodies, things, and others; turning them into emotions, feelings, thoughts, minds, and cultures; making them a matter of wishes and prayers. Suffering wraps itself around perceptions, conceptions, and memories. It associates with smells, sounds, sights, and colors; it shapes paths, creates landscapes, erects wall, and decorates palaces and gardens.[7] And who writes narratives without relaying stories of suffering?[8] Without law or rule, suffering is truly archaic and ontological. It embeds us in contexts and configurations and provokes juxtapositions and contrarieties. It fuses minds and spirits, individuals and circumstances, groups and times, and situations. Living with others turns on trust, loyalty, promise, and possibility, and with this comes failures and betrayal and, with each, inescapable forms of suffering.[9]

Sacrifice, First Exchanges, Cures, and Resolutions

First burials and cave paintings show that early humans (both Neanderthals and Cro-Magnons) expressed an awareness of their desire to carry on transactions with greater forces and spirits and their need to establish a better footing in existence. Moved by mixed and ambivalent emotions, fears, angers, images, and hopes, humans sought by flattery and even cajoling threat to enter into contacts and exchanges with elusive and fickle spirits and gods. Skirting a complex discourse of anthropology and archaeology, which turns on the origins, functions, and relations of decorations and representations, humans' use of symbols and languages long preceded civilization and expressed and manifested their awareness of their temporal, mutable, and vulnerable position in reality.

Magic, medicine, and religion and the rituals, myths, and rites with which they were associated have focused on diagnosing, explaining, overcoming, and curing suffering for tens of thousands of years, assuredly starting with burials, which reach back approximately one hundred thousand years. In turn, suffering in its multiple forms, from accidental pain to unwanted death, birthed and cradled experiences, relations, and languages. Associated with disequilibrium and disorders in individuals, groups, and nature and its seasons, suffering was conceived as having its source in notions of great powers and in spirits of earth, water, and sky. Feast and orgy, rite and myth began in conversations with divinities; with dance and masks, people enacted fears, wishes, expectations, hopes, and prayers.

Sacrifice, which transformed the suffering and death of animals, strangers, first born, and oneself into declarations and gifts to higher powers, formed the principal means for groups to bring themselves into accord with the proper order of being, reproduction, and life. In myriad forms, sacrifice established groups in place, time, and being. Through select acts of suffering (abnegation and ordeal, which amounts to the pain of doing without or undergoing hurt), human groups expiated themselves for wrong, validated their earnestness, and sealed their prayers, as needs and wishes, to higher powers and divinities. They used sacrifice to secure rebirth; solidify and purify social orders of wrongs, crimes, and sins; and renew broken human and divine relations. Sacrificial gifts expressed adoration, indebtedness, gratitude, respect, and loyalty.[10] Ordeals and fasts conferred ordination and special powers for their shamans, priests, and kings.

Blood validated human transactions. Blood joined body and spirits in suffering and through death. The eating of sacrificial flesh, of victim animal and person, established transcendent alliances and formed irrevocable covenants. Victims of ritual murders—be they animals, virgins, or first-born children—propitiated the gods, removed curses, secured the blessings of nature, and sent kings to their everlasting kingdoms. On the stone pyramid altars, Aztecs cut out the hearts of other tribes by the thousands with their surgically keen flint knives to satisfy their insatiably blood-thirsty gods. Sacrifices accompanied the establishment of the foundations of walls and temples. As historian Fustel de Coulanges points out, the classical city established and made right its walls by interring the dead and the earth of the mother city under their foundations.[11] A sacrificial gift, be it in victims or the payment of money (e.g., a *wergild*), paid for wrongs, purchased initiation into manhood and entrance into the warrior society and the shaman cult, and launched an expedition and its ships. Human victims were highest coin of exchange with arbitrary, powerful, and invisible powers. Suffering in the form of sacrifice made places and people sacred, in accord with its Latin roots of *sacer* ("holy") and *facere* ("to make").

Suffering itself, which etymologically carries with it the sense of undergoing pain, also carries, as bioethicists must recognize in their valorization of a patient's suffering, an individualizing and internalizing significance when identified and transmitted as self-sacrifice. Sacrifice of self professes a person's earnestness and wish to transact with another, or others, the deepest dedication and intention of the self. It can formalize and dramatize one's call to another in praise and thanks or as an open or concealed request for forgiveness and mercy. Of course, the coin of claimed suffering and sacrifice was, and is, spent in all human markets. Sacrifice can be claimed for any action, from ordinary tasks and abnegations to testing ordeals. In our world, the ordinary discourse of suffering in most things—that of mother and father for family or friend for friend or stranger—is ignored; only the most heroic, tragic, and officially recognized suffering receives public validation and is understood of human discourse in life, being, and transcendence.

Suffering characterized all facets of life in the world of yesteryear. Greek myth and literature recognized that suffering came to shore in boats of all sizes. It was inherent to risk, contingency, action, and life itself. Optimism belonged only to the naïve. Of the singular case of tragic rich king Croesus, who in the very end lost kingdom and son, Herodotus wrote, "No man is happy until he is dead." Suffering, as Homer and the Greek tragedians elaborated in their fundamental works, was the price for being out of place and out of harmony with one's self, among one's neighbors, or under the jealous and scrutinizing stare of the gods' fickle eyes. It fell to the prophets or prophetesses—the blinder they were, the more accurate their divinations—to identify fatal inheritances, condemning transgressions, or yet mistaken transmissions.

Pity and the Greeks

With civilization in the East, the Near East, and Greece came systematic reflection and formal teaching. But neither philosophy nor religion explained suffering, and sacrifices were still required to carry on vital transactions with higher powers. In the face of events and tragedies, human emotions had to be ritualized and disciplined. All traditions must both permit and yet moderate therapeutic wailing and mourning, yet for the sake of the living. Individuals, families, communities, and soldiers could not be allowed to go to pieces in the face of the suffering experienced and wrought. (At Pien, there was a man who on the death of his mother wept with the abandon of a child. Master K'ung said, "Grief! This is indeed grief. The difficulty is to keep on like this."[12])

In the course of civilizing themselves, living in sedentary villages and then specialized cities, humans had to learn to tame and regulate their interactions and associated emotions and impulses. This meant selective expression, repression, and disguising. Despite coming to this perennial but delicate task with hundreds of thousands of years of learning, human minds remained filled with impulses, urges, and ambivalent feelings. The face and body of the other provoked and stimulated reactions. Always in play—right on the very surface of interactions—the presence, condition, and gestures of the other as sympathetic or hostile, suffering or threatening, signaled care or threat and the likelihood of respect or insult. At the same time the other (as singular or group, old or young, identical or opposite gender, cast, and class) affirmed one's own superiority or inferiority by virtue of strength, well-being, and status.

Perceived, conceived, or simply imagined weaknesses called forth a whole band of spontaneous and learned reactions. The ruling hand of the rich or the soliciting hand of the beggar activated inner compasses. With immediacy and deliberation, humans are alerted to one another's conditions. Felt sympathy, arrogance, and cunning artifices shape the matrices of responses. Recognitions of a fellow person or group in debilitating pain and under the weight of crushing suffering can elicit and mingle fellow feelings of kindness, concern, affection, pardon, and love, yet disdain, disgust, and even aggression.

Pity, mercy, and love have been idealized since early civilization as the highest human forms of fellow feelings. Philanthropy has been considered a high road to the highest road of justice and the true way to gods. Books of aphorisms accumulated long lists of quotations suggesting that mercy stands higher than justice and our pity for and love of another wins God's love and pity, although they also record pity in the service of meaner motives; and books of quotations place fellow feelings in service of meaner causes: I feign pity to win it for myself or yet to robe myself in piety. In the *Oxford Book of Aphorisms,* in the sections "Friends and Foes" and "Sympathies and Antipathies," we read the eighth-century B.C. ancient Hesoid, in his *Work and Days*: "Potter bears a grudge against potter, and craftsman against craftsman, and beggar is envious of beggar, and bard of bard." And there, from the modern and self-reflective aphorist Pascal, we read: "Men naturally hate each other. We have used concupiscence as best we can to make it serve the common good, but this is a mere sham and a false image of charity, for essentially it is just hate." In his *Treatise of Human Nature,* 1739, Hume went a step further, anticipating the most violent modern individualistic thinkers: "Pride and hatred invigorate the soul; and love and humility enfeeble it."[13]

Early religions and philosophies took up pity as a question of man's disposition to man and god's to man. At stake was the elemental question of who looks upon whom, how and why. Pity, no doubt plastic in nature and diverse in form, can flood souls with affinities for all suffering perceived—one thinks of the telling phrase, "my heart goes out to you." At the same time, pity can be feigned, malleable, and even stifled by senses of superiority, repugnance, and fear of contagion and contamination. Every language has words stemming from pity.[14] In classical and New Testament Greek, the single word for pity, *Ëleos,* bridges to calls for mercy, clemency, grace, and even forgiveness. At the same time, another line of pity, a first aperture to pain and suffering, can be associated with shared fellow and even animal feelings. The Greek roots for "matching feeling' form *sympathy*; are voiced in the Latin offering of *condolence* (with shared pain), and, to choose but one more language, are echoed in the German words *Mitleid* (with joined suffering) and *Mitgefühl* (with participating feeling).

Like phenols for ants, which help them distinguish between what is living and what is dead, pity, which scents the varied topography of human pain, suffering, and tragedy, can signal association and affinity by similar emotions, sorrow, and pathos. It can join humans together in suffering experienced and remembered. Expressions of human grief—wailing, keening, and lamentation—can instantly evoke the pity of all with the reach of its expression. Our body and its movements give rise to emotions in others. The crying child, the sorrowing mother, and the moans of the dying person—as seen or yet experienced in images, sounds, gestures, and even aesthetic expression—reverberate within and call up primary responses. The entire social landscape can elicit pity, crossing boundaries between individuals and groups, humans, animals, and nature, and even mutually embrace the living, the dead, and their gods.

With great variance, individuals, societies, cultures, philosophies, and religions express pity and react with pity. Suffering can call for pity, even when the person who suffers does not want pity in any form. In some cases, only the keenest heart perceives suffering, whereas in others, suffering presents itself in such a horrid and overwhelming way that it awakens a fear of contagion. The leper of old knew himself in rotting flesh to be too grotesque to solicit pity, a kind touch from any hand.

In the old world, suffering ever threatened to wash over village and valley with the flood of disease, famine, and plague. It could not be staved off, isolated, or quarantined. There were more sick than could be cared for—dead than could be buried. Moaning and lamentations went up like smoke. Suffering exceeded pity's cup. Prayers could not compass the suffering. To find anything similar in modern, developed society, we must turn to modern mass war, as witnessed in the American Civil War, when great battlefields could not be traversed in the wake of battle without stepping on abandoned corpses.

For us in the West, the Greeks singularly explored suffering and pity with their tragedies, which were preoccupied with the pitiful fate of royal families. Revealed to have killed his father and married his mother, King Oedipus blinds himself and wanders in his incurable woe outside all walls and embrace of human emotions. The epics of Homer and the histories of Herodotus and Thucydides also explore fate as culminated and dramatized in overwhelming suffering and the pity it evokes.

At center of the tragedy is the protagonist's transgression of the order of things and gods, and a resulting nemesis. With pride, jealousy, and vengeance, gods scrutinized human gifts and deeds. And when gods and humans intermingle, there are always tragic consequences. Indeed, their taboo relations produce monsters such as the incest-conceived Minotaur of Crete's labyrinth and the satyrs, the goat-men who chummed with Pan and Dionysius.[15]

The Greeks viewed polis and cosmos through suffering and pity. They narrated life, nature, and the gods under the rubric of tragedy. The Greeks built a literature on wrongs and resulting curses and punishments. Divining the source of afflictions gave rise to shrines and temples like the island of Delos. Greek medicine and healing did not exclude the search for deeper causes of suffering in the violation of the law, the breaking of a code, flaws of character, the anger and jealousy of the gods, and the precarious moral order of being.

The Greeks and Romans used elaborate tools and potions to treat and cure patients, and with the Greek Hippocratic Oath codified medical practice. At the same time, Greeks sought therapy elsewhere. Aristotle found healing for participating audiences in the great tragedies of the fifth century B.C. According to his *Poetics,* the tragedies gathered their audience into the pitiful suffering of the tragic protagonists, and in conclusion to the story's unraveling plot and its climatic suffering came cathartic relief, a purging and purifying cleansing of soul. The audience was afforded a temporary relief from threatening and engulfing suffering that netted all life.

The Greeks and Romans also turned to philosophy to cope with suffering. With a type of naturalism (most illustratively found in first-century poet and atomist B. C. Lucretius's *De Rerum Natura*), classical philosophers sought to free thoughtful minds from any investment of entangling feelings in the twists and turns of precarious life. They counseled that fate and fortune arose beyond the ken of human thought and action. There was no release from unforeseeable accidents and the path of blind laws. Stoics, in particular, argued one could do no more than meet and practice one's duties with dignity. With less stern prescriptions, not dissimilar to so much contemporary self-help literature, Epicureans proposed a regime of moderate pleasures of body and the most lasting pleasures of friendship and good conversation. Concern with the wills of arbitrary gods, the fear of implacable death, and dreams of the afterlife only enchained the soul in worry and illusion.

Covenants of Suffering

The Old and New Testaments contradicted both the tragic and therapeutic responses of the classical world. For Jew and Christian, suffering tested and perfected faith. It prepared the believer for God's love and redemption. Suffering came with original sin, the wages of which were death and mortality. Both faiths concurred that an all-powerful and merciful God alone answered human suffering. The

Lord of creation took pity. Suffering delivers all those who truly lament, supplicate, and yearn for justice, forgiveness, and love to God, ultimately loved and cherished beyond all else in creation. Out of the bounty of his love, God formed a covenant with man and, by Christian faith, allowed his divine self to enter into and dwell within the incarnate flesh of humans as Jesus Christ. He thereby secured his creatures' salvation and history with his resurrection and redemption.

By Abraham's willingness to sacrifice his only and long-awaited son, God reciprocated. He irrevocably committed himself to his creature across time and promised to turn his healing countenance to pitiful and woeful humankind, who stood in need of grace, mercy, and forgiving pardon. In turn, he insisted on human reciprocity—that humans fully open their hearts to God. In turn, God pledged to respond to humans' prayers—their endless complaints, lamentations, and supplications that conveyed a constant need for help, forgiveness, and renewal.

The Psalms, which praise and glorify God, increasingly and repeatedly make requests. In Psalm 120, the believer cries out, "In my distress, I cry to the Lord, and he may answer me," and in Psalm 116, he declares gratitude for having been heard:

> Because he inclined his ear to me,
> therefore I will call on him as long as I live. . . .
> For Thou has delivered my soul from death
> My eyes from tears,
> My feet from stumbling;
> I walk before the Lord
> in the land of the living.

Christianity, which belonged to the Old Testament by the premise of an absolute, personal, and merciful God, at least from one point of view culminated the pledge of a redemptive God. The covenant of the New Testament joined believers, in Paul's words, to the faith of Abraham, who believed in the God "who gives life to the dead and calls into existence the things that do not exist"—who believed "in hope against hope that he should become the father of many nations."[16]

For Christians, God wondrously expanded the covenant. With the sacrifice of his own son, God turned away from retribution and promised the final transformation of humanity—and offered examples and promises of endless miracles of body, spirit, and heart. In profound disagreement with philosophies and religions that found their answers in transformations of mind, and antithetical to enlightened and secular moderns whose faith is in the powers of the praxis and works of science, technology, and medicine, Christ anchored faith in redemptive history and the hope of his cross.

Christ's sheep were those who were the humble, rejected, and afflicted—those who cried out for life, miracles, and justice. Christ called believers beyond themselves. They had to make his sacrifice, pity, mercy, and clemency their own. They had to turn themselves—body, spirit, suffering, and community—into a reciprocal sacrifice to God. In this way, a Christian was required to transform his or her suffering into self-abnegation, love, and sacrifice to God.[17] Paul created a theology of hope through the embrace of suffering:

> Through him we have obtained access to this grace in which we stand and we rejoice in the hope of sharing the Glory of God. More than that we rejoice in our sufferings, knowing that suffering produces endurance and endurance produces character, and character produces hope, and hope does not disappoint us because God's love has been poured into our hearts through the Holy Spirit which has been given to us.[18]

Christian wisdom was, in sum, not of power of words but the glory and the hope of the saving cross of Christ.[19] It was not the search for reason nor for an enlightenment that dissolved the self and its connection to the body and the endless cycle of reincarnation. It was neither the Stoics' rational autonomy of law and authority nor the Epicureans' garden of select and moderated pleasures, and it stands in contradiction to multifaceted contemporary equations that reduce happiness to suffering, suffering to pains, and pains to curable and resolvable wrongs, conditions, and problems of the mind, the body, and society.

By faith, Christians were called to make themselves a living altar. The church became a community of suffering. It expressed itself in sacraments, the lives of saints, and images and icons focused on sacrifice and grace: the crucifixion, the sufferings of Mary, the wounded virgins, and the martyred saints. The church's mission lay in the incorporation of its believers into the life and teachings of Christ. Watered by the blood of martyrs, the church was an active repository of the grace pooled from Christ's suffering and suffering endured, faithfully embraced, and glorified. Ideally, the church carried the cross and the hope for the community of the living and the dead to the end of time. Prayers to and for the dead and the saints, pilgrimages great and small, crusades holy and profane, and other doctrines and practices (associated especially with early church and medieval and Orthodox Christianity), such as purgatory, indulgences, and the communion of saints, resonated the faith that the church was the guardian and the mediator of the grace of Christ.

Earth, creatures, and humanity radiated the grace of creation. God's forms were embodied in all things, and humanity, the knowing form of forms—to use a formula borrowed from the scholastics—occupied a special place in creation by virtue of participating with knowledge in the essential forms of other forms. Humanity's incarnation and freedom placed it higher than the angels. In all the kingdoms of being, there was an unmatched glory to the human body and mind. Human powers and potential conferred on humanity rights to build and rule the animals of the world. Laws, societies, and cities expressed humanity's power to build and create. Philosophy, science, and theology manifested its capacity to think. The ministrations of its schools, hospitals, orphanages, and alms-giving illustrated its capacity to put its thought and action in the service of fellow humans. Its defects and sufferings in one part occurred through the failure to realize its whole potential in mind.

Under the intellectual influence of Greek and Roman and Jewish and Arab thought, medieval Christians extended their mastery of matter nature, and society. They advanced philosophy, logic, science, algebra, and technological innovation. And with premises that all men, women, and children—poor, serf, and slave—had a dignity in creation and a potential destiny with Christ, they elaborated educational, social, and charitable institutions and articulated rights, traditions, authorities, doctrines, and institutions that helped establish foundations for individual rights and political freedom. Self-sacrifice constituted individual vows, penance, and sacrifices, and in imitation of and participation in the afflictions, agonies, and sufferings of Christ, Mary, and the saints, innocent suffering elicited pity and called for charity, repented sin merited forgiveness, and the miracles and ministry of Christ warranted duplication by the church.

The Reformation saw Protestants and Catholics engaged in murderous war against one another. It also saw principalities battling principalities and unified states opposing corporations, principalities, and empires. More than a century of devastating war brought participants begrudgingly, reluctantly, and far from wholeheartedly to the utility of tolerance and freedom. At the same time, as Lord Acton argues, the Reformation and early modern history saw evidence that the advance of individual autonomy and the independence of institutions furnished practices, concepts, and agencies that promoted freedom, but also created abstract justification for eliminating enemies of the truth.[20]

Assuming that suffering came with incarnate flesh, neither Catholic nor Protestant enrolled in Francis Bacon's belief that emergent science and its empirical way of understanding and application held hope for "the relief of man's estate." As much as individual Christian thinkers joined and even helped define the broad aspirations of the Enlightenment as a progressive improvement of the human condition, they did not, however, enroll in an ultimate triumph over pain and suffering divorced from the Christian promise of salvation and redemption. As much as the Christian populate flocked to medicine as well as traditional folk cures, magic, and superstitions—whatever promised relief from daily pain and crushing fate—experience joined them to orthodox Christian theology in ruling out earthly happiness.

The Great Fissure

Both flowing from and advancing with and by the momentum of the mass technological, commercial, and political transformation of society, whose main material roots were founded in the second half of eighteenth-century western Europe, secularism offered an entirely new and unprecedented set of premises about the human condition and the very ends of history. First, it assumed that suffering could be reduced to calculable and ultimately curable units of human experience, into quantifiable and treatable pains. With an equally revolutionary somersault it considered even prayers for divine pity and its mercy degrading to the dignity of human power, autonomy, and self-perfection. Rallying its energies around a perfectible human, a creature of earthly potential and realization, it idealized humanity and future perfection and happiness and reserved its most cherished sentiments—as still echoed in contemporary political platforms—for dreams of human fulfillment for all. Secularism, as first fully articulated by the varied range of eighteenth-century French and western European Enlightenment thinkers, directed hope and activities to relieving humans of their ignorance and superstitions and of cruel and arbitrary dictatorship. In its most radical expressions, it preached freedom, democracy, and even equality.

This belief had its roots in improved material conditions. It grew out of improved agriculture, technology, applied arts, manufacturing, finance, and transportation. It was heralded by multiplying governmental reforms undertaken by monarchies (especially but not exclusively enlightened monarchies) and embryonic republics in, for example, the Declaration of Independence and the U.S. Constitution, and yet the millenarian and revolutionary aspirations of the French Revolution. It did not die but in measure continued with Napoleonic transformations of France and old Europe and formed the core of utopian and messianic quests of post-Napoleonic politics. Under an ongoing systematization of human affairs, multiplying sectors of the eighteenth century's elite took up the banner of humanity as a self-realizing and self-redeeming species. Identified as physiocrats, deists, rationalists, atheists, and yet collectively as *philosophes*, these secular thinkers articulated a multidimensional faith in progress as foreseen by a belief in free markets, technological improvement, social advancement, efficient institutions, and scientific knowledge. Classic stoicism, epicureanism, and skepticism buttress their faith in the autonomy of human reason and action. Nurtured by an earlier antireligious tradition wearied of religious wars and theological debates that went with the Reformation, Enlightenment thinkers affirmed the rectifying beneficence of skepticism and materialism.[21] Their idealized conception of humanity's progress did not speak to the common lot of human plagued by sickness, irrationality, evil, death, and tragedy.

The philosophers offered what twentieth-century American historian Carl Becker ironically titled *The Heavenly City of the Eighteenth Century Philosophers* (1932). Constituting a new climate of ideas, what Becker termed, the "second Middle Ages," they reset north on the compass of history. Within the spiritual matrix of their idealized city, in which modern medicine and contemporary bioethics largely operates, reason displaces revelation; science does away with magic; technical agencies and policies leave the dead, prayer, and transcendental hope out of therapeutic equations; and human works, anchored in a broad philanthropy, supersede charity and acts of love. They set aside pity and mercy for visions and programs of improvement and reform. They stripped suffering of transcendental meaning significance, equating it with earthly pains to be defeated.

The Enlightenment formed the progressive narrative that shaped nineteenth-century confidence. Paramount eighteenth-century philosopher Immanuel Kant set forth the Enlightenment's first tenet when he declared that humanity had come of age. One of the age's sympathetic historians, Peter Gay, contends that the Enlightenment did nothing less for posterity than join rationality, reformism, freedom, cosmopolitanism, and progress in a quest for a new human order.

Suffering Revalidated

Conservatives and reactionaries, contemporary thinkers and ideologues, were spawned in contradiction to the humanizing Enlightenment and the "godlessly proud and bloody" French Revolution and its hegemonic propagator, Napoleon's France. By their lights, especially those of French-speaking Savoyard philosopher, writer, lawyer, and diplomat, Joseph DeMaistre (1753–1821), authority and suffering ultimately belonged to human fate, God, and his providence.

In the same period, in the early decades of the nineteenth century, romanticism dramatically reinterpreted suffering and generated a new sympathy for it. With origins deep in eighteenth-century literature and sentiment—led by German, English, and French thought—romanticism opened and cultivated emotional and imaginative apertures to suffering. It transformed the human literary mind from a mirror into a lamp, to echo the title of M. H. Abrams's mid–twentieth-century classic, *The Mirror and the Lamp: Romantic Theory and the Critical Tradition* (1953). It endowed the writer with the presumption of a reaching empathy that opened itself to the ineffable suffering of the solitary individual and the unique communities and people of emergent nations. Romantic literature found rich and bridging metaphors between self and other, self, nature, and God.

Romantics aestheticized suffering into a badge of individuality and a claim to possessing a distinct fate. They made dramatic, self-lacerating, and even demonic suffering a matter of pride. The nimbus of suffering framed singularity. Forming the redemptive pole of romantic literature, the suffering of the pure heart stood in opposition to the dark, diabolic, and solitary soul. Master romantic writer and great psychologist of the inner life of pride, sacrifice, and suffering, Dostoevsky, across his writings from *Notes from the Underground* to *Crime and Punishment* to *The Brothers Karamazov,* transformed the polarity of innocent, Christ-like, kenotic suffering and Luciferian pride into the great contesting duality of spiritual existence.[22]

For the romantic, suffering sanctified a group's history and established its claim to a transcendent end. The long-suffering homeless Poles became by romantic provenance the Christ of nations. The deprived, the abandoned, the downtrodden and enslaved, with all their suffering, were transformed into hallowed subjects worthy of a redemptive narrative.

Elevating romantic preoccupation with struggle and strife, philosopher Georg Wilhelm Hegel (1770–1831), whose early theory was forged in the kiln of Christian theology in the 1790s, used suffering to fashion a logical, dialectical, and metaphysical discourse about the strife-laden history and the dramatic course of justice, truth, and self-consciousness across time. Suffering played a vital role for Hegel in the dialectical process of thesis, antithesis, and synthesis—assertion, negation, and unification, or conflict and resolution—by which humanity crossed history. For Hegel, the philosopher of time, history was the story of humanity's long, arduous journey to full being, ideal society, and godlike consciousness.

Inverting Hegel's moral and metaphysical spirit of history into a material history of human energy and the means of production, Karl Marx, at one time one of Hegel's most ardent disciples, put the suffering proletarian at the center of his narrative of the ultimate liberation and fulfillment of humanity. The proletariat, the last of history's oppressed classes, suffered all abuse at the hands of the capitalist and his industrial mode of production. They lost family, village, tradition, God, and the fruit of their own hands and the energy and life of their own individual and collective body. As Marx states, "[He] does not ever reckon labour as part of his life, it is rather the sacrifice of his life."[23] The proletariat, both the archetypical and singular historical victim, was emptied of being itself. Like the kenotic Christ, the proletariat formed the hallowed vessel into a new species of humanity. The proletariat was Prometheus ready to spring into revolt and bring forth a saving revolution.

In one sense, Marx (1818–1883), though several generations younger, was an ally of the founder of utilitarianism, Jeremy Bentham (1748–1832), who sought to reestablish social ethics and the law in terms of a purported felicific calculus whose governing principle was choosing the greatest happiness (most pleasures) or the least suffering (minimal pains) for the majority. Sharing the main premises of the Enlightenment, Marx and Benthan were secular to the bone. Neither found an ounce of transcendence in human suffering.[24] In counter distinction to Bentham, however, Marx not only sided with the early radical French socialists but also internalized the German romantic spirit of *Sturm und Drang* (storm and stress) and absorbed the class conflict inherent in the French Revolution, the total war of Napoleon, and the spontaneous European revolts and revolutions of 1820, 1830, and 1848. For Marx, the Industrial Revolution foretold the penultimate stage of suffering and conflict that would ultimately be resolved with the full realization and completion of humanity.

Intellectual leadership turned on defining suffering. Not without pertinence to the role of contemporary intellectuals and bioethicists, intellectual historian Roy Porter suggests that early nineteenth-century intellectuals formed a new priesthood, either as enlightened thinkers who would reduce suffering to calculable and curable pain or as romantic thinkers who enshrined suffering and made it messianic.[25] The message of the latter, be it on behalf of nation, democracy, socialism, or even technocratic control, constituted a full secular gnosticism: to know the right truth was to be on the right and inevitable side of history.

Hardening Hearts and Naturalizing Suffering

In the second half of the nineteenth century, determined by reactions to the failed revolutions of 1848, European thought hardened. Progress, no longer universal to humanity, was considered exclusive of possession of nation and class. The future turned on street war and military battles. These harsh militant premises—typified by Marxian socialism predicated on class warfare and by German unifier Bismarck's equation of power and right—found intellectual validation in the spread of the blind materialism of physics, empirical and positivist sociology and Darwinian science. They collectively suggested that nature ran by pain and suffering (tooth and claw) and by the survival and reproduction of the fittest.

Although conservatives and liberals contended that laws deduced from nature should not hold because society, institutions, values, and minds were the fruit of human history, not the result of nature—its blind laws and its inevitable violent and random course—the closing decades of the nineteenth century saw more and more thinkers assenting to the premise that humans, animals among animals or yet a collection of atoms in a field of forces, were irrational and destined to suffer. Humanity operated by inner powers and laws beyond its full cognizance and the prescriptive diameter of its values. Extreme neo-romantics like Friedrich Nietzsche (1844–1900) idealized energy, life, will, and even violence. Nietzsche attacked Greek philosophy—the "one-eyed monster" of enervating Socrates and abstract and stultifying Plato, the elemental vitality of myth, rite, and tragedy. He attacked Christianity for its subverting praise of the humble and the meek. Assimilating to his classical training, Darwinism, cynicism, and a philosophy of heroism, Nietzsche consistently loathed his times for its pseudo-rationalism, sentimental philanthropy, liberal and social reformism, vulgar and coarse nationalism, tasteless democracy, and leveling socialism. For Nietzsche, suffering, which could be brutal, blind, and yet cruel and stupid, had no redemptive value unless it fed the agony of the creative and heroic life.

Sigmund Freud (1856–1939) was another turn-of-the-century thinker who turned humanity over to the control of harsh ineluctable laws of nature. The founder of psychoanalysis, Freud located inescapable conflict, tension, guilt, anxiety, repression, and suffering at the core of human experience. He gave little importance to pity, sympathy, and fellow feelings and to our need to account in some way or another for one another's suffering. For Freud, the very genesis of self was born out of a triangular conflict between the undifferentiated and primordial energy of the all-wanting id; the parental, cultural, judging, and repressive superego, ever restraining want, wish, and fantasy; and finally but never perfectly, the balancing and controlling ego, which precariously, agonizingly, and often with lasting trauma sought to negotiate the conflicting claims between the body and the mind, taboo sexual desires and internalized discipline, and the nurturing mother and the law-giving father, and to live out a productive life of mind and work between excessive pleasure and inhibiting pain. As if to privatize the release of the cathartic Greek tragedy, he offered prolonged individual therapy sessions between patient and therapist. In their course, patients recognized and, thus in measure, freed themselves from the emotional traumas that formed the history of their common but conflict-laden and repressed minds. Understanding did not end their suffering but instead freed them from debilitating pains. In later writings, Freud extended his theory of repression and channeled his observations about these sufferings and energies into conceptions of society, culture, the state, and the arts.

Multiplying offshoots of this sort of naturalism and social Darwinism, which inspired and legitimatized economic, social, and political theory, rooted human advances in biological evolution and material development. From this perspective, suffering went with life. In the hardest doctrines of capitalism, racism, and eugenics, the laws of survival and competition displaced sympathy, philanthropy, and notions of mutual advantage and cooperation. Translated into the service of late nineteenth-century doctrines of nationalism and militarism, Darwinism, in one of its multiple variants, sponsored arms races, global imperialism, and the rush to annex the resources and peoples of North and South America, Africa, the Pacific, Asia, and China.

Despite great technological advances, by the nineteenth century's end, the dark language of twentieth-century existentialism—which we identify with dread, angst, separation, loneliness, and absurdity—had begun to seed the contemporary mind. Doctrines of racism, imperialism, and national hegemony abounded, contradicting internationalism, pacifism, and humanitarian socialism and exposing idealists' impotence before engulfing storms of what was to become the gateway of twentieth-century European life; and by the first decade of the twenty-first century, humanity had traveled down the deepest corridors of irrationality, war, and destruction. The engines of progress—be they the nation, the state, science, technology, or global commerce—still threatened disorder, chaos, and even destruction at every turn. At the 1893 World's Fair in Chicago, patrician Henry Adams saw the energy-creating dynamo as an engine driving humanity to an unprecedented stage when the potency and glory of human self-making put human fate in balance. As the primary symbol of contemporary humanity, the impersonal dynamo displaced the loving and merciful Virgin Mary, who was at the center of the medieval answered pray and supplication.

Remorselessly and mercilessly, the First World War mobilized soldier, machine, resources, industry, society, government, and regimentation for victory in what proved a consuming and exhaustive total war. World War I was the gate through which history entered our contemporary world. It turned the engines of progress—technology, industry, democracy, and nationalism—into efficient and mass-killing machines. Victory meant depletion, exhaustion, and the defeat of the enemy, its population, its society, and its industry. The war unfolded as remorseless but ultimately futile attacks and counterattacks. Propaganda generated hate. Cannons, machine guns, barbed wire, and a parade of new weapons—airplanes, tanks, and poison gas—sought surrender before pity and mercy were offered. Justice, human dignity, and progress were put on hold. Nation-states proved all-powerful and merciless sacrificial priests.

Competing visions for the future, including Wilson's and Lenin's, filled the ideological dockets of postwar Europe and the world at large. They offered entirely different agendas for power, reasons, and values. They centered on wronged victims and rights of vindication and millenarian missions requiring suffering and heroic collective sacrifice. The Bolshevik Party, which in 1917 captured, defeated, and devastated Russia, recomposed the nation around the party's absolute control of government and its exclusive representation of the narrative of the victim in the form of the international proletariat. It made the proletariat the ideological justification for the revolution, a succession of purges, and ruthless tyranny at home and in its global policies. The Fascists in Italy and the Nazis in Germany wove aggressive narratives of a nation's past suffering and humiliation, its sacrifice and mission in the present, and its justifiable future vindication and fulfillment. In the name of the betrayal of soldiers on the front and the German people after World War I, Hitler preached revenge against middle-class idealism, pacifism, and money. Nazis translated this worldview biologically, historically, and ethically into a racism that attributed its violation, shame, and suffering to contamination and betrayal by ongoing and active conspiracies of the financial, alien, international Jew. On the grounds of national, party, and racial purification at home and abroad, they destroyed, killed, and eliminated Jews, Romanis, and whole classes and groups of peoples deemed inferior. They also purged, imprisoned, and executed communists and socialists, national conservatives and traditionalists, and Christians who were considered impediments to Nazi rule. Offering bioethics extreme cases of medicine and science in the service of the nation, the Nazi regime used doctrines of biological evolution and racial purity to justify mass extermination, to strip the physically and mentally disabled of all rights, and to use twins and prisoners as subjects of widespread medical experiments.

Anticipated by ideological conflicts and wars in Europe and across the globe, World War II magnified and generalized World War I. Aside from putting the most advanced science, technology, and means of national production and mobilization into the service of a global war, the war's conclusion, with atomic bombs dropped on Japan, put contemporary humanity under the shadow of nuclear obliteration and raised the most challenging ethical questions about what means states could use in the defense of their lands and freedom. The United States and the Soviet Union armed themselves to wage a mutually destructive war that might coincidentally end planetary life and afflict pain and suffering beyond measure.

Great but Ambivalent Hopes

Of all the theaters of twentieth-century science, medicine and public health best exemplified progress. They validated in part and promised beyond all past earthly hopes a longer, fuller, and better life. There is no room here for a complete catalog of all their accomplishments during the nineteenth and twentieth centuries. It would require surveying the nineteenth-century introduction of fresh water and public sanitation, public education, food and work regulations, and improved housing and nutrition. It would demand reference to improvements in surgery, starting with Napoleon's doctors' amputations, new prosthetics during the Civil War, pain-killing anesthesia and antiseptics, and finally the hospital itself as a saving rather than a killing institution. Medicine's advance went forward with inoculations and quarantining and the expansion of charitable and public hospitals, poor houses, and other specialized medical and social institutions, schools, and asylums.

Twentieth-century medicine reached into the deep habitats of pain and suffering. It came with intrusive machines for diagnosis. X-ray machines anticipated scanning devices that peered deeply into organs and ultimately cells themselves. In a different sector, laboratory diagnostic tests, thanks to chemistry's mastery of molecules and biology, brought knowledge of the germ—bacteria and viruses. What were perennially mystifying killer diseases—for instance, small pox, typhoid, anthrax, tuberculosis, and elusive polio—were deciphered and defeated. Sulfur and then penicillin constituted unprecedented offenses against infection, while mass-manufactured aspirins and capsules of every sort eased everyday maladies and miseries.

Matching the ministration of everyday treatments were life-saving appendectomies, tonsillectomies, and assisted breach births. Surgery successfully invaded brains, eyes, ears, and hearts. As scopes increasingly probed and cured, immunizing injections and blood and liquid transfusions saved lives. Transplantation of corneas, hands, livers, kidneys, hearts, and lungs rewrote humans' fates. Now, in the twenty-first century, cell and stem cell implants promise at last cures for body-killing and mind-stealing diseases, and genetic research has given rise to the possibility of embryonic design and a dream of human beings constructed by choice.

Bioethics must now face an utterly extraordinary breaching of all limits in nature. Philosophical and religious questions of every sort are raised by humanity's place in nature, creation, and history. There are no clear signposts about what can, must, and should be promised to humans suffering and in pain. Beyond such difficult but comparatively prosaic questions as to what medicine can deliver to whom, by whom, with what means, and at what cost, there are unfolding sets of moral, ethical, and legal questions about the rights of human and animal life.

Innovations, however great, do not advance us beyond elemental questions. Suffering, however diagnosed, belongs inseparably to body and mind over a single day and the course of a lifetime. It belongs to wish and worry, memory and hope. As long as humans are in flesh and spirit, they know discontent. They forever precariously exist in anguish over exchanges, gifts, and sacrifices. They bounce between past ways, present potentials, and possible future consequences. As much as rationalizing and systematizing institutions and companies and advertisements promise otherwise, no exact calculus exists to diminish suffering and augment happiness. Suffering cannot be reduced to hierarchies of quantifiable pains and marginalized to treatable conditions. As much as pharmacologically, surgically, and psychologically treatable pains direct medicine's everyday practices, bioethics must recognize that suffering belongs to the less quantifiable realms of interpretation and judgment, social and cultural orders, and philosophy and religion.

Contemporary medicine and medical institutions can misinterpret and prejudicially apply sources and treatments for pains and types of suffering. They can degrade patients to their maladies and their treatment. On behalf of making them well, they can steal their dignity. When legislation and government equate suffering with class, race, and gender, politicians become the doctors of the national body. They distort sciences and cure along lines of official and ideological victims. This dramatizes and moralizes suffering as in vogue and, on that basis, channels pity, compensation, and research.[26]

Beyond this, global interdependency, which grows by leaps and bounds, delivers us collectively to profound ambivalence and divisions. Who knows how to calculate their fellow feelings and responsibility for seven billion other humans? As much as science and technology have expanded our potential as well as our increased food supply, social communication, and health care, do we see a corresponding and unilateral improvement in human well-being? Indeed, do we not find an equation between enhanced material progress and the diminishment of reproduction in the Western world and massive gender imbalance in China, where abortion results in the elimination of females? Progress, from any view, does not consistently bring increased happiness or even enhanced physical well-being.[27] Beyond such disputatious matters as the social use of euthanasia, medically assisted suicide, and abortion as either a woman's right or the destruction of life, acute arguments turn on governmental rights and duties to serve rights and goods as well as allay maladies and suffering. These arguments raise questions about the claims of the future against the present and the effectiveness and the means of national and international agencies to envision and secure a better collective future. In play are types of dichotomies between the reality of largely limited, ineffective, and ideologically driven international and humanitarian organizations and more powerful, though often ruthless, nation-states that withdraw benefits, suppress rights, deny democracy, accumulate weapons—including nuclear, chemical, and biological—and sanction the destruction of whole peoples, regions, cultures, and nature.

Beyond concerns for contemporary means and goals of medicine, technology, and the life sciences, bioethics is increasingly pushed beyond the limits of moral imagination. Questions raised by stem cell and genetic research raise issues about the control, mutations, and creation of human life itself.[28] Current advances in psychotropic drugs, alternative reproductive technologies, personalized genetic medicine, preimplantation genetic diagnosis, genetic engineering, end-of-life issues (palliative care), and stem cell technologies force bioethicists to confront elemental matters. They must ask whether sectors of contemporary science disregard all tradition values in their quest to modify themselves. They force us to ask whether humanity will turn its increasing biogenetic capacity into a eugenic racism based on self-selection, genetic testing, and abortion. On this count we feel guilty by our very capacity to act, or cite the relevant French refrain, *tout capable est tout coupable.*

From another quarter comes an additional question. How does such a subjective and protean creature, always whimsical and ever powerful, and, at times, stupid and brutish, proceed wisely, consistently, and benignly? What bounds and regulates our subjective quest for happiness and our flippant and outrageous attempts to eliminate suffering, defects, and all imagined bodily and psychological impediments? Can any person or society, despite what it protests, find authority, order, or stability independent of tradition, religion, and embodied community? From what or whom will this artificially invented and self-willed creature find solace and receive mercy? Where will it find hope? On what terms could a creature who believes it can medically and psychologically engineer its being write tragedies and offer any kind of transcendent narrative to its adventure in time?

Already pushed on all fronts by a relativism based on real differences of singular individuals, distinct groups, and autonomous culture, what basis is there for predicating a universal notion that one day humans collectively will eliminate all pain and suffering? And, equally problematic, without conceding that suffering, though profoundly personal, is a universal human experience, with what philosophic, metaphoric, and mythic currency will persons and communities valorize their experiences and lives and carry on mutual moral correspondence? Through love, pity, pardon, and mercy, suffering leads the self to associations, responsibilities, memories, and communal services and prayers. With what substance other than self-abnegation and self-sacrifice do individuals and groups profess their allegiances, pay the prices of sins or wrongs, and thereby merit a renewed standing in community? Defiant of every philosophy proposed on the achievement of painless happiness and undisturbed enlightenment, suffering as self-subsuming sacrifice validates freedom and responsibility, with pacts and agreements of trust and love. Beyond all that medicine, science, and technology mark out in the conquest and promise of conquest of pain, personal suffering and sacrifice transcend individual selves and offer unions of lasting value.[29]

Beyond History and Ethics

Suffering proves a knife's edge for bioethics. Medical dialogues must walk the edge of identifying the suffering and pains to be negated and defeated and those to be acknowledged and left to exist and even embraced and reverenced. As concentrated suffering, discipline and sacrifice validate person and community. Suffering arises from the deepest quarters of conscience, freedom, and value and our capacity to dedicate lives and suffering to others and purposes. Suffering permits no escape from ambivalence, paradox, and tragedy. For as much as we wish to escape the crushing gravity of pain, illness, accident, and work and all the ills that accompany poverty and tyranny, we cannot pay for contemporary medicine and technology at the cost of suffering and sacrifice that give values to freedom, truth, faith, and alliance.

Bioethics can charge medicine, science, technology, and institutions and professions with the duty to protect human dignity. It can offer analytical and imaginative discussions of the dignity of personal suffering, especially in the last stages of life, and its relation to law and public policy. But it cannot precisely or definitively place humans in being, nature, and history. It cannot fathom the human spirit or know what events will reveal. Prophecy is forever contradicted by surprise and doubt. And as the walls of past cities and civilizations vanished, so, too, will the grounding assumptions and encircling certitudes of this age vanish.

I agree with contemporary philosopher Isaiah Berlin that moral identities, truly diverse and differentiating and rooted in culture, religion, freedom, and aspirations, are formed around the values by which we live and for which we suffer. By suffering we bear full witness and testimony; we martyr ourselves, to rely on the telling Greek etymology of the verb *maptúpomai.* Morals cannot be empirically traded away. They drive those who wish humans well to the assumption that "the first public obligation is to avoid the extremes of suffering," which can include the destruction of values and freedom. Revolutions, wars, and assassinations paradoxically became primary instruments to achieve collective goals in the therapeutic and utopian twentieth and twenty-first centuries. A pragmatist and supporter of freedom, Berlin cautions that surgical amputations invite infection, cures can have doleful outcomes, and judgments are frequently contingent, precarious, and even dead wrong. The supposed good always threatens with the unimaginable bad.[30]

In democratic times, states still turn fickle and cruel, majorities give way to frenzy and go mad, and the intentions of the best measures go violently astray. Finally, and simply, there is no certain social calculus; the utilitarian measure—the greatest good for the greatest number (or the least pain for the fewest)—cannot *not* be clearly defined or applied, even if it is all we often have in matters of democratic legislation. However sincere motives are to help and cure pain and remove forms of suffering, limits exist in knowledge, the irreconcilable divisions of ethics, and the coarseness of agencies of reform and justice. The bioethicist must chart a course in the winds of stunning innovation, advance ever in the teeth of the surprise of unexpected events, and not capsize given list and tilt with shifting ballasts of want and aspiration. And the bioethicist, having taken counsel from the historian, might suggest that persons and communities cannot be severed from what they take to be the value of their suffering and sacrifice. And because of this, they must listen to expressions of pity, mercy, and hopes and prayers that exceed the chapels of science, technology, and medicine.

Notes

1. Just midway in the twentieth century, the unprecedented historical revolution of science, technology, and medicine led French philosopher and biologist Jean Rostand to ask with the title of a book, *Can Man Be Modified?* (New York: Basic Books, 1959).

2. Wilfred McClay, *"Beyond the Right to Life": A review of Ramesh Ponnuru, The Party of Death* (Washington, DC: Regnery, 2006) in *The New Atlantis* Fall, no. 14 (2006), 73, 79.

3. This definition and location of bioethics was borrowed from the syllabus of Cathy Gere's "The History of Bioethics" (Cathygere@cantab.net).

4. Michael Palma, *Begin in Gladness* (Scottsdale, AZ: Star Cloud Press, 2011), 19.

5. For a discussion of how surfaces give first perceptions and establish conceptions, see Joseph A. Amato, *Surfaces: A History* (Berkeley: University of California Press, 2013).

6. Montaigne cited in Jeffrey Martin Greet, "Montaigne's Critique of Cicero,' *Journal of the History of Ideas* 36 (1975), 595–612.

7. The color black has come to have in our society a special, though not exclusive, association with suffering and death. White, blue, and purple also resonate passion, sadness, and mourning involved in death and dying; browns and yellows can indicate fall, autumn light, and the death of nature; bright red can stand for flowing blood and dark red for congealed and caked blood. For additional discussions of colors and their relation to suffering, see Philip Ball, *Bright Earth: Art and the Invention of Color* (Chicago: University of Chicago Press, 2003) and Michel Pastoreau, *Black, The History of a Color* (Princeton, NJ: Princeton University Press, 2008).

8. I found in*Jacob's Well: A Case for Rethinking Family History* (St. Paul, MN: Minnesota Historical Society Press, 2008). I could not tell my own family history without reconstructing stories of ordeals, travail, and suffering. I discovered in *When Father and Son Conspire* (Ames, IA: Iowa State University Press, 1988)that I could not reconstruct a 1983 Minnesota murder of two bankers without analyzing the stories a father and son told each other about the wrongs they suffered and intend to vindicate. Lies formed the motive that both led and justified the murder they carried out.

9. The other is treated as an ontological pole of the self-defining individual not just in modern psychology and sociology but also in contemporary phenomenology. For the ontological power and presence of the other for the self, see Adriaan Peperzak, Simon Critchley, and Robert Bernasconi, eds., *Emmanuel Levinas: Basic Philosophical Writing* (Bloomington, IN: Indiana University Press, 1996), esp. 5–31; and Roger Scruton, *The Face of God* (London: Continuum, 2012), esp.73–112.

10. For a discussion of sacrifice and gifts and exchanges, see Joseph A. Amato, *Guilt and Gratitude: A Study of the Origins of Contemporary Conscience* (Westport, CT: Greenwood Press, 1982), esp. 22–35; and Joseph A. Amato, *Victims and Values: A History and a Theory of Suffering* (New York: Praeger, 1990), esp. 23–43. For a notion of sacrifices of renewal, see Mircea Eliade, *Cosmos and History: The Myth of the Eternal Return* (New York: Harper & Brothers, 1959), 35–36. For sacrifice as a way to maintain and restore order, see René Girard, *Violence and the Sacred* (Baltimore: The John Hopkins University Press, 1977), esp. 258–259 and 314–315.

11. Numa Denis Fustel De Coulanges, *The Ancient City* (Baltimore: The John Hopkins University Press, 1980), esp. 134–142.

12. Quotation is found in Confucian T'an Kung Li'C i, T'an Kung I, 2, ed. E. R. Hughes, *Chinese Philosophy in Classical Time* (London: Everyman's Library, 1942), 31.

13. The above quotations were taken from John Gross, ed., *The Oxford Book of Aphorisms* (Oxford, UK: Oxford University Press, 1983), 133, 138, 139, 142, 144.

14. In Latin, pity gives rise to the Italian *pieta*. In Russian, pity (*zhalost*) has a large range of connotations. It is rooted in *zhal*, which can indicate pain, express shame, or be a

matter of regret. The rich verb *zhalets* can mean to feel sorry for, to declare regret, to give mercy, or to spare someone. Although *zhaloba* and its verb *zhalovatsa* mean complaint and to complain, and the very common *pazhalista* (for the pain of it) means please, *zhalkee* means pitiable, miserable, or wretched, and connotes other forms of suffering that might merit compassion or evoke disgust and justify disdain.

15. Walter Burkert, *Greek Religion* (Oxford, UK: Blackwell, 1985), 64–66, passim.

16. Romans 4:16.

17. As most developed in the Russian Orthodox faith, Christianity sponsors a kenotic faith; suffering, including death by violence, empties the soul of illusions of self and earth. Christianity extends pity to all suffering: my suffering is yours, and ours is Christ's.

18. Romans 5:2–5.

19. Paul's theology can be read as coming out of the interplay of suffering and hope. In Romans, Chapter 8, we read, in verse 8, "If we be dead with Christ we believe we shall live with him, that we suffer with him that we may also be glorified with together." In verses 23 and 24, "The spirit of the faithful is to groan within ourselves waiting for adoption" And this invisible hope teaches, in verse 36, "for thy sake we are killed all day long, we are accounted as sheep led to the slaughter." And in verses 37 and 38, "neither life, nor death; nor height, nor depth—separate us from the love of God, which is in Christ Jesus our Lord."

20. For a short discussion of Lord Acton's problematic position on the Reformation, see Gertrude Himmelfarb, *Lord Acton: A Study in Conscience and Politics* (Chicago: University of Chicago Press, 1952), 43–47. Two pertinent Acton essays, "The History of Freedom in Christianity" and "The Protestant Theory of Interpretation," are found in his *Essays on Freedom and Power*, ed. Gertrude Himmelfarb (New York: Meridian, 1955), 53–81 and 113–140, respectively.

21. Jonathan Israel seeks to turn radical secularism into the true Enlightenment in *A Revolution of the Mind: Radical Enlightenment and Intellectual Origins of Modern Democracy* (Oxford, UK: Oxford University Press, 2010), reviewed by Joseph A. Amato, "A Revolution of Mind? A Purge of the Enlightenment," *Modern Age* 53, no. 22 (2011), 54–57.

22. I explore the theme of innocent and proud suffering in Joseph A. Amato, "Dostoevsky," in *Ethics, Living or Dead* (Portals Press/Crossing Press, 1982), esp. 35–52.

23. Karl Marx, *Labour and Capital* (1849), cited in Amato, *Victims and Values*, supra note 10, 116.

24. Amato, *Victims and Values,* supra note 10, 114.

25. Roy Porter, *Flesh in the Age of Reason* (New York: W. W. Norton, 2003), 474.

26. For a historical treatment of suffering as a value and the moral axis of the political and rhetorical definition of victim, see Amato, *Victims and Values*, supra note 10, esp. 137–208.

27. For an examination of the condition of twentieth century ethics, see Amato, *Ethics, Living or Dead*, supra note 22, esp. 111–118.

28. A useful introduction to the issues involved genetic and stem cell research is provided by Leo Furcht and William Hoffman, *The Stem Cell Debate: Beacons of Hope or Harbingers of Death* (New York: Arcade, 2008).

29. Views of life and person as a matter of suffering and sacrifice, risk and embodiment, are found across twentieth century thought and were notably developed by the French Catholic tradition of personalism as articulated by Emmanuel Mounier

and a set of thinkers gathered around his journal *Esprit*, Joseph A. Amato, *Mounier and Maritain: A French Catholic Understanding of the Modern World* (Tuscaloosa, AL: University of Alabama Press, 1975; reissued by Sapienta Press, in Ypsilanti, MI, 2002, with preface by Thaddeus Radzilowki.) The importance of sacrifice as part of discourse of self and world is keenly elucidated by philosopher Michael A. Weinstein, *Structure of Human Life: A Vitalist Ontology* (New York: New York University Press, 1979).

30. Isaiah Berlin, "In the Pursuit of the Ideal," *New York Review of Books*, March 17, 1988), 18.

PART TWO

Suffering in Biology

5

Social Neuroscience Meets Philosophy: Suffering, Empathy, and Moral Cognition

Jean Decety

The experience of suffering is often represented as deeply personal and highly contextual. However, to some extent other people have access to our internal affective states. Humans are social creatures, and our survival is largely dependent on our interactions with others. Brain mechanisms evolved to perceive and respond with care to others when they are in distress, whether this distress is the result of physical injury, social loss, social rejection, or longing for a loved one.

The long history of mammalian evolution shaped our brains to recognize and respond with care to signs of suffering of others. In fact, evidence from a wide range of academic disciplines, including recent work in social neuroscience, converges to suggest that social pain and physical pain operate through common neurophysiological mechanisms.[1] Evolutionarily, in mammalian species, physical and social pain were both necessary to promote survival and motivate defensive and protective behaviors. In addition, they likely played a critical role in the development of care-based morality in humans. This representation of these different types of pain as sharing common neurophysiological mechanisms further supports the principle of neural reuse theories.[2] Instead of giving rise to brand new systems, most evolutionary changes involve the differentiation of a current system to produce a new outcome. Neural circuits established for one purpose can be exapted (exploited, recycled, redeployed), without losing their original functions. The fact that the physical pain and the social pain-distress systems both alert organisms to the presence of a noxious environmental stimulus makes it likely that they would share the same neural circuitry, possibly with the circuit for physical pain gradually expanding to include that of social pain/distress.

The primary goal of this chapter is to integrate evolutionary biology with research in social neuroscience on empathy and morality to clarify the interactions between the affective processes involved in the experience and perception of physical, social pain, and suffering and their relationship to moral cognition. The chapter begins by examining how sensitivity to signs of suffering has evolved

TABLE 5.1

Definition of the Concepts Used

- Empathy is the natural ability to share and understand emotional and affective states of others without a confusion between self and other.
- Empathic concern is another-oriented emotional response and motivational state congruent with the perceived welfare of someone in need.
- Event-related potentials (ERPs) are a noninvasive method of measuring brain activity during cognitive processing. The transient electric potential shifts (so-called ERP components) are time-locked to the stimulus onset (e.g., the presentation of a word, a sound, or an image). Each component reflects brain activation associated with one or more mental operations.
- Genetic polymorphism the recurrence within a population of two or more discontinuous genetic variants of a specific trait in such proportions that they cannot be maintained simply by mutation.
- Hypothalamic-pituitary-adrenal axis (HPA axis) is a complex set of direct influences and feedback interactions among the hypothalamus, the pituitary gland, and the adrenal glands. The HPA axis is a major part of the neuroendocrine system that controls reactions to stress and regulates many body processes, including digestion, the immune system, mood and emotions, sexuality, and energy storage and expenditure.
- Social pain is the experience of pain as a result of interpersonal rejection or loss, such as rejection from a social group, bullying, or the loss of a loved one.
- Autonomic nervous system is the part of the peripheral nervous system that is responsible for regulating involuntary body functions, such as heartbeat, blood flow, breathing, and digestion. This system is further divided into two branches: the sympathetic system and the parasympathetic system. The sympathetic division of the autonomic nervous system regulates the flight-or-fight responses. The parasympathetic division of the autonomic nervous system helps maintain normal body functions and conserves physical resources.

in the context of parental care in mammalian species and which neurobiological mechanisms support its operation. Next, the neurodevelopment of morality is discussed with reference to early signs of the ability to perceive sensitivity and fairness and exhibit concern for others, abilities posited as precursors to a more mature understanding of morality. Then, neuroimaging studies focusing on the perception of others' physical and social distress are presented in support of the role of empathic arousal in moral judgment. Finally, the chapter will address a number of emotion-processing dysfunctions in psychopathy to further illustrate how the lack of sensitivity to others' suffering contributes to a callous disregard for the welfare of others and amoral conduct. See Table 5.1 for a list of the concepts used in this chapter and their definitions.

The Neuroevolution of Our Sensitivity to Others' Distress

As a species, humans are highly social mammals that depend on other conspecifics for survival and reproduction. The ability to model the emotions of nonrelatives and react appropriately when interacting within a social group probably confers a number of evolutionarily advantageous skills (e.g., better able to communicate and detect distress in group members and protect them). Furthermore, positive social behaviors, such as caregiving, are essential for both reproduction and survival. Most mammals, including humans, are motorically immature at birth, and caregiving is necessary to compensate the infant's undeveloped motor and autonomic nervous systems.[3] Many of the same neurophysiological and endocrine systems that permit birth, lactation, and parental behavior have been implicated in the giving and receiving of positive experiences.[4] However, these processes are not limited to mother–infant interactions. Biologically unrelated individuals may express and experience concern for others and caregiving.[5] This suggests that the motivational system that originally developed to promote care for offspring was co-opted and used to facilitate positive relationships between biologically unrelated group members. For example, in humans, our relationships with spouses, friends, and coworkers are highly valued despite requiring vast amounts of psychological resources to maintain. In fact, perceiving such relationships as threatened engenders profound emotional and physiological stress responses.[6] Conversely, feeling well connected with and supported by friends and family provides a strong behavioral and psychological buffer that can actually diminish stress responses and result in improved health.[7] This provides strong evidence for the repurposing of motivational components of prosocial behaviors such as empathy that originally developed to motivate parental care as invaluable tools for the formation and maintenance of strong social bonds between unrelated individuals.

Animal research demonstrates that the ability to share and be affected by others' emotional states, an ability integral to maintaining the social relationships important for survival, is organized by basic neural, autonomic, and endocrine systems subserving attachment-related processes, including the brainstem, the preoptic area of the thalamus, and paralimbic areas, as well as the autonomic nervous system.[8] These systems underlying attachment appear to exploit the strong, established physical pain system, borrowing aversive signals associated with pain to indicate when relationships are threatened.[9] Moreover, higher-level cortical structures have been proposed to reflect a system involved in detecting, processing, and reacting to the occurrence of salient events regardless of the sensory modality through which these stimuli are conveyed. Therefore, just as the physical pain system alerts organisms to the presence of a noxious environmental stimulus, so, too, does the social pain system: the experience of social pain alerts an individual to potential threats in the social environment and can induce various coping strategies to attempt to mitigate the threats (e.g., increase motivation to strengthen relationships).[10]

Converging evidence from animal behavior,[11] functional neuroimaging studies in typically developed individuals,[12] and lesion studies in neurological patients[13] indicates that empathy and caring for others employ a large array of brain structures and systems extending beyond the cortex (amygdala, hypothalamus, insula, anterior cingulate cortex and orbitofrontal cortex) and also involve the autonomic nervous system (ANS), hypothalamic-pituitary-adrenal axis (HPA), and endocrine systems that regulate bodily states, emotion, and reactivity (Figure 5.1).

A large number of studies have provided compelling evidence implicating neuropeptides in the regulation of sociality, emotion, and the ANS. In particular, oxytocin, which is both a hormone and a neuromodulator, is causally related to caring

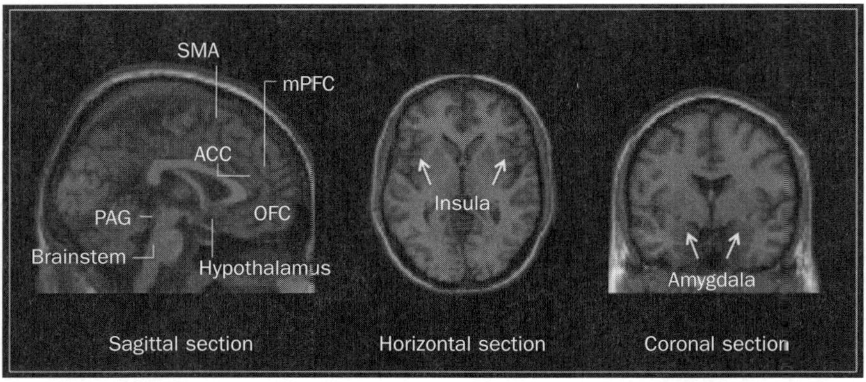

FIGURE 5.1 Interconnected set of brain regions that play a crucial role in the experience of empathy and caring for others labeled on sagittal, horizontal, and coronal sections of a structural magnetic resonance image. Functional imaging studies revealed that the anterior insula and the anterior cingulate cortices are conjointly activated during the perception or even the imagination of someone in physical or social distress. The insula provides a foundation for the representation of subjective bodily feelings, which substantiates emotional awareness. The anterior cingulate cortex (ACC) can be divided anatomically based on cognitive (dorsal) and emotional (ventral) components. The dorsal part of the ACC is connected with the prefrontal cortex and parietal cortex as well as the motor system, making it a central station for processing top-down and bottom-up stimuli and assigning appropriate control to other areas in the brain. By contrast, the ventral part of the ACC is connected with amygdala (a structure involved in assigning affective significance to stimuli), ventral striatum, hypothalamus, and anterior insula and is involved in assessing the salience of emotion and motivational information. The orbitofrontal cortex (OFC) is involved in sensory integration, in representing the affective value of reinforcers, and in moral decision making. In particular, the OFC is thought to regulate planning behavior associated with sensitivity to reward and punishment and is closely connected to the anterior insula and amygdala. The hypothalamus, especially the medial preoptic area, is involved in regulating basic motivational states and is essential for parental behavior and caregiving. This region is heavily interconnected with the ACC and the OFC, as well as the amygdala and periaqueductal gray (PAG). mPFC medial prefrontal cortex; SMA, superior mesenteric artery.

behavior and stress regulation and has receptors throughout the maternal caregiving circuit.[14] There is increasing evidence for the role of oxytocin in human social cognition, empathy, and prosocial behavior. Oxytocin administration by nasal spray decreases neurophysiological responses to social stress.[15] Intranasal administration of oxytocin, compared with placebo, reduces amygdala activation and modulates its coupling with brainstem regions that are involved in automatic fear reactivity.[16] In a double-blind placebo-controlled study, a single dose of oxytocin or placebo was randomly given to male participants 50 minutes before playing the trust game.[17] The results showed that investors receiving oxytocin displayed more maximum sharing behavior and had a significantly higher median and higher average transfers of monetary units. When controlling for the possibility that oxytocin just increased risk taking and not trust in particular, a risk game was used. Results showed that the oxytocin group did not significantly differ from the control group in risk taking. Additionally, a single dose of intranasally administrated oxytocin is sufficient to cause a substantial increase in an individual's ability to accurately identify affective states on a test relying on the detection of subtle affective facial expressions.[18] A more nuanced role of oxytocin in social behavior was documented in a study which found that normal variance in baseline social-cognitive competence moderates the effects of oxytocin. In that study, oxytocin improved empathic accuracy only for individuals with lower social-cognitive competence.[19]

There is evidence that a naturally occurring genetic variation of the oxytocin receptor relates to both empathy and stress profiles. This was discovered in a study that tested how the rs53576 polymorphism of the oxytocin receptor relates to empathy and stress reactivity.[20] Compared with individuals homozygous for the G allele of rs53576 (GG), individuals with one or two copies of the A allele (AG/AA) exhibited lower behavioral and dispositional empathy. Furthermore, AA/AG individuals displayed higher physiological and dispositional stress reactivity than GG individuals, as determined by heart rate response during a startle anticipation task and an affective reactivity scale. Another study reported that individuals with two G alleles of OXTR rs53576 exhibited more sensitive parenting behavior.[21]

These results concur with animal research suggesting a critical role for oxytocin in prosocial approach behavior and reactivity to social stress. It has also been proposed that the interaction between oxytocin and dopamine enhances reward from social encounters, promoting engagement in social interactions.[22] One significant difference that must be taken into account in human research is the fact that, in humans, high-level cognitive abilities such as executive function, language, and theory of mind are layered on phylogenetically older social and emotional capacities. These evolutionarily newer aspects of information processing expand the range of behaviors that can be motivated by empathy, such as caring for and helping out-group members and even members of a different species.[23] These newer levels, however, depend on evolutionarily older levels of organization and should not be viewed as independent of or conflicting with one another.

The Development of Empathy and Care-based Morality

Human babies enter the world ready to attend to social stimuli and engage in social interactions. Newborns look significantly longer at a happy facial expression than a fearful one, indicating that this preference reflects experience acquired over the first few days of life[24] In addition, neonates contagiously cry in response to the distress of conspecifics in their proximity,[25] a reaction heightened in response to another's crying compared with the child's own crying.[26] Contagious crying's specificity and characteristics of affect sharing have prompted the hypothesis that it is one of the earliest forms of empathic arousal. Subcortical pathways connecting the brainstem, superior colliculus, hypothalamus, pulvinar, and amygdala, all of which develop very early in fetal brain development, mediate this affect sharing in neonates.[27] As infants develop and learn, they are increasingly able to evaluate their social surroundings and even differentiate agents based on their social actions toward each other. For example, 3-month-olds preferentially attend to a character who had previously acted in a prosocial (versus antisocial) manner,[28] suggesting a partiality toward those that "do good things." By 6 months of age, this visual preference has expanded to behaviors, with participants not only selectively attending to prosocial agents (when paired with antisocial or neutral characters) but also selectively approaching them.[29] Further, by 15 months of age, some infants are able to evaluate the fairness of an agent in a third-party situation. In a recent study examining the relationship between a visual violation of expectation task and infants' sharing behaviors, it was found that infants who shared a toy they preferred (over a nonpreferred toy or no toy at all) also attended significantly longer to a third-party interaction in which the allocation of resources among conspecifics was unequal.[30] This suggests that those infants who behaved altruistically also expanded their prosocial expectations to the interactions of others.

Prosocial behaviors in the form of helping, sharing, and consoling emerge shortly after the first year of life. Early signs of helping behavior are reported in the toddler years, with 14- to 18-month-olds fetching objects of desire that appear out of reach for an experimenter[31] and helping to complete household chores.[32] Early other-oriented empathic responding to the distress of another was observed from 8 to 16 months and continued to increase gradually into the second year.[33] Children between the ages of 1 and 2 years exhibit increased comforting behaviors toward individuals in distress[34] and may even give up their own favorite objects in an empathetic gesture.[35] Furthermore, toddlers have been found to exhibit more concern toward the victim of a moral transgression than the transgressor, even if the victim did not show any behavioral markers of distress.[36] This suggests that 18- to 25-month-olds are reacting not simply to emotional displays but also to the intentions and desires of others. Taken together, this evidence indicates that children younger than 2 years already respond in socially appropriate ways while viewing others in distress or pain.

Pain facilitates evolved protective social functions, not only warning the person suffering it that something is awry, but also providing the understanding that another conspecific is at risk and inducing expressive behaviors that attract the attention of others and motivate prosocial behavior. In support of this, when exposed to their infants' cries (compared with neutral sounds), first-time mothers who were breast-feeding reported higher ratings of sadness and desire to help for their infants' cries than control sounds.[37] As stated previously, human infants are biologically predisposed to emotionally resonate with the basic affective (positive and negative) states of others, the first step in the experience of empathy.[38] Given the adaptive value of emotional contagion—the infant gains rapid insight into the emotional states of those around her—this ability should not come as a surprise.

When another individual is in distress or pain, empathic arousal is the process by which the perceiver becomes vicariously distressed.

One developmental study combined neurophysiological measures, including functional magnetic resonance imaging, eye-tracking, and pupillary response, with behavioral measures assessing affective and moral judgments across age.[39] Participants aged between 4 and 37 years viewed scenarios depicting intentional versus accidental actions that caused harm or damage to people and objects. Morally salient scenarios evoked stronger empathic sadness in young participants and were associated with enhanced activity in the amygdala, insula, and temporal poles. While intentional harm was evaluated as equally wrong across all participants, ratings of deserved punishments and malevolent intent gradually differentiated with age. As age increased, participants punished an agent who damaged an object less severely than an agent who harmed a person. Furthermore, age-related increases in activity were detected in the ventromedial prefrontal cortex (vmPFC) in response to intentional harm to people, as well as increased functional connectivity between this region and the amygdala. In all participants, irrespective of their age, perceived intentional harm to people (as opposed to accidental harm) was associated with increased activation in brain regions sensitive to the perception, prediction, and interpretation of others' intentions such as the right posterior superior temporal sulcus,[40] as well as regions processing the affective consequences of these actions, namely the temporal poles, insula, vmPFC, and amygdala. The more participants reported being upset about harmful actions, the higher the activity in the amygdala. The younger the participants were, the greater their empathic sadness for the victim of harm. Ratings of sadness for the victim correlated with activity in the insula, thalamus, and subgenual prefrontal cortex. This latter region has extensive connections with circuits implicated in emotional behavior and autonomic-neuroendocrine response to stressors, including the amygdala, lateral hypothalamus, and brainstem serotonergic, noradrenergic, and dopaminergic nuclei.[41] Damage to this region, especially if it occurs during early childhood, is associated with abnormal autonomic responses to emotional experiences and impaired comprehension of the adverse consequences of pernicious social behaviors.[42]

Together, these studies show that the pattern of developmental change in response to the perception of others' distress and suffering is indicative of a gradual shift from the monitoring of somatovisceral responses in young children to a more cognitive evaluative level associated with executive control of higher-order emotion and empathic concern in older participants.

Perceiving Others in Distress is Influenced by Social Context and Relationships

Because of the importance of perceiving other conspecifics in distress to survival and its adaptive value, human infants are biologically predisposed to be sensitive to others' emotional expressions, especially when the expressions are vocalized.

Neonates appear to possess a neural mechanism for discriminating vocalizations associated with emotions. For instance, they exhibit a mismatched electroencephalographic response over the right hemisphere in response to emotionally laden syllables (happy or fearful vs. neutral) within the first few days of life.[43] In 3- to 7-day-olds, another person's sad vocalizations are associated with a selective increase of neural activity in brain regions involved in processing affective stimuli, such as the orbitofrontal cortex and insula.[44] These results suggest remarkably early functional specialization for processing negative emotions expressed in the human voice.

Numerous functional neuroimaging studies revealed that, when individuals are presented with stimuli conveying another person's distress and physical and social pain, reliable activation of a neural network involved in the first-hand experience of pain, including the anterior midcingulate cortex, anterior insular cortex, supplementary motor area, and periaqueductal gray area, occurs. Activation in this network has been reported in response to facial expressions of pain, injury of body parts, imagining the pain of others, being socially excluded, or simply observing a signal indicating that someone will receive painful stimulation.[45] These activations in the neural circuit involved in the first-hand experience of pain from passive viewing of others in pain may not be specific to the sensory qualities of pain. Instead, they might be associated with more general survival mechanisms such as aversion and withdrawal when exposed to danger and threat.[46]

Importantly, this brain response to signs of suffering is highly dependent on social relationships, and various social and contextual factors moderate the experience of empathy. Empirical work with both nonhuman animals[47] and humans has shown that empathy can be moderated by how the target person is perceived, including how similar[48] or likable that person is to the observer,[49] and by group membership.[50] This affects information processing of the different components of empathy such as affective arousal, emotion understanding, and motivation to care.[51] Neuroimaging studies have documented that the neural network associated with the perception of others' distress is modulated by various social, contextual, and interpersonal factors. For instance, one functional magnetic resonance imaging (fMRI) study demonstrated that empathic arousal is moderated early during information processing by a priori attitudes toward other people.[52] In that study, participants were significantly more sensitive to the pain of individuals who had contracted AIDS as the result of a blood transfusion, evidenced by significantly higher pain and empathy ratings and significantly greater hemodynamic activity in areas associated with pain processing when they viewed videos of facial expression of pain, as compared to individuals who had contracted AIDS as the result of their illicit drug addition (sharing needles). Another fMRI study found evidence for the modulation of empathic neural responses by racial group membership.[53] Notably, the neural response in the ACC to perception of others in pain decreased remarkably when participants viewed faces of racial out-group members being pricked by a needle relative to racial in-group members. Furthermore, activity in the pain network was enhanced when people viewed their loved ones in physical pain compared with strangers[54] and reduced if the person in pain had been unfair in a prior interaction.[55]

To the extent to which affective arousal promotes empathic concern and helping behavior one might expect perceivers to experience reduced concern for out-group victims as well. Recent research provides support for this hypothesis. Soccer fans in one study observed either another fan of their favored team (in-group) or a fan of their rival team (out-group) experiencing painful shocks.[56] Participants showed increased empathy for in-group over out-group targets, reporting higher pain ratings and showing greater activation in the anterior insula for in-group targets. Participants also reported feeling more empathic concern for in-group targets, and they were more likely to volunteer to help by sharing the pain of in-group than out-group targets. Moreover, the difference in anterior insula activation when viewing in-group versus out-group members in pain predicted group differences in helping behavior. Another neuroimaging study demonstrated that the failures of an in-group member are painful, whereas those of a rival out-group member give pleasure—a feeling that may motivate harming rivals.[57]

Individuals' personal context also modulates affective arousal, as demonstrated by two functional neuroimaging studies showing that physicians do not react to the pain of others in the same way as nonphysicians do. One study compared the neuro-hemodynamic response in a group of physicians and a group of matched control participants while they viewed short video clips depicting hands and feet being pricked by a needle (painful situations) or being touched by a cotton bud (nonpainful situations). The results demonstrated activation of the pain matrix in controls when they attended to the painful situations relative to the nonpainful ones. However, when physicians watched painful procedures, a different pattern of activation was observed, with cortical regions underpinning executive function and self-regulation (dlPFC and mPFC) and executive attention (precentral, superior parietal, and pSTS/TPJ) activated.[58] Unlike in the control group, no signal increase was detected in the pain matrix in the physicians. A second study recorded event-related potentials (ERPs) from physicians and matched controls while they were presented with the same visual stimuli.[59] The results showed early signal change 110 milliseconds after stimulus presentation, which differentiated between pain and no pain over the frontal cortex, reflecting negative arousal, as well as late P3 over the centroparietal regions in control participants. In contrast, no such early ERP response was detected in physicians, indicating that affect regulation has very early effects, inhibiting the bottom-up processing of negative arousal from the perception of painful stimuli.

Affective arousal in response to another's distress seems to be a necessary part of normal empathic and moral development. This affective response is present as early as childhood, increasingly subject to modulation and regulation by higher-order neural regions with age, which is also influenced by individuals' own specific experiences with and the context in which they view pain and distress.

The Lack of Sensitivity to Others in Psychopathy

Psychopathy, a neurodevelopmental personality disorder believed to affect approximately 1 percent of the general population, epitomizes the process through which a lack of sensitivity to another's distress or suffering contributes to callous disregard to others.[60] Individuals with psychopathy demonstrate stunted emotional development and a general lack of empathy exhibited through specific individual traits. Psychopathy has been associated with an uncommitted mating behaviors, increased sexual coercion, lack of parental investment, increased number of sexual partners, and increased sexual promiscuity. Psychopaths are often callous, shallow, and superficial. They do not fear punishment, have difficulty regulating their emotions, and do not experience insight into or empathy for the effect of their behaviors on others.

There is solid evidence that empathy deficits and a lack of regard for others may play a role in aspects of moral judgment, particularly those associated with care-based morality. Adult psychopaths fail to experience distress cues as aversive regardless of whether that observer is the aggressor or a bystander,[61] evidenced by work indicating that offenders with high levels of psychopathy show reduced autonomic arousal while viewing a confederate receiving electric shocks.[62] The ability to experience distress as aversive is critical for the development of moral emotions (e.g., guilt, empathy and remorse) because distress cues are assumed to activate tendencies to withdraw in any observer who processes them.

These abnormal responses to moral transgressions or the distress of others are evident as early as childhood. For example, children with psychopathic tendencies exhibit reduced electrodermal responses to distress cues (e.g., a crying face) and threatening stimuli (e.g., a pointed gun) relative to controls.[63] A study using electroencephalography recently examined this phenomenon by assessing how callous-unemotional traits in juvenile psychopaths are related to empathic arousal deficits.[64] In this study, juvenile offenders with high callous-unemotional traits, juvenile offenders with low callous-unemotional traits, and age-matched, typically developing adolescents were shown images of people in pain while electroencephalograms and ERPs were recorded. Results demonstrated that youth with high callous-unemotional traits exhibit atypical neural dynamics of pain empathy processing in the early stages of affective arousal. This abnormality was exemplified by a lack of the early EPR response (120 milliseconds), thought to reflect an automatic aversive reaction to negative stimuli, and was coupled with relative insensitivity to actual pain (as measured with the pressure pain threshold). Nevertheless, their capacity to understand intentionality was not impaired. This uncoupling between affective arousal and emotional understanding likely contributes to psychopaths' callous disregard for the rights and feelings of others.

Brain abnormality in a number of neural regions and circuits seems to account for the lack of affective arousal in individuals with psychopathic traits. Structural neuroimaging studies associate psychopathy with a host of morphological brain abnormalities, including reduced volume of the amygdala; reduced gray matter volume in the frontal and temporal cortex, especially in the right posterior superior temporal sulcus; and increased volume of the striatum. Furthermore, psychopaths often exhibit signs of reduced structural integrity of the uncinate fasciculus[65]—which connects parts of the limbic system in the temporal lobe (such as the hippocampus and amygdala) with the orbitofrontal cortex, a region necessary for moral decision making.

Further evidence of abnormalities in moral reasoning in individuals with psychopathy research indicates that individuals who score high on psychopathy evaluations understand moral norms but generally disregard them. For instance, a study that evaluated incarcerated offenders found no evidence that offenders high in psychopathy—as measured by total psychopathy score—were any worse at distinguishing moral from conventional transgressions than were low-psychopathy offenders.[66] These results are consistent with an fMRI study examining psychopathic responses to pictures depicting morally wrong social actions, unpleasant but not immoral social scenes, and neutral social scenes.[67] In this research, psychopathic and nonpsychopathic criminal offenders rated the severity of the moral violation depicted in each type of stimuli. Both groups rated moral violations significantly higher in moral severity than unpleasant but not immoral scenes, and no differences were observed between groups within any of the image conditions, suggesting equally accurate abilities to distinguish moral violations. Interestingly, brain activation recorded during the evaluation of moral violation pictures did detect differences in processing between psychopaths and nonpsychopaths. Atypical brain activity was detected in several regions involved in moral decision making, including reduced mora versus nonmoral picture distinctions in the vmPFC, amygdala, and anterior temporal cortex in psychopaths relative to nonpsychopaths. These results indicate that psychopaths use different brain regions when making moral decisions than do nonpsychopaths. Importantly, psychopaths have a dysfunction in the vmPFC—a critical region that supports the integration of emotional responses with moral decision making—which contributes to moral insensitivity and lack of empathic responses.

All together, the available evidence indicates that failures in moral knowledge or reasoning alone do not give rise to antisocial behaviors or callous disregard for others. Rather, these behaviors arise from an inability to combine this reasoning with aversive affective arousal. The atypical processing of negative emotional stimuli, such as perceiving others suffering or in pain, which is an important source for empathic concern, coupled with poor inhibitory control, may account for morally inappropriate behavior in psychopaths. Evidence for such deficiencies is found not only in behavior but also at the neural level of analysis. Dysfunction of the connectivity between the amygdala and vmPFC seems to partially explain low socioemotional responses to others' distress, although it is important to note that a lack of empathic arousal alone does not explain offensive behaviors. Behavior is motivated by rewards and discouraged by punishments, with the former influencing behavior more effectively than the latter in most individuals. Offending behavior exists and persists because it is rewarding, and these rewards in turn affect the activity of the mesolimbic dopamine system. For example, pathological reward seeking in individuals with impulsive-antisocial psychopathic traits increases their likelihood of engaging in behaviors that are dangerous to others and themselves.[68] A functional neuroimaging study of youth with aggressive conduct disorder found increased activation in the striatum and amygdala when adolescents watched people being intentionally hurt by others.[69] The extent of amygdala activation to viewing others in pain was positively correlated to the participant's number of aggressive acts and their ratings of daring and sadism scores. This suggests that increased activity in the amygdala, particularly when coupled with activation in the striatum, may reflect a general arousing effect of reward.[70] In keeping with this result, sadists relative to nonsadists showed greater amygdala activation when viewing an individual being physically injured.[71] They also rated pain pictures higher on pain severity than nonsadists. Sadists, but not nonsadists, showed a positive correlation between pain severity ratings and activity in the anterior insula.

Overall, neuroscience research with both healthy individuals and psychopaths supports the notion that emotion reactivity plays a central role in moral judgments and empathic concern for others.

Concluding Remarks

Our ability to perceive and respond with care to the suffering of others stems from evolutionarily ancient subcortical mechanisms (e.g., brainstem and hypothalamic circuitries) associated with affective sensitivity, attachment, and parental care for their young.[72] Empathy-related behaviors have co-opted more primitive homeostatic processes involved in reward and pain systems in order to facilitate various social attachment processes. One salient example of the evolutionary representation of neurobiological function is in the relationship between the neuropeptide oxytocin and mammalian social behavior. This evolutionary perspective is compatible with the nested brain–mind hierarchies model proposed by Panksepp,[73] which posits that, as in other mammalian species, human emotions spread across conspecifics, and, at times, these shared emotions facilitate empathic concern, promoting prosocial behaviors and altruism. Primary emotional processes, potential sources of empathy, coordinate with secondary processes, such as learning and memory mechanisms (i.e., knowing what others are feeling). Together, these then interact with higher mental processes, which exert a variety of top-down influences regulating empathic tendencies (i.e., desires to respond compassionately to others' distress).

To experience concern about another's welfare, an individual needs to be affectively and empathically aroused and able to anticipate the cessation of mutually experienced personal distress.[74] Without input from the affective system (empathic arousal), moral behavior is understandably difficult to develop. This is best exemplified in children who do not respond emotionally to others' suffering and in adult psychopaths, who understand what is right or wrong in a given situation but do not seem to care.[75] These individuals and others like them, who exhibit diminished aversive emotion processing, often display impaired moral judgment, suggesting that cognitive understanding alone is not sufficient for moral behavior. As evidenced in juvenile and adult psychopaths, a lack of empathic arousal, coupled with impaired emotion processing, contributes to impaired moral judgment.

The neural circuits underlying our sensitivity to others' suffering, empathic concern, and caregiving are deeply rooted in the evolution of parental care and living in social groups to ensure the individual's role in promoting the survival and reproductive success of other conspecifics. Far from being an automatic stimulus–response reaction, the perception of other people in distress and physical or social pain is influenced by a variety of factors, including genetic polymorphisms, internal physiological states, bonds with others, cognitive factors, and experiential influences throughout development. Because this sensitivity component is a requirement for activating caregiving motivation and prosocial behaviors, a comprehensive understanding of how interpersonal relationships interact with the neurobiological substrates of empathy and caring is critical to develop positive social interactions and tolerance across groups and nations.

Notes

1. Geoff MacDonald and Mark R. Leary, "Why Does Social Exclusion Hurt? The Relationship between Social and Physical Pain," *Psychological Bulletin* 131 (2005): 202–223.

2. Michael L. Anderson, "Neural Reuse: A Fundamental Organizational Principle of the Brain," *Behavioral and Brain Sciences* 33 (2010): 245–313.

3. Stephen W. Porges and C. Sue Carter, "Mechanisms, Mediators, and Adaptive Consequences of Caregiving," in *Moving beyond Self-Interest: Perspectives from Evolutionary Biology, Neuroscience, and the Social Sciences*, ed. Stephanie L. Brown, R. Michael Brown, and Louis A. Perner (New York: Oxford University Press, 2012), 53–71.

4. C. Sue Carter, "Neuroendocrine Perspectives on Social Attachment and Love," *Psychoneuroendocrinology* 23 (1998): 779–818.

5. Sarah B. Hrdy, Mothers and Others: *Evolutionary Origins of Mutual Understanding* (Cambridge, MA: Belknap Press, 2008).

6. Greg J. Norman et al., "Social Neuroscience: The Social Brain, Oxytocin, and Health," *Social Neuroscience* 7, no. 1 (2012a): 18–29.

7. Bert N. Uchino, John T. Cacioppo, and Janice K. Kiecolt-Glaser, "The Relationship between Social Support and Physiological Processes: A Review with Emphasis on Underlying Mechanisms and Implications for Health," *Psychological Bulletin* 119 (1996): 488–531.

8. Jaak Panksepp, Affective Neuroscience: The Foundations of Human and Animal Emotions (London: Oxford University Press, 1998).

9. Naomi I. Eisenberger, "Why Rejection Hurts: What Social Neuroscience Has Revealed about the Brain's Response to Social Rejection" in *The Oxford Handbook of*

Social Neuroscience, ed. Jean Decety and John T. Cacioppo (Oxford: Oxford University Press, 2011), 586–598.

10. Geoff MacDonald and Mark R. Leary, "Why Does Social Exclusion Hurt? The Relationship between Social and Physical Pain," *Psychological Bulletin* 131 (2005): 202–223.

11. Dale J. Langford et al., "Social Approach to Pain in Laboratory Mice," *Social Neuroscience* 5 (2010): 163–170.

12. Claus Lamm, Jean Decety, and Tania Singer, "Meta-analytic Evidence for Common and Distinct Neural Networks associated with Directly Experienced Pain and Empathy for Pain," *NeuroImage* 54 (2011): 2492–2502.

13. J. Hornak et al., "Changes in Emotion after Circumscribed Surgical Lesions of the Orbitofrontal and Cingulate Cortices," *Brain* 126 (2003): 1691–1712.

14. C. Sue Carter, "Neuroendocrine Perspectives on Social Attachment and Love," *Psychoneuroendocrinology* 23 (1998): 779–818.

15. Markus Heinrichs, "Social Support and Oxytocin Interact to Suppress Cortisol and Subjective Responses to Psychosocial Stress," *Biological Psychiatry* 54 (2003): 1389–1398.

16. Peter Kirsch et al., "Oxytocin modulates neural circuitry for social cognition and fear in humans," *Journal of Neuroscience* 25 (2005): 11489–11493.

17. Michael Kosfeld et al., "Oxytocin Increases Trust in Humans," *Nature* 435 (2005): 673–676.

18. Gregor Domes et al., "Oxytocin Attenuates Amygdala Responses to Emotional Faces Regardless of Valence," *Biological Psychiatry* 62 (2007): 1187–1190.

19. Jennifer A. Bartz et al., "Oxytocin Selectively Improves Empathic Accuracy." *Psychological Science* 114 (2010): 1426–1428.

20. Sarina M. Rodrigues et al., "Oxytocin Receptor Genetic Variation Relates to Empathy and Stress Reactivity In Humans," *Proceedings of the National Accdemy of Sciences* 106 (2009): 21437–21441.

21. Marian J. Bakermans-Kranenburg and Marinus H. van IJzendoorn, "Oxytocin Receptor (OXTR) and Serotonin Transporter (5-HTT) Genes Associated with Observed Parenting," *Affective Neuroscience* 3 (2008): 128–134.

22. Thomas R. Insel and Larry J. Young, "The Neurobiology of Attachment," *Nature Reviews Neuroscience* 2 (2001): 129–136.

23. Jean Decety, "The Neuroevolution of Empathy" *Annals of the New York Academy of Sciences* 1231 (2011): 35–45.

24. Teresa Farroni et al., "The Perception of Facial Expressions in Newborns," *European Journal of Developmental Psychology* 4 (2007): 2–13.

25. Grace B. Martin and Russell D. Clark, "Distress Crying in Neonates Species and Peer Specificity," *Developmental Psychology* 18 (1982): 3–9.

26. Marco Dondi, Francesca Simion, and Giovanna Caltran, "Can Newborns Discriminate Between Their Own Cry and the Cry of Another Newborn Infant?" *Developmental Psychology* 35 (1999): 418–426.

27. Jean Decety, "The Neurodevelopment of Empathy in Humans," *Developmental Neuroscience* 32 (2010a): 257–267.

28. J. Kiley Hamlin, Karen Wynn, and Paul Bloom. "Three-Month-Olds Show a Negativity Bias in Social Evaluation," *Developmental Science* 13, no. 6 (2010): 923–939.

29. J. Kiley Hamlin, Karen Wynn, and Paul Bloom, "Social Evaluation by Preverbal Infants," *Nature* 450 (2007): 557–559; and Hamlin JK, Wynn K, Bloom P, and Mahajan

N. How infants and toddlers react to antisocial others. *Proc Natl Acad Sci U S A* 108 (2011): 19931–19936.

30. Marco F. H. Schmidt and Jessica A. Sommerville, "Fairness Expectations and Altruistic Sharing in 15-Month-Old Human Infants," *PLoS ONE* 6, no. 10 (2011): e23223.

31. Felix Warneken and Michael Tomasello, "The Roots of Human Altruism," *British Journal of Psychology* 100 (2009): 455–471.

32. Harriet L. Rheingold, "Little Children's Participation in the Work of Adults, a Nascent Prosocial Behavior," *Child Development* 53 (1982): 114–125.

33. Ronit Roth-Hanania, Maayan Davidov, and Carolyn Zahn-Waxler, "Empathy Development from 8 to 16 Months: Early Signs of Concerned for Others," *Infant Behavior and Development* 34 (2011): 447–458.

34. Carolyn Zahn-Waxler et al., "Development of Concern for Others," *Developmental Psychology* 28 (1992): 126–136.

35. Margarita Svetlova, Sara R. Nichols, and Celia A. Brownell, "Toddlers' Prosocial Behavior: From Instrumental to Empathic to Altruistic Helping," *Child Development* 81 (2010): 1814–1827.

36. Amrisha Vaish, Malinda Carpenter, and Michael Tomasello, "Sympathy through Affective Perspective-Taking and Its Relation to Prosocial Behavior in Toddlers," *Developmental Psychology* 45, no. 2 (2009): 534–543.

37. Jeffrey P. Lorberbaum et al., "A Potential Role for Thalamocingulate Circuitry in Human Maternal Behavior," *Biological Psychiatry* 51 (2002): 431–445.

38. Jean Decety and Margarita Sveltova, "Putting Together Phylogenetic and Ontogenetic Perspectives on Empathy," *Developmental Cognitive Neuroscience* 2 (2012): 1–24.

39. Jean Decety, Kalina J. Michalska, and Katherine D. Kinzler, "The Contribution of Emotion and Cognition to Moral Sensitivity: A Neurodevelopmental Study," *Cerebral Cortex* 22 (2012): 209–220.

40. S. -J. Blakemore et al., "The Detection of Contingency and Animacy from Simple Animations in the Human Brain," *Cerebral Cortex* 13 (2003): 837–844.

41. Wayne C. Drevets et al., "Subgenual Prefrontal Cortex Abnormalities in Mood Disorders," *Nature* 386 (1997): 824–827.

42. Antoine Bechara et al., "Failure to Respond Autonomically to Anticipated Future Outcomes following Damage to the Prefrontal Cortex," *Cerebral Cortex* 6 (1996): 215–225.

43. Yawei Cheng et al., "Voice and Emotion Processing in the Human Neonatal Brain," *Journal of Cognitive Neuroscience* 24 (2012): 1411–1419.

44. Anna Blasi et al., "Early specialization for voice and emotion processing in the infant brain," *Current Biology* 21 (2011): 1–5.

45. See Lamm, supra note 12, for a meta-analysis.

46. Jean Decety, "To What Extent Is the Experience of Empathy Mediated by Shared Neural Circuits?" *Emotion Review* 2 (2010b): 204–207.

47. E.g., see Langford et al., supra note 11.

48. C. Daniel Batson, Shannon Early, and Giovanni Salvarani, "Perspective Taking: Imagining How Another Feels versus Imagining How You Would Feel," *Personality and Social Psychology Bulletin* 23 (1997): 751–758.

49. E.g., Megan N. Kozak, Abigal A. Marsh, and Daniel M. Wegner, "What Do I Think You're doing? Action Identification and Mind Attribution," *Journal of Personality and Social Psychology* 90 (2006): 543–555.

50. E.g., Yanelia Yabar et al., "Implicit Behavioral Mimicry: Investigating the Impact of Group Membership," *Journal of Non-verbal Behavior* 30 (2006): 97–113.

51. Stephanie Echols and Joshua Correll, "It's More than Skin Deep: Empathy and Helping Behavior across Social Groups," in *Empathy–From Bench to Bedside*, ed. Jean Decety (Cambridge, MA: MIT Press, 2012), 55–71.

52. Jean Decety, Stephanie C. Echols, and Joshua Correll, "The Blame Game: The Effect of Responsibility and Social Stigma on Empathy for Pain," *Journal of Cognitive Neuroscience* 22 (2009): 985–997.

53. Xiaojing Xu et al., "Do You Feel My Pain? Racial Group Membership Modulates Empathic Neural Responses," *Journal of Neuroscience* 29 (2009): 8525–8529.

54. Yawei Cheng et al., "Love Hurts: An fMRI Study," *NeuroImage* 51 (2010): 923–929.

55. Tania Singer et al., "Empathic Neural Responses are Modulated by the Perceived Fairness of Others," *Nature* 439 (2006): 466–469.

56. Grit Hein et al., "Neural Responses to Ingroup and Outgroup Members' Suffering Predict Individual Differences in Costly Helping," *Neuron* 68 (2010): 149–160.

57. Mina Cikara, Matthew M. Botvinick, and Susan T. Fiske, "Us versus Them: Social Identity Shapes Responses to Intergroup Competition and Harm," *Psychological Science* 22 (2011): 306–313.

58. Yawei Cheng et al., "Expertise Modulates the Perception of Pain in Others," *Current Biology* 17 (2007): 1708–1713.

59. Jean Decety, Chia-Yan Yang, and Yawei Cheng, "Physicians Down Regulate Their Pain Empathy Response: An Event-Related Brain Potential Study," *NeuroImage* 50 (2010): 1676–1682.

60. Robert D. Hare, Without Conscience: The Disturbing World of the Psychopaths among Us (New York: Guilford, 1999).

61. R. James R. Blair, "A Cognitive Developmental Approach to Morality: Investigating the Psychopath," *Cognition* 57 (1995): 1–29.

62. Albert S. Aniskiewicz, "Autonomic Components of Vicarious Conditioning and Psychopathy," *Journal of Clinical Psychology* 35 (1979): 60–67.

63. E.g., R. James R. Blair, "Responsiveness to Distress Cues in the Child with Psychopathic Tendencies," *Personality and Individual Differences* 27 (1999): 135–145.

64. Yawei Cheng, An-Yi Hung, and Jean Decety, "Dissociation between Affective Sharing and Emotion Understanding in Juvenile Psychopaths," *Development and Psychopathology* 24 (2012): 623–636.

65. Michael Koenigs, Arielle Baskin-Sommers, and Joseph P. Newman, "Investigating the Neural Correlates of Psychopathy: A Critical Review," *Molecular Psychiatry* 14 (2010): 1–8.

66. Eyal Aharoni, Walter Sinnott-Armstrong, and Kent A. Kiehl, "Can Psychopathic Offenders Discern Moral Wrongs? A New Look at the Moral/Conventional Distinction," *Journal of Abnormal Psychology* 121 (2012): 484–497.

67. Carla L. Harenski et al., "Aberrant Neural Processing of Moral Violation in Criminal Psychopaths," *Journal of Abnormal Psychology* 119 (2010): 863–874.

68. Joshua W. Buckholtz et al., "Mesolimbic Dopamine Reward System Hypersensitivity in Individuals with Psychopathic Traits," *Nature Neuroscience* 13 (2010): 419–421.

69. Jean Decety, Kalina J. Michalska, Yuko Akitsuki, and Benjamin B. Lahey, "Atypical Empathic Responses in Adolescents with Aggressive Conduct Disorder: A Functional MRI Investigation," *Biological Psychology* 80 (2009): 203–211.

70. Elizabeth A. Murray, "The Amygdala, Reward and Emotion," *Trends in Cognitive Sciences* 11 (2007): 489–497.

71. Carla L. Harenski, "Increased Fronto-Temporal Activation during Pain Observation in Sexual Sadism," *Archives of General Psychiatry* 69 (2012): 283–292.

72. Don M. Tucker, Phn Luu, and Douglas Derryberry, "Love Hurts: The Evolution of Empathic Concern through the Encephalization of Nociceptive Capacity," *Development and Psychopathology* 17 (2005): 699–713.

73. Jaak Panksepp, "Empathy and the Laws of Affect," *Science* 334 (2011): 1358–1359.

74. Mark A. Barnett and Shannon Thompson, "The Role of Perspective Taking and Empathy in Children's Machiavellianism, Prosocial Behavior, and Motive for Helping." *Journal of Genetic Psychology 146* (2001): 295–305

75. See Cheng, Hung, & Decety, supra note 63.

6

Biology of Suffering

Daniel Krashin, Natalia Murinova,
Catherine Q. Howe, and Jane C. Ballantyne

The inadequacy of the words we use to describe pain and suffering are never more apparent than when outlining their biology. Although *pain* and *suffering* are not the same, we tend to use the words synonymously. When pain specialists encounter patients with chronic pain, they frequently report suffering. This suffering is expressed as physical pain, but its roots lie much deeper. These roots are created by past experiences and present fears, not found in the body or explained by pathology.[1] Modern imaging enables us to see most pathological causes of pain. Thus, we understand that two individuals with the same pathology on an image may experience this condition very differently. For one person, the physical pain becomes the focus for a life of suffering, while for another, the physical pain is sublimated, or even disappears.

This chapter will necessarily simplify human suffering in order to fit it into the biological model that we understand. First, we will describe the biological mechanisms that produce pain as a physical symptom. Next, the biological underpinnings of common psychiatric disorders will be examined. To complete the discussion, we will explore the relationships between physical and emotional pain.

Pain as a Physical Symptom

> Nature likewise teaches me by these sensations of pain, hunger, thirst, etc., that I am not only lodged in my body as a pilot in a vessel, but that I am besides so intimately conjoined, and as it were intermixed with it, that my mind and body compose a certain unity.

RENÉ DESCARTES, MEDITATIONS VI

In 1664, the French genius René Descartes upended previous pain theories when he proposed that pain was a disturbance that traveled along fibers from an origin

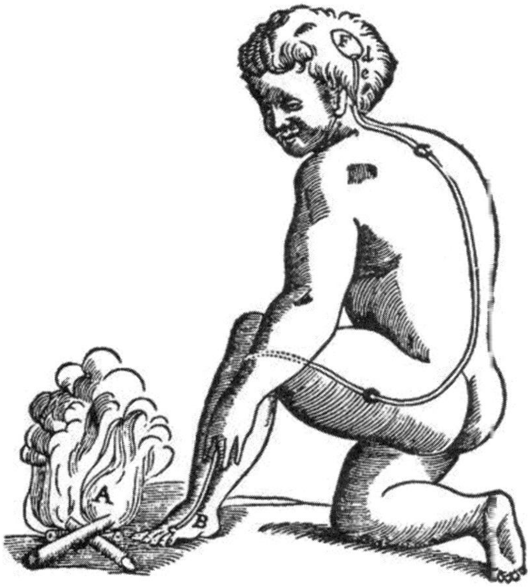

FIGURE 6.1 Descartes's model of pain, with a single line traveling from the burned foot to the brain, was the dominant scientific model of pain for centuries. (From Rene Descartes. *L'homme de René Descartes.* [Paris: Charles Angot, 1664]. John Liebeskind History of Pain Collection.)

(i.e., a burn) to the brain (Figure 6.1). Before this theory, pain was understood as a spiritual experience, imbued with mystery and mysticism. For example, it could be an external force that entered the body through an injury, or it could be seated in the heart. Contemporary science provides us a sophisticated understanding of the biological mechanisms of pain. When it comes to translating the experience of physical pain into the emotional state of suffering, we are left with much uncertainty. We focus here on the biological mechanisms. It is salutary to remember that medical remedies can be helpful in modifying pain transmission, but often fail to help persistent unexplained pain. This still poorly understood form of pain may be better understood and managed using more ancient concepts.

A LINE-LABELED SYSTEM

Since Descartes first proposed that a tubular system transmitted information from the periphery to the brain, an army of scientists—first anatomists and physiologists, later neurobiologists and others—have identified a complex nerve network for nociception. Nociception is the sensory detection of a potentially harmful event, anything from a pinprick to the searing touch of a hot iron. Nociception only refers to the nerve signal and must be distinguished from pain, which is a complex human experience. Pain can only be expressed in personal terms and involves sensory, psychological, and cognitive components (Figure 6.2). Nociception, more than pain,

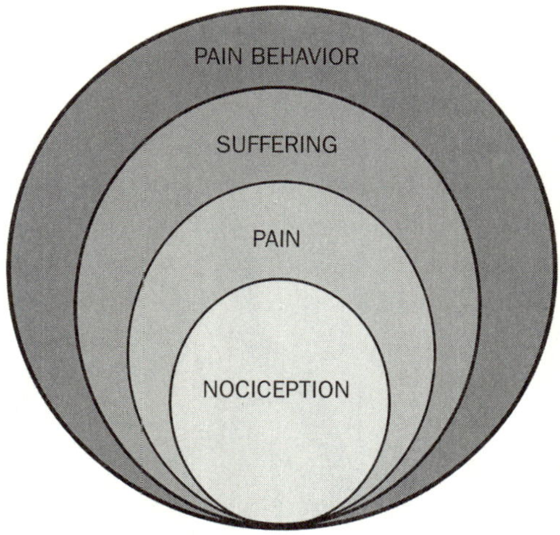

FIGURE 6.2 The Loeser "onion" model of pain consists of concentric layers. Unfortunately, doctors can only observe the outermost layer, pain behavior. (From Loeser, John D. "Pain as Metaphor." *Narrative, Pain, and Suffering* 34 (2005): 17.)

has a comprehensible neural and biological basis. Suffering may be the most important layer to understand. Unfortunately, doctors can only observe the outermost component of pain, pain-related behavior.

Neural Basis

The neural pain system broadly consists of nociceptors. A nociceptor is a nerve cell that detects potentially injurious stimuli and sends an alarm signal through the spinal cord to the brain. This activation of nociceptors activates the pain process (nociception). The human experience of pain is a combination of nociception plus higher brain activity. The nociceptors have free terminals at their lower ends, which are capable of transducing mechanical, thermal, and chemical signals. This transduction turns a specific stimulus into a nerve signal, which happens through specific receptors such as TRPV1 (transient receptor potential vanilloid family type 1) that responds to noxious heat as well as capsaicin.[2] Capsaicin is the active component of chili peppers. When capsaicin comes in contact with tissues, it activates the TRPV1 receptor, and this produces the familiar sensation of burning.

Most tissues in the body are innervated by nociceptors. There are subsets of nociceptors that perform separate functions and are sensitive to different stimuli. The nociceptors vary by diameter and presence of myelination. Myelin is an electrical insulator that wraps around the axon of a neuron. The more myelin, the faster the nerve can conduct signals and thus the faster the painful stimulus will travel. The largest myelinated A-delta fibers transmit rapidly, and they are involved in the initial well-localized pain. This pain is sometimes called *first pain*. Smaller unmyelinated C fibers transmit slowly and are involved in the later, more diffuse pain called *second pain*.

Nociceptors in the skin and other body parts below the neck transmit signals to the dorsal horn of the spinal cord. In the case of head and neck, the nociceptors send signals to special brain nucleus, the trigeminal solitary tract. From these way stations, ascending nociceptive tracts transmit nociceptive input from the dorsal horn or solitary tract to the pain centers of the brain. These ascending pathways send signals from the lower levels of the nervous system toward a higher level of the nervous system in the brain. The higher centers in the brain process the nociceptive signal and contribute the discriminatory, affective, motor, and other aversive responses to pain. These contributions help the brain understand the kind of pain, its location, how unpleasant it is, and even motor responses to the pain, such as flinching from a hot surface. These higher brain centers are also involved in creating the pain memory, which reminds us not to touch a hot stove the second time. Descending systems travel down from the higher centers to modify nociceptive input at multiple levels and can increase or decrease the perception of pain.[3]

The nociceptors that come from the body, called primary afferent nociceptors, synapse in the dorsal horn or solitary tract with the ascending nociceptive tracts. These way stations are an important site for further processing and integration of pain signals. A wealth of neurotransmitters can be released in the dorsal horn from the primary afferent neurons, descending neurons that modulate pain perception, and interneurons that tie the two systems together. The best-studied excitatory neurotransmitters, which stimulate neurons, include glutamate, aspartate, substance P, calcitonin gene–related peptide, neurotrophic factor and bradykinin. These excitatory neurotransmitters increase the perception of pain. Inhibitory neurotransmitters, which calm neurons, tend to decrease pain. These inhibitory neurotransmitters include endogenous opioids, γ-aminobutyric acid (GABA), and glycine. Endogenous opioids are similar to the opioid painkillers that doctors prescribe but are synthesized by the body in small amounts to regulate the nervous system, particularly pain perception.

The second-order neurons that come from the dorsal horn are dorsal horn projection neurons. The equivalent in the head and brain are cranial projection neurons. The second-order neurons are classified as high threshold, known as nociceptive-specific neurons, which carry information only from a specific kind of painful stimulus, or as wide dynamic-range neurons, which collect stimuli from a larger area and also integrate nonpainful sensory information with non-noxious (A-beta) neurons. The second-order neurons climb up the spinal cord predominantly in the spinothalamic tract, the largest and most important ascending pathway for pain transmission. This tract ends at the thalamus, the brain's largest and most important relay for pain signals to higher brain centers. The thalamus may be thought of as the "executive secretary" of the brain, in that it collects all the stimuli arriving at the higher level of the brain and routes them to the appropriate areas. Other dorsal horn neurons ascend in the spinobulbar tract, which sends projections to the brainstem and on to the thalamus and limbic structures.

The thalamus sends some pain signals to the primary somatosensory cortex. This pathway, termed the thalamocortical or discriminatory pathway, carries information about the intensity and location of the pain stimuli. The limbic, or emotional, pathway carries nociceptive signals to the limbic system, where the affective component of pain is processed. The memory of pain becomes the foundation for an individual's response to, and ability to cope with, pain in later life.[4]

The human sensation of pain is only experienced when both thalamocortical (sensory and discriminatory) and limbic (emotional) pathways are combined in the brain. Only then does the person know that something hurts, where it hurts, how it hurts, and how badly it hurts. It is only in the brain that pain takes on a meaning. In a complex process from these and other areas of the brain, descending signals can exert an excitatory or inhibitory influence, with a profound effect on the ultimate pain experience.[5]

Molecular Basis

Nociceptors are the specialized primary neurons that the body requires to perceive pain. The nociception begins by activation of different types of voltage-sensitive ion channels activated by different stimuli. The main stimuli include heat and cold, which activate temperature transient receptor potential (TRP) ion channel transducers such as TRPV1. There are also chemically sensitive ion channels and metabotropic receptors (TRPV1, P2X3), which are activated by acids, prostaglandins, and cytokines and other inflammatory factors.[6] Activation of these ion channel transducers ultimately leads to action potentials, which create nociceptive nerve signals, which travel to the dorsal horn.[7]

In the cell body of the dorsal horn nerve, action potentials produce an inrush of calcium and a synaptic release of glutamate, both highly stimulating. Glutamate quickly creates action potentials through AMPA-kainate ionotropic receptors, which are magnified by *N*-methyl-D-aspartate (NMDA) receptor ion channels. This process encodes information about the onset, intensity, quality, location, and duration of peripheral noxious events into the nerve signal that is transmitted to the higher centers.

The activity of both peripheral and central components of the pain system is not fixed. Some neurons fire in a frequency proportional to the intensity of the pain. The pain system activation can be altered by repeated peripheral stimulation. It can be affected by changes to the chemical milieu of the terminal and by other stimuli. An example of peripheral sensitization occurs when an action potential leads to calcium flooding into a nerve cell through TRPV1 ion channels, which activates the enzyme protein kinase C. Protein kinase C, in turn, activates the TRPV1 channel through phosphorylation. Other substances, such as prostaglandins, bradykinin, and 5-HT, can also sensitize nerves. These agents activate kinase enzymes within the cell that phosphorylate and thereby increase the activity of voltage-gated sodium channels through G-protein–coupled or tyrosine kinase receptors. In all these examples, the phosphorylated ion channels are more likely to activate the nerve, rendering it more sensitive to stimuli.

Repeated or prolonged peripheral stimulation also changes sensory processing in the dorsal horn, resulting in hypersensitivity—a process known as central sensitization. Central sensitization, also known as central augmentation, refers to changes that make the nervous system more sensitive and thus lower the pain threshold. Peripheral stimulation also increases processes within the cell that make it more sensitive to stimuli, including activation of protein kinase (PKA). These PKA enzymes increase the sensitivity and excitability of nerve membranes by phosphorylating NMDA and AMPA-kainite receptors. This sensitization amplifies responses to both noxious and non-noxious stimuli. These changes can spread to nearby synapses and cause other areas of the body that were not injured to also become sensitized (secondary hyperalgesia). Hyperalgesia is an increased response to a stimulus that is normally painful. After a peripheral injury, these changes in the spinal cord (central plasticity) are initially driven by peripheral input but later become self-sustaining because of induction of cyclooxygenase-2 in the dorsal horn, an enzyme that produces the inflammatory chemical prostaglandin E_2. Central sensitization is also driven by misfiring of injured nerve fibers. This misfiring, called ectopic activity, can create abnormal connections among neurons that lead to painful sensations in the absence of painful stimuli. Possibly, this leads to structural reorganization of the central nervous system. Many of these processes persist as chronic pain.[8]

The unraveling of neural and molecular pain mechanisms has played a significant role in redefining pain, its purpose, and its treatment.[9] Our present ability to understand and visualize the neuroanatomy of pain has led to many invasive treatments, including injections of anti-inflammatory steroids and local anesthetics and neuroablative and neurostimulation therapies. At the same time, the discovery of the molecular mechanisms underlying pain provided the basis for new pain drug development. These therapeutic advances, driven by our mechanical understanding of pain, have resulted in the biomedical approach to pain treatment that dominated most of the twentieth century. This therapeutic approach still has great relevance to the treatment of pain with a clear pathoanatomic basis, such as most pain caused by injuries, surgeries, and cancer. Yet it is essential to understand that the line-labeled system and the molecular systems we have described are only the scaffold upon which pain builds itself. The biology of suffering transcends this scaffold and can only be understood by taking into account the emotional factors that so often drive chronic pain, which arise from the brain's higher functions and are less amenable to biomedical treatment.

PAIN AS A MOTIVATIONAL STATE

While the Renaissance anatomists and later the Victorian physiologists busied themselves working out neural pain pathways and specificity theories based on the properties of nociceptors, many major insights into the nature and purpose of pain were only recently achieved. Endogenous (originating in our brain) opioid systems, critical in pain modulation, were imagined but not discovered until the 1970s.[10] That this system, so vital to the survival and evolutionary success of the species, should have been absent from the physiology texts merely decades ago is a constant reminder of how far we have come in recent years in understanding the biological basis of pain and suffering.

Wall and Melzack's gate control theory published in 1967 was a key advance in understanding pain modulation.[11] Thinking about pain was turned on its head by new concepts of neural plasticity. These concepts challenged the simplicity of prior theories. Wall's discovery was that vital relays in the spinal dorsal horn were subject to powerful control by supraspinal sites. Stimulation of large tactile fibers (A-beta fibers) was also found to affect such control. Later Reynolds, Liebeskind, and others showed that activation of the periaqueductal gray in the midbrain decreased pain responses in animals.[12] The periaqueductal gray receives input from the hypothalamus and limbic system. It controls nociceptive transmission through connections in the rostral ventromedial medulla and the dorsolateral pontine tegmentum, which in turn projects descending fibers to the spinal dorsal horn. Following this discovery, neurosurgeons were later able to produce clinically significant pain relief using midbrain stimulation. These discoveries demonstrated the ways that the brain modulated pain sensations and led to the development of stimulation techniques for the treatment of pain. These findings led to the concept that the body's pain systems exist most of the time in a neutral mode, providing "background noise" that can be brought to consciousness (or buried into unconsciousness) by thought and emotion—quite apart from their obvious role as a signal of injury.[13]

When we are comfortable, the subject of pain does not cross our minds. Only when pain and suffering do not allow us to continue in our life journey do we appreciate what we have lost. We take for granted our ability to modulate pain perceptions and are not aware of the remarkable systems within us that help manage pain.

It was not pain scientists, but rather addiction researchers, who discovered a system of endogenous opioids and opioid receptors in the 1970s. These discoveries were made about the same time as the discoveries of Wall, Melzack, and others concerning pain and central plasticity.[14] Although discovered separately, these systems are clearly linked, and the endogenous opioid system is now known to be crucial in pain processing and modulation.

Opioid receptors are found in abundance in all areas of the brain and spinal cord involved in pain processing.[15] The opioid system accounts in large part for the ability of phylogenetically advanced species to adapt to their environment. It thus contributes to their survival and evolutionary success. This is the link to addiction because survival behaviors, such as feeding, fighting, and sexual intercourse, all stimulate the reward centers of the brain through opioid receptors, and the pleasurable sensation produced is a powerful motivator that is sought out repeatedly. Through opioid mechanisms, pain can be suppressed (during battle or immediately after injury) or heightened (to enhance protective reflexes in the presence of injury, or when under threat), as suits the occasion. Endogenous opioid mechanisms can be usefully recruited to treat pain using, for example, exercise, acupuncture, or the placebo effect.[16]

A neuroscientist of our time, Howard Fields, has described pain as a motivational state. This motivational state is influenced by the state of opioid circuits and provides potent guidance to decision making.[17] The opioid circuits "can operate in both pain-inhibiting and pain-facilitating states," providing either aversive or appetitive motivation, which contributes to adaptive behavioral choice. The brain provides itself its own carrots and sticks. Circuit models of behavior are tested in animals by injecting agonists (such as opioid drugs) and antagonists (opioid blockers) into the nuclei that are part of the behaviorally defined circuit to see if they directly affect behavior. These can also be tested in humans using functional imaging and opioid antagonists. This circuit analysis has allowed researchers to define a sequence of events from molecular phenomena at synapses to human behavior and perception. The dual control so described arises from two neuronal subpopulations—"off" cells and "on" cells, which exhibit reciprocal firing preceding nociceptor-elicited withdrawal reflexes, as in the hand flinching from a hot stove.[18] These off and on cells provide descending control from the higher centers of the brain. Serotonin-producing neurons in the rostral ventromedial medulla provide additional state-dependent control of nociceptive transmission. Evolution has not only produced a precise and sensitive system for perceiving pain, it has also developed refined mechanisms for dynamically adjusting this system in response to events.

Suffering through Psychiatric Illness

Physical pain and psychological distress can cause significant suffering. However, a limited medicalized concept of pain ignores the broader significance of suffering. The stories of our lives are embedded in the story of the communities from which we derive our identity. Chronic pain results in loss of the valued self-image, without the creation of a new acceptable image. According to Charmaz, the end result is that these individuals suffer from leading restricted lives, experiencing social isolation, being discredited, and feeling like a burden on others.[19]

The onset of a mental illness changes the course of one's life, and the narrative of one's life changes as well. The future life one had hoped for may become unreachable. This aspect of suffering, like consciousness itself, is difficult to address with the tools of neuroscience and may be neglected for lack of objective measures. There is no comprehensive theory accounting for how the brain gives rise to the mind. Therefore, this section will consider the biology of mental suffering through the prism of two common and severe psychiatric disorders, major depression and post-traumatic stress disorder (PTSD), as representatives of mood and anxiety disorders. Both conditions commonly coexist with chronic pain.

The biology of psychiatric illness is complex, and our understanding of the brain's functioning is partial at best. Generally speaking, most psychiatric conditions have both a genetic and an environmental component. Their genetic components are usually complex patterns of traits associated with vulnerability for psychiatric conditions. Developmental and environmental stressors encountered in the womb and throughout life may act on these vulnerabilities and thus create illness. One important mechanism for this is epigenetic change. Epigenetic changes are modifications to the genetic material that affect which genes are expressed, without actually changing the genetic sequence. If genes are the recipes for life, epigenetic modifications are the hand-written notes in the cookbook that make the recipes unique.

MAJOR DEPRESSION

> But the Spirit of the Lord departed from Saul, and a distressing spirit from the Lord troubled him.
>
> 1 Samuel 16:14-23

Depression is a syndrome that can arise from multiple different disease processes and conditions, or it can occur spontaneously. The mood associated with depression is not always sadness and may be described as feelings of flatness or numbness, irritability, or worry. The prevalence of depression appears to be increasing, possibly owing to the modern lifestyle with its energy drain and disconnections. Consider the typical working day in the developed world: waking up tired, checking emails, skipping meals or eating at the desk, and working long hours in solitude with little social support. Many factors play into developing depression, including genetic risk factors, which are often reinforced by childhood stresses brought on by the parent's own issues.[20] Personal factors, such as low self-esteem, anxiety disorders, or substance use, play a large part in the development of depression. Trauma, psychosocial adversity, deaths of loved ones, or loss of employment can also set the stage for depression. Social support and education appear to build resilience and decrease the risk for depression but do not eliminate it entirely.

Research techniques have been directed toward the study of the brain of patients with depression for more than one hundred years. However, the question remains open of whether these differences in the brain are the cause of depression, the consequence of depression, or epiphenomena from the true causes of depression.[21]

Developmental Factors

Childhood abuse and neglect increase lifelong vulnerability to depression and other psychiatric illnesses. Severe stress in childhood may result in a lifetime of sensitivity to stress, decreased resilience, and increased risk for depression.[22] This may be mediated by long-lasting activation of the corticotropin-releasing factor cells in the hypothalamus, which lead to increased levels of cortisol, the stress hormone, and chronic stress responses. This is a prime example of an abnormality of the hypothalamic-pituitary-adrenal (HPA) axis, which is frequently implicated in mood disorders. Increased activity of the HPA axis and increased tonic release of glucocorticoids such as cortisol are common in depression.[23] Prolonged periods of high cortisol level are associated with decreased nerve cell growth and shrinkage of the hippocampus, the brain area responsible for memory formation.[24]

Abnormalities of multiple neurotransmitters have been identified in depression. The early monoamine hypothesis suggested that the depressed brain simply lacked serotonin and norepinephrine; however, this appears to be a gross oversimplification.[25] The role of serotonin is easily demonstrated by feeding subjects meals devoid of tryptophan, the amino acid that is converted into serotonin. This diet depletes the nervous system of serotonin, which makes susceptible subjects feel depressed and irritable.[26] A similar technique can be used to deplete the catecholamines dopamine and norepinephrine, producing depression in some patients.[27] Decreased dopamine transmission has been shown to be associated with depression in multiple types of studies in humans and animals.[28]

Both inhibitory and excitatory neurotransmitters show abnormalities in depression. Magnetic resonance spectroscopy, which is able to detect levels of specific neurotransmitters in a living brain, found increased levels of excitatory glutamate and decreased inhibitory GABA in the occipital cortex of patients with major depression.[29] Abnormal levels of glutamate, glutamine, and GABA were found in the prefrontal cortex of patients with untreated major depression.[30] The cingulate and prefrontal cortex of depressed patients who committed suicide have also been shown to have abnormal expression of receptors for both glutamate and GABA.[31]

Endogenous opioids have also been implicated in depression. Women with depression have lower opioid receptor–binding availability compared with nondepressed women, although this measure decreased in both groups when they were encouraged to think of their memories of sad events.[32] Intriguingly, this general opioid-binding deficit is also found in fibromyalgia, a pain condition with a very high rate of comorbid depression.[33] Animal models have further suggested that endogenous opioids acting at delta-opioid receptors help regulate the rewarding effect of dopamine at the nucleus accumbens, providing a direct link between opioids, motivation, and mood.[34]

The influence of genes on depression risk is highly individual. Gene expression is influenced by the environment, deprivation, and stress.[35] Thus, genes confer a vulnerability to depression that can be activated by the right combination of environment and development. The inheritance of depression is complex, and it is incorrect to speak of a "gene for depression."[36] However, some specific gene loci have been implicated in depression, particularly genes that regulate the endocrine and neurotransmitter systems. Polymorphisms in the *CRHR1* gene, which codes for regulation of cortisol release, appear to reduce the risk for depression in adults with abuse in childhood.[37] One variation of the serotonin transporter gene increases the impact of mild stress in raising the risk for depression.[38]

Environmental factors can result in epigenetic changes, which modify gene expression without changing the genetic sequence. Epigenetic changes can last a lifetime and even be inherited.[39] Epigenetic changes, such as methylation of DNA and modifications of histones, have been found in the frontal lobes of depressed patients who died by suicide.[40] Epigenetic changes have been found in the hippocampus in the gene sequence for the glucocorticoid receptor gene promoter in subjects who committed suicide who had suffered abuse as children. These changes were not found in controls without abuse histories.[41]

Depression does not exist in a vacuum, and all depressed patients exist in a social context, although it may be strained and frayed by the effects of depression. Social network effects have been studied, and peers prove to have a powerful influence: isolation from them, criticism from them, or depression in them can all increase the risk for depression.[42] Having depressed family members, friends, or even friends of friends can raise one's risk for depression.[43] Family members can contribute to the maintenance of the depressed state through criticism and emotional over involvement.[44]

POST-TRAUMATIC STRESS DISORDER

According to a *New York Times* article by Lizette Alvarez published in 2009, the Pentagon announced that the Purple Heart would be reserved for soldiers with physical injuries only and not given to soldiers diagnosed with PTSD. The Pentagon offered two reasons for declining to award the medal: PTSD is not intentionally caused by the enemy, and it is difficult to diagnose objectively.

Many combat veterans returning from Iraq and Afghanistan have been diagnosed with PTSD, with symptoms such as depression, nightmares, and suicidality. More than three hundred thousand veterans have been diagnosed with PTSD.[45]

Psychological trauma has always been a part of life: wars, disasters, and abuse have caused significant trauma, and throughout history, it has been noticed that some people seemed more resilient and able to move and grow despite these experiences, while others developed significant symptoms that impaired their lives after the stress. In her book, *Bend, not Break*, the China-born CEO of Geomagics Software Company, Ping Fu, describes a childhood caught up in the Chinese Cultural revolution, followed by exile and study in a foreign country while still a young woman. Her biography is a splendid example of resilience, and yet we cannot explain why she was able to thrive in such difficult circumstances.[46]

The question is analogous to the enigma of chronic pain: Why do some people suffer trauma and heal, while others suffer devastating complications that last for years and affect their whole life? The answer is complex and cannot be neatly defined but clearly involves genetics, epigenetics, and neurobiology, as well societal acceptance of people after trauma and the support of the society as whole.

PTSD, unlike any other psychiatric condition, requires a traumatic event as its genesis.[47] PTSD is defined as mental health condition triggered by a terrifying life event. The symptoms include intrusive recollections of the trauma, avoidance and emotional numbness in response to stimuli reminiscent of the trauma, and hyperarousal symptoms such as excessive startle response. The typical features of PTSD, including intrusive memories, recurrent dreams, and flashbacks, imply changes to the brain's ability to handle traumatic memory.[48] Most of us have experienced trauma, but few of us will develop PTSD.[49]

PTSD takes time to develop and is often chronic. Current theories of PTSD involve changes in neural plasticity that affect mood and behavior.[50] Neural plasticity refers to lasting alterations of neural pathways and synapses as a result of changes in behavior, environment, and neural processes. PTSD research has focused on a few specific brain areas, which are associated with memory processing and trauma response. Shrinkage in the size of the hippocampus, the main memory processing area, has been observed. The hippocampus is part of the limbic system and is important for the creation of short- and long-term memory. The prefrontal cortex is the anterior part of the frontal lobes, just behind the forehead. It is responsible for executive function and self-control. The anterior cingulate cortex (ACC) plays a role in rational cognitive functions. Finally, the amygdala is a small almond-shaped brain area that is activated in response to threat and produces emotions of anxiety or rage.

As in depression, the HPA axis is affected in PTSD, but in the opposite direction, resulting in tonically low cortisol release. The low cortisol level promotes the re-experiencing of traumatic memories. This deficit in the stress hormone results in uncontrolled adrenaline release. It is conjectured that the prefrontal cortex and ACC, which are normally responsible for emotional regulation and rational responses to the environment, are unable to control the amygdala's threat response, resulting in hypersensitivity and overreaction. This process of sensitization and re-experiencing of trauma over time changes the body's response to stress.[51] This can create a vicious cycle because the body becomes more prone to stress reactions at the same time that the brain is becoming less able to manage constructive responses to stress.

Liberzon measured regional cerebral blood flow in PTSD with single-photon emission computed tomographs,[52] which show the function of the brain, unlike magnetic resonance images, which show only the structure of the brain. These studies showed activation in the amygdala and nucleus accumbens that was seen only in the PTSD patients. The amygdala plays a primary role in the processing of memories and emotional reactions. The amygdala is considered part of the limbic system. Nucleus accumbens is considered a critical component of the brain's pleasure center. Studies of patients who were visualizing combat scenes while hearing a narrative of traumatic events showed increased activation of the amygdala and ACC.[53] This evidence strongly suggests the involvement and possible overactivation of limbic structures in PTSD.

The search for what causes some people exposed to trauma to develop PTSD has included study of genetic predisposition. Polymorphisms at some particular gene loci appear to predispose patients to developing PTSD.[54] Polymorphisms in biology occur when two or more phenotypes exist in the same population, the occurrence of more than one form (morph). A polymorphism of the *FKBP5* gene is involved in cortisol receptor regulation. COMT polymorphisms are associated with PTSD and other anxiety and pain disorders. COMT stands for catechol-methyltransferase, an enzyme that breaks down monoamine neurotransmitters. Polymorphisms that cause COMT to be less active, such as the COMT val158met polymorphism, are associated with less ability to tolerate stress and greater risk for developing PTSD after trauma. The *CHRNA5* gene is associated with nicotine dependence and tobacco abuse as well as PTSD, and the *CRHR1* gene in the context of early life trauma influences HPA axis function.

Recent work in behavioral epigenetics has suggested that this mechanism may play an important role in developing and maintaining PTSD symptoms after trauma.[55] An environmental change, such as a traumatic event, could serve as an epigenetic modifier, changing the function but not the structure of a gene. The epigenetic changes can turn genes on or off. Once completed, these epigenetic changes can be long lasting and even be transmitted across generations.[56] One mechanism of epigenetic change that has been observed in PTSD, glucocorticoid gene methylation, durably changes the activity of the gene and hence the activity and reactivity of the HPA axis. This could then change the individual's ability to respond to further stresses. This may be a biological explanation for the psychological phenomenon of survivorship in PTSD: even after treatment and successful adjustment, patients may not feel that they have returned to their premorbid state. The *FKBP5* gene mentioned previously has been found to be subject to DNA demethylation in patients with history of childhood trauma. Since this gene helps regulate the glucocorticoid system, this changes the responsiveness of the stress hormone system and the body's ability to control stress responses and catecholamine levels.[57]

The endogenous (internal brain) opioid system is thought to also play a role in maintaining PTSD. The common symptoms of stress-induced analgesia and numbness and dissociation may be mediated by endogenous opioid activity.[58] Chronic PTSD creates permanent changes on every level, from gene expression to levels of neurotransmitters to the balance of adrenaline and cortisol, the stress hormone. These alterations have a lasting effect on the sufferers' experience of everyday life, their ability to interact in social situations, and their ability to handle the stresses of everyday life.

Shared Neurobiological Substrates for Physical and Emotional Pain

In its everyday use, the word *suffering* usually has both physical and emotional connotations. Indeed, it would be difficult to find instances of physical suffering or pain without accompanying emotional experience. Extensive epidemiological evidence also indicates the common co-occurrence of chronic physical pain conditions and emotional distress in the forms of diagnosable psychiatric disorders.[59] It therefore should not be particularly surprising that physical and emotional pain states share multifaceted connections on the neurobiological level.

NEUROTRANSMITTER SYSTEMS

The endogenous opioid system is arguably the most intriguing neurochemical system that has complex involvement both in pain modulation and in the neural network that regulates emotion, motivation, reward, and social attachment. The euphoria-provoking and reward-producing nature of endogenous opioid peptides (i.e., endorphins) was described soon after their discovery in the 1970s.[60] Endorphins are thought to bind mu-opioid receptors on the ventral tegmental dopaminergic neurons and induce the release of dopamine.[61] Dopamine binds to dopamine receptors in the pleasure–reward circuitry of the brain, maintaining a hedonic tone and producing a sense of reward. Abnormalities in endogenous opioid activity were found in patients with depression, in patients with schizophrenia,[62] and in suicide victims.[63] Animal models also confirmed the role of the opioid system in emotional regulation. Mice genetically altered to lack delta-opioid and mu-opioid receptors, respectively, showed changes in anxiety and depressive behaviors.[64]

More recently, evidence pointed to the role of mu-opioid receptors in forming social attachment. Attachment behavior is characterized by special bonding with the primary caregivers.[65] Forming an attachment relationship with at least one primary caregiver is thought to be crucial for the normal emotional development of an infant. Mouse pups lacking the mu receptor gene were found to be deficient in attachment behavior in ways similar to autistic human infants.[66] They seemed indifferent to maternal absence. These findings seem to underscore the importance of the endogenous opioid system in social and emotional development.

A group at the University of Michigan used positron emission tomography (PET) to study the in vivo regulation of pain and emotion by the endogenous opioid system.[67] Activation of the endogenous opioid system was measured by the binding of a selective mu-opioid receptor radiotracer. Either a prolonged painful state or sadness was induced in the experimental subjects as they underwent PET imaging. The pain and sadness challenges were associated with changes in mu-opioid neurotransmission in various brain regions. They elicited similar effects on mu receptors in the ventral basal ganglia, including the nucleus accumbens and ventral pallidum, and in the amygdala. The sadness challenge was noted bilaterally, in contrast to the pain stimulus, which was only seen unilaterally. In a more recent study, the experimenters compared the endogenous opioid response to the sadness challenge in patients with major depression to the response in healthy volunteers.[68] The results showed significant alteration of mu-opioid neurotransmission in depressed patients compared with healthy controls. Taken together, these findings point to the overlapping and differential endogenous opioid pathways involved in pain and emotional distress regulation.

Besides endogenous opioids, a number of other neurotransmitter systems are also implicated in the dual roles of regulating pain and emotional state. The glutamate-NMDA system, for example, is thought to enhance signal transmission in the nociceptive circuitry and therefore contribute to *central sensitization*, the amplification of pain signals within the central nervous system.[69] As noted earlier, abnormalities in the glutamate-NMDA system are also involved in the pathogenesis of depression. It thus makes logical sense that intravenous infusion of the NMDA receptor antagonist ketamine has been shown not only to decrease pain in certain chronic pain syndromes[70] but also to exert a rapid antidepressant effect.[71] Other neurotransmitters, such as serotonin and norepinephrine, are important inhibitory transmitters in the descending pathways that modulate the spinal transmission of nociceptive input.[72] The overlapping roles of these neurotransmitters in pain modulation and in depression explain the analgesic and antidepressant efficacies of amine uptake inhibitors,[73] which serve to increase the levels of serotonin and norepinephrine.

NEUROANATOMICAL PATHWAYS

A series of elegant experiments by the Eisenberger group at University of California, Los Angeles highlighted the shared neuroanatomical substrates for physical and emotional pain.[74] Participants in the studies played a virtual ball-tossing game (Cyberball) while undergoing functional magnetic resonance imaging. The game was designed such that the participants were led to believe that they were excluded by other players during the game, and these other players were, without the knowledge of the participants, simulated by a preset computer program. Self-reported emotional distress as a result of the social rejection was measured and correlated with functional magnetic resonance imaging findings. The first study of the series showed that social rejection activated both the dorsal anterior cingulate cortex (dACC) and the anterior cingulate (AI), two areas that are typically activated by physical pain.[75] The ACC is composed of cognitive (dorsal) and emotional (ventral) components. The ventral part of the ACC is connected with the amygdala, nucleus accumbens, hypothalamus, and anterior insula and is involved in assessing emotion and motivation. The ACC is important in tasks that require learning and problem solving. The activity in the dACC was also found to correlate with the degree of self-reported social distress. The overlap of brain regions involved in the experience of social rejection and of physical pain was confirmed by a separate study using a different experimental paradigm in which subjects received two challenges.[76] In one challenge, they were asked to think back to the experience of a recent unwanted breakup of a romantic relationship. In the other, they received painful heat stimulation. Both the physical pain and emotional pain activated the dACC and AI in the same individual subjects. Furthermore, the areas of dACC and AI have also been shown in other studies to be activated by emotionally painful experiences other than social rejection, for instance, grief.[77]

Given the apparent overlap in the neural substrates for physical and social pain, the Eisenberger group went on to test several predictions derived from this finding. First, they asked if individuals more sensitive to one kind of pain (physical or social) are also more sensitive to the other. In one study, they measured the subjects' baseline sensitivity to painful heat stimuli and then had them complete a round of the Cyberball game. Subjects who had greater baseline pain sensitivity indeed reported higher levels of social distress after the game.[78] In a second study, they identified subjects who carried a mu-opioid receptor polymorphism, which had been linked to greater sensitivity to physical pain. Compared with normal controls, these subjects demonstrated greater social rejection sensitivity and had increased activity in the dACC and AI with social exclusion.[79]

Next, they asked if factors that modulate one type of pain influence the other type of pain experience. Since inflammation is known to increase physical pain, they examined the effect of endotoxin, a proinflammatory agent, on the feeling of social rejection. Participants who received endotoxin versus placebo had greater feeling of social disconnectedness after completing the Cyberball game,[80] and those who had the largest increase in blood interleukin-6 level as a result of the endotoxin also had the greatest activation in the dACC and AI in response to social rejection.[81] On the other hand, subjects who took acetaminophen, a painkiller, had significant reduction in self-reported hurt feelings as well as significantly less activity in the dACC and AI in response to the Cyberball game compared with subjects who took a placebo.[82] The authors justifiably concluded that acetaminophen seemed to act as a "social painkiller" as well as a physical painkiller. In sum, factors that altered one type of pain did have a parallel effect on the other type of pain and also a corresponding effect on the common neuroanatomical substrates for physical and social pain, namely the dACC and AI.

A UNIFYING BASIS FOR PHYSICAL AND EMOTIONAL PAIN

Taken together, evidence emerging from the genetic, biochemical, and anatomical levels all point to substantial overlap in the biology of physical pain and emotional distress. That there exists a unifying biological basis for the two types of suffering is consistent with the epidemiological data that one type, exemplified by chronic pain, seldom exists without the other (which can usually be codified into various psychiatric illnesses), and vice versa. Ultimately, it is also congruent with our own subjective human experience that when we suffer, we rarely suffer one without the other.

Conclusion

In an era when our understanding of pain mechanisms is becoming increasingly sophisticated, we still have difficulty treating pain and addressing emotional suffering. We know only some of the biological pathways involved in pain and some of the molecular processes, and we are at the beginnings of genetic and epigenetic research. At our present level of knowledge, we are unable to remove chronic pain and emotional suffering. The biomedical approach to pain treatment has pervaded much of the past several decades. Current medicine training addresses structural disorders such as tumors. Our efforts to reverse pain by injecting or ablating nerves or using drugs has been less successful, however, because we are trying to amend the function of the brain, not fix the brain structure.

Pain is a survival mechanism to help us escape injury, but when it becomes chronic, it can affect all aspects of life for those affected, as well as their loved ones. Pain affects lifestyle, personal relationships, productivity, and finances. It can cause extreme personal suffering.

The increased use of opioid pain killers during the past 15 years to treat chronic noncancer pain and the opioid epidemic that followed provide a particularly sobering illustration of the complexity of the neurobiological adaptations underlying chronic pain and emotional suffering and of how targeting physical pain without recognizing or adequately treating the accompanying emotional issues can lead to detrimental results. Because of its euphoric effect, the "opium cure" had been used to treat depression in the late-nineteenth to the mid-twentieth centuries until nonaddictive antidepressant drugs became available.[83] The risk for addiction had limited the use of opioids for chronic noncancer pain until the 1990s, when their use became more liberalized and when increasingly more patients with chronic pain started to receive long-term opioid therapy.[84] This trend was followed by an alarming rise in the rates of opioid abuse and overdose deaths, which paralleled the increase in opioid sales in the years between 1999 and 2010; opioid deaths more than tripled between 1999 and 2009.[85]

Common psychiatric disorders, such as depression, anxiety, and PTSD, which frequently co-occur with chronic pain, have likely contributed to the rise in the use of opioid therapy for chronic pain and the increase in adverse outcomes. Several epidemiological studies have shown that patients with mental health diagnoses are more likely to receive long-term opioid therapy for their pain and at higher doses compared with those without a psychiatric diagnosis.[86] Given what was discussed earlier about the roles opioids play in social affiliation, it is possible that in patients with both chronic physical pain and emotional distress, opioids may have been used as the de facto remedy to alleviate existential suffering and as a substitute for the rewards of social connection. Unfortunately, evidence so far suggests that opioids do not promote functional recovery or return to work.[87] Furthermore, comorbid mental health issues have been found to increase the risk for adverse outcomes, such as opioid overdose, misuse, and abuse among patients receiving long-term opioid treatment for chronic pain.[88] Thus, whatever neurobiological adaptations occur with prolonged exposure to exogenous opioids seem to belie the simplistic nociception model of pain.

Getting to know the neurobiological connections between physical pain and emotional suffering has been important in understanding why pain is necessary, why pain is inexorably linked to pleasure and mood, and how pain and suffering are powerfully amenable to central control. Such understanding also helps explain why there would be neurobiological adaptations to chronic pain and its treatments that could render the treatments themselves less useful than the underlying natural processes that can be vigorously recruited either consciously or unconsciously.

BIOETHICS OF PAIN AND SUFFERING IN LIGHT OF THESE NEUROBIOLOGICAL INSIGHTS

As we have discussed, pain and suffering are customarily combined, but they are not synonyms. Pain may exist when the person is not suffering, and people can suffer in the absence of pain. Bioethics in the past often used abstract and idealized problems, not real life situations, and ignored real moral issues. Pain is a subjective experience. The findings on physical examination, radiographs, and laboratory tests cannot predict the degree of pain experienced, and many chronic pain patients, such as sufferers of headache, fibromyalgia, and low back pain, have no unique findings that would explain their symptoms and their suffering. The traditional reaction of Western medicine to these facts has been to divide pain into different groups, with pain that is attributed to physical disorders being deemed more legitimate and pain that cannot be attributed to such physical disorders, or that seems excessive for the objective findings, falling under suspicion. The medical lexicon is replete with terms for this inexplicable and disorderly pain: psychosomatic, embellished, functional, and hysterical. This class of pain patients is inevitably stigmatized and labeled as drug seeking, malingering, or needy. These beliefs, when held by health care providers, interact with widely held prejudices in Western society, resulting in the observed tendencies to offer less pain treatment to ethnic minorities and women.

The collective behavior of pain patients and their providers has manifest effects on society. The economy is affected through the loss or gain of productive work hours and the provision of expensive care. Chronic pain plays a sizable role in health care and productivity, with growing rates of health care utilization and disability. The treatment of pain also affects the public health field and the criminal justice system through the prescription of opioids, which may be abused, stolen, or sold for a profit. Thus, pain treatment is not solely a matter for the triangle of provider, patient, and insurer but also is an arena in which many public and private interests contend.

The provider's primary allegiance should remain to the patient. Pain is a potent cause of suffering and one of the greatest ills that besets the human condition. C. S. Lewis named his examination of theodicy "The Problem of Pain," in recognition of the uniqueness of pain, stating that pleasure may be disregarded but that "pain insists upon being attended to."[89]

The key principles of bioethics that have been commonly discussed in recent Western medical philosophy include beneficence, nonmaleficence, respect for autonomy, and justice. This list is certainly somewhat arbitrary and might include many virtues, and it is noteworthy that the common interest is not recognized in this short list, reflecting the Western tradition of individualism. This tradition has strengthened in the past few decades, such that autonomy, informed consent, and civil liberties are emphasized in clinical care.

In the field of pain treatment, this emphasis has shifted the clinical calculus; the "patients first" approach has led to such worthy initiatives as perceiving pain as the "fifth vital sign" and seeking heroic measures to treat pain. The pursuit of benefit to the patient and reflecting the patient's wishes have led to patient-centered care and many quality improvements. However, some critics feel that this approach devalues the special expertise and responsibility of the health care provider. Whereas the physician might formerly have had the primary responsibility in finding the proper balance between risk and benefit, thus fulfilling the mandates of beneficence and nonmaleficence, decision making is now a group task, to be shared by the provider, the patient, and possibly other family members or advisers.

Specifically in the field of pain medicine, this raises concerns about overtreatment and inappropriate treatment. Patients suffering pain may feel compelled to pursue any treatment that offers a scrap of hope, while the provider may feel that these treatments are too risky, inappropriate, or unlikely to be helpful. Thus, clinicians are in a complex position, required to provide information and give their best advice to the patient, guided by the patient's own stated preferences. Although the importance of patient satisfaction and the dictates of patient care will surely influence the clinician's choices, the final responsibility lies with the clinicians to try to maximize benefit and steer the patient away from the gravest dangers and worst outcomes.

Many pain treatments have proved to have less benefit than was initially perceived, such as the many treatments that have been proposed for discogenic back pain. Others have proved to be helpful in relatively few patients, such as back surgery for pain. And many pain treatments have proved to be much riskier than was initially thought; the primary example of this, of course, must be chronic opioid therapy for noncancer pain. The risks and ethical dilemmas are greatly reduced for the clinician treating either acute pain or pain in cancer patients and palliative care patients; in these cases, the pain is temporally limited, and an extraordinary effort is warranted in the expectation that it will resolve soon.

In patients with chronic noncancer pain and in cancer survivors, pain treatment must be safe and sustainable. Prescription opioids currently represent a public health issue in the United States. These medications are associated with an increase in the rates of accidental overdose and admissions to substance abuse treatment programs.[90] Accidental overdoses caused 27,658 deaths in 2007, of which 11,499 were a result of prescription opioids. The rate of death from overdose and the amount of prescription opioids prescribed both more than tripled from 1999 to 2009.[91]

Careful attention must be paid to risk factors and addiction. It is very common to find both physical and mental forms of suffering, and it is not considered ethical to deny treatment for these. Pain specialists should be skilled in the assessment and diagnosis of pain and in the selection of treatment. Although the decision about whether to prescribe opioids rightly receives much careful attention, it is equally important to offer nonopioid medications and to address the psychological and psychiatric factors that contribute to suffering in chronic pain. Some patients are likely to be made worse by treatment with opioids, but opioids should not be arbitrarily denied for nonmedical reasons.

Clinicians striving to offer their patients the best possible pain care are faced with many obstacles. As noted earlier, the state of the art of pain treatment is not very satisfactory, with a 40 percent reduction in pain severity considered successful (by researchers—the patients would prefer a much more robust decrease). Procedures and surgery have narrow indications and sometimes only temporary benefit. Medications for pain are mostly nonspecific, and clinicians have limited ability to predict which medication will be effective for which condition in which patient. Many medications are limited in their efficacy as well by side effects, particularly sedation and fatigue.

In the absence of objective signs of pain and suffering, clinicians must rely on clinical acumen and standardized assessments. Clinical acumen is restricted by all the limits of empathy and imagination—it is difficult to empathize with the sick when one is well, and still more difficult when the suffering patient is from a different class, culture, or background. Nonetheless, the clinician must treat pain one patient at a time, letting the patient partner in determining what is effective and what is tolerable.

The bioethics of pain treatment must reflect the complicated and ambiguous current understanding of pain and suffering. Ethicists, like clinicians, make their job too easy if they only attend to some part of the clinical dilemmas and focus on the importance of patient autonomy, for example, to the exclusion of other issues. Robust principles to guide clinicians in balancing their clinical responsibilities and their respect for the patient's autonomy are not well developed in the ethical or legal realms. Bioethics must also consider the ethical imperatives of public health and utilization. We do not, it is commonly said, ration medical care at the bedside. In fact, rationing of medical care is in general highly controversial and often unsystematic. However, this issue is particularly relevant in pain management, where the needs of patients are insistent, and treatment options continue to proliferate.

Glossary

Action potential: the change in electrical charge of a nerve cell that is associated with the nerve cell firing and sending a message along its length.

Agonist: a molecule that binds to a receptor and turns it "on."

Antagonist: a molecule that binds a receptor without turning it on, in effect blocking it.

Ascending nociceptive tracts: the nerve pathways that transmit nociceptive signals from the relay stations in the spinal cord and brain nuclei to the higher centers of the brain.

Central sensitization: changes in the spinal cord and brain that make them more sensitive to nociceptive stimulus and can even produce pain without nociceptive stimulus.

Cortical centers of the brain: regions of the outermost layer of the brain specialized for specific functions, such as perception or movement.

Descending systems: nerve pathways that travel "down" from the higher brain to the relay stations and can modulate them to be more or less sensitive.

Ectopic activity: spontaneously generated painful nerve impulses that arise elsewhere in the pain pathways than the nociceptors. See *central sensitization*.

Endogenous opioids: peptide molecules produced in the body that are similar to opioid drugs and that help regulate many body functions, including pain and suffering.

Epigenetic changes: changes in a cell's biology that influence the expression of genes without changing the underlying DNA sequence.

Excitatory: tending to increase the rate of firing of a nerve; turning a nerve "on."

Gate control theory: the theory that both thin and thick nerve fibers can carry pain information to the relay stations in the dorsal horn of the spinal cord, and that these pain signals can interfere with each other, closing the "gate" to the brain.

Hyperalgesia: increased sensitivity to pain.

Hypothalamic-pituitary-adrenal (HPA) axis: the system running from the hypothalamus and pituitary in the brain to the adrenal glands, which controls the release of cortisol, a stress hormone.

Inhibitory: tending to decrease a nerve's rate of firing; turns nerve "off."

Limbic pathway: the pain pathway that sends pain signals from the spinal cord to the limbic system and helps the brain determine the unpleasantness of the pain stimulus and its emotional reaction to the pain. Contrast with thalamocortical pathway.

Limbic system: a complex network of brain regions that lie around and above the thalamus and help regulate emotion, behavior, and memory.

Metabotrobic receptor: a receptor that sits on the outer membrane of cells and, when activated, activates a second messenger system, which can affect a variety of other cell functions. Contrast with *voltage-gated ion channel*.

Neuroablative: a form of pain treatment involving the temporary or permanent destruction of nerve function, typically by heat, cold, chemicals, or surgery.

Neurostimulation: a form of pain treatment that uses pulsed electrical stimuli to interfere with pain transmission in nerves or the spinal cord.

Neurotransmitter: molecules produced by the body that bind to receptors on nerves and make them more or less likely to fire.

Nociception: the process of communicating noxious stimuli through nerve signals. Nociception does not count as pain until the brain has responded to it and treated it as a painful stimulus.

Nociceptive-specific neuron: nerve that usually responds only to stimuli that would be intense enough to cause injury to the body, e.g., a red-hot stove but not a warm one. Also known as a "sleeping" or "silent" nociceptor.

Nociceptor: any of a variety of nerves that respond to noxious stimuli; the human body has nociceptors for heat and cold, mechanical pressure, and chemical irritants. Also, the specific receptors that detect these noxious stimuli.

Periaqueductal gray: the gray matter around the cerebral aqueduct in the midbrain that sends descending modulation to the spinal cord to influence pain perception. See *descending systems*.

Peripheral sensitization: the phenomena by which peripheral nerves become overly sensitive after nerve injury, sometimes causing hyperalgesia.

Polymorphism: mutations of specific locations in the genetic code. Also known as "point mutations," these can cause changes to the functioning of cells or the entire organism, especially when the patient has mutations in both of their copies of that gene.

Primary afferent: the sensory nerves traveling from receptors or sensory organs in the periphery toward the central nervous system.

Primary somatosensory cortex: the higher cortical region of the brain that allows the brain to map the location of an incoming stimulus, letting the patient know that the pain is in the big toe, for example.

Spinothalamic tract: the main pain pathway in the spine traveling from the dorsal horn of the spinal cord to the thalamus.

Thalamus: a brain region on top of the brainstem that sits between the lower brain and the cortical regions and helps direct stimuli from the body and lower brain to the appropriate cortical regions.

Thalamocortical pathway: the pathway from the thalamus to the cortical brain centers that lets the brain know the location, nature, and intensity of the pain stimulus (but not its unpleasantness). Contrast with limbic pathway.

Transduction: the process of converting physical stimuli (such as heat or a touch) to nerve signals that can be transmitted to the brain.

Voltage-gated ion channel: A receptor that sits on the membrane of a cell and opens a channel when the voltage potential of that membrane reaches a certain point. Usually the channel then lets a flood of ions through the membrane, further changing the voltage potential. This is one way that nerves generate action potentials.

Wide dynamic-range neuron: the most common type of neuron, which arises from the dorsal horn of the spinal cord. These neurons respond to different kinds of stimuli and to a wide range of different-intensity nerve signals.

Notes

1. C. Heim et al., "The Link between Childhood Trauma and Depression: Insights from HPA Axis Studies In Humans," *Psychoneuroendocrinology* 33 (2009): 693–710; A. D. Craig, "How Do You Feel—Now? The Anterior Insula and Human Awareness," *Nature Reviews Neuroscience* 10 (2009): 59–70; N. I. Eisenberger. "The Pain of Social Disconnection: Examining the Shared Neural Underpinnings of Physical and Social Pain." *Nature Reviews Neuroscience* 13 (2012): 421–434.

2. C. L. Stucky, M. S. Gold, and X. Zhang, "Mechanisms of Pain," *Proceedings of the National Academy of Sciences of the United States of America* 98 (2001): 11845–11846; C. A. Ufret-Vincenty et al., "Localization of the PIP2 Sensor of TRPV1 Ion Channels,"

Journal of Biological Chemistry 286 (2011): 9688–9698; S. E. Jordt, D. D. McKemy DD, and D. Julius, "Lessons from Peppers and Peppermint: The Molecular Logic of Thermosensation," *Current Opinions in Neurobiology* 13 (2003): 487–492.

3. H. L. Fields, *Pain Mechanisms and Management*, 2nd ed. (New York: McGraw-Hill, 2002); H. L. Fields, M. M. Heinricher, and P. Mason, "Neurotransmitters in Nociceptive Modulatory Circuits," *Annual Review of Neuroscience*, 14 (1991): 219–245; T. L. Yaksh and T. A. Rudy, "Narcotic Analgestics: CNS Sites and Mechanisms of Action as Revealed by Intracerebral Injection Techniques," *Pain* 4 (1978): 299–359.

4. C. Heim et al., supra note 1.

5. H. L. Fields, M. M. Heinricher, and P. Mason, supra note 3; F. Porreca, M. H. Ossipov, and G. F. Gebhart, "Chronic Pain and Medullary Descending Facilitation," *Trends in Neuroscience* 25 (2002): 319–325; M. O. Urban and G. F. Gebhart, "Supraspinal Contributions to Hyperalgesia," *Proceedings of the National Academy of Sciences of the United States of America* 96 (199): 7687–7692; M. Zhuo M and G. F. Gebhart, "Characterization of Descending Facilitation and Inhibition of Spinal Nociceptive Transmission from the Nuclei Reticularis Gigantocellularis and Gigantocellularis Pars Alpha in the Rat," *Journal of Neurophysiology* 67 (1992): 1599–1614; M. J. Neubert, W. Kincaid, and M. M. Heinricher. "Nociceptive Facilitating Neurons in the Rostral Ventromedial Medulla," *Pain* 110 (2004): 158–165.

6. C. A. Ufret-Vincenty et al., supra note 2.

7. C. F. Woolf and M. W. Salter, "Neuronal Plasticity: Increasing the Gain in Pain," *Science* 288 (2000): 1765–1769.

8. Ibid.; P. J. Siddall and M. J. Cousins, "Persistent Pain as a Disease Entity: Implications for Clinical Management," *Anesthesia and Analgesia* 99 (2004): 510–520.

9. C. J. Woolf and I. Decosterd, "Implications of Recent Advances in the Understanding of Pain Pathophysiology for the Assessment of Pain in Patients," *Pain* Suppl. 6 (1999): S141–S147; S. H. Sindrup and T. S. Jensen, "Efficacy of Pharmacological Treatments of Neuropathic Pain: An Update and Effect Related to Mechanism of Drug Action," *Pain* 83 (1999): 389–400.

10. C. G. Pert and S. H. Snyder, "Opiate Receptor: Demonstration in Nervous Tissue," *Science* 179 (1973): 1011–1014; J. Hughes et al., "Identification of Two Related Pentapeptides from the Brain with Potent Opiate Agonist Activity," *Nature* 258 (1975): 577–580.

11. R. Melzack and P. D. Wall, "Pain Mechanisms: A New Theory," *Science* 150 (1965): 971–979; P. D. Wall, "The Laminar Organization of Dorsal Horn and Effects of Descending Impulses," *Journal of Physiology* 188 (1967): 403–423.

12. D. V. Reynolds, "Surgery in the Rat during Electrical Analgesia Induced by Focal Brain Stimulation," *Science* 164 (1969): 444–445; D. J. Mayer et al., "Analgesia from Electrical Stimulation in the Brainstem of The rat," *Science* 174 (1971): 1351–1354.

13. H. L. Fields, M. M. Heinricher, and P. Mason, supra note 3; R. Melzack, P. D. Wall, and T. C. Ty, "Acute Pain in an Emergency Clinic: Latency of Onset and Descriptor Patterns Related to Different Injuries," *Pain* 14 (1982): 33–43; H. K. Beecher, "The Measurement of Pain: Protoype for the Quantitative Study of Subjective Responses," *Pharmacological Review* 9 (1956): 59–209.

14. C. G. Pert and S. H. Snyder; J. Hughes et al., supra note 10.

15. M. Eguchi, "Recent Advances in Selective Opioid Receptor Agonists and Antagonists," *Medical Research Reviews* 24 (2004): 182–212.; H. Akil et al., "Endogenous Opioids: Overview and Current Issues," *Drug and Alcohol Dependence* 51 (1998): 127–140.

16. H. K. Beecher, "The Powerful Placebo," *Journal of the American Medical Association* 159 (1955): 1602–1606.; R. de la Fuente-Fernandez, M. Schulzer, and A. J. Stoessl, "The Placebo Effect in Neurological Disorders," *Lancet Neurology* 1 (2002): 85–91; P. Petrovic et al., "Placebo and Opioid Analgesia—Imaging a Shared Neuronal Network," *Science* 295 (2002): 1737–1740.

17. H. Fields, "State-Dependent Opioid Control of Pain," *Nature Reviews Neuroscience* 5 (2004): 565–575.

18. M. J. Neubert, W. Kincaid, and M. M. Heinricher, supra note 5; M. M. Heinricher, Z. F. Cheng, and H. L. Fields, ":Evidence for Two Classes of Nociceptive Modulating Neurons in the Periaqueductal Gray," *Journal of Neuroscience* 7 (1987): 271–278; H. L. Fields, A. Malick, and R. Burstein, "Dorsal Horn Projection Targets of on and off Cells in the Rostral Ventromedial Medulla," *Journal of Neurophysiology* 74 (1995): 1742–1759.

19. K. Charmaz, "Loss of Self: A Fundamental Form of Suffering in the Chronically Ill," *Sociology of Health and Illness* 5 (2008): 168–195.

20. J. G. Green et al., Childhood Adversities and Adult Psychiatric Disorders in the National Comorbidity Survey Replication I: Associations with First Onset of DSM-IV Disorders," *Archives of General Psychiatry* 67 (2010): 113–123.

21. M. aan het Rot, S. J. Mathew, and D. S. Charney, "Neurobiological Mechanisms in Major Depressive Disorder," *Canadian Medical Association Journal* 180 (2009): 305–313.

22. J. G. Green et al., supra note 20.

23. S. A. Vreeburg et al., "Major Depressive Disorder and Hypothalamic-Pituitary-Adrenal Axis Activity: Results from a Large Cohort Study." *Archives of General Psychiatry* 66 (2009): 617–626; C. F. Gillespie and C. B. Nemeroff CB, "Hypercortisolemia and Depression," *Psychosomatic Medicine* 67, Suppl. 1 (2005): S26–S28

24. R. H. Belmaker and G. Agam, "Major Depressive Disorder," *New England Journal of Medicine* 358 (2008): 55–68.

25. D. J. Nutt et al., "Consensus Statement and Research Needs: The Role of Dopamine and Norepinephrine in Depression and Antidepressant Treatment." *Journal of Clinical Psychiatry* 67, Suppl. 6 (2006): 46–49.

26. P. L. Delgado et al., "Tryptophan-Depletion Challenge in Depressed Patients Treated with Desipramine or Fluoxetine: Implications for the Role of Serotonin in the Mechanism of Antidepressant Action," *Biological Psychi*atry 46 (1999): 212–220.

27. P. L. Delgado et al., "Monoamines and the Mechanism of Antidepressant Action: Effects of Catecholamine Depletion on Mood of Patients Treated with Antidepressants," *Psychopharmacology Bulletin* 29 (1993): 389–396.

28. B. W. Dunlop and C. B. Nemeroff, "The Role of Dopamine in the Pathophysiology of Depression," *Archives of General Psychiatry* 64 (2007): 327–337.

29. G. Sanacora et al., "Reduced Cortical Gamma-Aminobutyric Acid Levels in Depressed Patients Determined by Proton Magnetic Resonance Spectroscopy," *Archives of General Psychiatry* 56 (1999): 1043–1047.

30. G. Hasler et al., "Reduced Prefrontal Glutamate/Glutamine and Gamma-Aminobutyric Acid Levels in Major Depression Determined Using Proton Magnetic Resonance Spectroscopy," *Archives of General Psychiatry* 64 (2007): 193–200.

31. P. V. Choudary et al., "Altered Cortical Glutamatergic and Gabaergic Signal Transmission with Glial Involvement In Depression," *Proceedings of the National Academy of Sciences of the United States of America* 102 (2005): 15653–15658.

32. S. E. Kennedy et al., "Dysregulation of Endogenous Opioid Emotion Regulation Circuitry in Major Depression in Women," *Archives of General Psychiatry* 63 (2006): 1199–1208.

33. R. E. Harris et al., "Decreased Central Mu-Opioid Receptor Availability in Fibromyalgia," *Journal of Neuroscience* 27 (2007): 10000–10006.

34. E. M. Jutkiewicz and B. P. Roques, "Endogenous Opioids as Physiological Antidepressants: Complementary Role of Delta Receptors and Dopamine," *Neuropsychopharmacology* 37 (2012): 303–304.

35. K. S. Kendler et al., "A Swedish National Twin Study of Lifetime Major Depression," *American Journal of Psychiatry* 163 (2006): 109–114; P. F. Sullivan, M. C. Neale, and K. S. Kendler, "Genetic Epidemiology of Major Depression: Review and Meta-Analysis," *American Journal of Psychiatry* 157 (2000): 1552–1562.

36. P. F. Sullivan et al., "Genome-Wide Association For Major Depressive Disorder: A Possible Role For The Presynaptic Protein Piccolo," *Molecular Psychiatry* 14 (2009): 359–375.

37. R. G. Bradley et al., "Influence of Child Abuse On Adult Depression: Moderation by the Corticotropin-Releasing Hormone Receptor Gene," *Archives of General Psychiatry* 65 (2008): 190–200.

38. A. Caspi et al., "Influence of Life Stress on Depression: Moderation by a Polymorphism in the 5-HTT Gene," *Science* 301 (2003): 386–389; K. S. Kendler et al., "The Interaction of Stressful Life Events and a Serotonin Transporter Polymorphism in the Prediction of Episodes of Major Depression: A Replication," *Archives of General Psychiatry* 62 (2005): 529–535.

39. P. O. McGowan et al., "Epigenetic Regulation of the Glucocorticoid Receptor in Human Brain Associates with Childhood Abuse," *Nature Neuroscience* 12 (2009): 342–348; E. W. Fish et al., "Epigenetic Programming of Stress Responses Through Variations in Maternal Care," *Annals of the New York Academy of Sciences* 1036 (2004): 167–180.

40. M. Schroeder et al., "Epigenetics and Depression: Current Challenges and New Therapeutic Options," *Current Opinion in Psychiatry* 23 (2010): 588–592.

41. P. O. McGowan et al., supra note 39.

42. H. Hayhurst et al., "Expressed Emotion and Depression: A Longitudinal Study," *British Journal of Psychiatry* 171 (1997): 439–443; E. Paykel, *Life Events: Effects and Genesis. Psychological Medicine* 33 (2003): 1145–1148.

43. B. W. Dunlop and C. B. Nemeroff, "The Role of Dopamine in the Pathophysiology of Depression," *Archives of General Psychiatry* 64 (2007): 327–337.

44. H. Hayhurst et al., supra note 42.

45. L. Alvarez L. Purple Heart Is Ruled Out for Post Traumatic Stress Disorder. *New York Times* (2009 January 8).

46. P. Fu and M. Fox, *Bend, not Break: A Life in Two Worlds* (New York: Portfolio/Penguin, 2013).

47. D. T. Acheson, J. E. Gresack, and V. B. Risbrough, "Hippocampal Dysfunction Effects on Context Memory: Possible Etiology for Posttraumatic Stress Disorder," *Neuropharmacology* 62 (2012): 674–685.

48. I. Liberzon et al., "Brain Activation in PTSD in Response To Trauma-Related Stimuli," *Biological Psychiatry* 45 (1999): 817–826.

49. R. C. Kessler et al., "Posttraumatic Stress Disorder in the National Comorbidity Survey," *Archives of General Psychiatry* 52 (1995): 1048–1060; J. A. Boscarino and R. E. Adams, "PTSD Onset and Course Following the World Trade Center Disaster: Findings

and Implications for Future Research," *Social Psychiatry and Psychiatric Epidemiology*, 44 (2009): 887–898.

50. Chambers RA, Bremner JD, Moghaddam B, et al. "Glutamate and Post-Traumatic Stress Disorder: Toward a Psychobiology of Dissociation," *Seminars in Clinical Neuropsychiatry* 4 (1999): 274–281.

51. J. A. Boscarino, "Posttraumatic Stress Disorder, Exposure to Combat, and Lower Plasma Cortisol among Vietnam Veterans: Findings and Clinical Implications." *Journal of Consulting and Clinical Psychology* 64 (1996): 191–201.

52. I. Liberzon et al., supra note 48.

53. S. L. Rauch et al., "A Symptom Provocation Study of Posttraumatic Stress Disorder Using Positron Emission Tomography and Script-Driven Imagery," *Archives of General Psychiatry* 53 (1996): 380–387; L. M. Shin et al., "Visual Imagery and Perception in Posttraumatic Stress Disorder: A Positron Emission Tomographic Investigation," *Archives of General Psychiatry* 54 (1997): 233–241.

54. J. A. Boscarino et al., "Higher FKBP5, COMT, CHRNA5, and CRHR1 Allele Burdens Are Associated with PTSD and Interact with Trauma Exposure: Implications for Neuropsychiatric Research and Treatment," *Neuropsychiatric Disease and Treatment* 8 (2012): 131–139.

55. R. Yehuda and L. M. Bierer, "The Relevance of Epigenetics to PTSD: Implications for the DSM-V," *Journal of Traumatic Stress* 22 (2009): 427–434.

56. M. J. Meaney and M. Szyf, "Environmental Programming of Stress Responses Through DNA Methylation: Life at the Interface between a Dynamic Environment and a Fixed Genome," *Dialogues in Clinical Neuroscience* 7 (2005): 103–123.

57. T. Klengel et al., "Allele-Specific FKBP5 DNA Demethylation Mediates Gene-Childhood Trauma Interactions," *Nature Neuroscience* 16 (2012): 33–41.

58. C. Heim and C. B. Nemeroff, "Neurobiology of Posttraumatic Stress Disorder," *CNS Spectrums* 14 (2009): 13–24.

59. I. Elman, J. K. Zubieta, and D. Borsook. "The Missing P in Psychiatric Training: Why It Is Important to Teach Pain to Psychiatrists," *Archives of General Psychiatry* 68 (2011): 12–20.

60. J. D. Belluzzi and L. Stein, "Enkephalin May Mediate Euphoria and Drive-Reduction Reward," *Nature* 266:556–558, 1977.

61. P. L. Tenore, "Psychotherapeutic Benefits of Opioid Agonist Therapy," *Journal of Addictive Diseases* 27 (2008): 49–65.

62. D. Naber et al. "Endogenous Opioid Activity and Beta-Endorphin Immunoreactivity in CSF of Psychiatric Patients and Normal Volunteers," *American Journal of Psychiatry* 138 (1981): 1457–1462.

63. R. Gross-Isseroff et al., "Regionally Selective Increases in Mu Opioid Receptor Density in the Brains of Suicide Victims," *Brain Research* 530 (1990): 312–316.

64. D. Filliol et al. "Mice Deficient for Delta- and Mu-Opioid Receptors Exhibit Opposing Alterations of Emotional Responses," *Nature Genetics* 25 (2000): 195–200.

65. J. Bowlby, *Attachment*, 2nd ed. (New York: Basic, 1983).

66. A. Moles, B. L. Kieffer, and F. R. D'Amato. "Deficit in Attachment Behavior in Mice Lacking the Mu-Opioid Receptor Gene," *Science* 304 (2004): 1983–1986.

67. S. C. Ribeiro et al., "Interface of Physical and Emotional Stress Regulation through the Endogenous Opioid System and Mu-Opioid Receptors," *Progress in Neuropsychopharmacology and Biological Psychiatry* 29 (2005): 1264–1280.

68. S. E. Kennedy et al., supra note 32.

69. M. Costigan, J. Scholz, and C. J. Woolf, "Neuropathic Pain: A Maladaptive Response of the Nervous System to Damage," *Annual Review of Neuroscience* 32 (2009): 1–32.

70. M. J. Sigtermans et al., "Ketamine Produces Effective and Long-Term Pain Relief in Patients with Complex Regional Pain Syndrome Type 1," *Pain* 145 (2009): 304–311.

71. C. A. Zarate Jr. et al., "A Randomized Trial of an *N*-methyl-d-Aspartate Antagonist in Treatment-Resistant Major Depression," *Archives of General Psychiatry* 63 (2006): 856–864.

72. W. Rahman, R. D'Mello, and A. H. Dickenson, "Peripheral Nerve Injury-Induced Changes in Spinal Alpha(2)-Adrenoceptor-Mediated Modulation of Mechanically Evoked Dorsal Horn Neuronal Responses," *Journal of Pain* 9 (2008): 350–359.

73. R. H. Dworkin et al., "Pharmacologic Management of Neuropathic Pain: Evidence-Based Recommendations," *Pain* 132 (2007): 237–251.

74. N. I. Eisenberger, "The Neural Bases of Social Pain: Evidence for Shared Representations with Physical Pain," *Psychosomatic Medicine* 74 (2012): 126–135.

75. N. I. Eisenberger, M. D. Lieberman, and K. D. Williams, "Does Rejection Hurt? An fMRI Study of Social Exclusion," *Science* 302 (2003): 290–292.

76. E. Kross et al., "Social Rejection Shares Somatosensory Representations with Physical Pain," *Proceedings of the National Academy of Sciences of the United States of America* 108 (2011): 6270–6275.

77. H. Gundel et al., "Functional Neuroanatomy of Grief: An fMRI Study," *American Journal of Psychiatry* 160 (2003): 1946–1953; A. Kersting et al., "Neural Activation Underlying Acute Grief in Women after the Loss of an Unborn Child," *American Journal of Psychiatry* 166(2009): 1402–1410; M. F. O'Connor et al., "Craving Love? Enduring Grief Activates Brain's Reward Center," *NeuroImage* 42 (2008): 969–972.

78. N. I. Eisenberger et al., "An Experimental Study of Shared Sensitivity to Physical Pain and Social Rejection," *Pain* 126 (2006): 132–138.

79. B. M. Way, S. E. Taylor, and N. I. Eisenberger, "Variation in the Mu-Opioid Receptor Gene (OPRM1) Is associated with Dispositional and Neural Sensitivity to Social Rejection," *Proceedings of the National Academy of Sciences of the United States of America* 106 (2009): 15079–15084.

80. N. I. Eisenberger et al., "Inflammation and Social Experience: An Inflammatory Challenge Induces Feelings of Social Disconnection in Addition to Depressed Mood," *Brain, Behavior, and Immunity* 24 (2010): 558–563.

81. N. I. Eisenberger et al., "An fMRI Study of Cytokine-Induced Depressed Mood and Social Pain: The Role of Sex Differences," *NeuroImage* 47 (2009): 881–890.

82. C. N. Dewall et al., "Acetaminophen Reduces Social Pain: Behavioral and Neural Evidence," *Psychological Science* 21 (2010): 931–937.

83. P. L. Tenore, supra note 61.

84. J. C. Ballantyne, "Safe and Effective When Used As Directed: The Case of Chronic Use of Opioid Analgesics," *Journal of Medical Toxicology* 8 (2012): 417–423.

85. Centers for Disease Control and Prevention, "CDC Vital Signs: Prescription Painkiller Overdoses in the US. 2011," accessed May 21, 2013, http://www.cdc.gov.offcampus.lib.washington.edu/vitalsigns/PainkillerOverdoses/index.html.

86. J. Breckenridge and J. D. Clark, "Patient Characteristics associated with Opioid versus Nonsteroidal Anti-Inflammatory Drug Management of Chronic Low Back Pain," *Journal of Pain* 4 (2003): 344–350; M. D. Sullivan et al., "Regular Use of Prescribed Opioids: Association with Common Psychiatric Disorders," *Pain* 119 (2005): 95; M. D. Sullivan et al., "Association between Mental Health Disorders, Problem Drug Use, and Regular Prescription Opioid Use," *Archives of Internal Medicine* 166 (2006): 2087.

87. M. Noble et al., "Long-Term Opioid Management for Chronic Noncancer Pain," *Cochrane Database System Review* (2010): 1.

88. M. J. Edlund et al., "Risks for Opioid Abuse and Dependence among Recipients of Chronic Opioid Therapy: Results from the TROUP Study," *Drug and Alcohol Dependence* 112 (2013): 90–98; J. Park and R. Lavin, "Risk Factors associated with Opioid Medication Misuse in Community-Dwelling Older Adults with Chronic Pain," *Clinical Journal of Pain* 26 (2010): 647–655; J. A. Boscarino et al., "Risk Factors for Drug Dependence among Out-Patients on Opioid Therapy in a Large US Health-Care System," *Addiction* 105 (2010): 1776–1782.

89. Lewis, C S. *The Problem of Pain.* New York: Macmillan, 1940. Print.

90. S. Okie, "A Flood of Opioids, a Rising Tide of Deaths," *New England Journal of Medicine* 363 (2010): 1981–1985.

91. Centers for Disease Control and Prevention, supra note 85.

7

What Is Suffering and What Sorts of Beings Can Suffer?

David DeGrazia

Everyone who is reading this chapter has experienced suffering and knows that suffering is a bad thing. It is bad in the sense that, just considered in itself, it makes things go worse for the subject. Suffering decreases one's experiential welfare or quality of life for as long as it persists—even if it sometimes has longer-term benefits such as growth of character or perspective. Assuming for the moment that animals can suffer, suffering is the object of the interest that is most straightforwardly attributed to them: an interest in avoiding suffering. Whether animals have an interest in remaining alive (as opposed to having a good quality of life while alive), in being free (independently of freedom's effects on quality of life), or in engaging their natural capacities (again, independently of effects on quality of life) is somewhat controversial because one might hold that their good or well-being consists entirely in experiential welfare. Yet, even if that reductionist view of animal well-being is correct, the avoidance of suffering is unquestionably a central interest of animals—a central aspect of their welfare. Suffering is intrinsically bad for any subject who can suffer.

But what, exactly, is suffering? And what sorts of creatures are capable of suffering? This essay addresses these questions. It opens with a conceptual investigation of suffering and distinguishes broad and narrow conceptions. The section that follows addresses what sorts of beings can suffer in the narrow, more restrictive sense of the term. It is argued that if we provisionally set aside radical skepticism about animal consciousness (a position addressed later), there is a strong empirical case for the proposition that many animals, and not only mammals, are capable of suffering in this restricted sense. But insofar as the broader conception of suffering

A draft of this paper was presented at a conference entitled "Animals, Ethics, and the Law" at the University of Tennessee, Knoxville. A second draft was presented to my colleagues in the Department of Philosophy, George Washington University. I would like to thank attendees of both talks—especially Colin Allen, Tad Zawidzki, and Eric Saidel—for their helpful feedback. Thanks also to Jacqueline Drayer for research assistance on the topic of nociceptors and to Ron Green and Nathan Palpant for editorial suggestions that greatly strengthened the paper.

proves fundamental for moral purposes, the paper proceeds in the next two sections to ask what sorts of creatures can suffer in this sense. In the first of those two sections, a substantial empirical case is sketched for the thesis that animals from a wide array of species (at least mammals, birds, reptiles, amphibians, and some fish) are sentient, or have the capacity for consciousness, and are therefore capable of suffering in the relevant sense. In the next section, a radical skeptical challenge invoking a higher-order thought theory of consciousness is presented and rebutted. The conclusion is that there is ample reason to believe, and little reason to doubt, that animals representing a wide range of species are capable of suffering in the broad sense of this term. A brief coda considers implications for bioethics.

Before proceeding, it might be helpful to say more about the motivations for this paper. One motivation, purely intellectual, is to help clarify a concept whose meaning may be unclear because of varying uses of the term *suffering* and the subtle relationship between suffering and other mental states and capacities. A second, more practical motivation is to combat two types of intellectual mischief that can interfere with the important objective of reducing animal suffering. The types of intellectual mischief that I want to neutralize are (1) emphasizing a distinction between suffering and pain, and claiming that (a) animals cannot suffer and (b) pain without suffering is trivial; and (2) contending, more radically, that animals entirely lack conscious life and therefore cannot even feel pain. The intended result is that commonsense attributions of morally significant experiences to animals will be seen to enjoy the support—rather than the opposition—of science and philosophy.

What Is Suffering?

To determine what sorts of beings can suffer, we have to know what we're looking for. So, what is suffering? There is no simple answer to this question because the term is used in different ways. In what we might call the objective sense of the term, suffering is roughly equivalent to misfortune. More precisely, the verb *to suffer* is treated as transitive: one suffers a misfortune. Now, one can suffer a misfortune without being aware of it, say if one's house is destroyed while one is away on vacation; and such a possibility highlights the distinction between this objective sense of suffering and the subjective sense that will be our topic. In the subjective sense, *to suffer* is an intransitive verb: one suffers, period, rather than suffering something. Such suffering is subjective in the sense of mind dependent: suffering is a type of mental state or occurrence. Moreover, suffering is consciously experienced, which is why it automatically lowers one's quality of life while it occurs. If suffering could occur without one's feeling it, it would not have this tight conceptual tie to experiential welfare.

Suffering in this subjective sense (the only sense I will discuss for the remainder of this paper) is an *unpleasant* mental state. What more can be said in unpacking the concept? That depends on the specific conception one embraces.

On a broad construal of the concept articulated by Jamie Mayerfeld, to suffer is, roughly speaking, to feel bad.[1] Refining the concept, he proposes that suffering is a disagreeable *overall* feeling—where the qualification is included to account for the fact that good and bad feelings can occur in a subject simultaneously.[2] One might, say, feel elated upon receiving good news despite having just painfully bumped one's knee; here, presumably, one would not suffer. But our ordinary concept of suffering suggests that mild disagreeable feelings, even overall disagreeable feelings, such as slight boredom or slight impatience, do not amount to suffering. Thus, Mayerfeld proposes that suffering be understood (for most purposes) as a *more-than-mild* disagreeable overall feeling; yet, for other purposes, such as thinking about where an individual falls on a hedonic scale of overall feeling, he employs the term *suffering* to cover the entire negative portion of the scale.[3] We therefore have two relatively broad conceptions of suffering. According to one, suffering is any more-than-mild disagreeable overall feeling. According to the other, suffering is *any* disagreeable overall feeling. An even broader conception is possible: suffering is any disagreeable feeling, period. On this broadest of conceptions, any pain or feeling of discomfort, nausea, or distress would count as suffering. Although the breadth of this conception clearly exceeds that of our ordinary concept of suffering, it is useful in considerations of welfare to have an umbrella term for the entire range of disagreeable or unpleasant experiences. Suffering, on this conception, covers any experience that registers negatively for the subject just on account of how it feels.

In contrast to these broad conceptions, suffering is often construed more narrowly as an experience that is intense, attributable to the subject as opposed to a body part (unlike sensory pain and bodily discomfort), and more emotional than sensory.[4] One might claim that suffering is not really an emotion because it does not orient the subject for a particular type of adaptive action (as, say, fear orients one to escape danger and anger orients one to retaliate).[5] Addressing that matter would require defending a particular theory of emotions, something I am reluctant to do. In any case, it seems accurate to say that suffering in a relatively narrow sense is *an emotional state*. By this I mean that, in suffering, the subject makes a cognitive appraisal of her overall situation in evaluative terms.[6] Although such evaluative terms are relatively sophisticated in the case of some emotions, such as guilt ("I did something wrong") and anger ("He wronged me [or someone I care about]"), in the case of suffering, the evaluative terms may be quite primitive, involving only reference to the subject's own welfare ("This is terrible for me") or to the present situation ("This is terrible"), which affects his welfare. If I am correct in conjecturing that prelinguistic human beings are capable of having such thoughts in nonlinguistic form, then lack of linguistic capacity does not preclude one's having emotional states.

Along the lines of what I am calling a narrow conception, Eric Cassell has influentially defined suffering as a "state of severe distress associated with events that threaten the integrity of [a] person."[7] He explicitly states his view regarding what sorts of subjects are capable of suffering: "Only persons suffer."[8] Cassell's analysis is motivated by such observations as the following. Whether and how much one suffers—in this narrower sense that clearly distinguishes suffering from (sensory) pain—can vary in accordance with attitudes or expectations about whatever pain or distress one is in and the context in which it occurs. Even the pain of a mild headache can lead to great distress and suffering if the pain endures with no end in sight, or if the subject believes the headache to be a sign of impending physical collapse. Conversely, soldiers have sometimes received major injuries yet apparently suffered little because of the relief of anticipated removal from battle or positive attitudes about the heroic context in which injuries were incurred. Distance runners who experience pain and discomfort in a race may or may not suffer, or may suffer more or less, depending on such psychological factors as how they evaluate their performance and whether they are confident or fearful about the remainder of the race. Thus, any *meanings* one assigns to one's situation, as well as one's expectations for the future, are critical determinants of whether and how extensively a subject suffers.

When Cassell speaks of threats to integrity, he uses "integrity" in the sense of wholeness. The idea is that suffering involves a response to a sense that *the subject herself* is threatened in a substantial way—as when a persisting headache is understood to threaten physical doom or psychological collapse, or a troubled effort in a competition is taken to mean that one may well fail.

Suffering bears a close relationship to distress. Distress, which includes a wide variety of psychological phenomena, may be understood as a typically unpleasant emotional response to the perception of environmental challenges or to equilibrium-disrupting internal stimuli.[9] It may be caused by such diverse phenomena as the sight of a predator, the belief that one may fail, or diarrhea. The precise relationship between distress and suffering is a subtle matter. Perhaps suffering is a form of severe distress, as Cassell claims. Or maybe suffering is distinguishable from distress but closely associated with it, as in the idea that one can suffer in response to distress. One might be nervous, notice one's heartbeat, and fly into a panic attack. We might describe this as suffering (the panic attack) as a response to distress (nervousness). I suppose we could equally well describe it as mild distress growing into severe distress, consistent with the idea that suffering is a form of distress. In any case, the conceptual difference between these two ways of specifying the relationship between distress and suffering will have no significant bearing on our investigation.

In addition to having some close relationship to distress, suffering is also closely related to pain, even if (on the present, narrow conception of suffering) it is clearly distinguishable from pain. In a helpful summary statement, Cassell notes that "... people in pain frequently report suffering from pain when they feel out of control, when the pain is overwhelming, when the source of the pain is unknown, when the meaning of the pain is dire, or when the pain is apparently without end."[10] Suffering here involves an emotional response to the experience of pain. To be a response to pain, of course, requires being distinct from pain. Authors who underscore this distinction often claim that suffering requires self-awareness.[11] If suffering necessarily involves attitudes towards the future—in particular, one's own future—it makes sense to specify that suffering requires *temporal* self-awareness, an awareness of oneself as persisting over time. If we add to this claim the traditional assumption that only *persons* are self-aware, we arrive at Cassell's thesis that only persons suffer.

Later, I will consider evidence suggesting the great implausibility of this thesis. For now, it is worth considering what the thesis—which some, like Cassell, build into the very definition of suffering—implies. Assuming the concept of a person is defined in terms of psychological capacities, and in such a way as to exclude all or nearly all nonhuman animals, then a person is (roughly) a being who has the capacity for relatively complex forms of consciousness as found in normal human beings of, say, two years or older.[12] With this understanding of personhood, the thesis that only persons can suffer implies that a human infant on whom scalding water is poured does not suffer. Nor does the dog who is left unanesthetized during hours-long surgery or who is slowly tortured by a sadist. I find these implications very hard to believe. But the empirical evidence bearing on this question will prove indispensable to any confident judgment.[13]

In delineating the narrow conception of suffering, it seems fairly plausible to say that all and only beings capable of highly unpleasant emotional states can suffer. Whether the assignment of meaning is necessary for suffering is a question we may leave open. For those who do assign meaning to their circumstances, this factor plays a major role in whether and to what extent they suffer. But perhaps the assignment of meaning is not a necessary condition. Insofar as it may be possible for a young infant devoid of temporal self-awareness to suffer from scalding water or the like, it is also debatable whether any temporal self-awareness is necessary for suffering.[14] At the same time, such self-awareness may be necessary for particular types or manifestations of suffering, such as miserable remorse for a past action or agonizing dread of a future possibility. A being devoid of temporal self-awareness cannot have suffering related to remorse or dread yet may be capable of suffering in a more cognitively primitive way—although, again, even the latter claim is disputable.

One thing that is clear is that suffering, in the narrow sense under consideration, requires strong affect. This is consistent with Cassell's characterization of suffering as a state of *severe* distress. And it is consistent with the observation that mild pain typically doesn't occasion suffering and that even great pain doesn't if the subject does not become very emotional or distressed. I therefore suggest this working definition: *suffering is a highly unpleasant emotional experience associated with significant pain or distress*. Saying "associated with" bypasses the conceptual issue of whether suffering *is* a form of distress. Mentioning pain is worthwhile insofar as pain so often occasions suffering. Requiring that either pain or distress must be significant accurately accommodates our judgments about when suffering (in the narrow sense) occurs. For example, while it is true that one can suffer from even mild pain if it is sufficiently long-lasting, or is interpreted as signifying one's doom, it is also clear that in such a case, one's distress would be significant.

Having now analyzed suffering both in a very broad sense and in a narrow sense, we may turn to the question of what sorts of creatures can suffer, beginning with suffering in the narrow sense just sketched.

What Sorts of Beings Can Suffer in the Narrow Sense?

What sorts of creatures can suffer in the sense of experiencing a highly unpleasant emotional state associated with significant pain or distress? My contention is that if we bracket radical skepticism about animal consciousness in general (a position I will address later), there is a strong case that many animals can suffer in this narrow sense. I have in mind at least all mammals, probably birds, and quite possibly other vertebrate species. Of course, to say that these nonhuman animals can suffer in this sense is not to claim that all beings capable of suffering can suffer in precisely the same ways (or to the same degree). Perhaps a relatively broad range of animals, as well as human infants, can suffer in being miserable in some cognitively uncomplicated way. Only those beings with temporal self-awareness can suffer in a way involving guilt or dread. Presumably only persons can suffer existential angst at the possible nonexistence of a deity or the likely eventual extinction of the human race. Thus, to claim that a certain type of creature can suffer in the narrow sense is simply to claim that that type of creature can suffer in *some* way that meets the relevant criteria. The same point applies to suffering in the broad sense, which we will consider later.

What considerations support my assertion that many nonhuman animals can suffer in the narrow sense? First, it is a plausible thesis that many animals experience emotions. (Remember that suffering in this sense is an emotional state.) While the emotional life of animals may be impoverished in comparison with ours, there are strong grounds for believing that many animals experience fear at the perception of a threat, anxiety in unfamiliar settings in which vigilant alertness is adaptive, and surprise when expectations are suddenly dashed and reorienting one's perceptions is the thing to do.[15] Some social animals apparently experience sadness at the loss of close associates and a sort of primitive anger when they or their dependents are harmed or threatened by others against whom retaliation is possible. On the positive side of the emotional spectrum, the behavior of some animals gives the irresistible impression of expressing contentment, gladness, sometimes even joy. To focus our discussion, let us concentrate on fear, which may be the most primitive and widely experienced emotion among animals.

Along with anxiety, anger, sexual arousal, and several other states, fear is associated with the autonomic sympathetic nervous system, which is designed for action (or preparation for action, which may involve temporary inhibition) in what might broadly be called *emergency* situations. Fibers in this nervous system increase heart rate and general arousal while decreasing digestion and other processes associated with rest. Also implicated is the limbic system, comprising a relatively primitive group of structures that are essential to emotion and motivation. Fear is clearly adaptive for animals unable to get by on simple stimulus–response routines. It motivates appropriate, focused, and often flexible responses to perceived dangers.

The adaptive value of fear is evident, providing one reason to think that natural selection might have conferred this emotional capacity on many animals. There is also the fact that much animal behavior appears to be fearful, for example, attempts to flee at the perception of danger. But consideration of behavior, even in the context of careful reflection on natural selection, is not sufficient to attribute fear—or any other emotion—to animals. An unconscious state that functions similarly to an emotion might generate the behavior and confer the adaptive functioning favored by natural selection. We need to consider further evidence.

What, then, about the physiology and neuroanatomy of fear? Nearly all vertebrates—specifically, all jawed vertebrates—have an autonomic sympathetic nervous system, and at least most vertebrate taxa feature a limbic system.[16] Indeed, benzodiazepine receptors, which are believed to be part of the neurochemical substrate that mediates *anxiety*, have been found in nearly all vertebrate species investigated.[17] (The exception was a cartilaginous fish; the three bony fishes studied had the receptors.) I am assuming that evidence for the capacity for anxiety would a fortiori count as evidence for the capacity for fear. Of course, to say that a particular animal such as an amphibian experiences fear or anxiety is not to say that its fearful or anxious states are as cognitively complex as corresponding human or even mammalian states; it is, however, to say that the attributed emotional states are consciously experienced.

How confident should we be that the presence of these systems and apparently fearful behavior in animals indicate actual fear, a consciously felt emotion? In a later section, I will address radical skepticism about animal consciousness. For now, it is worth noting a few further points about neuroanatomy. First, all mammals have a neocortex, the very thin six layers of gray matter that surround the deeper white matter of the cerebrum. Many experts believe that the neocortex is critical to consciousness in humans and, presumably, other mammals. While only mammals have a neocortex, birds, reptiles, and to some extent amphibians have a type of cortex (sometimes called a *pallium*), which may play a role in the conscious processing of their experiences. My present claim is not that the experience of fear requires a cortex, a claim that might be doubted in the view of the possibility of different neural structures playing this role in animal taxa (not to mention the presence of benzodiazepine receptors in bony fishes). My point is simply that, even if fear is impossible without a cortex, many vertebrate species possess this piece of equipment.

The forgoing observations suggest that many animals experience fear. Presumably, among these animals, many experience some other emotions. Thus, the fact that suffering in the narrow sense is an emotional state does not present a conceptual or empirical obstacle to the claim that many animals can suffer.

Then again, suffering in the narrow sense is a *highly unpleasant* emotional experience. That means that a subject must be capable of strong affect to be able to suffer. Perhaps some animals who have emotional lives experience only weak or dim affect. The dimmer their conscious experiences in general, the more likely this is the case. So, there may be animals who can experience mild fear, say, but nothing affectively strong enough to call suffering.

But consider this. Among animals who experience emotions, it would be adaptive to experience them to different degrees, roughly corresponding to the extent of urgency in a given situation, so as to motivate behaviors to different degrees. For example, an immediate threat of mortal danger should occasion great fear, whereas a more remote threat of moderate danger should occasion less because it may not be adaptive to react right away in the latter case if one is, say, nursing a child or eating. And, if some animals can be mildly afraid, moderately afraid, or terrified, it is fairly plausible that they can experience distress of different degrees and, when distress is significant, suffering.

It is worth remembering in this context that pain varies in degree and often occasions suffering. In humans, pain perception involves a *sensory dimension*, which informs a subject of the location and intensity of a noxious stimulus, and an *affective-motivational dimension*, which motivates adaptive behavior. It is believed that the anterior cingulate cortex (ACC), a portion of the neocortex, is implicated in the experience of the affective dimension of pain,[18] which is associated with suffering.[19] All mammals have an ACC, strengthening the case that at least they can suffer.

At this point, however, I would like to suggest that suffering in the narrow sense, while very important insofar as it involves *highly* unpleasant experiences, is not the only kind of suffering that should concern us. All unpleasant experience is, by definition, disagreeable or aversive to its subject; all such experience is disliked for the way it feels. So, suffering in the broad sense that covers all unpleasant experience is, in a way, more fundamental than suffering in the narrow sense. I am assuming that there is *some* reason not to cause anyone needless pain or distress regardless of its intensity. (Because pain has not only a sensory dimension but also an affective dimension, I assume that all pain is at least slightly unpleasant.) Pain—even without suffering (in the narrow sense)—matters.

Some may find my insistence that pain matters overly solicitous and perhaps maddeningly impractical. Yet even they should admit that it is far more difficult to attribute *degrees* of unpleasantness than to attribute the occurrence of unpleasant experiences. Thus, we should be interested in knowing what sorts of subjects are sentient and therefore capable of experiencing pleasant and unpleasant experiences.

And, in the world as we know it, the best way to approach this issue is to ask what sorts of subjects have the capacity for consciousness.

Evidence for Consciousness in Animals

Before we consider evidence for consciousness in animals, we should illuminate our target, for "consciousness" has several meanings. First, consciousness is often distinguished from the state of being asleep or comatose. That one is awake or conscious in this sense—which has been called *creature consciousness*—does not directly entail any subjective mental states because even patients in a persistent vegetative state have sleep–wake cycles. By contrast, what Ned Block dubbed *access consciousness* involves the ability of a creature to detect salient features of its environment or body and use the information in responding appropriately—that is, in a coordinated, non–self-defeating way—in behavior or speech.[20] A fish, for example, may visually perceive a predator, gaining access consciousness of its presence, stop eating, and swim away. But the type of consciousness that is most important in this discussion—and the type that philosophers have in mind when using the unqualified term *consciousness*—is *phenomenal consciousness*, which involves subjective, qualitative experiences and not just the processing and coordinated deployment of salient information (as in access consciousness) or the state of being awake (as in creature consciousness). To employ Nagel's immortal phrase, when one is conscious in this sense, *there is something that it is like* to be one at that time.[21] It is not part of the concept of phenomenal consciousness that the subject be self-conscious or aware of herself; it is sufficient to be conscious of *anything* in the sense of having subjective, qualitative experiences of something.

The concept of phenomenal consciousness is central to our investigation, and some readers may find Nagel's definition less helpful than I do, so let me offer a few further remarks in an effort to clarify. Rocks are obviously not conscious in this sense. Neither are plants, which lack a brain or anything functionally similar to a brain. Some, but not all, animals—most obviously, normal human beings—have the capacity for consciousness. Now imagine some sort of animal endowed with a brain that can integrate lots of information about the environment, allowing the animal to respond to environmental contingencies in coordinated ways that enhance its prospects for survival and reproduction. This creature has access consciousness. What more is required to have phenomenal consciousness? The relevant information processing must generate *subjective experience*, which *feels like something*, for the creature to be phenomenally conscious at a given time. (Note that in this context, *feels* and related terms such as *feeling* do not imply affect or emotion; these terms simply offer another way of conveying qualitative, subjective experiences.) Now consider artificial intelligence. Imagine a robot that can move around, take in and integrate information of different kinds about its environment and body, and use that information in performing tasks and avoiding damage from objects in the environment. What would have to be the case for this robot to have phenomenal consciousness? The robot's information processing would need to generate *subjective experience*, which *feels like something or has qualitative features*. What occurs within the robot, therefore, could not be described in purely quantitative terms. Some qualitative description (e.g., "painful," "fascinating," "familiar seeming") would be necessary to describe its experiences.

Because consciousness in this sense is essentially subjective, it is more difficult to demonstrate rigorously that a creature is phenomenally conscious than it is to show that he is awake or that he has access consciousness. Difficult or not, the attribution of phenomenal consciousness is our primary concern because only this kind of consciousness is closely tied to the suffering in the broad sense—that is, unpleasant experiences. I assume here that something cannot be pleasant or unpleasant unless it is actually *felt*—consciously experienced—and that any creatures endowed with phenomenal consciousness are capable of having at least some pleasant and unpleasant feelings. In other words, I assume that in our world (not all possible worlds), sentient creatures and creatures with the capacity for consciousness are the same set of creatures.

So, how can we know whether animals are phenomenally conscious (hereafter, *conscious,* for short)? One might simply appeal to common sense. If we were to poll the public—asking, "Do you believe that animals are conscious, that they not only react to stimuli, and interact with the world, but typically have subjective experiences in doing so?"—I am fairly sure that nearly everyone would answer affirmatively for a broad class of animals that includes at least the vertebrates. Certainly, our spontaneous perceptions of the behavior of most, if not all, animals incorporate the assumption that they are conscious: we perceive their feeding, walking, interacting, and so forth as conscious behavior—as involving feeling or subjective experience. One might take this to settle the matter, as John Searle more or less does,[22] and say that we know that, say, the dog is conscious in chasing the ball because we just see that she is.

While this may sound dogmatic, I confess to having *some* sympathy for this approach—in fact, quite a lot of sympathy when it comes to animals as closely related to us as mammals. Yet, this "I just see that a wriggling fish is conscious" approach is inadequate for our purposes. Natural selection has apparently endowed us with an innate tendency to read animal behavior as conscious[23]; and it is surely conceivable that this perceptual tendency was adaptive, in terms of predicting animals' behavior, without being accurate about animal minds with respect to the *full range* of animals whose behavior we perceive as conscious. Thus, further work is required.

At the same time, to deny that, say, mammals are conscious is so violently contrary to common sense—which ought to count for something—that those who endorse such a radical denial shoulder a burden of proof. In the next section, I will argue that the most promising effort to carry this burden is unsuccessful. What about animals whose consciousness is less obvious than that of mammals? As noted in the previous paragraph, our instinctive attributions of consciousness are fallible. So, we need to consider evidence. My contention is this: what we ought to believe, given available evidence, is that at least mammals, birds, reptiles, amphibians, and the members of some fish species are conscious creatures. There is also considerable reason to believe that, among the invertebrates, cephalopods (octopi and squid) are conscious creatures.

Let us begin with a chart compiled by Gary Varner, who collated information from four publications that addressed, in relatively comprehensive ways, evidence for animal consciousness—more specifically, pain.[24] Varner identified six indicators that are reasonably considered relevant in attributing pain to animals: (1) the presence of nociceptors (neural end organs that detect noxious stimuli); (2) possession of a central nervous system; (3) whether the nociceptors are connected to the central nervous system; (4) the presence of endogenous opioids (e.g., endorphins, enkephalins); (5) whether the creature's behavior in response to noxious stimuli is modified by analgesics; and (6) whether its responses are analogous to human responses. I will add a further indicator, which is relevant to the attribution of anxiety and fear: (7) the presence of benzodiazepine receptors. On the basis of the collated findings, Varner maintained the following: mammals and birds satisfied all these criteria. Herpetafauna (reptiles and amphibians) and fish satisfied most of them, but it was somewhat doubtful that they had nociceptors, and it was unknown whether their responses were modified by analgesics. The cephalopods, uniquely among the invertebrates, scored the same as herpetafauna and fish, except that for cephalopods, it was also unknown whether they had endogenous opioids.

The data on which Varner relied are now somewhat old. More recent findings confirm that reptiles and teleost fishes (a classification that includes most extant fish species) have nociceptors and are responsive to analgesics.[25] I am willing to assume the same about amphibians, who lie evolutionarily "between" fish and reptiles. Meanwhile, I am unaware of further data that significantly clarify the case of cephalopods.[26] As for the indicator that I added to the list—presence of benzodiazepine receptors—we have seen that mammals, birds, reptiles, amphibians, and some fish species make this grade.

Of course, other sorts of evidence are also relevant, but most of them have not been so thoroughly investigated across animal taxa. One might suggest, however, that we add this indicator to our list: the presence of some sort of cortex. That addition would strengthen the case for mammals, birds, and reptiles, weaken the case for fish and invertebrates, and leave amphibians somewhere in between. But the relevance of this putative indicator is highly debatable—and debated. In an influential discussion, James Rose has argued that fish are incapable of conscious experience.[27] Advancing a spirited argument that a functioning neocortex is necessary for consciousness in mammals, he underscores the absence of a neocortex in fish (and other nonmammalian species). Not surprisingly, this reasoning has been challenged. According to Chandroo and coauthors, available evidence indicates that the fish forebrain, even without a neocortex, may have evolved to support conscious experience.[28] And we have already noted that teleost fish have nociceptors and demonstrate relief from analgesics. It seems highly possible that convergent evolution permitted the independent emergence of consciousness in more than one evolutionary line with somewhat differing neural substrata. Indeed, there is now some reason to doubt that a functional cortex is strictly necessary for consciousness *even in humans*.[29] So, I will decline to add the presence of a cortex to the list of indicators of consciousness.

It may be worthwhile to mention some other sorts of evidence, even if they have been sought in a limited range of species. Some of this evidence is discussed by Adam Shriver.[30] To elaborate on a point made earlier, experts believe that pain in humans involves two largely (but probably not entirely) discreet systems: a sensory-discriminatory system, which conveys information about the bodily location and intensity of a noxious stimulus to the somatosensory cortex; and an affective-motivational system, which makes the experience unpleasant and motivates adaptive action by projecting signals through the anterior cingulate cortex to the frontal lobe.[31] To a significant extent, the systems can be dissociated—for example, hypnosis or morphine can shut down the affective-motivational system while the sensory-discriminatory system is working. In rats, lesioning the ACC results in persistence of a withdrawal reflex in the presence of a noxious stimulus but less effort to get away. In monkeys, damage to the insular cortex—which, like the ACC, is part of the affective-motivational system—yields similar behavior. These findings strongly suggest that rats and monkeys normally experience both the sensory and the affective dimensions of pain, and at least the affective dimension would entail consciousness.

But pain behavior is not the only sort of behavior that can be suggestive of consciousness. For example, as Colin Allen notes, monkeys whose primary visual cortex has been damaged show impairments that resemble those of human blindsight patients, who apparently have partial, unconscious visual perception.[32] Normal humans have conscious visual experiences that allow for normal responses to visual stimuli; damage to the striate cortex can destroy conscious vision apparently without destroying partial, unconscious vision—causing blindsight. Because monkeys with similar brain damage seem to have visual limitations similar to those of human blindsight patients, it is reasonable to infer that normal monkeys, like normal humans, also have conscious visual experience.

Most of the present discussion of evidence for consciousness across animal taxa has focused on Varner's synthesis of the findings of various studies, supplemented by some updates about nociceptors and analgesic response as well as consideration of benzodiazepine receptors. Let me here mention another systematic review of evidence, which incorporates more discussion of animal behavior than does Varner's synthesis, while focusing on just two nonmammalian types of animals: birds and cephalopods. Edelman and coauthors review the various types of evidence at a level of detail that would be excessively space consuming to summarize here, so let me just note their conclusion. They argue that there is a strong case for consciousness in birds, while the case for cephalopods remains open.[33] Their findings are consistent with what I have argued.

My thesis, again, is that we should believe on the basis of available evidence that at least mammals, birds, reptiles, amphibians, and members of some fish species are conscious creatures, that they are capable of having (phenomenal) consciousness; we should also be very open to the possibility that cephalopods are among this group. But let us not rest here. There is a theory of consciousness that can reintroduce skeptical doubts into our investigation. Although I consider this theory and its implications intellectual mischief, I have been impressed at how seriously some philosophers take this theory. And philosophers of mind and cognitive sciences often influence the conceptual scaffoldings deployed by comparative psychologists and ethologists. Meanwhile, the findings of these scientists sometimes influence public opinion. So, this theory deserves consideration and a response.

The Higher-Order Thought Theory of Consciousness

In discussing consciousness as a necessary condition of suffering, we refer to phenomenal consciousness, which involves subjective, qualitative experiences. Nowadays, as a result both of the Freudian revolution in psychology and all its intellectual progeny and of contemporary cognitive psychology, we are comfortable with the proposition that some mental states are unconscious. The problem of *state* consciousness is to distinguish mental states that are (phenomenally) conscious from mental states that are not. Higher-order theories of consciousness agree on this general claim: a mental state is conscious if and only if a creature is conscious of that mental state in some suitable way.[34] So, for example, having pain does not entail that one feels it, that is, experiences it consciously. Conscious pain occurs when the creature not only has pain but also is conscious of having it in some way specified by the theory. A creature whose pain and other mental states were always unconscious would never suffer.[35]

Among higher-order theories of consciousness, there are two broad types: *inner sense theories*, which ascribe to each creature capable of having conscious states an inner monitoring mechanism that tracks mental states, and *higher-order thought (HOT) theories*. Only the HOT approach will concern us here because it furnishes the most developed grounds for skepticism about animal consciousness. According to this approach, as it is commonly formulated, a mental state is conscious if and only if a creature has a thought about it. One feels one's pain, on this view, only if one thinks about it. Without the higher-order thought about pain, pain doesn't feel like anything.

This approach does not automatically imply that nonhuman animals lack conscious experiences and therefore suffering. After all, many animals may be capable of thinking. And perhaps they sometimes think not only about their environment and about what to do but also about their mental states, such as their pain, hunger, or sensory perceptions. If so, they can experience these states consciously. (Again, throughout this section, I am using the term *conscious* as short for "phenomenally conscious.") Now, one might insist that only creatures with full-blown language can have such thoughts, perhaps on the grounds that thinking implicates concepts, the possession of which requires sophisticated language. One would then have to contend with the rather incredible implication that ordinary human infants have no conscious feelings at all. But intuitive plausibility is not the only theoretical desideratum, and some HOT theorists accept this implication.

In discussions of animals' mental life, the HOT theory that has received the most attention, by far, is that of Peter Carruthers. In a recent article, Carruthers states that he doubts there would be any need for a creature to evolve the capacity to monitor its own mental states unless the creature could think about them.[36] This motivates a focus on higher-order *thoughts* rather than inner sense or a monitoring mechanism (lest anyone think we were neglecting the type of higher-order theory that posits an inner sense). Specifically, Carruthers holds that a state is conscious for a creature if and only if it's *available to be thought about* by that creature. He believes that there is no compelling evidence that any nonhuman animals are capable of having HOTs and therefore expresses skepticism that any animals have conscious states.[37] Why does he think there is such a close connection between phenomenal consciousness and HOTs? His view is that the latter evolved alongside so-called theory of mind: the ability to have beliefs and attitudes about other individuals' mental states. Theory of mind evolved to allow a highly social type of creature, hominids, to interpret each other's behavior more accurately: in other words, to engage in fine-grained behavior reading through "mind reading." If another hominid is vocalizing at you, you can better predict and respond to his behavior if you have a sense of what he thinks, wants, and intends. Because we know that humans typically have a theory of mind, and because (Carruthers believes) there is no compelling evidence that any nonhuman animals have a theory of mind, we may responsibly conjecture that animals' mental states are devoid of (phenomenal) consciousness. They do not feel like anything or have any qualitative, subjective features. So, animals can't suffer.

I believe that Carruthers's view of animal minds verges far from the truth and fails to motivate responsible skepticism about animal consciousness. Let me advance several rebuttals.

First, it is extremely hard to believe that neither apes, nor dolphins, nor elephants can feel anything or be conscious of anything. Anyone who does not sincerely doubt that these complex creatures have conscious experiences should not embrace the HOT view that generates this implication. Now, there is a lively debate about whether some nonhuman primates have higher-order thoughts and a theory of mind, so a HOT theorist might say that her theory can accommodate the intuitive judgment I've invoked: that these animals have conscious experiences. But our intuitions are not much less insistent that cats and dogs also have conscious experiences, yet there is no compelling evidence that they have higher-order thoughts. Any theory that implies that cats and dogs are incapable of consciousness bears a burden of proof. Carruthers, while perhaps accepting this burden, would assert that our intuitions on the matter of cats and dogs are erroneous. Presumably, he would say the same about young human children before they achieve a theory of mind: these children have no conscious experiences. Since episodic memories, memories of particular experiences, are impossible unless one was conscious when one had the relevant experiences, those of us who believe that we have memories of our toddler days must all be mistaken. Or else we acquired a theory of mind very young. Or else Carruthers's view is incorrect.

Consider a second problem. Higher-order thought is supposed to make a mental state conscious. Presumably, in most cases, the HOT is not *itself* conscious. If it were—as perhaps it is in cases of introspection—there would have to be an even higher HOT that made it, the first HOT, conscious. In any case, to avoid an infinite regress of HOTs, some HOT must be *unconscious* in rendering conscious the mental state it's about. The problem is one of explanatory mystery: How can an unconscious state, an unconscious thought, make another mental state conscious?[38] How does this work? This request for an explanation is not, of course, a devastating argument. But it adds to the sense that the theory is a very odd one with more difficulties—in terms of raising questions and bearing intuitive costs—than advantages.

Third, a thought experiment suggests that the theory omits a necessary condition for consciousness. Imagine a robot equipped with sophisticated light-pattern sensors, which function as eyes, and other sensors. The robot can move around in response to environmental conditions and process information about its sensory data in ways that provide information about its own perspective or state (e.g., its location, its physical condition). All this seems compatible with an unconscious robot. Yet this robot, we have imagined without any conceptual or empirical absurdity, has experiences (unconscious ones) that are available to be thought about (unconsciously). The availability to HOT and even the occurrence of such thoughts do not seem to entail that this robot has conscious states. Carruthers, it seems, has failed to capture some necessary condition of what it is to be conscious. I think the necessary condition is simply this: that the state is felt or subjectively experienced.

One might charge me here with a double standard. For I say that the robot, despite such and such behavior and information processing, might be unconscious, while I also claim that various animals, who feature such and such behavior and information processing, ought to be judged conscious. But my position does not reflect a double standard. In the case of animals, I emphasize not only behavior and information processing but also physiology and neuroanatomy in the context of evolution. Of course, I know nothing about what hardware would be needed to enable a robot to have HOTs. But such a cognitive feat does not seem terribly complicated and would not seem to demand hardware (whatever it might be) that would generate consciousness.

A fourth difficulty has been noted by Colin Allen.[39] Carruthers's thesis that hominids evolved phenomenal consciousness as a means of better interpreting each other's minds, which underlies the HOT theory, is poorly motivated. On Carruthers's view, if my auditory experience of your vocalizations and my visual experience of your bodily movements are conscious, then they are available for me to think about, which allows me to manage interactions with you better than if I couldn't think about what I hear and see. So far, so good. But this account fails to explain our conscious experiences more generally. As Allen puts it, "there seems little to interpret regarding others' mental states in the way they smell or taste to us, nor in the way our stomachs feel when we have not eaten for a while."[40] Much of our conscious life has nothing to do with the ability to interpret other people. Moreover, we are never consciously aware of other people's pheromones, yet our unconscious perception of them affects our interpersonal behavior. So, it seems that there is no tight connection between consciousness and behavior-guiding systems, even in highly social, mind-interpreting animals like us. Considering the overall oddity of Carruthers's view, he owes us some very compelling grounds for accepting the theory despite its oddity. In my judgment, he has not provided such grounds. He has not carried his considerable burden of proof.

Meanwhile, there are some promising functional accounts of consciousness that would support its attribution to many animals. One conjecture is that consciousness evolved to enable creatures to manage complexity in unfamiliar situations.[41] Consider processes that, in humans, can occur either consciously or unconsciously—such as placing your feet while running. These processes work better unconsciously in familiar settings (say, running on smooth terrain) but work better consciously in the presence of novelty or unpredictability (say, running amid pot holes). Perhaps, then, consciousness increases our capacity to manage complexity. Another conjecture, motivated by a variety of experimental results, is that consciousness plays a significant role in learning to avoid noxious stimuli—rather than repeatedly encountering and withdrawing from them—and in correcting one's own perceptual errors.[42] This conjecture coheres well with the speculation that consciousness helps an agent to manage complexity and novelty. Those are the sorts of circumstances in which learning and self-correction are adaptive. A third conjecture is that the evolutionary function of phenomenal consciousness is to enable, or at least enhance, access consciousness, with which the brain integrates information available to distinct sensory and cognitive systems, thereby directing coordinated, effective behavior.[43] A fourth account—which partly overlaps with the second—focuses on (conscious) pain in particular. I find it elegant in its simplicity as well as plausible:

> All animals face hazards that cause tissue damage and most have nociceptive reflex responses that protect them from such damage. However, some taxa have also evolved the capacity for pain experience, presumably to enhance long-term protection through behavior modification based on memory of the unpleasant nature of pain.[44]

Unpleasantness, which is motivating, is impossible without (phenomenal) consciousness.

All these accounts provide more plausible stories about why consciousness might have evolved than Carruthers's mind-reading story. Further, these more promising accounts do not generate the sorts of problems that Carruthers's theory has. Thus, I conclude that Carruthers's HOT theory of consciousness furnishes no compelling grounds for turning a skeptical eye toward what has been marshaled as evidence for consciousness in animals. Many animals have phenomenal consciousness. They can suffer in the broad sense of the term, and a significant subset can also suffer in the narrow sense.

Some Implications for Bioethics

What implications do our findings about suffering have for bioethics? In briefly addressing this question, I will assume that (intentionally or negligently) causing suffering—whether in the weak or the strong sense—to any being we have good reason to believe is capable of suffering is *pro tanto* wrong. That is, causing suffering tends to be wrong and requires special justification in order to be permissible. This is because beings who are capable of suffering in at least the broad sense have interests, and beings who have interests have moral status.

This has implications for human beings who are sentient—that is, have the capacity for consciousness—but whose personhood or full moral status is contested. Infants, late fetuses, and deeply demented individuals who have yet to lapse into a coma all have moral status and a morally important interest in avoiding suffering. This implication leaves open whether such human beings have full or only partial moral status. And it certainly doesn't settle important questions about how these individuals may be treated. But the acknowledgement of moral status for these nonparadigm (yet sentient) human beings should terminate any discussions that tacitly assume that these individuals lack moral importance in their own right. Their capacity to suffer must not be overlooked.

Turning now to animals, we can draw the implication that animal research is morally permissible only if (to state just one necessary condition) it does not impose unnecessary suffering on its subjects. What counts as "necessary suffering" will turn on various considerations, including one's view about how much moral status animals have. However one answers it, though, the present point applies to nearly all research animals. It does not apply to insects, horseshoe crabs, and other invertebrate species regarding which there is little evidence of consciousness. But it applies to all vertebrate species (except perhaps some fish species) and cephalopods. Moreover, because there is an overwhelming case that mammals can suffer in the narrow sense and a strong case that birds can as well, the research community should assume that many harms caused to these animal subjects have the potential to be experienced as extremely aversive.

I also suggest, though I cannot defend the thesis here, that the capacity of animal subjects to suffer—and the moral status based on this capacity—means that we should reverse presumptions about animal research. The tendency within the biomedical research community is to presume that animal studies should precede human studies that involve risks for their subjects. I believe that the morally correct presumption leans in the opposite direction: we should presume that proposed animal studies are impermissible unless a persuasive justification is advanced, case by case, in their favor.

In addition, the field of bioethics ought to take animals far more seriously than it does at the present time. Bioethics conferences rarely schedule talks on ethical issues pertaining to animals, while journals rarely publish articles in the area. At a more personal level, hardly any bioethicists I know (at least in the United States) can be bothered to abstain from meat produced in factory farms, and surprisingly few of them even register any moral concern about the issue. A greater awareness of and seriousness about ethical issues as they pertain to animals would be a welcome development in American bioethics. I believe the facts about animal suffering recommend such a development.

Finally, to return to the "intellectual mischief" I have attempted to undermine in this paper, bioethicists should accept that the capacity to suffer is very well established among a wide array of animal species. Neither appeals to ignorance nor appeals to HOT theories of consciousness should be understood as justifying skepticism about animal consciousness and the capacity to suffer. The virtue of open-mindedness should not be confused with the vice of obtuseness, especially when the latter may serve to rationalize the mistreatment of sensitive creatures.

Notes

1. *Suffering and Moral Responsibility* (New York: Oxford University Press, 1999), 11.

2. Ibid., 14.

3. Ibid.

4. In speaking of "sensory pain" and "bodily discomfort," I do not mean to suggest that any sort of pain or discomfort is *entirely* sensory or bodily. On the contrary, I believe that all pain and discomfort have an affective component: unpleasantness. The reason for the modifiers "sensory" and "bodily" is that what is sometimes called "emotional pain" and "emotional discomfort" may not be sensory or bodily in the relevant sense at all.

5. See Peter Moskowitz, "A Theory of Suffering," *The Pain Practitioner* 16 (2006): 74–81, at 76.

6. For good discussions of emotions as involving evaluative appraisals, see Patricia Greenspan, *Emotions and Reasons* (New York: Routledge, 1988) and Nancy Sherman, "Emotions," in *Encyclopedia of Bioethics*, 3rd ed., Stephen Post, ed. (New York: Macmillan, 2004), 2:740–745.

7. *The Nature of Suffering and the Goals of Medicine* (New York: Oxford University Press, 1991), 33. See also Cassell, "Pain and Suffering," *The Encyclopedia of Bioethics*, 2nd ed., Warren Reich, ed. (New York: Macmillan, 1995), 1963.

8. Ibid.

9. For elaboration, see my *Taking Animals Seriously: Mental Life and Moral Status* (Cambridge, UK: Cambridge University Press, 1996), 116–117.

10. *The Nature of Suffering and the Goals of Medicine*, 36

11. See, e.g., Daniel Dennett, *Brainchildren* (Cambridge, MA: MIT Press, 1998), 347; and Michael Tye, *Consciousness, Color, and Content* (Cambridge, MA: MIT Press, 2000), 182.

12. For fuller discussions, see my "Great Apes, Dolphins, and the Concept of Personhood," *Southern Journal of Philosophy* 35 (1997): 301–320; and *Human Identity and Bioethics* (Cambridge, UK: Cambridge University Press, 2005), 3–7.

13. At a workshop in Amsterdam a few years ago, Cassell acknowledged in conversation with me that animals, not only persons, can suffer. His written statements reflect an earlier-held view.

14. Even if temporal self-awareness is necessary for suffering, perhaps because the former is necessary for experiencing emotional states, there is, I think, a strong case that many animals have such self-awareness. See my "Self-Awareness in Animals," in *The Philosophy of Animal Minds*, Robert Lurz, ed. (Cambridge, UK: Cambridge University Press, 2009), 201–217.

15. I discuss the evidence in *Taking Animals Seriously*, chap. 5.

16. Regarding the latter, less well-known point, see L. L. Bruce and T. J. Neary, "The Limbic System of Tetrapods: A Comparative Analysis of Cortical and Amygdalar Populations," *Brain Behavior and Evolution* 46 (1995): 224–234; and Guenther Stockinger, "Human Limbic System = Fish Telencephalon," *Spiegel Online* (11 March 2011).

17. M. Nielsen, C. Braestrup, R. F. Squires, "Evidence for a Late Evolutionary Appearance of a Brain-Specific Benzodiazepine Receptor," *Brain Research* 141 (1978): 342–346.

18. See Colin Allen, Perry Fuchs, Adam Shriver, and Hilary Wilson, "Deciphering Animal Pain," in *Pain: New Essays on Its Nature and the Methodology of Its Study*, Murat Aydede, ed. (Cambridge, MA: MIT Press, 2005), 351–366.

19. Moskowitz argues that the ACC and its connections with certain other brain parts "play an important, if not central, role in the experience of suffering," ("A Theory of Suffering," 78).

20. "On a Confusion about a Function of Consciousness," *Behavioral and Brain Sciences* 18 (1995): 227–247.

21. See, e.g., Nagel, "What Is It Like to Be a Bat?" *Philosophical Review* 83 (1974): 435–450.

22. "Animal Minds," *Ethica & Animali* 9 (1998): 37–50.

23. For valuable reflections on this matter, see Adam Arico et al., "The Folk Psychology of Consciousness," *Mind & Language* 26 (2011): 327–352.

24. Gary Varner, *In Nature's Interests?* (New York: Oxford University Press, 1998). The studies Varner cites are Jane Smith and Kenneth Boyd, ed., *Lives in the Balance* (New York: Oxford University Press, 1991); David DeGrazia and Andrew Rowan, "Pain, Suffering, and Anxiety in Animals and Humans," *Theoretical Medicine* 12 (1991): 193–211; Patrick Bateson, "Assessment of Pain in Animals," *Animal Behavior* 42 (1991): 827–839; and Margaret Rose and David Adams, "Evidence for Pain and Suffering in Other Animals," in *Animal Experimentation*, Gill Langley, ed. (New York: Chapman and Hall, 1989): 42–71.

25. See Craig Moseley, "Pain and Nociception in Reptiles," *Veterinary Clinics of North America* 14 (2011): 45–60; Lynne Sneddon, Victoria Braithwaite, and Michael Gentle, "Do Fishes Have Nociceptors? Evidence for the Evolution for a Vertebrate Sensory System," *Proceedings of the Royal Society of London* 270 (2003): 1115–1122; and Lynne Sneddon, "Evolution of Nociception in Vertebrates: Comparative Analysis of Lower Vertebrates," *Brain Research Reviews* 46 (2004): 123–130.

26. Regarding invertebrates more generally, Robert Elwood, who stresses behavioral evidence such as avoidance learning and responsiveness to analgesics, argues that such evidence is consistent with the thesis that crustaceans and mollusks (which include cephalopods) experience pain but is, at yet, inconclusive ("Pain and Suffering in Invertebrates?" *ILAR Journal* 52 [2011]: 175–84).

27. "The Neurobehavioral Nature of Fishes and the Question of Awareness and Pain," *Reviews in Fisheries Science* 10 (2002): 1–38.

28. Kristopher Chandroo, Stephanie Yoo, and Richard Moccia, "An Evaluation of Current Perspectives on Consciousness and Pain in Fishes," *Fish and Fisheries* 5 (2004): 281–295.

29. See Bjorn Merker, "Consciousness Without a Cerebral Cortex: A Challenge for Neuroscience and Medicine," *Behavioral and Brain Sciences* 30 (2007): 63–81. See also the open peer commentary on this article (*Behavioral and Brain Sciences* 30 [2007]: 81–134).

30. "Minding Mammals," *Philosophical Psychology* 19 (2006): 433–442, at 435–438.

31. While perhaps exaggerating the discreetness of these two systems, V. G. Hardcastle has influentially characterized them and many of the relevant empirical data (*The Myth of Pain* [Cambridge, MA: MIT Press, 1999]).

32. "Animal Consciousness," *Stanford Encyclopedia of Philosophy*, Edward Zalta, ed. (plato.stanford.edu/entries/consciousness-animal; entry published 12/23/95), sect. 5.1.

33. David Edelman, Bernard Baars, and Anil Seth, "Identifying Hallmarks of Consciousness in Non-Mammalian Species," *Consciousness and Cognition* 14 (2005): 169–187.

34. This is helpfully explained in David Rosenthal, "Higher-Order Theories of Consciousness," in *The Oxford Handbook of Philosophy of Mind*, Brian McLaughlin, Ansgar Bekermann, and Sven Walter, ed. (Oxford, UK: Clarendon, 2009), 239–252, at 240.

35. Here, for ease of reference, I use the term *pain* such that it is conceptually possible for there to be unconscious pain, even though this conflicts with my usual use of the term.

36. "Animal Mentality: Its Character, Extent, and Moral Significance," in *The Oxford Handbook of Animal Ethics*, ed. Tom Beauchamp and R. G. Frey (New York: Oxford University Press): 373–406, at 375.

37. Ibid.

38. Cf. Mark Rowlands, "Animals that Act for Moral Reasons," in *The Oxford Handbook of Animal Ethics*, ed. Tom Beauchamp and R. G. Frey (New York: Oxford University Press, 2011): 519–546, at 538–539.

39. "Animal Pain," *Nous* 38 (2004): 617–643, at 629–631.

40. Ibid., 630.

41. See my *Taking Animals Seriously*, 103–105; and Marian Stamp Dawkins, *Through Our Eyes Only? The Search for Animal Consciousness* (Oxford, UK: Freeman, 1993), 171–172.

42. See Colin Allen and Marc Bekoff, *Species of Mind* (Cambridge, MA: MIT Press, 1997), chap. 8 and Allen et al., "Deciphering Animal Pain," 355–361.

43. Shaun Nichols and Todd Grantham, "Adaptive Complexity and Phenomenal Consciousness," *Philosophy of Science* 67 (2000): 648–670. Their approach allows that access consciousness and phenomenal consciousness are logically distinct and separable in principle. The present conjecture is that in natural selection as it actually occurred, the two types of consciousness are closely connected and possibly the same phenomenon.

44. Elwood, "Pain and Suffering in Invertebrates?" 175.

PART THREE

Suffering in Policy and Law

8

Individual and Social Callousness toward Human Suffering

Daniel B. Hinshaw, Peter D. Jacobson, and Marisa P. Weisel

Human beings can be a fickle lot. They are capable of great generosity and may often demonstrate profound empathy for the distress of other members of their own species. Indeed, they may even invest deep emotion and lavish great attention upon other living creatures, which often become personal pets.[1] How is it possible that the human person can harbor such tender concern for the welfare of some while not infrequently exhibiting an apparently unfeeling response to or lack of awareness of the vulnerability and suffering of others? Those who have been drawn through altruistic impulses to enter the healing professions do not appear to have gained immunity to these paradoxical reactions to human need and suffering by their choice of profession.

Even this may be an overly optimistic viewpoint. In an essay titled *On Cruelty,* Montaigne said, "I fear that Nature herself has attached to Man something which goads him on towards inhumanity."[2] If callousness toward other human beings is inherent in the human condition, so are rationalizations for the behavior. We need only think about the searing debates over whether waterboarding constitutes torture and, even if it does, whether the ends (evidence gained that protects against further harms) justify the means. More to the point, human indifference or callousness toward suffering, or even the variable capacity of human beings to recognize and respond to suffering, can take on a life of its own if unchecked through law, professional ethics, or cultural norms.

Over time, this has been a particular concern for medical practice and, specifically, medical research. In this chapter, we will explore a number of factors that in their convergence may help elucidate and account for not only individual but also even societal callousness toward human suffering in the context of medical practice and research. In particular, we will highlight the role of medical research by examining the historical roots underlying the tragedy of the Tuskegee syphilis experiment, which exposed individuals and groups deemed to be subhuman or unworthy of society's protection to systematic abuse. If Montaigne is correct, human institutions will never eliminate the intentional or unintentional infliction of suffering (or the rationalizations), but they can certainly reduce its incidence and scope. Therefore, we posit that the post-Tuskegee reforms, put in place in the United States through the Belmont Report, have significantly reduced the scope and scale of suffering in medical practice and research. We also contend that a parallel cultural shift through the palliative care movement will further extend the Belmont Report's contributions. While hardly a panacea, these reforms have made it highly improbable that another Tuskegee will be tolerated.

Conflicting Goals in Medicine

A rapid shift of medicine's primary goal from relieving human suffering to diagnosing and treating disease accompanied the emergence of scientific medicine in the nineteenth century. For instance, work in anatomic pathology and germ theory established a scientific basis for understanding human illness, which led to new and often effective treatments for diseases. In turn, this created a revolution in health care. Newer treatments targeting specific diseases could be directly linked to dramatic relief of human misery, insofar as the diseases were sources of symptoms underlying a patient's suffering. Unfortunately, as medicine's emphasis shifted from relieving suffering to treating disease, physicians frequently neglected individual persons experiencing distress. Instead, physicians' primary focus became the diseases their patients harbored. As medicine became more scientific, practitioners of the healing art who still engaged primarily on a human level with their patients were increasingly viewed with suspicion; compassion might be a cover for ignorance and incompetence.

Two examples from the nineteenth century illustrate these issues within their cultural context. The first is a short story by the Russian author, Turgenev, entitled the *Living Relic*. In the story, a young peasant woman named Lukeria has a freak accident and falls while dancing. As a result, she develops a form of spastic paralysis, wastes away, and eventually is placed in a back corner of a large country estate. The estate's young male heir is the story's narrator. He has been out on a hunting trip resulting in a visit to the estate and comes upon Lukeria who is lying very still on a pallet looking like an icon of suffering. His first reaction is to propose taking her to a hospital: "Who knows, but maybe they can still cure you?" Her response underscores the radical changes in the medical approach to human suffering already emerging by the mid-nineteenth century: "Oh, no, master," she says in an agitated whisper, "don't send me to a hospital, let me alone. I'll only have to endure more agony there. There's no good in trying to cure me! Once a doctor came here and wanted to have a look at me. I said to him, begging him: 'Don't disturb me, for Christ's sake!' What good was it! He started turning me this way and that, straightening and bending my legs and arms and telling me 'I'm doing this for learning, that's why. I'm one who serves, a scientist! And don't you try to stop me, because they pinned a medal on me for my contributions to science and it's for you, you dolts, that I'm working so hard.' He pulled me about and pulled me about, named what was wrong with me—and a fine name it was! and with that he left."[3] In the search for the diagnosis, and the hunt for the disease, there can be an increasing blindness to persons who are suffering.

The second is a humorous piece from the British magazine *Punch,* which purports to record the conversation between two women about a physician one of them has just encountered:

> Lady visitor: "Oh that's your doctor, is it? What sort of a doctor is he?" Lady patient: "I don't know much about his ability but he's got a very good bedside manner."[4]

As the professional ideal for physicians evolved to that of dispassionate medical scientist, there was almost an overreaction in the opposite direction away from a "good bedside manner." William Osler, one of the founding professors at Johns Hopkins University Medical School and, later, Regius Professor of Medicine at Oxford University in the early twentieth century, served as a model of the ideal physician for several generations of young medical students In his now classic *Aequanimitas*, he cautions physicians about the dangers of displaying emotional responses to patients: "The physician who ... shows in his face the slightest alteration expressive of anxiety or fear ... is liable to disaster at any moment."[5] However, the line separating a dispassionate demeanor from frank callousness may be quite difficult to discern at times, especially from the perspective of a frightened patient who is suffering.

With the rapid increase in useful medical knowledge based on a scientific understanding of illness as abnormal anatomical or physiological processes, physicians, as medical scientists, made extraordinary gains in prestige and power. The inequality in the relationship between doctor and patient, which had long been an inherent aspect of the therapeutic encounter, was now becoming a large gulf. For even though the average practitioner might still be plagued by uncertainty and ignorance, a powerful, unconquerable ally in the form of *progress*—irresistible, relentless, scientific progress—was now on the side of the medical profession. Who could plausibly deny that it would only be a matter of time before most major causes of human disease and misery would be forced to capitulate before the advances of medical science?

As a consequence (though perhaps more accurately an aspirational goal), human progress through scientific discovery rapidly supplanted relief of individual human suffering as medicine's primary goal. The role of physicians for eons had been to attend to human distress, usually one person's suffering at a time. With the advent of scientific medicine, practitioners and researchers had the opportunity to relieve suffering on a massive scale through eliminating the proximate causes of suffering by identifying effective treatments for diseases. The same altruistic impulses that had been driven by witnessing individual human suffering could now be directed at attacking and destroying the causes of suffering for countless individuals.

But with the scientific revolution in medicine came an inevitable conflict between physician scientists' traditional role of caregiver and advocate for suffering individuals and their newer role in the pursuit of knowledge. Both are important and worthy medical objectives. In the abstract, medical progress, in relieving suffering for countless individuals, is a superior alternative to relieving suffering one patient at a time. Yet physicians have ethical, professional, and legal obligations to the individual patient. The search for medical progress cannot distort responsibilities to individual patients. Instead, they must be in equipoise.

Medical scientists understand that knowledge gained through experimentation might relieve future suffering, but not necessarily that of their experimental subjects. By the same token, experimental subjects knowingly or unknowingly accept their own suffering on behalf of others who might actually benefit in the future from any discovery made through their participation. Whenever experiments take precedence over the persons serving as subjects of the investigation, temptations inevitably arise. Abuses of human subjects in medical experimentation frequently arise when the knowledge to be gained trumps the concerns and needs of individual study subjects, as was the case in the Tuskegee syphilis experiment (discussed further later). Thus, although a majority of practitioners may still perceive the relief of suffering (along with other goals such as health maintenance and conquest of disease) as a major goal of medicine in the twenty-first century, the growth of scientific medicine has added complexity to the vision of how suffering is to be relieved and its priority within health care policy.

Indeed, the cure of disease has become such a powerful motivating force in medicine that even during the AIDS epidemic, priorities have always been given to finding a cure and then to delivering antiretroviral agents.[6] Relieving pain and distressing symptoms of those currently suffering and dying from the disease have become secondary or tertiary concerns. This apparent imbalance in priorities is most poignantly identified with regard to the lack of adequate pain relief and palliative care in both the developed and developing world. "In September 2008, the World Health Organization (WHO) estimated that approximately 80 percent of the world population has either no or insufficient access to treatment for moderate to severe pain and that every year tens of millions of people around the world, including around four million cancer patients and 0.8 million HIV/AIDS patients at the end of their lives suffer from such pain without treatment."[7]

This raises an important question that lies at the crux of the relationship between medical practice, including research, and suffering: Has the focus of modern medicine on curing diseases produced a blindness or callousness within the profession toward current suffering in favor of relieving some distant future suffering through the conquest of disease? Human suffering is centered in persons and their relationships.[8] Dame Cicely Saunders, founder of the modern hospice movement, coined the term *total pain* to describe the intersecting domains of distress (physical, psychological, social, and spiritual) that in their totality constitute the experience of suffering.[9] Ameliorating suffering requires careful assessment and management of the individual patient's symptoms while recognizing the unique meaning of a given symptom for the patient. Symptoms, beyond being major clues for diagnosing diseases, are also major clues to understanding the suffering that may be present. It is the meaning attached to a given symptom that may identify the underlying suffering.[10] For example, recurrent pain at the site of a cancer that has been in remission following treatment may be almost unbearable, regardless of its actual intensity, because it signifies the return of the cancer and that death is imminent. As will become evident later in this chapter, the Belmont Report, the corresponding development of institutional review boards (IRBs), and the palliative care movement have established that patients and subjects of human experimentation are persons who can suffer and that participation in research should not exacerbate their suffering, certainly not without their informed consent.

CONFLICTS OF INTEREST

In the current health care system, conflicts of interest compound the problem of conflicting goals. To be sure, medical care has always posed potential conflicts between a physician's professional obligations to the patient and financial incentives, especially in the research context. For instance, in *Moore v. Regents of the University of California*,[11] a physician took excess tissue samples to use in developing a pharmaceutical product without providing informed consent. The patient sued to recover a share of the profits, but the court ruled for the physician on restitution (though ruling against the physician for failing to obtain consent).

Yet physicians now face far more pervasive conflicts of interest than ever before. Most important, there is an increasing tension between the physician's economic interests and treatment recommendations. For instance, the complex web between pharmaceutical manufacturers and physicians, especially physicians conducting clinical trials for new pharmaceuticals, is so rife with suspicious incentives that it is the subject of numerous Inspector General opinions on illegal kickbacks and questions regarding adequate IRB oversight. An equally intractable issue now is about physician ownership of specialty hospitals. Not only do these specialty hospitals compete with general hospitals for the most profitable medical services, but they also force physicians to choose between their economic investment and what is best for their patients.

In general, the fee-for-service health care reimbursement system creates conflicts of interest for health professionals. This payment method creates incentives for providers to increase their own salaries; it rewards providers for recommending a greater number of more expensive services. As a result, health professionals may need to choose between increasing their own financial well-being (providing more services) and promoting their patients' health (providing an efficient number of services). Many cost-containment measures are designed to correct this particular conflict of interest. For example, episode-based payment models reimburse providers for all services delivered during a defined episode of care,[12] and pay-for-performance models create financial incentives to improve health outcomes within a given range of services.[13]

And finally, another contentious series of conflicts is over conscience clauses (i.e., the right of a health care provider to refuse certain services based on his or her moral beliefs). States such as Michigan are drafting legislation to provide a broad right for providers to refuse services for almost any reason. The issue remains unresolved but threatens to drive a wedge between patients and their physicians.[14]

PAIN MANAGEMENT

Another aspect of modern health care delivery that has tempered the attention to human suffering is inadequate pain management, which has become a major concern in the United States. Regulatory oversight of controlled substances, ethical concerns about terminal sedation, and general insensitivity to acute and chronic suffering have combined to constrain medical personnel from providing adequate pain management. As recently as 2001, one observer noted that: "Human dignity requires and demands that unnecessary and treatable pain be relieved.... If the importance of pain relief and the ethical obligation to relieve pain are so widely recognized, why do we continue to neglect treatable pain?"[15]

Nonetheless, recent reports of an epidemic of deaths related to misuse of prescription opioids[16] will likely contribute to neglecting pain treatment for many years to come, especially when combined with the potential for more aggressive prosecution of physicians who liberally prescribe opioids for chronic pain unrelated to terminal illness. Efforts to better educate physicians in the proper and safe use of opioids as part of the U.S. Food and Drug Administration risk evaluation and mitigation strategy[17] will be important measures to ameliorate the problem. But many physicians may interpret these efforts as additional burdens beyond the already complex requirements to maintain specialty certification, hospital credentialing, and licensure. In turn, over-regulating the risk for prescription abuse may lead to reducing the number of physicians who are willing to prescribe opioids for pain relief. In effect, well-intended public health efforts to ensure public safety may inadvertently contribute to callousness toward suffering at a systemic level.

The Healer's Encounter with Suffering: Understanding the Sources of Callousness

The recognition of suffering by physicians and other health professionals first requires their awareness that each patient, including those serving as subjects in research studies, is a person who can and does suffer. Health professionals are often called upon to perform painful and invasive procedures on their patients as part of standard medical care. For example, the first time a young surgeon in training is invited to make an incision in the operating room, cutting another person, even with the noblest of intentions, creates powerful and often conflicting emotions. On a cognitive level, the physician knows that the operation is intended to heal the patient, but there may still be an intense mix of emotions ranging from sheer excitement to horror that one is capable of cutting another human being. To function as a surgeon, the young physician must develop some degree of equanimity and emotional control in the operating room regarding what in any other context would be a terrible act.

To release this tension, health professionals sometimes use so-called gallows humor as a coping mechanism in the face of futility and intense suffering. Although such practices have been strongly discouraged in recent years, it was common for many generations of medical students to objectify their cadavers with various kinds of pranks to avoid deeper reflection on mortality and the person represented by the corpse they were dissecting.[18] Humor is clearly a powerful coping mechanism for humans under stress, and it may, under some circumstances, be a source of healing and health. However, cultural norms may also define the content of humor, such that a given group may have its own inner language of humor and its own context for what is humorous. Thus, in the context of being confronted with the horror and futility of death secondary to massive trauma or other equally distressing situations, medical professionals may cope with their own fears and feelings of helplessness with dark humor. As Decety and others have shown, physicians actually feel less empathy for the pain of others than their nonphysician counterparts. In fact, research in cognitive neuroscience has shown that physicians can regulate emotion in ways that dampen their own negative perceptions of others' suffering.[19] Without frequent, careful, and self-conscious reflection regarding their need for this form of coping, it seems that health professionals who engage in this type of humor may be at risk for developing an emotional and even spiritual or existential callousness to the suffering of others.

THE RESIDUAL EFFECTS OF SLAVERY

The historical and cultural roots of individual and social callousness toward suffering that facilitated the tragedy of the Tuskegee syphilis experiment are, in our view, a direct consequence of the attitudes that perpetuated slavery. It may be speculative to argue that Tuskegee could not have occurred without the cultural background of slavery and the Jim Crow era that followed.[20] To understand the origins of the insensitivity toward the poor black men of Macon County who became the subjects for the Tuskegee scientific inquiry, we need to review the attitudes and perceptions regarding enslaved Africans within the dominant white culture, both North and South, in antebellum America. Doing so may lend perspective to why experiments like Tuskegee occurred, and could happen again, absent appropriate institutional responses to the historical record.

While chattel slavery withered in the Northern states of the early republic, it flourished in the South primarily for economic reasons.[21] It was rare for any individual, even for those of abolitionist leanings, to insist on the inherent equality of blacks and whites. Although enslavement of Africans had been a part of the economic system of America from early colonial times, there had also been significant ambivalence about the institution even among the slaveholders. This ambivalence and anxiety about the institution of slavery was no more clearly expressed than in a letter written by Thomas Jefferson, a slaveholder himself, at the time of the Missouri Compromise in 1820: "... I can say with conscious truth that there is not a man on earth who would sacrifice more than I would, to relieve us from this heavy reproach, in any *practicable* way. The cession of that kind of property, for so it is misnamed, is a bagatelle which would not cost me in a second thought, if, in that way, a general emancipation and *expatriation* could be effected: and, gradually, and with due sacrifices, I think it might be. But, as it is, we have the wolf by the ear, and we can neither hold him, nor safely let him go. Justice is in one scale, and self-preservation in the other."[22]

By the 1830s, anxiety rapidly replaced this ambivalence as the economic rewards from the sale of cotton reached peak levels and the abolitionist movement in the North began to create an intense defensiveness among slaveholders. The discovery of an apparent slave insurrection plot in Mississippi in the wake of the Nat Turner slave rebellion in Virginia only served to further enhance slaveholders' concerns about loosening their grip on the "wolf's ear." Fortunately for these slaveholders, the churches and southern medical science provided the theological and scientific justifications for preserving the institution of slavery. It had long been felt among whites that by virtue of the ease with which they were enslaved, Africans had proved their inherent inferiority as a race. While southern churchmen found references to the "curse of Canaan"[23] as the basis for an alleged Biblical sanction of African slavery, southern physicians sought to confirm and demonstrate African inferiority from anatomic and physiologic differences between the races.[24]

In the 1850s, Professor Cartwright from the University of Louisiana integrated scientific expertise and theological erudition in explaining that "... the revelations of anatomy, physiology, and history were a mere re-writing of what Moses wrote. A knowledge of THE GREAT PRIMARY TRUTH that the negro is a slave by nature, and can never be happy, industrious, moral or religious, in any other condition than the one he was intended to fill.... It is this defective hematosis, or atmospherization of the blood combined with a deficiency of cerebral matter in the cranium and an excess of nervous matter distributed to the organs of sensation and assimilation, that is the true cause of that debasement of mind which has rendered the people of Africa unable to take care of themselves."[25]

TUSKEGEE: AM I NOT A MAN AND BROTHER?[26]

Professor Cartwright had his detractors within the southern medical establishment of the time, but few disputed his essential claim of Negro inferiority. It should be no surprise that the prevailing assumption of antebellum America regarding the increased "sensuality at the expense of intellectuality," purported to be a defining characteristic of people with African ancestry, persisted into the twentieth century and influenced the thinking of United States Public Health Service (USPHS) scientists who planned and executed the Tuskegee Syphilis experiment between 1932 and 1972.[27] Not only did these attitudes affect notions of perceived "Negro promiscuity," but they likely also influenced the USPHS investigators' central hypothesis that blacks and Caucasians would respond in fundamentally different ways to the same pathogens.

Tuskegee thus serves as an example of the medical community's willingness to collaborate with the larger dominant culture in providing support and scientific sanction of attitudes initially driven by self-interest that later acquire the cloak of philanthropy. Other egregious and horrific examples of similar collaborations between medicine and the larger culture in disparaging the value of a group of human beings could also be cited, such as the Holocaust. Remarkably, the USPHS physicians conducting the Tuskegee syphilis experiment were well aware of and horrified by the atrocities the Nazis committed against the Jews and other minorities, and yet did not see any connection between their experiment and the Nazis' activities. We are highlighting the connections between slavery and the Tuskegee experiment because of the residual and continuing racial health disparities in the United States that reflect the very strong and persistent influence of the antebellum attitudes to African Americans that still remain as a subtext within our culture.

The famous question, "Am I not a man and a brother?" was inscribed with the image of an African slave on his knees raising his chained hands in supplication on antislavery medallions produced by the ardent eighteenth century English abolitionist, Josiah Wedgwood. The more than four hundred African American men who were duped into participating in the notorious Tuskegee syphilis experiment from 1932 to 1972 were unable to ask this fundamental question of the USPHS physicians who organized the experiment. Although this rhetorical question, written as part of the polemics of antislavery campaigning in the late eighteenth century, may seem at first blush to be unrelated to the USPHS experiment, we contend that it is at the heart of the experiment's moral dilemma and resulting callousness to suffering. As already noted, the callous disregard for the humanity and suffering of the African American men of the Tuskegee experiment[28] has its roots in the American culture of racism engendered by the South's Peculiar Institution of slavery.

In 1972, former USPHS employee Peter Buxtun, acting as a whistle blower, leaked the horrifying story of the Tuskegee experiment to the press. What had originally been planned to be a short-term prospective study of the effects of syphilis in untreated African American males had evolved into a long-term study of the natural history of undertreated and untreated syphilis. At the time of the project's initiation in 1932, syphilis was a major U.S. public health concern. There was much interest among experts in venereal diseases in the natural history of the disease among different racial groups. An earlier study[29] from Norway of untreated syphilitics conducted between 1891 and 1910 provided considerable information about the disease in Caucasians, but there was little known about potential differences in how the disease might be manifested in persons of African ancestry. In the early part of the twentieth century, white physicians commonly assumed that there were high rates of sexual promiscuity among African Americans. Many of the USPHS physicians in the Division of Venereal Diseases shared this assumption, which led to the general perception among white physicians of "syphilis as the quintessential black disease."[30]

For the study, the USPHS targeted a rural county in Alabama because of the high concentration of poor, uneducated black men who would likely have untreated syphilis in various stages of progression. In fact, many of the study subjects would not previously have seen a physician for any treatment. The study's subjects were recruited by offering "free health care" directed at identifying and treating "bad blood." Among the rural blacks of Alabama, this vague term referred to a host of different conditions, including syphilis. The study's white investigators capitalized on being authority figures, whom rural blacks were quite accustomed to obeying. From the beginning, there was never any pretense of informed consent. The initial experiment planned to conduct an in depth study of untreated syphilis over several months to investigate the hypothesis that syphilis evolved in fundamentally different ways in blacks and whites, despite having the same etiological agent.[31]

At the study's outset, the USPHS consciously wrote protocols to undertreat subjects found to have syphilis because they could not afford to provide them the standard year-long medication regimen for treating the disease. To create further support for the project within the local community, the white USPHS investigators convinced the Tuskegee Institute's black leadership and its affiliated hospital to participate in the project. A most critical addition to the project was the hiring of a black nurse, Eunice Rivers, who served as liaison between the study and the subjects. Ms. Rivers added enormous credibility from the subjects' perspective because she treated them with compassion as *patients*.

As the initial study neared completion, the onsite investigator, Dr. Vonderlehr, was enthusiastic about continuing the research. Based upon the hypothesis that advanced syphilis produced predominately cardiovascular manifestations in blacks, compared with what were thought to be more common neurologic manifestations in whites, Vonderlehr and his USPHS superiors were excited to use their initial experimental subjects to identify a large cohort of males with cardiovascular complications of syphilis.

To control for the possibility of occult neural syphilis in their experimental patients, the investigators needed to examine the subjects' spinal fluid. At the time, spinal taps were quite painful and often complicated by severe headaches. There was no plan to provide treatment with the taps; they would only be of diagnostic value. Dr. Vonderlehr used gross deceit to recruit subjects for the spinal taps, offering "... YOUR LAST CHANCE FOR SPECIAL FREE TREATMENT. . ."[32] in an official letter from the Macon County Health Department. Dr. Vonderlehr then made the fateful proposal to extend the study of "untreated" syphilis for many more years. (This ignored the fact that the majority of the subjects had received some, albeit inadequate, treatment for syphilis, a major contaminating element in the study design. Not only was the study unethical, it was also bad science.) When Dr. Vonderlehr later became the director of the Division of Venereal Diseases, he was able to continue the study without external review. Even when penicillin emerged as a very effective treatment for syphilis,the USPHS investigators overseeing the study intervened to make sure that their study subjects would not receive penicillin because "... treatment would have ended the Tuskegee study."[33] Dr. Heller, who succeeded Dr. Vonderlehr as director of the Division of Venereal Diseases, later commended the study, stating: "The longer the study, the better the ultimate information we would derive."[34]

When Dr. Heller was asked about his views regarding the human experimentation conducted by the Nazi scientists, he responded, "I, like most everybody else, was horrified at the things that were practiced upon these Jewish people, such as doing experiments while patients were not only alive but doing such things as would cause their deaths.... All of these sorts of things were horrendous to me and I, like most everyone else, deplored them."[35] Yet, he was unable to see any connection between the Tuskegee experiment and the actions of the Nazi scientists, "... because to me there was no similarity at all between them."[36] Certainly, Dr. Heller and his colleagues could protest that any harm the subjects in the Tuskegee syphilis experiment suffered was on a much smaller scale, not even comparable to the large-scale madness and sadistic brutality exhibited by the Nazi scientists. Nonetheless, the ability of this subtler, yet pervasive "blindness to persons"[37] to taint and even poison human interactions, especially in the unequal relationship between physician and patient or medical scientist and experimental subject, should not be underestimated.

It is very difficult, if not impossible, to eliminate completely any element of self-interest from the medical ideal of actions motivated purely by disinterested compassion. Indeed, self-interest can penetrate both the actions that focus on the care of a single suffering patient and the thoughtful direction of human experimentation to gain useful knowledge for helping others. The potential for personal financial gain or academic glory is the more obvious temptation to manifest one's self-interest that can shift the primary focus away from the suffering patient to the practitioner's clinical skill or the scientist's intellectual curiosity. Without a conscious and persistent effort to search out and recognize the person who is also a clinical or experimental subject, this blindness to persons can rapidly become the default mode of perception for the physician or medical scientist. When this flawed human response becomes normalized and is at times linked to larger, communal perceptions driven by prejudice or ideology, the blindness to persons can translate into monstrous behaviors.

The Slippery Slope of Rationalization

An important aspect of understanding the callousness toward suffering is the process of rationalization. With the Tuskegee and slavery episodes we discussed previously, the imposition of suffering can only be justified through pretext. How else can we explain slavery's existence, survival, and cruelty despite its evident moral perversion? What else could account for maintaining the Tuskegee experiment far beyond any reasoned justification? Slavery progressed as a malevolent and institutionalized form of evil; Tuskegee continued through rationalization and callousness toward the subjects' suffering. The key question from the historical record is: What can we learn about how rationalization perpetuates suffering and what mechanisms are needed to penetrate the pretext?

The apparent inevitability and perpetual character of slavery within antebellum American culture demanded a process of rationalization to bolster and support its continued existence because it otherwise contradicted all that was sacred to Americans. Only a rare individual among the slaveholding class would openly state the most obvious reason for slave ownership—greed in the forms of cheap labor and increased personal gain. Greed and self-interest can become powerful motivators to transform humans into objects for manipulation, whether this may be in the egregious form of chattel slavery or in more subtle forms of abuse in our own day's fee-for-service medicine and human experimentation. If slaves make fortunes for their owners, slavery must be justified, along with whatever means are necessary to perpetuate the institution, including violence as well as intellectual and moral rationalization.

A more typical rationalization was the 1818 statement by the first congressman from the new state of Mississippi, George Poindexter, who said, "It is not with us a matter of choice whether we will have slaves among us or not: we found them here, and we are obliged to maintain and employ them. It would be a blessing, could we get rid of them; but the wisest and best men among us have not been able to devise a plan for doing it."[38] Thus, the first rationalization for slavery was that "we had no choice," which was not essentially different than the Nazi defense that "we were only following orders." Here, good men confronted evil that they could not (or would not) eliminate, an evil whose perpetuation was also in their own personal interests. And yet, it was immodest for gentlemen to take advantage of such an opportunity, so the opportunity itself became a difficult burden they inherited—one they bore with the most grace they could muster under the circumstances.

The second rationalization was to blame others for slavery's existence. Writing with this in mind, one Yankee turned Mississippi master struggled with the inherent cruelty of slavery in a letter to his brother: "That slavery is a great evil, there can be no doubt—and it is an unfortunate circumstance that it was ever introduced into this, or any other country. At present, it is a necessary evil, and I do not think admits of a remedy.... The sin of the business lies at the doors of those who first introduced slavery into the country. The evil now is too deep-rooted to be eradicated."[39] The contention that "the evil is too deep-rooted to be eradicated" further compounds the rationalization because it places greater emphasis on pragmatism (i.e., slavery as a necessary evil) instead of on the moral injustice to be eradicated.

Through minimizing the evils of slavery in his state, this particular slaveholder engaged in a form of denial, which is a related and third type of rationalization of an activity that he has no intention of ending, in his thinking that the real evils of slavery exist somewhere else. Denial is indicative of indifference or callousness toward an individual's suffering, a factor we will discuss later in the context of current medical practices.

As the slaveholders struggled to rationalize slavery, there was an additional difficulty. As freedom-loving democrats, how could they accept the responsibility and burden of enslaving others when this was clearly not in keeping with the ideals enshrined in the Declaration of Independence? Frederick Law Olmsted recognized the fundamental dilemma posed by the need to treat human beings as both property (things) and persons: "It is difficult to handle simply as property, a creature possessing human passions and human feelings, however debased and torpid the condition of that creature may be; while, on the other hand, the absolute necessity of dealing with property, as a thing, greatly embarrasses a man in any attempt to treat it as a person."[40]

It was this dilemma that underlay the frequent, necessary cruelties used to keep persons who were also property in subjection to their masters' authority. This was where Professor Cartwright and his colleagues provided the fourth rationalization—that Africans were essentially subhuman and would benefit from the slave owners' benevolence. Because they were fundamentally inferior, Africans were destined to be slaves. The concern that enlightened masters felt on their slaves' behalf could then be expressed in ways that uniquely reflected this rationalization based on enslavement as an act of benevolent kindness. In other words, slavery was actually a better alternative than the savage lives they would otherwise live.

The fifth rationalization emerges from the Tuskegee syphilis experiment itself. Abstract concepts, like scientific progress and hypothetical benefits for future generations, are not substitutes for the needs of the suffering person in the present moment. Yet, the idea of scientific progress may be one of the most powerful excuses for inflicting suffering; this idea continues to be used today to justify priorities in expenditures for both medical research and health care in general. To the extent that those in distress become less persons and more objects in this process of setting priorities, an institutionalized form of callousness toward human suffering has gradually and subtly altered the original goals of health care. For example, a recent review[41] of research in the United States directed toward the relief of physical distress and suffering in persons with advanced illnesses highlighted the very limited support that is currently provided; in fiscal year 2009, only 0.098 percent of the budget of the National Institutes of Health was committed for funding research in this area. This underscores the dominant priority funding agencies give to studying the mechanisms of disease rather than the direct relief of human suffering.

Not surprisingly, the consequences of these rationalizations followed former slaves even after emancipation and then directly led to the callousness toward suffering inherent in the Tuskegee experiment. Once the emancipated slave was no longer considered property, even the solicitous concern for their welfare (as for one's prized possessions) was quickly lost. In reviewing the smallpox epidemic, which killed so many refugee freedmen displaced during the chaos of slave emancipation late in the Civil War, it was noted that, "Despite the medical and public knowledge that smallpox could be easily transmitted through contact with an infected person, medical and governmental officials interpreted the growing number of cases of smallpox as consequences of the 'dirty habits' and immoral behavior of former slaves. . ."[42]

The ability of any white man with full legal sanction to torture, maim, and even kill fugitive slaves with essentially no accountability (and potentially receipt of a reward for one's efforts) in the antebellum era[43] helped establish a dominant white culture in which attitudes and approaches to Negroes were cruel in the extreme. Equally important, the rationalizations underlying the institution of slavery provided the historical and cultural antecedents that blinded the USPHS investigators to the major ethical deficiencies of the Tuskegee syphilis experiment. Take, for example, the rationalization justifying the continuation of slavery that relied on the weight of history's inertia to not admit any possibility for change. This appeal to duration was also a growing rationalization for perpetuating the suffering of participants in Tuskegee as the experiment extended beyond its original scope. In another sense, historical inertia has been a major factor inhibiting meaningful reform directed at creating equal access to health care in the United States.

Likewise, Olmsted's very perceptive analysis of the inherent difficulty for someone with philanthropic intentions to own another person as a piece of property is central to understanding the parallel issues at the heart of Tuskegee's horribly flawed medical experimentation. The USPHS investigators' initial interest for controlling syphilis in the black community may have represented true philanthropic concern. Unfortunately, it was tainted with unchallenged assumptions of African American inferiority that the investigators inherited not only from the larger American culture but also from American medical culture. Even as recently as the early 1950s, a respected scientist within the academic community in the United States speculated about the genetic differences among Africans that might make their enslavement more likely: "Our biological knowledge makes it seem inescapable that different ethnic groups possess inborn characteristics (aside from color) which are distinctive. It seems probable, for example, and in accord with general observation that American Indians, among whom there is wide diversity, are on the basis of inborn temperament sufficiently different from African Negroes so that slavery was feasible (and temporarily profitable) in one case and not in the other."[44]

Our two historical examples of callousness toward suffering set the stage for second-class health care, manipulation of research subjects, and lack of concern for informed consent. Although both of these examples involve African Americans, the implications go far beyond any identified group. For instance, a dramatic example of the tension between scientific progress and individual suffering was seen in the diffusion of high-dose chemotherapy with autologous bone marrow transplant (HDC-ABMT) for high-risk and metastatic breast cancer patients in the late 1980s.[45] Patients and their oncologists recognized the absence of feasible treatments and were willing to opt for unproven experimental procedures. Despite the lack of scientific evidence, entrepreneurial oncologists encouraged patients to try HDC-ABMT. At a cost of untold billions of dollars and intense suffering, often with shortened lives, HDC-ABMT was a debacle.

Individuals experience the type of suffering we are concerned about in this chapter in the context of relationships, especially in the clinical encounter and medical research. If one reduces another person to the status of an object, a thing, whether it is as a piece of property or as a research subject who no longer enjoys the dignity of recognition as a patient capable of suffering, the essential effect is the same. Public health officials may even state the obvious when they reminded one of the authors (DBH) that humans have always experienced pain and have suffered, with the implied question: "What's the hurry?"

Have the lessons learned from slavery and Tuskegee been translated into policies that will prevent such episodes from recurring? To the extent that the current regime governing clinical research in countries endorsing policies like those in the Belmont Report is operational, as we discuss later, we believe that the regime now governing medical research makes it highly unlikely that systematic episodes of callousness toward suffering in medicine and medical research will recur.

Medical Research Oversight

Tuskegee was not the only incidence of questionable medical research conducted without adequate oversight. In 1966, Dr. Henry Beecher published an alarming article in *The New England Journal of Medicine* to shed light on twenty-two examples of unethical or questionably ethical studies that were published in American peer-reviewed journals.[46] Although Beecher stated that his examples were not meant to present the worst cases, it is noteworthy that three of the listed examples involved experimentation on children, including the notorious scandals at the Willowbrook State School for disabled children in Massachusetts.[47]

Despite an increasing public awareness of questionable research practices in the 1960s, health professionals continued to use human subjects in unethical ways. During the Cold War (1944–1974), clinicians participated in federally sponsored human radiation experiments. A U.S. Advisory Committee on Human Radiation Experiments report released in 1995 showed that physicians conducted research involving plutonium injections and total-body irradiation (TBI) in adults, as well as research that tested the use of radioactive tracers in institutionalized children.[48] These experiments frequently risked the safety of individual patients for what was thought to be the common good. Despite being aware that TBI treatment was not likely to help (and could certainly harm) some participating cancer patients, the investigators still exposed these subjects to TBI to determine the effects that varying doses of radiation would have on military personnel. The U.S. Advisory Committee found little documentation supporting informed consent for these experiments; the few documents they did find contained insufficient information about potential risks and side effects. The report recommended "steps to improve three elements of the current federal system for the protection of the rights and interests of human subjects" in terms of oversight mechanisms to examine outcomes and performance of the system for protection of human subjects, appropriateness of sanctions for violations of human subjects protections, and extension of human subjects protections to non–federally funded research

Fortunately, medical research involving human subjects today looks much different than it did during the time of the Tuskegee syphilis experiment. In part because of the Tuskegee disclosure and ensuing furor, and in part as a reaction to Nazi Germany's horrific medical experiments, it became clear that the United States needed a more robust mechanism to oversee medical research.

In 1947, during the Nuremburg War Crime Trials, the Allies drafted the Nuremburg Code[49] to prevent the ghastly medical experiments that Nazi doctors performed on human subjects. The Nuremburg Code outlined ten ethical principles under which medical experiments could justifiably be performed on humans, and this outline was used to draft the World Medical Association's Declaration of Helsinki in 1964.[50] In response to these documents, Congress passed the National Research Act in 1974 to govern the rules of human subjects research both funded and conducted by the federal Department of Health, Education, and Welfare (now the Department of Health and Human Services).[51]

In 1978, after nearly four years of deliberation and study, the National Commission for the Protection of Human Subjects of Biomedical and Behavioral Research (the Commission) issued what is commonly known as the Belmont Report, which outlined the basic ethical issues relevant to human subjects research. The Commission identified three principles—respect for persons, beneficence, and justice—to assist both scientists and subjects in resolving the inherent ethical problems that are present when human subjects are used in research.[52] According to the Commission, respect for persons requires "that individuals should be treated as autonomous agents, and ... that persons with diminished autonomy are entitled to protection," and this principle can be applied to the use of informed consent in human subjects research. Similarly, the principle of beneficence demands that, "Persons are treated in an ethical manner not only by respecting their decisions and protecting them from harm, but also by making efforts to secure their well-being." This principle can be applied to the use of systematic risk and benefit assessments when designing and conducting research. Through the identification of justice as an ethical principle, the Commission examined questions related to fairness and the distribution of both the benefits and burdens of research, and they stipulated that the principle of justice must be used when selecting research subjects.

The Belmont Report represented a fundamental shift in the moral framework guiding medical research. For one thing, the ethical principles outlined in the Belmont Report formed the basis for constructing the legal framework under which human subjects research now operates in the United States. Codified in Title 45, Part 46 of the Federal Regulations,[53] the Federal Health and Human Services Policy for Protection of Human Subjects, also known as the Common Rule, describes the basic provisions for human subjects research conducted with funding from the Department of Health and Human Services. (Additional regulations regarding the use of human subjects in research are codified by fourteen other federal agencies and departments.[54])

For another, these rules stipulate the mechanism for ensuring the ethical conduct of medical research—namely, the use of IRBs to oversee the entire human experimentation process, and the use of informed consent before any research can be approved and conducted. At the core of the Belmont Report's ethical framework is the concept that individuals must be fully informed about the nature of the research and what an individual's participation will involve. No research may be conducted without the individual subject's knowing and voluntary consent. The informed consent agreement defines the terms of the research project, states the risks and benefits of participation, and explains what recourse the subject has if there are any concerns. When clinicians conduct formal experiments involving human subjects, the law is very clear: investigators must work with IRBs to create studies that minimize risk to subjects, including risks for psychological harm, relative to the potential benefits of the study while using sound research design that equitably selects subjects and seeks to maximize informed consent.[55] In this sense, the Belmont Report represents a holistic approach to human subjects, similar to the emphasis in palliative care.

Within the scope of clinical work, physicians are given considerable leeway to use interventions and therapies that they believe will improve the health of individual patients. Just as physicians may prescribe drugs for off-label use, surgeons are permitted to attempt new techniques in the operating room. (This is the process that allowed oncologists to use the HDC-ABMT procedure described earlier.) Physicians and their IRB administrators are responsible for determining the fine line between the practice of medicine and the use of patients in research. Accordingly, the Belmont Report notes that, "When a clinician departs in a significant way from standard or accepted practice, the innovation does not, in and of itself, constitute research. The fact that a procedure is experimental, in the sense of new, untested or different, does not automatically place it in the category of research."[56] When clinicians engage in true experimentation and research, the relationship between investigators and patients is contractual in nature, based on voluntary informed consent.

Arguably, the Belmont principles merely codify physicians' existing ethical obligations to their patients. The physician's oath to do no harm is reflected in professional and ethical norms of respect for patients and to act in a patient's best interests. And this certainly applies equally to their research subjects—to conduct research activities that are based on the patient's voluntary and informed consent. Yet, as discussed previously, physicians have used rationalizations to conduct experiments that should never have occurred.

CRITIQUES OF THE BELMONT REPORT

As the recurring issue of conflicts of interest suggests, the Belmont principles are not a panacea for eliminating all research abuses. In fact, many observers have offered withering critiques of the resulting IRB process.[57] For example, David Hyman cynically argues that, "There is no empirical evidence that IRBs have any benefit whatsoever."[58] Hyman critiques the IRB process as being costly and inefficient and as providing inconsistent protection to human subjects across IRBs. Other observers note similar concerns, such as informed consent documents that get longer and more complex over time; some IRB processes that seem to go beyond what Belmont intended (i.e., that minimal risk research projects should not be reviewed at all); excessive IRB paperwork requirements that may discourage some projects from moving forward; institutional conflicts of interest that may exist between IRB members and their colleagues; general underfunding of IRBs; and the potential difficulty of enticing researchers to serve as IRB members.[59] Many who believe that the existing review boards cannot adequately protect human subjects have candidly condemned IRBs, as well as the laws and regulations governing their existence.[60]

Critics rightly point to IRB failures and abuses, such as the death of a research subject in a University of Pennsylvania gene-therapy clinical trial[61] and the Kennedy-Krieger lead paint experiment in Baltimore[62] (though the study has its defenders). But the critics ignore one positive aspect of the process: it is difficult to point to systematic failures on the scale of Tuskegee that have occurred since the Belmont principles were codified. Indeed, the most striking aspect of the critiques is that they call for modest reforms, not repeal. After listing a litany of criticisms, Professor Riley concluded that, ". . . despite these continuing systematic problems, at least for the academic research model. . ., IRBs likely accomplish what they were designed to do. There are very limited reports of research participants suffering major injury."[63] We can infer, therefore, that the Belmont Report has largely succeeded in reducing the probability of the systematic failures that led to the new moral framework, even if individual failures remain.

Necessary, but Not Sufficient

For good reason, the United States places considerable faith in physicians and government officials to practice the basic ethical principles outlined in the Belmont

Report. We expect physicians and researchers to recognize the simultaneous need to protect individual patients from undue suffering when pursuing knowledge that may reduce needless suffering for future populations. Nevertheless, our laws and ethical norms are sufficiently flexible to recognize that clinicians and IRBs need to balance potential suffering for individual research participants with preventing suffering of future patients. The ongoing effort is how to balance this tension.

Laws and regulations to protect human subjects and physicians' dedication to professional ethics are necessary. But neither is sufficient to ensure that human subjects and patients are treated ethically in the course of research activities. In the United States today, we have implemented laws and regulations that mitigate a research professional's ability to inflict systematic suffering on a group of patients. Thus, we have progressed significantly from the days of the Tuskegee syphilis experiment, when an act of commission and purposefully inflicted suffering was generally accepted as the norm within the research community. Today, our rules make acts of commission nearly impossible, but they leave room for acts of omission.

But acts of commission still occur. As a cautionary warning to relaxing our vigilance based on the positive post-Belmont developments, we must consider how tenuous the gains can be when the rationalizations for imposing suffering overwhelm the legal and moral constraints. A good recent example is the role that physicians played in the systematic degradation and torture at Guantanamo and Abu Ghraib. As many accounts have described, some physicians willingly participated in waterboarding and other abusive interrogations after the 9/11 attacks.[64] According to Bloche and Marks (2005), physicians were complicit in designing the interrogation methods, including sleep deprivation and other strategies to coerce testimony, and shared detainees' medical records with military interrogators.

The rationalization for physicians' participation is reminiscent of the excuses for slavery and Tuskegee: "Physicians who did such work tend not to see these practices as unethical. On the contrary, a common understanding among those who helped to plan interrogations is that physicians serving in these roles do not act as physicians and are therefore not bound by patient-oriented ethics."[65] In this rationalization, the Hippocratic Oath does not apply because physicians act as combatants, not as detainees' physicians, akin to forensic psychiatrists. While acknowledging the ethical "conflict between the medical profession's therapeutic and social purposes," Bloche and Marks leave no doubt but that medical personnel who participated in these interrogations breached their ethical obligations, a position we share.

Similar questions have been raised about medicine's participation in implementing the death penalty. Medical participation in the death penalty regime has been rationalized as helping to put other humans to death in a more humane way. This suggests that medical personnel are still willing to inflict suffering for particular reasons; rationalizations for inflicting suffering have hardly been eliminated.

Moving Forward: The Role of Palliative Care

If we are correct that the Belmont Report has substantially reduced the probability of systematic abuses that inflict suffering, how can medicine ensure that physicians move beyond their training of "first do no harm" to focus on easing their patients' suffering? Moving forward, medicine must undergo a cultural shift. Our medical professionals must be trained in a way that highlights the importance of palliative care that eases individual patients' suffering. This education has the potential to create norms under which all medical personnel will be trained in self-reflection to combat callousness toward their patients and research subjects. Under this norm, researchers will make easing suffering their highest priority, with their own research goals as secondary considerations.

The Belmont Report guided the development of IRBs and human studies committees that have been absolutely essential correctives in limiting the potential for another Tuskegee syphilis experiment to occur. However, Belmont alone has not (and probably cannot) address the basic underlying problem of a blindness to persons that so often afflicts human beings when they acquire authority and power over others or perceive others through the lens of self-interest. The individual prejudices that blinded the USPHS physicians conducting the Tuskegee syphilis experiment to the persons who were also their research subjects grew out of the dominant white culture of antebellum America. The problem is fundamentally one of culture and must therefore be solved at a cultural level. Only a truly transformative phenomenon at the level of the larger culture can effectively address such a problem. The palliative care movement may qualify as such a phenomenon.

The World Health Organization has defined palliative care as "... an approach that improves the quality of life of patients and their families facing the problems associated with life-threatening illness, through the prevention and relief of suffering by means of early identification and impeccable assessment and treatment of pain and other problems, physical, psychosocial and spiritual. Palliative care:

- provides relief from pain and other distressing symptoms;
- affirms life and regards dying as a normal process;
- intends neither to hasten or postpone death;
- integrates the psychological and spiritual aspects of patient care;
- offers a support system to help patients live as actively as possible until death;
- offers a support system to help the family cope during the patient's illness and in their own bereavement;
- uses a team approach to address the needs of patients and their families, including bereavement counseling, if indicated;
- will enhance quality of life, and may also positively influence the course of illness;
- is applicable early in the course of illness, in conjunction with other therapies that are intended to prolong life, such as chemotherapy or radiation

therapy, and includes those investigations needed to better understand and manage distressing clinical complications."[66]

The palliative care movement began with care of the imminently dying in the context of hospice. As health care providers, policy makers, and, most important, the general public have recognized the great value of person-centered care focused on relief of suffering, palliative care's role is expanding upstream across diverse health care settings to address suffering wherever and whenever it is found. Palliative care has the potential to bring balance back to the therapeutic encounter so that any patient in need of treatment will be recognized as a person whose suffering must also be addressed. It also has the potential to play a major role in pain management at various stages of the therapeutic encounter. In particular, palliative care will help train more physicians to provide better basic pain management across a wider spectrum.[67] By the same token, identifying each potential subject of medical research first and foremost as a person with the capacity to suffer will strengthen and enervate the efforts of IRBs as well as motivate the actions of investigators.

As palliative care brings a greater awareness to the general public regarding the limitations of medical care when confronted by human mortality, the public may develop more realistic expectations of the health care system. In this sense, palliative care may help to reframe issues around death and dying in the same way that the Belmont Report has redefined the moral framework for medical research.

Conclusion

It would be both unfair and unrealistic to expect physicians to eliminate the world's suffering. To the extent that physicians as either clinical investigators or as members of the larger culture persist in having blindness to persons, their ability to relieve the suffering they encounter in the world will be compromised. This is true whether it results from ongoing subtle racism, professional self-interest (or professionally induced callousness), greed, apathy, or an obsessive commitment to an abstraction (i.e., the future progress of humanity to the exclusion of concern for the individual person in the present). Individuals will experience suffering as a result of disease, inequalities in resources (i.e., homelessness and lack of access to health care), poor health habits, "bad luck,"[68] and callousness toward those who suffer. In the United States, the residual role of race remains prominent in the ongoing struggle to alleviate racial disparities in health care that inflict unnecessary suffering. To return to Montaigne's thought that suffering is inherent to the human condition, we are under no illusions that indifference to human suffering can ever be eliminated. But we strongly believe that changes in cultural norms, stimulated by the palliative care movement and improvements to the Belmont reforms, will lead to new ethical frameworks that will significantly reduce the insensitivity to human suffering.

Notes

1. Michel de Montaigne, "On Cruelty," in *The Complete Essays* (London: Penguin Books, 2003), 488. "We owe justice to men: and to the other creatures who are able to receive them we owe gentleness and kindness."

2. Michel de Montaigne, "On Cruelty," in *The Complete Essays* (London: Penguin Books, 2003), 485.

3. Ivan Turgenev, "Living Relic," in *Sketches from a Hunter's Album*, trans. Richard Freeborn (Middlesex, UK: Penguin Books, 1972), 218.

4. *Punch*, March 15, 1884.

5. William Osler, *Aequanimitas* (London: HK Lewis, 1920).

6. This observation is based on Dr. Hinshaw's experiences in sub-Saharan Africa and other developing nations. Admittedly, this is a sensitive issue. Nonetheless, Dr. Hinshaw observed that nongovernmental organizations deliver antiretroviral agents and some level of social support (e.g., food, money) to assure compliance with the antiretroviral therapy. But they offer very little attention, training, or resources for treating or caring for the suffering (especially physical pain) of the infected persons.

7. Human Rights Watch, *"Please, Do Not Make Us Suffer Any More…": Access to Pain Treatment as a Human Right*, March 9, 2009, accessed March 9, 2014, http://www.hrw.org/en/reports/2009/03/02/please-do-not-make-us-suffer-any-more-0.

8. E. J. Cassel, "The Nature of Suffering and the Goals of Medicine," *New England Journal of Medicine* 306, no. 11 (1982): 639–645; Eric J. Cassell, *The Nature of Suffering and the Goals of Medicine*, 2nd ed. (Oxford, UK: Oxford University Press, 2004), 34.

9. Cicely M. Saunders and Nigel Sykes, *The Management of Terminal Malignant Disease*, 3rd ed. (London: Hodder and Stoughton, 1993).

10. E. J. Cassel, "The Nature of Suffering and the Goals of Medicine," *New England Journal of Medicine* 306, no. 11 (1982): 639–645.

11. Moore v. Regents of the University of California, 793 P.2d (Cal. 1990).

12. Robert E. Mechanic, "Opportunities and Challenges for Episode-Based Payment," *New England Journal of Medicine* 365, no. 9 (2011): 777–779.

13. Sally Trude, Melanie Au, and Jon B Christianson, "Health Plan Pay-for-Performance Strategies," *American Journal of Managed Care* 12, no. 9 (2006): 537–542.

14. This is a complex issue that is beyond the scope of this chapter. It has the potential for physician callousness toward the patient's total pain in the guise of moral opprobrium.

15. Sandra H. Johnson, "Relieving Unnecessary, Treatable Pain for the Sake of Human Dignity," *Journal of Law, Medicine & Ethics* 28, no. s4 (2001): 11–12, 11.

16. Centers for Disease Control and Prevention. "CDC Grand Rounds: Prescription Drug Overdoses—a U.S. Epidemic." *Morbidity and Mortality Weekly Report* 61, no. 01 (2012): 10–13.

17. See U.S. Food and Drug Administration REMS website for more information, accessed March 9, 2014, http://www.fda.gov/Drugs/DrugSafety/PostmarketDrugSafetyInformationforPatientsandProviders/ucm111350.htm.

18. Katie Watson, "Gallows Humor in Medicine," *Hastings Center Report* 41, no. 5 (2011): 37–45.

19. Y. Cheng et al., "Expertise Modulates the Perception of Pain in Others," *Current Biology* 17 (2007): 1708–1713; J. Decety, C. Y. Yang, and Y. Cheng Y. "Physicians Down

Regulate Their Pain Empathy Response: An Event-Related Brain Potential Study," *NeuroImage* 50 (2010): 1676–1682.

20. C. Vann Woodward, *The Strange Career of Jim Crow* (Oxford, UK: Oxford University Press, 1955).

21. Kenneth M. Stampp, "Profit and Loss," in *The Peculiar Institution: Slavery in the Ante-Bellum South* (New York: Vintage Books, 1956), 383–418.

22. Library of Congress. "Letter from Thomas Jefferson to John Holmes," accessed March 9, 2014, http://www.loc.gov/exhibits/jefferson/159.html.

23. The patriarch Noah cursed the children of Ham who exposed his nakedness in Genesis 9:25–27: "Cursed be Canaan, slave of slaves shall he be to his brothers.... Bless, O Lord, the tents of Shem; may Canaan be his slave. May God extend Japheth's bounds, let him dwell in the tents of Shem, may Canaan be their slave." *The New English Bible* (New York: Cambridge University Press, 1971). *Canaan* became synonymous with people of African ancestry in the minds of southern theologians who used this passage of scripture as a basis for enslavement of Africans.

24. For a review of southern medical perspectives and attitudes toward slaves and their health, see J. S. Haller Jr., "The Negro and the Southern Physician: A Study of Medical and Racial Attitudes 1800–1860," *Medical History* 16, no. 3 (1972): 238–253.

25. Fredric Law Olmstead, *A Journey in the Back Country* (New York: Mason Brothers, 1861), 64, accessed March 9, 2014, http://babel.hathitrust.org/cgi/pt?id=hvd.hn2c84;seq=9;view=1up;num=iii.

26. Inscription on antislavery medallion created by Josiah Wedgwood in 1787; for more information and an image of the medallion, see http://www.britishmuseum.org/explore/highlights/highlight_objects/pe_mla/a/anti-slavery_medallion,_by_jos.aspx, accessed March 9, 2014.

27. The Tuskegee Syphilis Study Ad Hoc Advisory Panel, *Final Report of the Tuskegee Syphilis Study Ad Hoc Advisory Panel* (Washington, DC: United States Department of Health, Education, and Welfare, Public Health Service, 1973), accessed March 9, 2014, http://www.thebereanchronicles.com/indepth_news/research_pages/tuskegee_experiment/tuskegee_pdf_files/final_report_01.pdf.

28. The description of the Tuskegee syphilis experiment that follows is primarily dependent on the classic account written by James H. Jones, *Bad Blood: The Tuskegee Syphilis Experiment*, New and expanded ed. (New York: Free Press, 1993).

29. Ibid., 92–93. The original research was published in German by E. Bruusgaard in *Archive fur Dermatologie und Syphilis* 157 (1929): 309–332.

30. Ibid., 24.

31. Ibid., 106.

32. Ibid., 127.

33. Ibid., 179.

34. Ibid., 179.

35. Ibid., 179, 180.

36. Ibid., 180.

37. An expression developed in Eric J. Cassell, "Diagnosing Suffering: A Perspective," *Annals of Internal Medicine* 131, no. 7 (1999): 531–534.

38. George Poindexter quoted in Charles S Sydnor, *Slavery in Mississippi* (Gloucester, MA: Peter Smith, 1965), 239.

39. George Lewis Prentiss, *A Memoir of S. S. Prentiss*, vol. 1 (New York: Charles Scribner's Sons, 1891), 107–108, accessed March 9, 2014, http://books.google.com/books?id=sNlqSZhA9c8C&pg=PA109&source=gbs_toc_r&cad=4#v=onepage&q&f=false.

40. Olmstead, *A Journey in the Back Country*, 64, supra note 25.

41. Sean R. Morrison, "The Status of Palliative Care Research in the U.S. and Opportunities for Collaboration" (National Palliative Care Research Center), accessed March 9, 2014, http://www.eapcnet.eu/LinkClick.aspx?fileticket=M_bV2rd5WbA%3D&tabid=752. For additional information, please see Laura P. Gelfman and R. Sean Morrison, "Research Funding for Palliative Medicine," *Journal of Palliative Medicine* 11, no. 1 (2008): 36–43.

42. Jim Downs, *Sick from Freedom: African-American Illness and Suffering During the Civil War and Reconstruction* (New York: Oxford University Press, 2012), 100.

43. For an extensive discussion of how slaves were subjugated, see Kenneth M. Stampp, "Chapter Four: To Make Them Stand in Fear," in *The Peculiar Institution: Slavery in the Ante-Bellum South* (New York: Vintage Books, 1956), 141–191.

44. Roger J. Williams, *Free and Unequal: The Biological Basis of Individual Liberty* (Austin, TX: University of Texas Press, 1953), 124.

45. Richard A. Rettig et al., *False Hope: Bone Marrow Transplantation for Breast Cancer* (Oxford, UK: Oxford University Press, 2007).

46. Henry K. Beecher, "Ethics and Clinical Research," *New England Journal of Medicine* 274, no. 24 (1966): 1354–1360, accessed March 9, 2014, http://www.hhs.gov/ohrp/archive/documents/BeecherArticle.pdf.

47. Ibid. See example 4, example 6, and example 16.

48. United States Advisory Committee on Human Radiation Experiments, *Advisory Committee on Human Radiation Experiments: Final Report* (Washington, DC: The Committee; Available from Supt. of Docs., U.S. G.P.O., 1995).

49. Archived Materials, Department of Health and Human Services, "The Nuremberg Code," accessed March 9, 2014, http://www.hhs.gov/ohrp/archive/nurcode.html.

50. World Medical Association, *Declaration of Helsinki—Ethical Principles for Medical Research Involving Human Subject* (Helsinki, Finland, 1964), accessed March 9, 2014, http://www.wma.net/en/30publications/10policies/b3/.

51. National Commission for the Protection of Human Subjects of Biomedical and Behavioral Research, *The Belmont Report: Ethical Principles and Guidelines for the Protection of Human Subjects of Research* (Washington, DC: Department of Health, Education, and Welfare, 1978), accessed March 1, 2012, http://www.hhs.gov/ohrp/humansubjects/guidance/belmont.html.

52. Ibid.

53. Code of Federal Regulations, *Protection of Human Subjects, "To What Does This Policy Apply?"* Title 45, Part 46, Section 101.

54. Department of Health and Human Services, "Federal Policy for the Protection of Human Subjects ('Common Rule')," accessed March 9, 2014, http://www.hhs.gov/ohrp/humansubjects/commonrule/index.html.

55. Code of Federal Regulations, *Protection of Human Subjects*, "*Criteria for IRB Approval of Research*" Title 45, Part 46, Section 111.

56. Ibid.

57. Full disclosure. Jacobson has been a member of the RAND Corporation's IRB for more than 20 years and has a more nuanced view of the process than Professor Hyman.

58. David A. Hyman, "Institutional Review Boards: Is This the Least Worst We Can Do?" *Northwestern Law Review* 101, no. 2 (2007): 749–774.

59. See, e.g., Steven Joffe, "Revolution or Reform in Human Subjects Research Oversight," *Journal of Law, Medicine & Ethics* 40, no. 4 (2012): 922–929; Margaret Foster Riley, "Federal Funding and the Institutional Evolution of Federal Regulation of Biomedical Research," *Harvard Law and Policy Review* 5 (2011): 265–287.

60. See, e.g., Timothy M. Straight, "Clinical Research Regulation: Challenges to the Institutional Review Board System," *Clinics in Dermatology* 27, no. 4 (2009): 375–383; Laura Stark, "Victims in Our Own Minds? IRBs in Myth and Practice," *Law & Society Review* 41, no. 4 (2007): 777–786.

61. For a recent commentary on this case, see Robin Fretwell Wilson, "The Death of Jesse Gelsinger: New Evidence of the Influence of Money and Prestige in Human Research," *American Journal of Law & Medicine* 36, no. 2/3 (2010): 295–325.

62. See, e.g., Robert M. Nelson, "Appropriate Risk Exposure in Environmental Health Research," *Neurotoxicology and Teratology* 24, no. 4 (2002): 445–449; Joanne Pollak, "The Lead-Based Paint Abatement Repair and Maintenance Study in Baltimore: Historic Framework and Study Design," *Journal of Health Care Law & Policy* 6, no. 1 (2002): 89–108.

63. Margaret Foster Riley, Federal Funding and the Institutional Evolution of Federal Regulation of Biomedical Research, *Harvard Law and Policy Review* 5 (2011): 265–287, at 284.

64. See, e.g., M. Gregg Bloche and Jonathan H. Marks, "When Doctors Go to War," *New England Journal of Medicine* 352, no. 1 (2005): 3–6.

65. Ibid., 3.

66. *National Cancer Control Programmes: Policies and Managerial Guidelines*, 2nd ed. (Geneva: World Health Organization, 2002), accessed June 23, 2011, https://apps.who.int/dsa/justpub/cpl.htm.

67. Timothy E. Quill and Amy P. Abernethy, "Generalist Plus Specialist Palliative Care—Creating a More Sustainable Model," *New England Journal of Medicine* 368 (2013): 1173–1175.

68. Most attributions of individual or large-scale suffering to "bad luck" fail to reflect deeper issues and causes that are unseen or not fully understood.

9

Human Rights and the Moral Obligation to Alleviate Suffering

Roberto Andorno and Cristiana Baffone

If happiness—understood as deep existential fulfillment—is the ultimate goal of life, then suffering contradicts in the most direct manner this basic aspiration of every individual. Suffering is the most painful and annihilating condition in human existence; it invades every corner of our being, tends to destroy any hope, and puts at risk our sense of integrity. Accordingly, suffering has been defined as "the state of severe distress associated with events that threaten the intactness of the person."[1]

Although suffering may overlap with physical pain, it extends beyond the bodily domain. Certainly, physical pain, at least when it rises above a certain level of intensity and duration, usually entails suffering, but both notions are not synonymous. First, there are other sources and varieties of suffering besides physical pain (e.g., moral suffering resulting from severe humiliation, injustice, discrimination, the breakdown of one's family, the death of a loved one, and solitude; metaphysical or existential suffering, which is caused by the loss of meaning in a person's life); second, a person's degree of suffering is not always directly correlated with the intensity of pain.[2] Several factors that affect the perception of somebody's pain can amplify or diminish the person's suffering. These factors include whether the pain is perceived as of short duration or, on the contrary, as a condition that the person will endure for a long period of time or even until the end of the person's life; whether the pain is regarded as absurd and meaningless, especially if it is the result of the malevolent will of other people (e.g., torture, inhuman punishment) or, on the contrary, as the result of an act of heroism or personal accomplishment (e.g., the pain suffered by the firefighter who succeeds in saving other people's lives, or by the mother at childbirth).

Assuming that the first moral principle, from which all others are derived, is that *good is to be done and evil avoided*, and admitting that suffering is an intrinsic evil, it is reasonable to conclude that *there is a moral duty to prevent human suffering.* This duty is, however, not absolute because it can be overridden or trumped by higher moral considerations. Using W. D. Ross's terminology, it can be said that the duty to prevent suffering is a "prima facie duty"[3] because it is not absolute but can be overridden, for instance, by the duty not to kill. A terminal and seriously ill man could indeed be relieved from his suffering by being killed, but such a killing might still be wrong because of the intrinsic value that we attach to human life. This is precisely the reason why active euthanasia is legally forbidden in virtually all countries, and instead it is recommended to facilitate access to palliative care to address this terminal distress.

The duty to prevent suffering can also be overridden, not by a rival *duty,* but by a rival *permission.*[4] For instance, a sentence to a long-term imprisonment as the result of a serious crime is usually a source of deep suffering for the convicted individual, but this inevitable distress can be justified by a requirement of justice (the punishment of crime and the prevention of further crimes).

The scope of this chapter is, first, to explore to what extent human rights can be conceptualized as a social response to human suffering; second, to investigate whether suffering could be regarded as the foundation of human rights; and finally, to analyze how three concrete forms of human suffering are addressed by human rights instruments: torture, starvation, and terminal illness.

Human Rights as a Social Response to Human Suffering

Former United Nations (U.N.) Secretary General Dag Hammarskjöld said in 1954 that "the United Nations was not created in order to bring us to heaven, but in order to save us from hell."[5] Paraphrasing this statement, it could be said that the human rights system was not conceived to make people happy but *to prevent—or at least to alleviate—their suffering.*

From a moral perspective, happiness and suffering are not just two sides of the same coin; they are morally asymmetrical notions.[6] As stated by Karl Popper: "human suffering makes a direct moral appeal, namely, the appeal for help, while there is no similar call to increase the happiness of a man who is doing well anyway."[7] This is one of the reasons why the dominant focus of human rights is preventing the most serious harms to people's physical and moral integrity rather than guaranteeing the perfect fulfillment of their well-being. Human rights are "much more concerned with avoiding the terrible than with achieving the best."[8] In the words of Shue, human rights have more to do with the "lower limits on tolerable human conduct" than with "great aspirations and exalted ideals."[9]

Certainly, giving a response to human suffering is not the only goal of human rights. Neither are human rights the only response, nor always the most efficient one, to the problem of human suffering. Many forms of distress, especially those of an existential nature and those resulting from our permanent exposure to disease and death, fall far beyond the legal domain.

Yet the human rights movement has from the very beginning been closely associated with suffering. Moreover, their formal recognition by the international community in the aftermath of the Second World War was a direct response to the Holocaust, which would become the symbol of extreme human suffering for postwar generations. If the twentieth century, especially in its second half, has been often described as the Age of Human Rights, it is, paradoxically, because that same century witnessed, in its first half, some of the most massive and systematic atrocities committed against human beings in history. The human rights movement was precisely motivated by those horrors and aimed to prevent "barbarous acts which have outraged the conscience of mankind" from ever happening again.[10]

The content of the Universal Declaration of Human Rights of 1948 (hereafter, UDHR) was to large extent informed by the full discovery, during the Nuremberg trials, of the atrocities committed in Auschwitz and the other concentration camps. The historian and bioethicist Robert Baker does not hesitate to claim that "the details revealed daily at Nuremberg gave content to the rights recognized by Articles 4 through 20 of the Declaration."[11] These articles concern the freedom from slavery and servitude (Article 4); the freedom from torture and cruel, inhuman, and degrading treatments or punishments (Article 5); the right to be recognized as a person before the law (Article 6); the right to equal protection under the law (Article 7); the right to access to justice and to a fair trial (Articles 8 and 10); the freedom from arbitrary arrest and imprisonment (Article 9); the rights to be presumed innocent until proved guilty and to be prosecuted only for acts that were legal offences at the time they were committed (Article 11); the right to privacy (Article 12); the right to freedom of movement (Article 13); the right to asylum (Article 14); the right to a nationality (Article 15); the right to marry and to found a family (Article 16); the right to property (Article 17); the right to freedom of thought, conscience, and religion (Article 18); the freedom of opinion and expression (Article 19); and the freedom of association (Article 20).

The disregard of all these rights is certainly a cause of suffering for the victims of such violations, although the degree of distress is obviously not the same in all of them. The practices that more directly, brutally, and seriously infringe on the physical and moral integrity of individuals and ultimately deny their intrinsic value as "persons" (e.g., torture and inhuman and degrading treatments and punishments, arbitrary imprisonment, sexual assaults) are cause of a much deeper suffering than the disregard of, say, the right to property or the freedom of association.

Arguing that human rights are primarily focused on preventing the worst forms of suffering does not necessarily entail denying the importance of those rights that extend beyond physical cruelty, or supporting a minimalist conception of human rights. All rights are important in the sense that there is a mutually reinforcing dynamic between them, and the fulfillment of one of them often depends on the fulfillment of the others. For instance, the right to freedom of speech and the right to education also significantly contribute to the realization of human dignity through the satisfaction of people's basic intellectual and psychological needs. In addition, history shows that the fight against torture, arbitrary arrests, and inhuman treatments or punishments may be significantly aided when people enjoy freedom of speech and have a better education.

The point we want to stress is that the degree of suffering caused by the violation of the different human rights is not the same but rather significantly varies from right to right. Therefore, if suffering is a paramount evil, one may conclude that it is more urgent for any society to ensure compliance with those rights that more directly aim to prevent or reduce extreme suffering—even if they concern a small portion of the population—than to promote the maximal well-being of the majority of people.

It is not by chance that, while most human rights are couched in positive terms ("Everyone has the right to. . ."), there are a few, those that aim to prevent the most severe forms of deliberately inflicted suffering, that are formulated in *negative* terms, as prohibitions: "No one shall be held in slavery or servitude"; "no one shall be subjected to torture or to cruel, inhuman or degrading treatment or punishment" (Articles 4 and 5 of the UDHR, respectively). The difference is not merely semantic but rather has significant practical implications: the rights framed in negative language are regarded as *absolute,* in the sense that they are not subject to any exceptions, while most rights can be limited in certain circumstances, provided that restrictions are necessary and are a proportionate way of achieving a legitimate purpose.[12]

This is to say that the relief of the most severe forms of suffering has *moral priority* over the promotion of the fulfillment of the general well-being of the population. A few cases of torture in which State officials are involved or a few cases of seriously degrading working conditions or starvation resulting from State inaction are more degrading for a society than, say, its lack of ability to ensure a more efficient public transportation system or better cultural offers for the majority of people. Suffering not only is the factor that motivated the emergence of human rights in modern times but also is the parameter that determines the degree of urgency in the implementation of the various rights.

Is Suffering the Foundation of Human Rights?

Theorists of human rights have traditionally paid little or no attention to the problem of suffering as such. The term *suffering* is hard to find in the subject index of most academic writings on human rights; it is also rarely present in human rights instruments. This does not mean that there is little connection between human rights and suffering. As mentioned earlier, human rights have to a large extent emerged in the midst of the twentieth century as a response to human suffering. However, the notion of suffering as such has not been traditionally regarded as a *legal* concept but rather merely as the implicit *psychological* underpinning of human rights violations.

It is only in the past few decades that a greater awareness has grown about the need to overcome an excessively formalistic conception of human rights, which tends to see human beings as disembodied right holders and forgets that people really suffer, both physically and mentally. In the words of Andrew Fagan, we are now beginning to realize that the "ethical imperative of human suffering"[13] must play a crucial role in our discussions about the form and content of human rights and that "the cornerstone of human rights must be a concern for human suffering."[14]

The greater importance we attach today to the role of suffering in human rights takes place simultaneously with the recent emphasis on vulnerability in ethical theory and on the crucial significance of empathy in the perception of ethical problems. Paradigmatic in this respect is the approach developed by Emmanuel Levinas, who claims that ethics rests upon an apprehension of the precariousness of life. In his view, ethics emerges primarily on the concrete level of person-to-person relationship and not on the level of purely theoretical knowledge. Levinas makes use of the "face" as a figure that communicates both the vulnerability of life and the incommensurable value of every individual. The relation to the face is "a relation with the other absolutely other, which I cannot contain, with the other in this sense infinite"[15]; the face of the other resists our power to assimilate them into mere knowledge. The face of the other silently remembers us the command: "you shall not commit murder."[16]

What are the implications of this emphasis on vulnerability for human rights theory? Does it entail that vulnerability can—or should—be regarded as the *foundation* of human rights? This is, for instance, the position of the sociologist Bryan Turner, who claims that human rights exist because "human beings share a common ontology that is grounded in a shared vulnerability."[17] In his view, the concept of human rights can be explained by the need to protect vulnerable human beings by social institutions, which in their turn pose threats to those human beings. The institutionalization of human rights is not but the attempt to resolve this dilemma in modern societies. According to Turner, human rights result from the observation that we are vulnerable beings, exposed to misuse, mistreatment, and exploitation. The historical circumstance that the modern human rights movement emerged as a response to the horrors of the Second World War shows well, in his opinion, that human rights are grounded on our vulnerable condition.

Although we sympathize with this view, we fear it is conceptually mistaken. We do not have rights *because* we are vulnerable but rather because we are *persons*, that is, because we possess inherent *dignity*. This is clear in international human rights law, which is grounded on the "recognition of the inherent dignity and of the equal and inalienable rights of all members of the human family" (UDHR, Preamble). In its first article, the Declaration emphasizes that "all human beings are born free and equal in dignity and rights." Human dignity is presented by this document as the bedrock of all the rights and freedoms set forth in the Declaration and, in particular, the basis for the prohibition of all forms of discrimination (Article 2), of slavery (Article 4), of torture, and of any cruel, inhuman, or degrading treatment or punishment (Article 5). Even more explicitly, the two major pillars of international human rights law after the UDHR, the International Covenant on Civil and Political Rights and the International Covenant on Economic, Social, and Cultural Rights of 1966, solemnly affirm in their Preambles that human rights "derive from the inherent dignity of the human person."

It is true that, historically, the development of international human rights norms after the Second World War was a direct consequence of the observation that we are vulnerable beings and exposed to any kind of misuse and cruelty. But human rights are not *grounded* on that observation. Vulnerability is a *condition,* not the *ground* of human rights. Vulnerability is a mere fact, which alone cannot have any normative effects. Vulnerability only becomes relevant for human rights after we have assumed that every human being has intrinsic dignity. In fact, both dignity and vulnerability play a role in the development of human rights. Human rights results as a confluence of both factors: one normative (the recognition of intrinsic worthiness of every individual), and one factual (the observation that human beings are vulnerable, fragile, and exposed to suffering):

Human dignity (normative element) + *Human vulnerability* (factual element) = *Human rights* (normative result)

In addition, there is another interesting interaction between vulnerability and human rights. When modern societies affirm that all human beings, even the most deprived, sick, and excluded ones, are worthy of respect and subject to inalienable rights, they assume that they are entitled to basic rights by the mere fact of being humans, and not by the circumstance of being healthy, or strong, or morally autonomous. This is to say that human dignity and its resulting human rights become paradoxically more visible in vulnerability than in self-sufficiency, in weakness than in power; they become especially patent in the most fragile human beings: in newborns, in small children, in the elderly, in the sick, in the poor. This is paradoxical because human dignity has been traditionally associated with the highest rational capacities, with the human power to dominate nature, with autonomous decision-making capacity. But in the most vulnerable, dignity is not hidden by intellectual or physical abilities, or good health, or beauty but rather appears in its pure state. This is clear in medical practice, which is constantly confronted with the human being in its nakedness, in its simple existence, and is required to discover the value of every patient in that context.[18]

Another approach that appeals to the concept of suffering to give new and more efficient responses to human rights problems is the one proposed by Richard Rorty.[19] The American philosopher claims that traditional—purely theoretical—understandings of human rights should be discarded in favor of an approach that he calls "sentimental education," by means of which people can learn about the details of others' lives—and particularly their suffering—in order to gain a better cross-cultural understanding of their needs and a more effective engagement in favor of human rights. It must be noted that Rorty does not address the issue of the human rights' foundation. Moreover, he argues that there is no theoretical foundation for human rights because there is no theoretical foundation for any value. His extreme skeptical, pragmatist view is focused on the practical ways of improving respect for human rights and discards any concern for their theoretical foundation. According to him, the cause of human rights does not require theory for its success but rather sympathy.[20]

The merit of Rorty's view consists in putting in evidence that purely theoretical arguments are insufficient to foster an effective response to human rights violations, and that we need to cultivate an affective personal experience of the suffering of our fellow human beings. The problem with this position is that, by exclusively focusing on "sentimental education" and by discarding any theoretical justification, it goes too far and ultimately eliminates reasoning. Rorty's approach amounts to ignore the fact that, as rational beings, we need reasons to support our actions, including our commitment in favor of human rights. Sympathy is an emotion, not a reason. Even acknowledging that emotions can play a valuable role in the promotion of human rights by helping to strengthen our sense of responsibility and concern for others, the need for a rational justification is, in the end, inescapable. As Michael Freeman rightly points out, "whether the action we take on the basis of our emotions is justified depends on the reasons for the action."[21] In other words, effective human rights promotion needs more than just a feeling of solidarity; it requires also a framework of general and universal principles that specify and characterize the rights to be protected and establish the procedural and organizational means necessary for the enforcement of those principles.[22]

The Paradigmatic Case of Intentionally Inflicted Suffering: Torture

When we think of intentionally inflicted suffering, torture is the first example that comes to mind. Torture is indeed "the paradigmatic case of suffering" because it is "a total assault on the psyche" and because during torture "all the signs point to destruction."[23] Being tortured is experienced by victims as a "living death."[24]

In the aftermath of the Second World War, as a result of the revelation that prisoners of concentration camps had been subjected to torture and other inhuman and degrading treatments, the international community felt it necessary to stress the absolute prohibition of torture, beginning with the UDHR of 1948, which states:

> No one shall be subjected to torture or to cruel, inhuman or degrading treatment or punishment. (Article 5)

Since then, uncountable global or regional human rights instruments have emphasized that torture cannot be accepted under any circumstances. The most significant documents are the Geneva Conventions relative to the Treatment of Prisoners of War, and to the Protection of Civilian Persons in Time of War of 1949, the International Covenant on Civil and Political Rights of 1966 (Article 7), the U.N. Convention against Torture and Other Cruel, Inhuman, or Degrading Treatment of 1984, the American Convention on Human Rights of 1969 (Article 5.1), the European Convention on Human Rights of 1950 (Article 3), and the European Convention for the Prevention of Torture and Inhuman or Degrading Treatment or Punishment of 1987.

Severe suffering is inherent to torture, and such suffering can be caused using either physical or psychological methods. This means that there can be torture without physical pain or injury. Widely accepted definitions of torture are explicit in this regard, such as the definition provided by the U.N. Convention Against Torture and other Cruel, Inhuman, or Degrading Treatment of 1984, which refers to torture as "any act by which severe pain or suffering, whether physical or mental" intentionally inflicted on a person for particular purposes, such as obtaining information, punishment, or intimidation (Article 1).

Torture is therefore not limited to acts causing physical pain but also includes those that aim at causing mental suffering. This point is crucial. After the reports of human rights abuses by the U.S. military in Guantánamo Bay, Iraq, and Afghanistan, questions have been raised as to whether certain harsh detention and interrogation methods amount to torture. A 2002 U.S. Justice Department Memorandum on torture argued that the use of waterboarding, prolonged sleep deprivation, and binding in stress positions might not be considered torture on the grounds that they do not cause *physical* injury.[25] To examine the validity of this claim, a study was carried out in 2007 with a population-based sample of survivors of torture from former Yugoslavia. According to the conclusions of this study, aggressive interrogation techniques or detention procedures involving deprivation of basic needs, exposure to aversive environmental conditions, psychological manipulations, humiliating treatment, and forced stress positions are not substantially different from physical torture in terms of the severity of mental suffering they cause, the underlying mechanism of traumatic stress, and their long-term psychological outcome.[26] Accordingly, the U.N. Committee against Torture issued a report in 2006 stating explicitly that harsh interrogation techniques such as those involving sexual humiliation, waterboarding, short shackling, and using dogs to induce fear constitute torture or cruel, inhuman, or degrading treatment or punishment and are therefore forbidden by international law.

The truth is that psychological torture can even be worse than torture mainly aiming at causing physical pain. While the physical injuries produced by torture are likely to heal, mental suffering is much deeper and likely to persist. As a physician from the International Red Cross states, "the worst scars [of torture] are in the mind."[27] The devastating psychological consequences of deep humiliation, threats, sleep deprivation, and solitary confinement are evident through the literature, observations of clinicians, and reports from victims.

Is there any significant difference between torture, on one side, and cruel, inhuman, or degrading treatment or punishment, on the other? The previously mentioned U.S. Justice Department Memorandum of 2002 used this distinction to argue that the latter practices may be justified under exceptional circumstances. It is true that the Convention against Torture and Other Cruel, Inhuman, or Degrading Treatment of 1984 introduced this distinction and, although it bans torture absolutely (Article 2), it imposes on States "only" the obligation to "undertake to prevent" cruel, inhuman, or degrading treatment (Article 16). However, other important legal instruments do not differentiate between the two notions. The foundational human rights instrument, the Universal Declaration of Human Rights of 1948, as well as the International Covenant on Civil and Political Rights of 1966 prohibit in absolute terms both torture and inhuman or degrading treatment (Article 5, and Articles 4 and 7, respectively). The same is true of the Geneva Conventions of 1949 and of the European Convention on Human Rights (Article 3).

As a matter of fact, the distinction between the two categories of ill practices is of degree, not of kind; it is based on the different intensity of the suffering inflicted to the victim, which varies depending on factors such as the duration of the ill treatment; its physical and mental effects; the sex, age, state of health of the victim; and the manner and method of execution. In this regard, torture can be said to be the highest form of inhuman or degrading treatment because it implies the infliction of more severe suffering or pain. Of course, determining whether a particular cruel or inhuman treatment qualifies as torture is a very subjective judgment. However, an interpretation in good faith of the relevant human rights instruments makes the distinction between these two notions legally irrelevant because the intention of the international community was clearly to prohibit both torture and inhuman or degrading treatment, and not to give governments an excuse to circumvent the absolute prohibition of torture by classifying methods as "cruel, inhuman, or degrading," rather than as "torture."[28]

Leaving aside the controversy around this distinction, the absolute prohibition of torture is sometimes criticized on the grounds that there could be situations in which this practice should be permissible. To this purpose, appeal is invariably made to the ticking bomb scenario: "Imagine that a terrorist has placed a powerful bomb somewhere in the middle of a city of 1,000,000 inhabitants, most of whom are likely to be killed or injured by the explosion; the man who planted the bomb has been arrested, he is the only who knows its location, and the artefact is programmed to explode within a few hours. If torturing the man is the only way for us to locate and deactivate to bomb, thereby saving hundreds of thousands of innocent people, then aren't we morally authorized—even required—to torture him?"

Several authors have stressed the fallacy of this scenario. They claim that it is unrealistic because it deceives us about the choices we face in the real world. As Mayerfeld points out, this scenario deceives us in two ways: first, by suggesting that the recourse to torture, if allowed, will be limited to such exceptional circumstances and never on innocent people; second, by suggesting that the ticking bomb situation is itself a realistic possibility, which it is not.[29] The fact is that the ticking bomb scenario is in practice invoked to allow torture in situations that have nothing to do with such unrealistic scenarios. The claim that torture should be permitted in exceptional cases corrupts the entire moral and political thinking in a society and must be rejected. In our opinion, the civilized nature of a society depends, among other indicators, on the absolute prohibition of this practice.

Certainly, torture is not only contrary to international human rights law but is also radically antithetical to the purpose of the medical profession, which is to alleviate the distress of fellow human beings, not to inflict pain on them. This is why any involvement of physicians in acts of torture, whether active or passive, either to judge what victims can endure, to suggest methods that will enhance suffering, or to falsify medical records, is condemned by international standards on medical ethics.[30] Unfortunately, almost seventy years after the trial of the Nazi doctors in Nuremberg, the involvement of physicians in torture is still a source of consternation. In 2004, the International Committee of the Red Cross, after an inspection of the U.S. prison in Guantánamo Bay, labeled the active role of physicians in physical and mental coercion of prisoners as "a flagrant violation of medical ethics."[31]

The primary consideration of health care professionals working in places of detention should always be to serve the best interests of detainees. Physicians may be asked to provide a medical opinion as to whether existing mental or physical health problems would preclude the individual from being questioned; they may also be requested to provide medical treatment to a person suffering a medical emergency during questioning. However, their role does not extend to ruling on the permissibility of any form of physical or psychological ill treatment.[32]

The complicity of physicians in acts of torture is hard to understand because it strikes at the heart of the medical profession. There seems to be a number of psychological characteristics, as well as social, cultural, and political factors that predispose physicians to participate in acts of torture.[33] Bloche and Marks, who conducted interviews with physicians involved in hard interrogation techniques in Guantánamo Bay and in Iraq, report the belief of some of the physicians "that physicians serving in these roles do not act as physicians and are therefore not bound by patient-oriented ethics."[34] What is clear is that new concerted efforts of intergovernmental and nongovernmental organizations are urgently needed in this area. As Grodin and Annas point out, "the re-emergence of physician complicity in torture presents an opportunity for the medical and legal professional organizations to work together transnationally to uphold both medical ethics and human rights."[35]

Suffering Caused by a State's Inaction: Starvation

Starvation is defined as "suffering or death caused by lack of food."[36] It is the most severe form of malnutrition, which at a certain point may become irreversible and lead to death. Prolonged starvation can cause permanent organ damage and, if complete, leads to death within 8 to 12 weeks in adults. In the final stages of starvation, a variety of neurological and psychiatric symptoms are experienced, as well as severe muscle atrophy and disturbances in heart rhythm.[37]

In children, chronic malnutrition is marked by weakness, greater exposure to disease, and growth retardation. Malnutrition is by far the biggest contributor to child mortality; it is a contributory factor in the death of 2.6 million children every year—one third of the global total of children's deaths.[38]

According to the Food and Agriculture Organization, about 925 million people around the world are chronically undernourished. This figure represents about 13.5 percent of the world population. Two thirds of the hungry live in just seven countries (Bangladesh, China, the Democratic Republic of Congo, Ethiopia, India, Indonesia, and Pakistan) and more than 40 percent live in China and India alone.[39]

Starvation represents a particularly dramatic expression of human suffering because it is related to one of the most basic, immediate, and inescapable human needs. Unfortunately, for many people, suffering because of hunger is an ordinary condition, which is mainly caused by poverty in addition to other factors such as civil war and natural disasters. The lack of nutrition leads to physical weakness, which affects the ability to work. Poor people suffer from hunger, and their starving condition traps them in their own poverty.

The human rights system has not ignored the drama of starvation because it challenges the satisfaction of one of the most basic and pressing human needs and, in the end, also puts at risk the fundamental right to life. The right to food is recognized in many international instruments, beginning with the UDHR of 1948, which states in Article 25:

> Everyone has the right to a standard of living adequate for the health and well-being of himself and of his family, including food, clothing, housing and medical care and necessary social services....

The right to food is also emphasized by one of the pillars of the human rights system, the International Covenant on Economic, Social, and Cultural Rights of 1966, which recognizes the "fundamental right of everyone to be free from hunger" (Article 11) and stresses that States have the obligation to take steps, individually and through international assistance and cooperation to the maximum of its available resources, to achieve progressively the full realization of the rights recognized in the Covenant, including the right to adequate food (Article 2.1).

The State's responsibility in this field encompasses three obligations: to take positive measures against the deprivation of people's food; to protect individuals from the violation of the right to food from third parties; and to facilitate and promote activities whose scope is to strengthen the access and the possibility of people to feed themselves.

In this regard, the right to food is defined through three elements, which are availability, accessibility, and adequacy[40]:

Availability refers to the possibility for people to feed themselves directly from productive land or other natural resources, or the existence of well-functioning distribution, processing, and market systems that can move food from the site of production to where it is needed.

Accessibility implies that both physical and economic access is guaranteed. Physical accessibility means that food must be within reach of everyone, including physically vulnerable individuals, such as children, elderly people, and physically disabled people. Economic accessibility implies that adequate food should be financially affordable without compromising other basic needs.

Adequacy means that food must satisfy the dietary needs of every individual at all stages throughout the life cycle and according to gender and occupation; it also entails that food must be safe and that adequate protective measures must be taken to prevent contamination of foodstuffs through adulteration or bad environmental or handling hygiene.

States fail to fulfill their obligation if they do not ensure the satisfaction of, at least, the minimal essential level required to be free from hunger.[41] A State can argue that, for instance, resources constraints make it unable to comply with this obligation, but it has to demonstrate that "every effort has been made to use all the resources at its disposal in an effort to satisfy, as a matter of priority, those minimum obligations" and that "it has unsuccessfully sought to obtain international support to ensure the availability and accessibility of the necessary food."[42]

Until the 1980s, the dominant academic view about world hunger was that it was simply caused by a lack of food in a particular society, that is, a problem of demand exceeding supply. However, since the end of the 1990s, the Indian economist and philosopher Amartya Sen has contributed to a better understanding of the problem, in particular, that the root of the hunger drama in the world does not merely lie in food production but also in inefficient food distribution and storage systems. He notices that the problem of hunger "involves much more than food" and that, "while much can be done through sensible government policy, it is important to integrate the role of the government with the efficient functioning of other economic and social institutions."[43]

Unfortunately, despite all the good intentions of international law, the right to food still remains largely unfulfilled today. In the words of Thomas Pogge, the right to a minimally adequate standard of living, including the right to food, is "by far the most under-fulfilled of all human rights" recognized by international law.[44]

Suffering Caused by Terminal Illness: Is There a Right to Die?

A terminal illness is a disease that cannot be cured or adequately treated and that is expected to result in the death of the patient within a short period of time (e.g., six months or less). Usually, the diagnosis of a terminal illness is devastating news for any patient. The world is turned upside-down as the goal of extended life vanishes. The individual is suddenly confronted with his or her own mortality in very realistic terms. This situation can be a source of deep suffering and depression, which could even lead some individuals to desire a hastened death.

According to Elisabeth Kübler-Ross, individuals who are confronted with an impending death experience a series of emotional stages: denial, anger, bargaining, depression, and acceptance. Of course, not everyone will experience all of these stages, or, if all are experienced, they will not necessarily occur in this particular order. Different people react in different ways; some move quickly into acceptance of their situation, while others become stuck in one stage or another.[45]

Those terminal patients who do not succeed in overcoming depression need special support. Palliative care plays a crucial role in such circumstances because it aims to improve the quality of life of terminally ill patients and to relief their suffering. In this regard, it is interesting to note that, according to several studies, depression, rather than pain, is the primary reason that some people may request assisted dying.[46] Personal psychological factors, the loss of body functions, poor family cohesion, and perceiving oneself as a burden to others are often the reasons why some terminally ill patients may become depressed and express a desire to accelerate their death. Not surprisingly, after depression is adequately treated, many terminally ill patients feel better, improve their quality of life, and relinquish their desire to hasten death.[47]

However, the question remains of what to do with those terminal patients who persist in their wish to die and request assistance with suicide. Do they have a "right to die"?

The expression *right to die* is not used here to mean the possibility for patients to refuse treatments or life support measures that they consider futile, burdensome, or disproportionate. In modern medical ethics and law, it is widely accepted that patients' right to informed consent includes the possibility for them to withhold and withdraw treatments, even if such decisions might adversely affect their health or even shorten their lives. Patients have even the right to make such decisions ahead of time by means of advance directives. Legal developments during the past two decades or so show, not only in the United States but also in Europe, a clear tendency toward the improvement of patients' self-determination regarding advance health care planning.[48]

The term *right to die* is used here to refer to the more controversial question of whether people have a right to obtain assistance with suicide or even to be mercifully killed by others (i.e., active euthanasia). It is important to note that having a *right* means having a claim against others that they act in a certain manner. Concretely, the existence of a "right to die" would mean that the State has a *positive obligation* to facilitate people with the necessary means to kill themselves or to be mercifully killed by others. Moreover, if there were such a right, the State should generally abstain from preventing people from committing suicide or from being killed by others at their request. Not surprisingly, there is consensus in the international community that there is not a "right to die" when it is understood in this sense. This seems to be valid even for those very few countries having decriminalized, under certain conditions, active euthanasia (The Netherlands, Belgium, and Luxembourg) and assisted suicide (Switzerland).[49]

In the United States, the Supreme Court ruled unanimously in 1997 in the cases of *Washington v. Glucksberg* and *Vacco v. Quill* that there is no constitutional right to assisted suicide. Similarly, in Europe, the European Court of Human Rights (ECtHR) has expressly denied the existence of a "right to die." The leading cases in this regard are *Pretty v. the United Kingdom* (2002)[50] and *Haas v. Switzerland* (2011).[51]

In *Pretty v. the United Kingdom,* the ECtHR ruled that "no right to die, whether at the hands of a third person or with the assistance of a public authority" can be derived from the provisions of the European Convention on Human Rights. The applicant in this case was Diane Pretty, a 43-year-old British woman, who was paralyzed from the neck down as a result of a progressive neurodegenerative disease. She had little decipherable speech, was fed through a tube, and had a short life expectancy. Her intellect and capacity to make decisions remained nonetheless unimpaired by the illness. Because, according to the English law, it is a crime to assist another to commit suicide [section 2(1) of the Suicide Act 1961], she sought a guarantee from the Director of Public Prosecutions that her husband, if he helped her to commit suicide, would be immune from prosecution. She claimed that the English law that prohibited assisted suicide infringed her rights under Articles 2 (right to life), 3 (prohibition of torture and of inhuman or degrading treatment), 8 (privacy), 9 (freedom of thought, conscience, and religion), and 14 (nondiscrimination) of the European Convention on Human Rights.

The Court's judgment rejects the argument that the Convention provides a ground for the recognition of a right to die. Regarding Article 2 on the right to life, the Court declares that this provision "cannot, without a distortion of language, be interpreted as conferring the diametrically opposite right, namely a right to die; nor can it create a right to self-determination in the sense of conferring on an individual the entitlement to choose death rather than life."[52] The judgment observes that in all the cases relating to Article 2 that were brought before the Court, the emphasis was always on "the obligation of the State to protect life."[53] For this reason, the Court is not persuaded by the applicant "that the right to life, guaranteed in Article 2, can be interpreted as involving a negative aspect" (namely, a right to die).[54] Neither is Article 3 (prohibition of torture and of inhuman or degrading treatment) regarded by the Court as relevant to the case because the "State has not, itself, inflicted any ill-treatment on the applicant. Nor is there any complaint that the applicant is not receiving adequate care from the State medical authorities."[55]

The ECtHR considers that only Article 8, recognizing the right to private life, falls within the applicant's claim.[56] But this does not mean that Article 8 has been violated. According to Paragraph 2 of this Article, interference with the right to private life can be lawful if it is "in accordance with the law" and is "necessary in a democratic society" for the aims mentioned in this provision. States have a considerable margin of appreciation of what is "necessary" to those purposes. In this regard, the Court holds that there are no particular reasons for claiming that "the blanket nature of the ban on assisted suicide is disproportionate."[57]

In 2011, in the case of *Haas vs. Switzerland,* the ECtHR confirmed that one cannot rely on the European Convention on Human Rights to claim a right to euthanasia or to assisted suicide. The applicant, Ernst Haas, a Swiss national, suffered from a serious psychiatric disorder and wanted to commit suicide with a lethal substance (sodium pentobarbital), which according to Swiss law, is only available on medical prescription. He did not qualify under this law because of his psychiatric disorder, so he vainly tried to obtain a dispensation in order to get the substance without prescription. He complained that this impossibility violated his right to privacy, guaranteed by Article 8 of the European Convention on Human Rights, and that the State should have provided him with the drugs to commit suicide.

The Court's judgment recognizes that "an individual's right to decide by what means and at what point his or her life will end... is one of the aspects of the right to respect for private life within the meaning of Article 8 of the Convention".[58] However, this is so provided that the individual is "capable of freely reaching a decision on this question and acting in consequence."[59] In other words, such a right only operates insofar as the action can be implemented by the individual, not with the help of a third party.[60]

The crucial point in the Haas case was whether States have a "positive obligation" to take the necessary measures to allow a dignified suicide.[61] For the Court to decide on this, it would be necessary to weight the different interests at stake, an exercise in which States enjoy a certain "margin of appreciation."[62]

The judgment also points out that the Human Rights Convention must be read as a whole; therefore, it is appropriate to refer in this case to Article 2, which creates for the authorities a "duty to protect vulnerable persons, even against actions by which they endanger their own lives."[63] For the Court, this latter provision obliges national authorities "to prevent an individual from taking his or her own life if the decision has not been taken freely and with full understanding of what is involved."[64]

The Court observes that the legal requirement of a medical prescription, issued on the basis of a psychiatric assessment, for obtaining a lethal drug pursues the legitimate aim of protecting individuals from making hasty decisions and to prevent abuse, especially in a country such as Switzerland, where the legislation and practice allow for relatively easy access to assisted suicide.[65] Therefore, the ECtHR does not endorse the claim according to which the State would have a positive obligation to take measures facilitating assisted suicide.

In summary, the suffering of terminally ill patients is addressed by legal systems through the promotion of palliative care and the recognition of the right to refuse treatments that patients may perceive as excessive, futile, or psychologically harmful. On the contrary, the recognition of a right to die (i.e., a right to assisted suicide or euthanasia) is not regarded by human rights law as a socially valuable solution to the problem posed by terminally ill patients.

Conclusion

There is a direct and inescapable connection between human rights and suffering. The human rights movement that emerged in the aftermath of the Second World War was an immediate response to the Holocaust, which would become the symbol of extreme human suffering for postwar generations. Despite this historical grounding, human rights theory has traditionally paid little attention to the problem of suffering as such, which has been usually regarded just as the implicit *psychological* underpinning of human rights violations, but not as a legally relevant concept in itself.

The classic framework for conceptualizing human rights tends to be excessively formalistic, ahistorical, and acontextual; it has a propensity to consider human beings as abstract rights holders, disregarding the fact that they are embodied beings who really suffer both physically and mentally as a result of human rights violations. It is only in the past few decades that greater awareness has developed about the need to take pain and suffering more seriously and explicitly into account in the implementation of human rights policy.

We are now realizing that the moral imperative to alleviate suffering is not just the historical factor that motivated the emergence of human rights in the midst of the twentieth century. It is, still today, though often implicitly, at the very heart of every serious human rights policy. Suffering is the parameter that determines the degree of urgency in the implementation of the various human rights. Moreover, the interpretation and implementation of human rights norms through the lens of suffering can contribute to develop compassion toward others and to promote a more effective and proactive commitment to human rights in the world.

Yet stressing the importance of suffering for human rights should not be understood as meaning that we can merely rely on a feeling of *empathy* to ensure their effective implementation. As rational beings, we also need *reasons* for action. The efforts oriented toward reducing suffering across the world need to be addressed through the use of practical reasoning and the guidance of a framework of universal principles that are grounded on the recognition of the inherent dignity of every fellow human being.

Finally, it is also important to remind that it is far beyond the scope of human rights –and of the law in general– to provide an efficient remedy to all forms of human suffering and to ensure happiness. The central scope of human rights law is much more modest: it attempts, above all, to give a response to those practices and situations that are a more severe source of human suffering. Returning to the Hammarskjöld's simile mentioned earlier, we can conclude that human rights are certainly unable to make our lives a paradise, but they can at least help to prevent many people's lives from becoming a hell on earth.

Notes

1. Eric J. Cassel, "The Nature of Suffering and the Goals of Medicine," *New England Journal of Medicine* 306, no. 11 (1982): 639–645.

2. Jamie Mayerfeld, *Suffering and Moral Responsibility* (New York: Oxford University Press, 1999), 24.

3. See William D. Ross, *The Right and the Good* (Oxford, UK: Oxford University Press, 1930).

4. Jamie Mayerfeld, supra note 2, 6.

5. Dag Hammarskjöld, "Address at the University of California Convocation: 13 May 1954," in *Public Papers of the Secretaries General of the United Nations*, Vol. II, ed. Andrew W. Cordier and Wilder Foote (New York: Columbia University Press, 1972), 301.

6. Jamie Mayerfeld, supra note 2, 128ff.

7. Karl Popper, *The Open Society and Its Enemies* (Princeton, NJ: Princeton University Press, 1950), 570.

8. James Nickel, "Human Rights," in *The Stanford Encyclopedia of Philosophy*, ed. Edward N. Zalta, 2013, accessed March 10, 2014, http://plato.stanford.edu/archives/spr2013/entries/rights-human/.

9. Henry Shue, *Basic Rights*, 2nd ed. (Princeton, NJ: Princeton University Press, 2006), 18.

10. Preamble of the Universal Declaration of Human Rights, 1948.

11. Robert Baker, "Bioethics and Human Rights: A Historical Perspective," *Cambridge Quarterly of Healthcare Ethics* 10, no. 3 (2001): 241–252.

12. "In the exercise of his rights and freedoms, everyone shall be subject only to such limitations as are determined by law solely for the purpose of securing due recognition and respect for the rights and freedoms of others and of meeting the just requirements of morality, public order and the general welfare in a democratic society" (UDHR, Article 29.2).

13. Andrew Fagan, "Back to Basics: Human Rights and the Suffering Imperative," *Essex Human Rights Review* 5, no. 1 (2008): 1–6.

14. Ibid.

15. Emmanuel Levinas, *Totality and Infinity* (The Hague: Nijhoff, 1969), 197.

16. Ibid., 199.

17. Bryan Turner, *Vulnerability and Human Rights* (University Park, PA: Pennsylvania State University Press, 2006), 6.

18. Roberto Andorno, "Four Paradoxes of Human Dignity," in *Menschenwürde und moderne Medizintechnik*, ed. Jan Joerden, Eric Hilgendorf, Natalia Petrillo, and Felix Thiele (Baden-Baden: Nomos, 2011), 131–140.

19. Richard Rorty, "Human Rights, Rationality and Sentimentality," in *On Human Rights. The Oxford Amnesty Lectures*, ed. Stephen Shute and Susan Hurley (New York: Basic Books, 1993), 112–134.

20. Ibid.

21. Michael Freeman, *Human Rights* (Cambridge, UK: Polity, 2002), 56.

22. Patrick Hayden, "Sentimentality and Human Rights: Critical Remarks on Rorty," *Philosophy in the Contemporary World*, 6, no. 3–4 (1999): 59–66.

23. Mayerfeld, supra note 2, 25.

24. David Sussman, "Defining Torture," *Case Western Reserve Journal of International Law* 37 (2006): 225–230.

25. U.S. Department of Justice, Office of Legal Counsel, *Memorandum for Alberto R. Gonzales. Counsel to the President. Re: Standards for Conduct for Interrogation under 18 U.S.C. 2340-2340A* (2002), accessed March 10, 2014, http://www.gwu.edu/~nsarchiv/NSAEBB/NSAEBB127/02.08.01.pdf.

26. Metin Başoğlu, Maria Livanou, and Cvetana Crnobarić, "Torture vs. Other Cruel, Inhuman, and Degrading Treatment: Is the Distinction Real or Apparent?," *Archives of General Psychiatry (*now: *JAMA Psychiatry)*, 64, no. 3 (2007): 277–285.

27. Hernán Reyes, "The Worst Scars Are in the Mind: Psychological Torture," *International Review of the Red Cross* 89, no. 867 (2007): 591–617.

28. Ibid.

29. Jamie Mayerfeld, "In Defense of the Absolute Prohibition of Torture," *Public Affairs Quarterly*, 22, no. 2 (2008): 109–128.

30. U.N. Principles of Medical Ethics relevant to the Role of Health Personnel, particularly Physicians, in the Protection of Prisoners and Detainees against Torture, General Assembly Resolution 37/194 of 18 December 1982; World Medical Association, Declaration of Tokyo: Guidelines for Physicians Concerning Torture and other Cruel, Inhuman or Degrading Treatment or Punishment in Relation to Detention and Imprisonment, 1975/2006.

31. Neil A. Lewis, "Red Cross Finds Detainee Abuse in Guantanamo," *New York Times*, November 30, 2004.

32. International Red Cross Committee, Report on the Treatment of Fourteen 'High Value Detainees' in CIA Custody," February 2007, 23, accessed March 10, 2014, http://assets.nybooks.com/media/doc/2010/04/22/icrc-report.pdf

33. Michael Grodin and George J. Annas, "Physicians and Torture: Lessons from the Nazi Doctors," *International Review of the Red Cross*, 89, no. 867 (2007): 635–654.

34. Maxwell Gregg Bloche and Jonathan H. Marks, "When Doctors Go to War," *New England Journal of Medicine*, 352, no. 1 (2005): 3–6.

35. Grodin and Annas, supra note 33, 654.

36. *Oxford English Dictionary*.

37. Rebecca J. Stratton, Ceri J Green, and Marinos Elia, *Disease-Related Malnutrition: An Evidence-Based Approach to Treatment* (Wallingford, CT: CABI, 2003), chap. 4.

38. Save the Children, *A Life Free From Hunger: Tackling Child Malnutrition* (2012), accessed March 10, 2014, http://www.savethechildren.org.uk/resources/online-library/life-free-hunger-tackling-child-malnutrition.

39. Food and Agriculture Organization (FAO), *Statistical Yearbook 2012. Part 2: Hunger Dimensions* (Rome: FAO, 2012).

40. U.N. Economic and Social Council, *General Comment 12: The Right to Adequate Food (Article 11),* May 12, 1999.

41. Ibid., para. 17.

42. Ibid.

43. Amartya Sen, "Hunger in the Contemporary World," in *STICERD Research Paper Series* (London: London School of Economics, 1997), accessed March 10, 2014, http://eprints.lse.ac.uk/6685/1/Hunger_in_the_Contemporary_World.pdf.

44. Thomas Pogge, "Poverty, Climate Change and Overpopulation," *Georgia Journal of International and Comparative Law* 38, no. 3 (2010): 525–542.

45. Elisabeth Kübler-Ross, *On Death and Dying* (New York: Simon & Schuster/Touchstone, 1969).

46. Maytal Guy and Theodore A. Stern, "The Desire for Death in the Setting of Terminal Illness: A Case Discussion," *Primary Care Companion to the Journal of Clinical*

Psychiatry 8, no. 5 (2006: 299–305; J. H. Brown, P. Henteleff, S. Barakat, and C. J. Rowe, "Is It Normal for Terminally Ill Patients to Desire Death?," *American Journal of Psychiatry* 143, no. 2 (1986): 208–211.

47. M. Guy and T. A. Stern, ibid.

48. Roberto Andorno, Nikola Biller-Andorno, and Susanne Brauer, "Advance Health Care Directives: Towards a Coordinated European Policy?," *European Journal of Health Law* 16, no. 3 (2009): 207–227; Roberto Andorno, "Regulating Advance Directives at the Council of Europe," in *Life, Death and Dignity: Regulating Advance Directives in National and International Law*, ed. Stefania Negri (Leiden: Brill Academic, 2012), 73–85.

49. This is especially the case in Switzerland, which is the only European country allowing nonphysician-assisted suicide and probably the only one in the world not requiring any particular medical condition for requesting assistance to commit suicide. This situation developed not as a result of a deliberate ultraliberal policy aiming to recognize a "right to die" or to "legalize" assisted suicide but instead as a consequence of an unintended gap in the Criminal Code. See Roberto Andorno, "Nonphysician-Assisted Suicide in Switzerland," *Cambridge Quarterly of Healthcare Ethics* 22, no. 3 (2013): 246–253.

50. ECtHR, *Pretty v. the United Kingdom,* Judgment of 29 April 2002, application no. 2346/02.

51. ECtHR, *Haas v. Switzerland,* Judgment of 20 January 2011, application no. 31322/07.

52. ECtHR, *Pretty v. the United Kingdom,* supra note 50, para. 39.

53. Ibid.

54. Ibid.

55. Ibid., para. 53.

56. Ibid., para. 65.

57. Ibid., para. 76.

58. ECtHR, *Haas v. Switzerland,* supra note 51, para. 51.

59. Ibid.

60. Despite using the term "right" in its judgment, the Court seems to employ it to mean a "liberty" rather than a claim-right (or right *stricto sensu).*

61. ECtHR, *Haas v. Switzerland,* supra note 51, para. 53.

62. Ibid.

63. Ibid., para. 54.

64. Ibid.

65. Ibid., paras. 57–58.

10

Exploring Interactions between Pain, Suffering, and the Law

Margaret Somerville

The law has a long, diverse and complex relation with suffering.

The Universal Declaration of Human Rights establishes, as part of international human rights law, that "[n]o one shall be subjected to torture or to cruel, inhuman or degrading treatment or punishment."[1] The Council of Europe's European Convention on Human Rights does the same transnationally for European countries.[2] And national constitutional law, for instance, the Canadian Charter of Rights and Freedoms, likewise prohibits the use of "any cruel and unusual treatment or punishment."[3] These are very important legal prohibitions on the intentional infliction of suffering on our fellow humans, especially at the hands of the state and its authorities.

The imposition of suffering is a major tool of the criminal law. Courts sentence convicted offenders on the basis of what is appropriate, from the viewpoint of justice, in terms of retribution and of punishment of the offender; specific and general deterrence—inhibiting that offender and the population, in general, respectively, from committing similar offences in the future; and rehabilitation of the offender.[4] In doing so, they can take into account victim impact statements, in which the victims of the crime describe their suffering, and award monetary compensation for that pursuant to "compensation of victims of crime" legislation.

In the private law context, I have explored elsewhere the courts' approaches to awarding damages for suffering[5] and the use of the law to try to reduce suffering.[6] Here, I will make only some general statements in those regards.

The Common Law has long been very wary of awarding damages for nonphysical injury, especially psychological trauma unaccompanied by physical injury, and still, today, refuses to award damages for the "normal vicissitudes of life," such as "normal" grief at the loss of a loved one. Perhaps that explains why the law speaks of "pain and suffering" collectively, although when both are present, it awards damages for both. When suffering is linked to the reality of pain arising from observable physical injury, the courts can be reassured that the claim for suffering is not frivolous or fraudulent, which is always one of their fears. This approach is consistent with the law's traditional stance that damages for "pain and suffering" were only legally compensable if they resulted from physical injury.

With the birth of modern psychiatry in the late nineteenth century, courts in Common Law jurisdictions recognized a tort action for the intentional infliction of mental suffering,[7] which, in American tort law, developed into the tort of outrageous conduct.[8] It was only in more recent times that damages for negligently inflicted "pure" nervous shock, that is, mental injury not resulting from physical injury, became recoverable on certain requirements being fulfilled.[9] One of these requirements is that the injured person suffers from a diagnosable mental illness as a result of the wrongful act.[10] Again, designated evidence of a certain kind is used to reduce the risk for frivolous or fraudulent claims, in short, is employed as a filtering device.

A late twentieth-century insight was that the law not only can inflict suffering but also, used in certain ways, can reduce it. The latter concept is encapsulated in the idea of "therapeutic jurisprudence."[11]

Even more recently, courts have been equating suffering to the loss of dignity, and vice versa. They define dignity as requiring that persons have control over what happens to them and, correlatively, equate the loss of autonomy and self-determination with a loss of dignity. This approach is consistent with American physician Eric Cassell's definition of suffering as having a sense of one's own disintegration and a loss of control over what happens to one.[12] Often, claims with regard to what respect for a person's dignity and autonomy requires are framed as respect for a right to choice. In short, allowing "choice" is put forward as the remedy for a loss of dignity and an appropriate means to relieve suffering.

At present, physician-assisted suicide and euthanasia are the most prominent and contentious issues in regard to which suffering and the proper approach of the law in dealing with it is a relevant consideration. The law already seeks to uphold or restore dignity by giving terminally ill, suffering persons who want to die control over what is done to them. Requirements for informed consent—which from the perspective of giving control over her treatment to the patient can be characterized as a "suffering reduction mechanism"[13]—and rights to refuse life-prolonging treatment are examples. However, pro-euthanasia advocates argue that the necessary and only sufficient control of suffering is to be able to choose death.

Pro-euthanasia advocates see euthanasia principally as a way to relieve people's suffering. They view suffering as the greatest evil and the relief of suffering as trumping almost all other values—the one exception is respect for individual autonomy. One of the challenges in responding to this argument in the euthanasia debate is that it's not easy to give meaning to suffering other than through religion, which is the way many people dealt with suffering in the past. But today, many people are not religious. When suffering cannot be given any worth or meaning and a person does not believe that there is anything inherently wrong in inflicting death on a suffering person, at least one who requests and gives informed consent to it—that is, they believe this is not unethical—it is very difficult to convince them that legalizing euthanasia is a bad idea.

This discussion also raises the philosophical claim that it is not the job or proper role of medicine or the law to relieve all suffering and that, in trying to do so, physicians and law makers are unjustifiably crossing boundaries that should be respected.[14] And that leads to the question I have been asked to address in this chapter: How, then, does and should the law deal with suffering?

In responding, I use as a template a first instance decision in a recent Canadian case, the *Carter* case,[15] in which a judge finds that prohibiting physician-assisted suicide is unconstitutional because it is necessary medical treatment for the relief of the suffering of people with disabilities who are unable to commit suicide without assistance.[16]

I would like, first, however, to describe briefly an important extralegal development that is likely to have impact on the law's approach to pain and suffering. This is the adoption in 2010 of the Declaration of Montreal,[17] the principles of which have recently been accepted by the World Medical Association.[18]

Law Responding to Pain

I became interested in the law's approach to pain and suffering because of my personal experience with pain and as a result of my father's experience of unrelieved excruciating pain when he first became terminally ill.[19] At his request, I started to write about the topic.[20] This led to speaking invitations.

One invitation was to address the Ottawa Medical Legal Society. I called the talk "Medicine or Murder"—it was about the connection between pain management and euthanasia. It was an evening event, and I noticed some people in the audience seemed to be "nodding off." So I stepped up the rhetoric and suggested that for physicians intentionally to leave a person in serious pain should be regarded as falling within the offence of criminal negligence causing bodily harm in the Canadian *Criminal Code*.[21] I continued that I regarded such conduct as so unethical that I personally would take a criminal prosecution against such a physician free of charge. (I used to teach criminal law, I'm a member of the Quebec Bar, and Canadian law allows private citizens to launch a criminal prosecution, although that is a rare event.) When I got to my office the next morning, there was bedlam. Unbeknown to me, a senior journalist from the Ottawa Citizen newspaper had been in the audience, and a headline on the front page of that day's Citizen read: "Ethicist recommends jailing doctors." Outraged physicians were calling from across Canada. But looking back, I'm not sorry I said what I did. Leaving people in pain is so horrible that we need to employ every wake-up call that we can to change that situation.

My work on ethical and legal aspects of pain and suffering elicited an invitation to speak at the International Association for the Study of Pain's meeting in Paris in 1993. I called the speech "Death of Pain,"[22] meaning to convey the double entendre message that we could kill the person with the pain or we could kill the pain. I'm adamantly against killing the person with the pain, that is, euthanasia, and passionately in favor of killing the pain.

So, I argued, among many other suggestions, that one way to implement that latter goal in practice would be to recognize that people in pain have a "fundamental human right" to have reasonable access to pain management and that unreasonable failure to provide such access was a *breach of their human rights.*

Others picked up that idea, in particular, an Australian pain specialist, Dr. Michael Cousins. He and his colleagues worked to create the Declaration of Montreal, which was approved at the meeting of the International Society for the Study of Pain in Montreal in September 2010.

THE DECLARATION OF MONTREAL

Here's part of what the Declaration of Montreal provides:

> Finding that pain management is inadequate in most of the world....
>
> And, recognizing the intrinsic dignity of all persons and that withholding of pain treatment is profoundly wrong, leading to unnecessary suffering which is harmful; we declare that the following human rights must be recognized throughout the world:
>
> *Article 1.* The right of all people to have access to pain management without discrimination.
>
> *Article 2.* The right of people in pain to acknowledgment of their pain and to be informed about how it can be assessed and managed.
>
> *Article 3.* The right of all people with pain to have access to appropriate assessment and treatment of the pain by adequately trained health care professionals.

Rights engender obligations. So, a human right to access to pain management means that health care professionals and health care institutions have ethical, and sometimes legal, obligations to offer patients such management. The Declaration of Montreal in formally recognizing these obligations will help to ensure that they are honored and not breached.

Sometimes, the Declaration will function as evidence to justify giving necessary pain relief treatment, when others would prevent that. In particular, it will help to overcome the harmful beliefs of some health care professionals who withhold pain management because they fear legal liability or that patients will become addicted. It will deliver a strong message that it's wrong *not to provide* pain management, not wrong to provide it.

The Declaration will also help Governments to understand that they have both domestic and international obligations, at the very least, not to unreasonably hinder either their own citizens' or other people's access to pain management. It is an outrage and a human tragedy that, in developing countries, many people in serious pain do not have access to opioids, including as a result of the conditions some countries attach to their foreign aid to these developing countries.

An egregious example of a lack of access to pain management in a developing country is documented in a report from Human Rights Watch. The vast majority of children dying from HIV/ AIDS in Kenya die with no pain relief treatment.[23]

The World Health Organization estimates that 5 billion people live in countries with low or no access to controlled medicines, which include all opioids, and have no or insufficient access to treatment for moderate to severe pain.[24]

We need to apply one of the most ancient and universally accepted maxims in making sure that everyone who needs pain management receives it: "Do unto others as you would that they would do unto you"—the Golden Rule. The Declaration of Montreal spells out what those "others" have a human right to expect when they are in pain.

Human rights, human responsibilities, and human ethics—which are three separate entry doors into the same reality of ensuring respect for all human beings[25]—all require that people are not abandoned when they are in pain and are provided with fully adequate pain management.

Law Responding to Suffering

I used to teach a course, "Ethics, Law, Science, and Society," to upper-year and graduate law students at McGill University, and one of the topics we discussed was euthanasia. I've researched euthanasia, physician-assisted suicide, the ethics and law of palliative care and pain relief treatment, decision making at the end of life, and related topics, for over three decades and published a 433-page book, *Death Talk: The Case against Euthanasia and Physician-Assisted Suicide*.[26] Yet, I came away from the class feeling that I had completely failed to communicate to most of my students what the problems with legalizing euthanasia were—that I was hitting a steel wall. This was not because of any ill will on their part; rather, they seemed not to see euthanasia as raising major problems—at least any beyond preventing its abuse—a reaction I found very worrying.[27]

So, I emailed my students explaining I felt "that I had not done a good job in presenting the euthanasia debate... [and] decided to see if I could work out why not by writing about it." I attached an early draft of my article setting out my thoughts in that regard and asked for comments; I received several, very thoughtful replies.

One student explained that she thought I was giving far too much weight to concerns about how legalizing euthanasia would harm the community and our shared values, especially that of respect for life, and too little to individuals rights to autonomy and self-determination and to euthanasia as a way to relieve people's suffering.

She emphasized that individuals' rights have been given priority in contemporary society, and they should also prevail in relation to death. Moreover, legalizing euthanasia was consistent with other changes in society, such as respect for women and access to abortion, she said.

I had suggested in my article that, among other causes of the move to legalize euthanasia, the vast exposure to death that we are subjected to in both current-affairs and entertainment programs might have overwhelmed our sensitivity to the awesomeness of death and, likewise, of inflicting it. But one of my students responded, "If anything, I think many of our reactions come not from an overexposure to death, but from an aversion to suffering, and an unwillingness or hesitancy to prolong pain."

The recent *Carter* case in British Columbia shows a trial court judge articulating, in great detail, both the same approach as the students took and the reasoning on which they based their approach. At 355 pages containing 137,000-plus words, the judgment of Justice Lynn Smith of the British Columbia Supreme Court in the *Carter* case[28] is rightly described as a tome. But it is one with potentially groundbreaking impact for Canadian society: if it is upheld on appeal, leaving aside abortion, it will represent the first step in our crossing the thousands-of-years-old line in the sand which establishes that we must not intentionally kill another human being (the only exceptions being when that is the only way to save human life, as in justified self-defense) or help them to kill themselves.

In striking down the prohibition of assisted suicide in section 241(b) of the Canadian *Criminal Code*[29] as unconstitutional, Justice Smith legalizes physician-assisted suicide and, where the person is incapable of committing suicide because of physical disability, euthanasia. One of the plaintiffs, Gloria Taylor, a woman suffering from amyotrophic lateral sclerosis (ALS or Lou Gehrig's disease) wanted to have a physician assist her in committing suicide at a time and a place of her choosing. Justice Smith legitimized and granted Ms. Taylor's wish, The judgment was appealed, but Ms. Taylor died of natural causes before the appeal judgment was rendered. The British Columbia Court of Appeal overruled Justice Smith's judgment on the grounds that it was contrary to the binding precedent of the Supreme Court of Canada's ruling in the *Rodriguez* case (discussed infra), in which a narrow majority held that the Canadian Criminal Code's prohibition of assisted suicide was constitutionally valid. The plaintiffs in the *Carter* case have now been granted leave to appeal to the Supreme Court of Canada, which is at liberty to overrule its previous precedent. It remains to be seen whether it will do so. Justice Smith's trial judgment provides, however, a rich and useful template for examining how, when faced with suffering, the law deals with it.

Read as a whole, Justice Smith's judgment gives a strong impression that she is far from neutral about physician-assisted suicide and euthanasia but, rather, favors these interventions in certain circumstances. In particular, with respect, the judgment gives undue weight to the evidence of witnesses in favor of legalizing physician-assisted suicide, while massively devaluing that of those who oppose it. Moreover, the judge's emphasis on the relief of suffering—the words "suffer" and "suffering" appear two hundred and twelve times in the judgment—gives rise to what appear to be philosophical and social biases being imposed by her upon the wealth of evidence submitted by both parties.

Thus, one can question Justice Smith's conclusions that physician-assisted suicide is not inherently unethical—that the availability of legalized physician-assisted suicide is necessary "medical treatment" for some people—and the very lengthy legal justification she constructs to allow her to implement her rulings to these effects. That justification is largely based on a selective application of *Canadian Charter of Rights and Freedoms*[30] jurisprudence and is established by distinguishing the precedent set by the Supreme Court of Canada in the *Rodriguez* case,[31] which found the prohibition of assisted suicide to be constitutional in a fact situation very similar to Ms. Taylor's. Below I examine, briefly, some of the issues related to suffering that the judgment involves and how they were dealt with.

THE PRIMARY GOAL OF PROHIBITING PHYSICIAN-ASSISTED SUICIDE

Central to the case, and Justice Smith's judgment, is whether protecting vulnerable people is the only purpose, or even the main purpose, of the prohibition on physician-assisted suicide. She rejects the Attorney General of Canada's argument that the purposes are more extensive, including upholding respect for human life and the integrity of the medical profession and "preventing negative messages about the value of human life, particularly the value of the lives of individuals with disabilities." [1187][32]

If the prohibition of assisted suicide were meant to uphold "respect for human life," in general, at the societal level, then, in all probability, it would not, in stark contrast to Justice Smith's rulings, be found to be unconstitutional on the grounds on which she relied, which focused only on individuals' rights. She ruled that the prohibition's harmful impact on people with disabilities such as Ms. Taylor, who want to commit suicide but need assistance to do so, was disproportionate and overbroad and impaired Ms. Taylor's *Charter* rights to "life, liberty and security of the person"[33] more than was necessary for the State to achieve its legitimate goal of protecting vulnerable people, and that it contravened Ms. Taylor's constitutional rights against discrimination on the basis of physical disability.[34] In other words, limiting the goal of the prohibition on assisted suicide to the protection of "vulnerable people" is essential to Justice Smith's reasoning that the prohibition is unconstitutional.

It is not surprising, therefore, that Justice Smith's conclusions do not take into account institutional or societal protections or needs, but rather are focused principally at the individual level and giving individuals' claims priority, which in Ms. Taylor's case was her claim of a right to access assisted suicide for the relief of suffering. In other words, Justice Smith accepts an individual's suffering as the principal justification for euthanasia, and rules its presence means an individual's request for "assisted death" trumps other claims and considerations.

There is a paradox here that Justice Smith's focus on individual persons' vulnerability, a focus meant to protect vulnerable people, is being used to place them at risk from assisted suicide by legitimizing it. The same reversal of an initial protective goal has occurred with the concept of quality of life. Initially "quality of life" was developed as a concept intended to protect and promote life through the argument that everyone had a right to the resources, especially health care resources, needed to maintain an acceptable "quality of life." Now the concept is often used to achieve the exact opposite outcome, namely, that a person's "quality of life" is so poor that they are better off dead or, at the least, don't merit the expenditure of resources needed to keep them alive.

Having decided that the ban on assisted suicide is intended primarily to protect vulnerable persons, Justice Smith then concludes that an absolute ban on it is not necessary to implement that goal and, moreover, that an absolute ban infringes Ms. Taylor's *Charter* rights as a disabled, suffering person and, by extension, those of other and similarly situated "vulnerable persons":

> In this case, I have found that the infringement [of the *Charter*] arises from the preclusion of physically disabled persons who are grievously ill and *experiencing intractable suffering* from ending their lives. Thus, it is the *absolute nature* of the prohibition against assisted suicide that requires justification, not the prohibition overall. In other words, the real question is whether the defendants have demonstrated justification for criminalizing the rendering of assistance in suicide to persons such as Gloria Taylor. (Emphasis added) [1171]

In reaching this conclusion, Justice Smith takes into account Ms. Taylor's own views that she does not need protection from assisted suicide as helping to establish that she does not. In other words, the judge gives priority to the value of individual autonomy in relation to a decision to commit suicide to avoid suffering. She rules that a safeguarded exception should be allowed and sets out the conditions for such an exception. Justice Smith envisions that the cases in which physician-assisted suicide or euthanasia is acceptable will be rare. But it is important to note that the method she sets out in her exception is broad and without the safeguards that might assure its application only in very restricted cases.

Because it is so unusual, I wish to note here the way in which Justice Smith interprets the right to life enshrined in section 7 of the *Canadian Charter of Rights and Freedoms*[35]:

> [The prohibition on assisted suicide in section 241(b) of the Criminal Code] infringes Ms. Taylor's right to life. [13]...[T]he legislation affects her right to life because it may shorten her life. Ms. Taylor's reduced lifespan would occur if she concludes that she needs to take her own life while she is still physically able to do so, at an earlier date than she would find necessary if she could be assisted. [17]

To say the least, this is a novel way to construct a breach of Ms. Taylor's *Charter* right to life. In effect, Justice Smith's reasoning converts the right to life to a right to death by physician-assisted suicide or euthanasia.

With respect to who are the suffering persons who may have access to physician-assisted suicide, in speaking about palliative care services in British Columbia, Justice Smith refers to "the end-of-life population" [692]. She does not define this term, which in the Royal Society of Canada Expert Panel Report on *End of Life Decision Making* encompasses a continuum beginning with a serious diagnosis or injury.[36] This expansion of a term that traditionally is used for those in the last days or weeks of life to all with chronic conditions resulting from illness and injury presages precisely the dangerous expansion along a "slippery slope" from the "limited" exception the judge proposes.

There is something chilling about Justice Smith's construction of an "end-of-life population" that is not present when we speak of "dying people," "vulnerable people," "terminally ill people," or, even, "the terminally ill." First, we do not know to whom it refers. But, if, as seems plausible, Justice Smith has accepted the approach of the Royal Society Expert Panel report, it may be all those with a serious diagnosis or injury that may be fatal in the course of time. And, of course, it is notoriously difficult to predict with any certainty the timing of death in relation to even obviously terminal illnesses for which no clinical treatment is possible.[37]

Just as troubling is the dropping of the word *people* or *person*. It is dehumanizing and depersonalizing and allows easier dis-identification from the person or people concerned. "The end-of-life population" is a term that marks off the people labeled as such from the general population. They become "them," in contrast to the "rest of us." It brings to mind author Susan Sontag's metaphor of the two "kingdoms," the kingdom of the well and the kingdom of the sick, but, if physician-assisted suicide or euthanasia were legalized, with even more alienating and frightening connotations:

> Everyone who is born holds dual citizenship, in the kingdom of the well and in the kingdom of the sick. Although we all prefer to use only the good passport, sooner or later each of us is obliged, at least for a spell, to identify ourselves as citizens of that other place.[38]

Justice Smith's depersonalized and undefined generalization of an "end-of-life population" also brings to mind the dystopic world imagined by P. D. James in her novel *The Children of Men,* in which elderly persons' duty to die is enacted through a form of mass suicide called the Quietus (quiet us).[39] And this disposal of the fragile through a "duty to die" was famously argued as policy by Colorado Governor Richard Lamm in the 1980s as well as by, in a modified form, ethicist and Hastings Center Fellow Daniel Callahan in the 1990s.[40]

The point, yet again, is that despite the promise of very restricted relaxation of the current legal prohibitions protecting persons, implicit in Justice Smith's decision is the invitation to expansion of physician-assisted death to many people not dying but diagnosed with a serious illness or disabled or, simply, suffering.

SUICIDE IS NOT A CRIME

Justice Smith focuses on the Canadian Parliament's repeal of the suicide and attempted suicide offences in 1972 and accepts, as she is bound to do by the precedent established by the Supreme Court of Canada in the *Rodriguez* case,[41] that this was not done to give a personal choice to die priority. She states:

> As to the objective underlying Parliament's repeal...the majority [in *Rodriguez*] held that the objective was not to recognize a consensus that the autonomy interest of those who might wish to kill themselves is paramount to the state interest in protecting the lives of citizens; rather, it was to recognize that attempted suicide did not mandate a legal remedy. [926]

With respect, I would explain the matter differently: the crimes were abolished to try to save the lives of suicidal people. It was hoped that if they were not threatened with the possibility of being charged with a criminal offence in seeking medical help to treat suicidal ideation, they and their families would be more likely to seek such assistance.

In coming to her conclusions about the acceptability of legally permitted assisted suicide, throughout the judgment Justice Smith relies heavily on the fact that it is not a crime to commit or attempt to commit suicide, and asks, why then is it a crime to assist it? She opines:

> [T]he law does not prohibit suicide. [15]...The plaintiffs...argue that there is no ethical distinction between the laws that permit suicide and those that prohibit physician-assisted suicide. [176]...What is the difference between suicide and assisted suicide that justifies making the one lawful and the other a crime, that justifies allowing some this choice, while denying it to others? [1010]

The answer is, as explained above, that decriminalizing suicide and attempted suicide is intended to protect life; decriminalizing assisted suicide does the opposite. We try to prevent suicide and, importantly, there is no right to commit suicide. If there were such a right, we would have a duty not to treat people who attempt suicide, in order to try to save their lives, and to let them die.

The difference between suicide and physician-assisted suicide is fundamental. Suicide is a solitary act that we may try to prevent but that is carried out by the individual, usually in despair. Physician-assisted suicide is a social act in which medical personnel licensed and compensated by the state are involved in the termination of the life of a person with the approval of the state. It asks not that we attempt to preserve life, the normal role of medicine and the state, but instead that we accept and act communally upon a person's judgment that his or her life is unworthy of continuance.[42] It is to see the infliction of death as an ethical, appropriate, and justified response to suffering. This is exactly the message that those trying to prevent suicide want to negate totally.

Assisted suicide thus involves a separate ethical enquiry that distinguishes it from suicide, an enquiry that is not undertaken in the judgment: this is the ethics of society's and a physician's complicity in helping people to kill themselves.

Legalized physician-assisted suicide involves both these forms of complicity: society is complicit in legalizing the procedure, and a physician, licensed by society and, in Canada, compensated by it, is complicit in carrying it out.

For this reason the value of respect for life, especially at the societal level of respect for human life in general, is differently impacted by assisted suicide compared with suicide. The former contravenes this value, and particularly at the societal level, in a way that the latter does not.

Justice Smith relies on the dissenting judgment of Chief Justice Lamer of the Supreme Court of Canada in the *Rodriguez* case to find that

> ...s. 241*(b)* of the *Criminal Code* creates an inequality by preventing persons physically unable to end their lives from having the option to choose suicide, while other members of the public have that option. He [Chief Justice Lamer] found that the inequality is imposed because of a physical disability, a personal characteristic among the grounds of discrimination listed in s. 15(1) [of the Canadian Charter]. He concluded, at 549-50, that the inequality constitutes a burden or disadvantage since it limits the ability of persons who are subject to the inequality to take and act upon fundamental decisions regarding their lives and persons; for them, "the principle of self-determination has been limited." Differing from the majority, he found that the infringement of s. 15 was not justified under s. 1 [of the Charter]. [1014]

But Justice Smith fails to mention that in order to rule to this effect the Chief Justice recognized a *right* to choose to commit suicide. The way in which the Chief Justice's ruling is summarized in the head note to the *Rodriguez* case throws a different light on the passage from his judgment upon which Justice Smith relies:

> "This inequality—*the deprivation of the right to choose suicide*—may be characterized as a burden or disadvantage, since it limits the ability of those who are subject to this inequality to take and act upon fundamental decisions regarding their lives and persons." (Emphasis added)[43]

Does such a right mean that we would have correlative obligations not to prevent people making that choice? Certainly, hospital emergency rooms and health care professionals faced with a patient who has attempted suicide do not, at present, act on that basis.

WEIGHTING THE EVIDENCE DISPROPORTIONATELY

Consistent with focusing on the risks and harms to individuals, the vast majority of the evidence to which Justice Smith gives credibility is empirical evidence. Correlatively, she dismisses or gives short shrift to evidence she labels as nonempirical. In fact, the word *empirical* appears with great frequency in the judgment—twenty-eight times in all. (It is paired with the words *studies, research, evidence, knowledge, data, foundation, work, proof,* and *precision*.) Suffering can be empirically established, although the evidence that demonstrates it is to a large extent subjective. In the *Carter* case, it was introduced in evidence by witnesses who described either their own circumstances of illness and disability, and explained why they wanted the option of physician-assisted suicide to be available, or those of loved ones, who had also wanted that option.

In contrast, the judge dismisses or gives little weight to most of the defendants' expert witnesses' testimony on the grounds that it's not empirically based. (See, for example, such references by the judge to the evidence of Dr. Jose Pereira, Baroness Ilora Finlay, and Dr. Herbert Hendin [664]) The problem here is that many of the risks and harms of legalized physician-assisted suicide and euthanasia, at levels other than the individual one, are metaphysical risks and harms (to values, beliefs, attitudes, norms, and so on), not physical risks and harms, the former of which are not necessarily assessable through empirical research, especially those that will occur in the future. The strong emphasis on empirical evidence, to the exclusion of other valid and accepted research methodologies, means that what can't be measured or counted is treated as unimportant or ignored.

In summary, almost all of the judge's analysis, in particular of the risks and benefits of physician-assisted suicide, is at the level of the individual suffering patient, who wants physician-assisted suicide. By focusing her analysis at this level and treating empirical evidence as the only relevant or credible evidence, Justice Smith, in effect, uses an exclusionary mechanism to eliminate the evidence of the defendant governments' experts against legalizing physician-assisted suicide. In doing so, she weighs the balance heavily in favor of the relief of suffering as the overriding value and a strong justification for physician-assisted suicide and euthanasia.

UNDERLYING ASSUMPTIONS AND PRINCIPLES

The judge makes assumptions that assisted suicide (and euthanasia) is not inherently wrong and, moreover, that access to such an intervention is morally required in certain circumstances, in particular, to relieve suffering. In all probability, she is doing the same as we find in the Royal Society Expert Panel Report[44] and the Quebec Legislative Assembly report,[45] both of which she admitted in evidence against the defendants' objections. This is simply to assume, without justifying doing so, that individual autonomy is the value that always takes priority. Like both those reports, her entire judgment is also consistent with the adoption of a philosophical base of moral relativism and an approach of utilitarianism, which favor seeing relief of suffering as an overriding justification for physician-assisted suicide.

In addressing the question of whether the principle of preservation of life has exceptions, Justice Smith, first, finds that it does, and then accepts the evidence of one of the plaintiffs' expert witnesses, Canadian philosopher Professor Wayne Sumner, to the effect that death is not a loss or bad, if there is no benefit in a continuing life—in other words, that a poor quality of life and suffering can justify such an exception. Here's her reasoning:

> With respect to the first question [Does a physician have an overriding duty to support the inviolability of life and refrain from intentionally causing death, or can it be ethical, in an individual case, for a physician to assist a competent and informed patient who requests hastened death?], I think that the real difference of opinion is not about the value of human life; no-one questions that the preservation of human life has a very high value in our society. Rather, the difference of opinion is about whether the preservation of human life is an absolute value, subject to no exceptions. [350]

Professor Sumner explores this point:

> Normally we assume that death is one of the worst fates that can befall us, which is why in both ethics and law the causing of death is taken to be such a serious matter. But what makes death such a bad thing in the normal case is what it takes away from us—the continuation of a life worth living. The disvalue of death is therefore a direct function of the value of the life thereby lost. This is the *deprivation account* of the badness of death: death is bad for us by virtue of depriving us of the goods of continued life. On this account showing that death would be bad for a person requires a comparison between two possible futures for that person: the one in which he dies and the one in which he lives on. If the goods of further life would outweigh the evils then it would be better for the person to continue living, and death would therefore be a harm to him since it would deprive him of this good future. (Emphasis in original) [351]

This is a *quality of life* argument couched in different terms, those of nondeprivation. The person's quality of life is seen as being so poor that she is not deprived of any benefit—indeed, pursuant to this reasoning, she might even be perceived as receiving benefit–by her life being taken.

Although the judge speaks of this approach applying "in an individual case," this same reasoning could readily be applied to babies with disabilities, people with dementia, and so on. Justifying the taking of or not maintaining the lives of such people on the basis of their poor quality of life and the suffering continued life involves is usually supported on the grounds they are "individual cases," and the cumulative effect of the decisions taken in those cases is ignored. But the cumulative effect is to wipe out the people with a specified characteristic as a group. For instance, in North America, at least 85 percent of babies with Down syndrome are now aborted. And recently, two bioethicists caused an international furor when they published a paper in a highly respected journal proposing "post birth abortion": parents who have a child with Down syndrome, whom they would have aborted if they'd known of its condition, should be allowed to have it killed after birth (legalized infanticide).[46]

It merits noting in the context of exploring the cumulative effect of legalizing physician-assisted suicide and euthanasia that both the Royal Society panel's report[47] and the Quebec Legislative Assembly Committee report[48] raise the issue of whether euthanasia should be available for mentally incompetent people, for instance, those with Alzheimer's disease. Neither report comes out against that being allowed, but rather they leave the question open, stating that this is an issue to be examined further at a later date. However, if physician-assisted suicide is medical treatment meant to relieve suffering, as supporters of it argue, then it would be discriminatory to offer it to mentally competent people and not to incompetent ones.

THE "NO DIFFERENCE" ARGUMENT

The essence of the "no difference" line of pro-euthanasia argument, which was accepted by Justice Smith, is that we already accept and practice interventions, such as withdrawal of life-support treatment or provision of necessary pain management, that result in death or could shorten life, respectively, and there is no ethical or moral difference between these, on the one hand, and physician-assisted suicide and euthanasia,[49] on the other, and there ought to be no legal difference. The reasoning is that the latter are of the same kind and have the same consequence as the former and legalizing them is just a further incremental step along a path that we have already taken and regard as ethically acceptable. Justice Smith puts it this way:

> That spectrum [of acceptable interventions at the end-of-life] already encompasses decisions where the likely consequence of the decision will be the death of the patient. [1240]

I call this strategy "legalizing euthanasia through confusion."[50] It depends on a misleading and, I would argue, false analogy. The issue in the "euthanasia debate" is not *if* we die—we will all die eventually—but the ethics and law of *how* we die. People who oppose physician-assisted suicide and euthanasia believe these are unethical ways to die and can be validly distinguished from the other ways in which life may be shortened and, consequently, the former should remain prohibited.

The essential ethically and legally relevant differences between the two kinds of interventions do not include that between an act and an omission, on which pro-euthanasia advocates, such as Canadian law professor, Jocelyn Downie, allege anti-euthanasia proponents rely.[51] Like the *acts* of physician-assisted suicide or euthanasia, an *omission*, for example, withdrawal of life-support treatment that results in a person's death, can be (but, unlike physician-assisted suicide or euthanasia, is not necessarily) ethically, morally, and legally culpable. The relevant differences between these two kinds of interventions lie in the primary intention with which they are undertaken and in causation of death.

The distinction between pain relief treatment and euthanasia hinges on the physician's primary intention in giving the treatment and the patient's need for the treatment given.

Pain relief treatment given with a primary intention to relieve pain and reasonably necessary to achieve that outcome is not euthanasia, even if it did shorten the patient's life (which is a very rare occurrence for correctly titrated treatment). Any intervention, including the use of pain relief drugs, carried out with a primary intention of causing the patient's death and resulting in that outcome, is euthanasia.

Acting with a primary intention to kill is a world apart from acting with a primary intention to relieve pain. And this is not a novel or exceptional approach. The law recognizes the relevance of such distinctions in intention daily. If we accidentally hit and kill a pedestrian with our car, it is not murder; if we deliberately run him down with our car intending to kill him, it is. It's the same act, but different intentions make the difference.

People in pain are among the most vulnerable persons, so the issue of adequate pain management has special application in relation to them. As Albert Schweitzer said, "Pain is a more terrible Lord of mankind than death itself." A person in pain can want to die by any means, rather than have to go on living in pain. Consequently, as I explained earlier in this chapter, we have serious ethical obligations—and I would argue legal obligations—to offer everyone fully adequate pain management.

An adverse consequence of equating pain management to euthanasia is that it can make people who reject euthanasia reject adequate pain management for ethical or religious reasons, or because of fear that if they consent to it, they will be euthanized. Experience in the Netherlands shows that the latter is not an unjustified fear: It's been alleged that Dutch physicians have interpreted patients' consent to pain management as consent to euthanasia.[52]

The *primary intention* is also different in withdrawing life-support treatment, on the one hand, and physician-assisted suicide and euthanasia, on the other. In withdrawing life-support treatment, the primary intention is to respect the patient's right to refuse all treatment or to remove medically futile treatment or that where the burden of the treatment for the patient outweighs any benefits. In physician-assisted suicide or euthanasia, the *primary intention* is to help the patient to kill himself or to kill him, respectively. The former intention is ethically and legally acceptable; the latter intentions are not.

Patients have a right to refuse treatment, even if that means they will die. Such a refusal is an exercise of their right to autonomy and self-determination, but the content of that right in such situations is a right not to be touched without their consent—a right to inviolability—not a right to die.

Pro-euthanasia advocates use recognition of the right to refuse treatment, even when it results in death, to argue that, likewise, patients should be allowed to exercise their right to autonomy and self-determination to choose death through lethal injection. As explained previously, they say that there is no morally or ethically significant difference between these situations, and there ought to be no legal difference.

They found their argument by wrongly characterizing the right to refuse treatment as a "right to die" and then generalizing that right to include euthanasia and physician-assisted suicide. But the right to refuse treatment is not a right to die and does not establish any such right, although death results from respecting the patient's right to inviolability. The right to refuse treatment can be validly characterized as a "right to be *allowed* to die," which is quite different from a right to be killed that euthanasia would establish.

This particular pro-euthanasia line of argument is just one more example of promoting euthanasia through deliberate confusion between interventions, such as acting on valid refusals of treatment, that are not euthanasia and those that are.

This brings us to the issue of causation, which also differentiates refusals of treatment that result in death from euthanasia.

In refusals of treatment that result in death, the person dies from her underlying disease—a natural death. The withdrawal of treatment is the occasion on which death occurs, but not its cause. If the person had no fatal illness, she would not die. And, moreover, sometimes patients, who refuse treatment and are expected to die, do not die. In contrast, in euthanasia, death is certain, and the cause of death is the lethal injection. Without that, the person would not die at that time from that cause.

The fact that the patient dies in both refusing treatment that results in death and in euthanasia is one of the causes of the confusion between the two situations. If we focus just on that outcome of death, we miss what the real point of distinction between the two situations is.

Here's how Justice Smith articulated the plaintiffs' expert witnesses' "no difference" arguments, which she endorsed. [See, for example, at 335, 339, 349]:

> [T]he plaintiffs argue that the current line drawn between permissible and impermissible end-of-life care is based upon distinctions that in reality have no practical ethical or moral force. They also argue that there is no ethical distinction between the laws that permit suicide and those that prohibit physician-assisted suicide." [176]...One of the main arguments for the proposition that physician-assisted death can be an ethical practice is that physician-assisted death is ethically indistinguishable from conventionally ethical end-of-life practices such as withholding or withdrawing treatment or administering palliative sedation." [186]...However, as set out in my review of the evidence with respect to safeguards, in the opinion of a number of respected ethicists and practitioners, physician-assisted death *in an individual case* is not ethically distinguishable from currently legal and ethically accepted end-of-life practices. (Emphasis added) [1369]

It's interesting to speculate why the judge, yet again,[53] limited her statement to "an individual case." Read in relation to the judgment as a whole, it is probably because she requires justification for physician-assisted suicide in each case and that would require that the person were "grievously ill" [1271], that is, suffering. But it could also be taken to mean such interventions are not able to be justified as a group or on the whole, because of their cumulative effect on important shared values, in particular respect for life, or at institutional and societal levels, issues that Justice Smith does not consider in any depth or at all. Or it could be that the judge wants to avoid setting a precedent that people with a certain disability are automatically identified by that disability as having a claim—or even a right—with respect to having access to physician-assisted suicide or euthanasia.

The judge continues:

> For physicians who see no ethical distinction between assisted death for grievously ill patients and certain current legal end-of-life practices, the law draws an arbitrary line and promotes a kind of hypocrisy. Removing it would permit physicians a more open relationship with their patients and support intellectual honesty in the ethical debate. Indeed, evidence from other jurisdictions suggests that physicians are able to provide better overall end-of-life treatment to patients at the end of their lives once the topic of assisted death is openly put on the table. [1271]

In considering the impact on physicians, patients, and palliative care of legalizing physician-assisted suicide, Justice Smith recognizes there will be both positive and negative effects but concludes the positive ones will outweigh the negative. [1270–1285] In her judgment, she considers the personal stories of people who recounted serious suffering because physician-assisted suicide or euthanasia was not available. Personal stories of those who oppose these interventions, while submitted, apparently were not a factor in her deliberations.

Yet, in contrast to her rulings to the contrary, Justice Smith notes that the Supreme Court of Canada recognized that there is a valid distinction between refusing life-support treatment and euthanasia:

> *Rodriguez* also summarized and clarified the law regarding the common law right of patients to refuse consent to life-sustaining medical treatment, and to demand that such treatment be withdrawn or discontinued. As I have earlier described, the majority [of the Supreme Court of Canada] accepted that there is a valid distinction between the role of physicians in those situations and the role of physicians in assisted suicide or euthanasia, based on the intention of the physician. [929]

In the context of considering the "no difference" line of reasoning, it merits noting that a common thread among all end-of-life interventions, and their goal, is the avoidance or relief of suffering. The pro-euthanasia argument is that such relief is the overriding priority and an end that justifies any necessary means of achieving it, including assisted suicide and euthanasia.

DISMISSING SLIPPERY SLOPES

In assessing the practical slippery slope—the risks for abuse if an absolute ban on physician-assisted suicide is not maintained and it's permitted under certain conditions—the Judge considers "life ending acts without explicit request" (LAWER) and the presence of mental illness in people wanting physician-assisted suicide. She extensively reviews "medically assisted dying" legislation in Oregon, the Netherlands, and Belgium and notes that prohibiting physician-assisted suicide and euthanasia doesn't prevent them from being carried out (see, e.g., 523). And, she again conflates pain relief and withdrawal of treatment, on the one hand, with euthanasia, on the other. [525]

The judge's reassuring conclusions about the effectiveness of safeguards in the jurisdictions she examines are, however, far from universally shared and evidence for the existence of both practical slippery slopes and logical slippery slopes—the expansion of justifications for physician-assisted suicide and euthanasia—is very convincing. In fact, her findings with regard to the practical slippery slope have been expressly rejected by the High Court of Ireland in *Fleming v. Ireland and others,*[54] after the court extensively reviewed the evidence on which Justice Smith relied. Here's how their finding is summarized:

> In that case [the *Carter* case], the Canadian court reviewed the available evidence from other jurisdictions with liberalised legislation and concluded that there was no evidence of abuse. This Court also reviewed the same evidence and has drawn exactly the opposite conclusions. The medical literature documents specific examples of abuse which, even if exceptional, are nonetheless deeply disturbing. Moreover, contrary to the views of the Canadian court, there is evidence from this literature that certain groups (such as disabled neonates and disabled or demented elderly persons) are vulnerable to abuse. Above all, the fact that the number of LAWER ("life-ending acts without explicit request") cases remains strikingly high in jurisdictions which have liberalised their law on assisted suicide (Switzerland, Netherlands and Belgium)—ranging from 0.4% to over 1% of all deaths in these jurisdictions according to the latest figures—without any obvious official response speaks for itself as to the risks involved.

A relatively recent chilling example of the logical slippery slope is the euthanizing, in December 2012, of 45 year old twins in Belgium. Deaf since childhood, Marc and Eddy Verbessem were facing the additional disability of blindness. Accepting that they were irremediably suffering, their physician euthanized them.[55]

Justice Smith rules that the nature of the risks of "medically assisted death" is no different from that of other end-of-life decisions. In other words, she again adopts the "no difference" approach, outlined previously, to reject the dangers of physician-assisted suicide opening up slippery slopes by accepting the plaintiffs' suggestion,

> that the very same risks exist with respect to current end-of-life practices [as with physician-assisted suicide]. A patient who chooses to withdraw from life-sustaining treatment may present exactly the same challenges to caregivers, who need to know if the patient is truly giving informed consent, is not suffering from untreated depression, or is acting under some kind of duress or coercion. [1237]

Justice Smith does not look at the logical slippery slope in the Netherlands constituted by the expansion of justifications for euthanasia, and she does not mention the major increase in the use of terminal/palliative sedation (the patient is sedated until he dies) in Belgium.[56] This can be euthanasia (terminal sedation), but is not in circumstances in which it is the only reasonable way to relieve serious pain and suffering (palliative sedation). We can ask why terminal sedation is being favored over "classic" euthanasia methods (lethal injections) that have been used up to the present in the Netherlands. Might palliative sedation make the patient's death seem more like a natural death? Might it reflect a moral intuition that there's something wrong in intentionally killing another human being and the killing is less obvious when a lethal injection is avoided? Or might it just be that administrative requirements, such as the requirement to report cases of euthanasia are inapplicable to terminal sedation?

PRIORITIZING AUTONOMY AND CHOICE

At its simplest, the euthanasia debate can be seen as a clash between the value of "respect for life" and the value of respect for individual autonomy, usually backed up by a "relief of suffering" argument and disagreement as to which should take priority. People who oppose euthanasia give priority to respect for life and point out that pain and suffering can be relieved without killing the person who suffers, including, where warranted, by palliative sedation.

In contrast, the value of "choice" or individual autonomy and self-determination is central to the pro-euthanasia argument and because it gives the person a sense of control is seen, in itself, as reducing suffering. Here are some examples of how that argument is expressed in the *Carter* judgment:

> No-one should be deprived of liberty, or *forced to suffer*, without adequate cause. Failing to respect an autonomous choice to die risks paternalism. (Emphasis added) [315]

For people with liberal values, paternalism is always a major harm.

Justice Smith rules:

> In my opinion, the law [prohibiting assisted suicide] creates a distinction that is discriminatory. It perpetuates and worsens a disadvantage experienced by persons with disabilities. *The dignity of choice* should be afforded to Canadians equally, but the law as it stands does not do so with respect to this ultimately personal and fundamental choice [to die]. (Emphasis added) [1161]

But, even assuming that there is a legally relevant distinction, in view of the fact that no one has a right to commit suicide and, where possible people who attempt it will be prevented from doing so, one can query whether the law creates a discriminatory distinction.

I also note here the use of the phrase "the dignity of choice," which I have not encountered before. Dignity is a complex and controversial topic in bioethics,[57] and choice is a neutral concept in the sense that some choices will enhance human dignity, others will harm it, and it's *what* we choose that makes a choice ethical or unethical, not just the presence of choice, itself.

JUSTIFYING PHYSICIAN-ASSISTED SUICIDE AND EUTHANASIA THROUGH RELIEF OF SUFFERING

As noted already, respect for individual autonomy and choice is one of the primary values for supporters of legalizing euthanasia; the other is the relief of suffering. Justice Smith links these values to each other and also gives priority to the relief of an individual's suffering over risks for harm to other individuals from the precedent set by the means used to relieve that suffering. She states:

> [M]y review of all the evidence shows that the ethical and practical arguments *in favour of* making physician-assisted death available to the limited category of patients described [include that]. . . . it is unethical to refuse to relieve the suffering of a patient who requests and requires such relief, simply in order to protect other hypothetical patients from hypothetical harm. [315(l)] . . . It must not be overlooked that what is at stake for someone in Gloria Taylor's situation is not merely autonomy, nor is it simply autonomy with respect to physical integrity. It is the *autonomy to relieve herself of suffering*. (Emphasis added) [1156]

The Attorney General of Canada argued that

> the Court must address whether the autonomy interests and suffering of some individuals are outweighed by the public benefits of promoting the value of every life, preserving life, protecting the vulnerable, preventing abuses, maintaining the physician-patient relationship and promoting palliative care. [1247]

But the judge rejects arguments that harm to society can outweigh individuals' rights to autonomy, although she requires the presence of suffering for those rights to extend to physician-assisted suicide and euthanasia. In doing so, the judge limits the scope of a person's autonomy to choose death, by requiring the presence of suffering. In other words, the presence of suffering is functioning as a limiting device on the exercise of a legal right to autonomy with respect to self-willed death and the assistance of a physician in implementing that goal.

Justice Smith also sees the presence of suffering at the end of life as differentiating suicide in that context from it in other contexts, and as a justification for the former:

> [The Attorney General of] Canada mistakenly presumes that Canadians do not see a difference between assisted death in response to intolerable suffering at the end of life, and suicide arising out of mental illness or transitory sadness. [1262]

The judge does not consider that many suicidal people also experience what they perceive as "intolerable suffering" and the likely impact of the message that this passage gives that suicide is an appropriate response to suffering, at least in some circumstances.

Suffering is a very difficult reality to deal with in postmodern democracies, such as Canada. Traditionally, we have accommodated suffering in our lives by finding meaning in it, but we largely did that through religion. In secular societies, it is much more difficult for many people to find such meaning. Yet it can be found, as many stories of deep suffering and bravery that move us profoundly attest.

ACCEPTING PHYSICIAN-ASSISTED SUICIDE AND EUTHANASIA AS MEDICAL TREATMENT

The judge appears to accept the argument that legalizing euthanasia enhances palliative care. [See, e.g., 584, 585, and 721] This goes some way, at the least, toward treating euthanasia as, as some have termed it, "the last act of good palliative care." It's also consistent with the "no difference among them" approach to a spectrum of end-of-life medical interventions that include euthanasia and physician-assisted suicide, discussed earlier. But my colleague, Donald Boudreau, a specialist physician, and I adamantly reject that euthanasia can ever be medical treatment because it is fundamentally incompatible with the healing role of physicians.[58]

Apart from other considerations, whether euthanasia is medical treatment matters in Canada for jurisdictional reasons. Governance of medical treatment is a provincial, not a federal, jurisdiction, which is one reason why the report, "Dying with Dignity," of the Quebec Legislative Assembly committee,[59] and the Quebec College of Physicians and Surgeons, which supports legalizing euthanasia, both argue that it is medical treatment. If it were, the Quebec Government would have the right to pass laws to regulate these "treatments" and physicians to administer them to patients.

But, were physician-assisted suicide and euthanasia to be legalized, should physicians or some other professionals carry them out? In other words, should we clearly separate those interventions from medical treatment?

It's a controversial suggestion, but I propose that if we were to legalize physician-assisted suicide and euthanasia, we should take the "medical cloak" off them, that is, physicians should not be the ones to carry them out.

One reason, among many, to take the medical cloak off physician-assisted suicide and euthanasia is that it causes people to fear physicians, accepting pain relief treatment, and hospice and palliative medicine and care.

As well, placing a medical cloak on physician-assisted suicide and euthanasia, yet again, causes confusion. It makes these interventions seem safe, ethical, and humane because those are the characteristics we associate automatically with medical care, when, in fact, we all need to question the ethical acceptability of legalizing physician-assisted suicide and euthanasia and physicians being authorized to carry them out.

One suggestion for alternative practitioners, which has shocked even people who are euthanasia advocates, is to consider having specially trained lawyers. I was giving a speech on euthanasia at a national medical association conference in Australia. I stated on two or three occasions that "we can't have physicians killing people." A pro-euthanasia palliative care physician in the audience leapt to his feet and shouted, "Margo, will you stop using that word killing; it's not killing, it's VAE [voluntary active euthanasia]."

Later in the speech, I addressed the issue of who should carry out euthanasia, if we were to legalize it. I argued against physicians because, as I explained earlier, that makes people frightened of consulting physicians and reluctant to accept pain relief treatment because they fear being euthanized. The solution I suggested would be to have a specially trained group of lawyers, which is not my original idea.[60] The justification put forward for this choice is that lawyers understand how to interpret properly and to strictly apply laws and, for pro-euthanasia advocates, ensuring that in order to prevent abuse is their major concern, not euthanasia itself.

The same physician who had objected to my using the word "killing" again jumped to his feet and this time loudly exclaimed, "Margo are you crazy? We can't have lawyers killing people." I agree wholeheartedly, and neither should we have physicians killing people. With the medical cloak on the act, it was not killing; with the cloak off, the same act was killing.

Justice Smith turns to the British Columbia Prosecutorial policy on assisted suicide for definitional assistance with respect to whether physician-assisted suicide is medical treatment:

> In the policy, "palliative care" is defined as "a qualified medical practitioner, or a person acting under the general supervision of a qualified medical practitioner, administering medication or other treatment to a terminally ill patient with the intention of relieving pain or suffering, even though this may hasten death." The policy states that that conduct, "when provided or administered according to accepted ethical medical standards, is not subject to criminal prosecution." [303]

In other words, the policy can be expansively interpreted as placing euthanasia in same category as other end-of-life treatment interventions that "may hasten death."

Justice Smith was deeply impressed with the evidence given by American philosopher and bioethicist, Professor Margaret Battin, an expert witness for the plaintiffs, who is a prominent advocate of legalizing physician-assisted suicide and euthanasia. She extensively reviewed and endorsed Battin's views about

> the core principles central to the [euthanasia] debate: liberty (also referred to as freedom, self-determination or autonomy) and mercy (compassion, or the right to be free from pain and suffering)... [and] a third core value for physicians, non-abandonment. [239]

The judge also extensively reviews research by Battin and her colleagues on euthanasia in the Netherlands and in Oregon and endorses their findings that abuses are within acceptable limits.[61] She approvingly quotes Battin to the following effect:

> Those who oppose physician aid in dying must show that the principles of liberty and *freedom from suffering* that are basic to an open, liberal and democratic society should be overridden. (Emphasis added) [241]

In short, a reversal of the burden of proof is justified on the basis of respecting liberty and implementing freedom from suffering.

LOOKING BEYOND THE INTENSE INDIVIDUALISM OF THE *CARTER* CASE

There is a radical difference between valuing only what we want in relation to our own life or also valuing the lives of generations to follow and deciding what we owe to them, and acting accordingly. Legalizing physician-assisted suicide or euthanasia in order to allow personal preferences concerning death to prevail, as Justice Smith does in the *Carter* case, is an example of the former. Rejecting physician-assisted suicide or euthanasia, because of the harm we believe it would do to individuals, our shared values, societal institutions, society, and future generations, is an example of the latter. Before we would legalize euthanasia, we need to ask ourselves, "If we do that, how might our great-great grandchildren die?" and answer honestly.

Physicians and nurses must be sensitive to patients' pain and suffering and meet it with great compassion, but that must be done without intentionally inflicting death. Suffering reduction and death infliction must never be equated.

Physicians' and nurses' absolute rejection of intentionally inflicting death is necessary to maintaining people's and society's trust in both their own physicians and the profession of medicine as a whole. This is true, in part, because physicians and nurses have opportunities to kill that are not open to other people.

Physicians and nurses need to continue to have a clear line that powerfully manifests to them, their patients, and society that they do not inflict death. Both their patients and the public need to know with absolute certainty—and be able to trust—that is the case. Anything that blurs that line, damages that trust, or makes physicians or nurses less sensitive to primary obligations to protect and respect life is unacceptable. Legalizing physician-assisted suicide or euthanasia would do all of these.

Moreover, it is a very important part of the art of medicine to sense and respect the mystery of life and death, to hold this mystery in trust, and to hand it on to future generations— including future generations of physicians. We must consider deeply whether legalizing physician-assisted suicide or euthanasia would threaten this art, this trust, and this legacy. I believe it would.

The "euthanasia debate" is a momentous one. It involves our individual and collective past (the ethical, legal, and cultural norms that have been handed down to us as members of families, groups and societies); the present (whether we will change those norms); and the future (the impact that this would have on those who come after us). We need a much broader analysis and a great deal more thought before we follow down the path that Justice Smith maps out in the *Carter* case.

The central issue in the *Carter* case is not just what compassion for Ms. Taylor might lead people, who do not have ethical or moral problems with physician-assisted suicide or euthanasia—who, it appears, include Justice Smith—to recommend. The central issue is whether we will abandon some of the most important foundational values of our Canadian society. If we are going to do that, at the least we should explicitly recognize that is what we are doing. With respect, the *Carter* judgment is a total failure in that regard.

Conclusion

In this chapter I have focused largely on the issues of physician-assisted suicide and euthanasia to explore the interaction of law and pain and suffering because I believe that what our societies decide about legalizing these interventions will be the defining event for each of them of the first half of the twenty-first century.

In making those decisions, we need to keep in mind an old saying in human rights: "Nowhere are human rights more threatened than when we act purporting to do only good." This warns us that the good that we hope to realize can blind us to the harms and risks also unavoidably involved in doing that good. When the good we seek is the relief of serious suffering, our moral intuition that it is wrong to intentionally kill another human being can be overwhelmed. Such intuitions are important guides in making good ethical decisions.[62] And while we ignore our feelings at our ethical peril,[63] our emotional reactions to an individual person's suffering need to become "examined emotions" if we are to avoid the danger of their misleading us ethically.[64]

By arguing against physician-assisted suicide and euthanasia, I am proposing that there are and should be ethical and legal limits to our freedom to alleviate suffering and that these interventions are not legitimate means of doing so. Just as the axiom "freedom in fetters" tells us that we must restrict freedom to some extent, to protect and maintain the conditions that make freedom possible, so we must restrict what we do to relieve suffering to ensure that we protect and maintain the shared values that are necessary if we are not to risk creating a society in which no reasonable person would want to live.

These limits mean that within bioethics and biolaw, we must position our moral and legal obligations to relieve suffering, such that they are consistent with upholding respect for human life, both at the level of the individual person and human life, in general, at the societal level. Fortunately, we have new tools to help us to achieve that balance. Often, the unprecedented powers of the new medicine and science face us with additional serious ethical difficulties. In relation to relieving pain and suffering, the opposite is true. Research is providing us with means never before possible to help those who need our help to relieve their pain and suffering.

For millennia, our kinds of societies have prohibited euthanasia and assisted suicide—why then, now, when there is nothing new about the circumstances in which these interventions are called for and there is so much more we can do to relieve suffering, do we think that intentionally inflicting death is a good response to suffering? A wise answer to that question requires much thought.[65] What would be the long-term impact of death by euthanasia becoming the norm? How would that affect the way in which we view and treat old, vulnerable, and disabled people? We must address these and many other questions before changing the law to allow the intentional infliction of death.

Just as we now realize our actions could destroy our physical ecosystem and we must hold it on trust for future generations, we must also hold our metaphysical ecosystem—the collection of values, principles, beliefs, attitudes, shared stories, and so on that bind us together as a society—likewise, on trust for them. That requires that we always react to pain and suffering with deep compassion and assistance to relieve it, but that we kill the pain and suffering, not the person with the pain and suffering.[66]

Notes

1. U.N. General Assembly, *Universal Declaration of Human Rights*, December 10, 1948, 217 A (III), accessed March 11, 2014. http://www.unhcr.org/refworld/docid/3ae6b3712c.html.

2. The European Convention on Human Rights (ECHR) (the *Convention for the Protection of Human Rights and Fundamental Freedoms*) Council of Europe, article 3.

3. *Canadian Charter of Rights and Freedoms, The Constitution Act, 1982*, being Schedule B to the *Canada Act 1982* (UK), 1982, c 11Section 12.

4. Margaret Somerville, "The Ethics of Pizza, Prison and Punishment," *The Globe and Mail*, January 4, 2013, accessed March 11, 2014, http://www.theglobeandmail.com/commentary/the-ethics-of-pizza-prison-and-punishment/article6928550/

5. Margaret Somerville, "Pain and Suffering at Interfaces of Medicine and Law," *University of Toronto Law Journal* 36 (1986): 286–317.

6. Margaret Somerville, "Death of Pain: Pain, Suffering, and Ethics," in *Progress in Pain Research and Management,* Vol. 2, Proceedings of the 7th World Congress on Pain, International Association for the Study of Pain, ed. Gerald F. Gebhart, Donna L. Hammond, and Troels S. Jensen (Washington: IASP Press, 1994), 41–58. Also published in Margaret Somerville, *Death Talk: The Case against Euthanasia and Physician-Assisted Suicide* (Montreal: McGill Queen's University Press, 2001), 433, chap.14, 218–230.

7. *Wilkinson v. Downton* [1897] 2 Q.B. 57.

8. *Samms v. Eccles*, 11 Utah 2d 289, 358 P.2d 344 (1961).

9. G.H.L. Fridman et al., *The Law of Torts in Canada*, 3rd ed. (Toronto: Carswell, 2010) 324–330.

10. Ibid., 325.

11. See David Wexler and Bruce J. Winick, *Law in a Therapeutic Key: Developments in Therapeutic Jurisprudence* (Durham, NC: Carolina Academic, 1996)

12. Eric Cassell, "The Nature of Suffering and the Goals of Medicine," *N Engl J Med* 36 (1992): 1440–1441.

13. Margaret Somerville, "Human Rights and Medicine: The Relief of Suffering," in *International Human Rights Law: Theory and Practice*, ed. Irwin Cotler and F. Pearl Eliadis. (Montreal: The Canadian Human Rights Foundation, 1992), 505–522. Also published in "Death Talk," supra note 6, chap. 13, 205–217.

14. See Daniel Callahan, "When Self-Determination Runs Amok," *The Hastings Center Report* 22, no. 2. (1992): 52–55.

15. *Carter v. Canada (Attorney General),* 2012 BCSC 886.

16. In *Carter v. Canada (Attorney General)* 2013 BCCA 435, a majority of the British Columbia Court of Appeal overturned the first instance judgment in the *Carter* case, which is currently on appeal to the Supreme Court of Canada.

17. International Association for the Study of Pain, accessed March 26, 2014 https://www.iasp-pain.org/Advocacy/Content.aspx?ItemNumber=1821

18. World Medical Association Resolution on the Access to Adequate Pain Treatment, Adopted by the 62nd WMA General Assembly, Montevideo, Uruguay, October, 2011,

accessed March 11, 2014, http://www.painaustralia.org.au/images/pain_australia/Declaration/WMA%20Resolution.pdf.

19. This section on pain management is a condensed version of a part of another text, Margaret Somerville, "Law, Marching with Medicine but in the Rear and Limping a Little": Ethics as "First Aid for Law," in *The Ethicalization of Law*, ed., Silja Voneky (Freiberg: Springer-Verlag, 2013).

20. Somerville, supra note 5.

21. *Criminal Code,* R.S.C., 1985, c. C-46 (as amended), sec. 221.

22. Supra note 6.

23. Human Rights Watch, *A Question of Life or Death: Treatment Access for Children Living With HIV in Kenya*, December 2008, accessed March 11, 2014, http://www.hrw.org/sites/default/files/reports/kenya1208webwcover.pdf.

24. Declaration of Montreal, supra note 17.

25. Margaret Somerville, "Human Rights and Human Ethics: Health and Health Care," in *Death Talk*, supra note 6, 327–343, 331.

26. Supra note 6.

27. This story about my students first appeared as part of an opinion article published as Margaret Somerville, "The Case against Euthanasia," *The Ottawa Citizen*, June 27, 2008.

28. Supra note 15.

29. Supra note 21.

30. *Canadian Charter*, supra note 3.

31. *Rodriguez v. British Columbia (Attorney General)*, [1993] 3 S.C.R. 519.

32. Numbers in square brackets refer to paragraphs in the *Carter* judgment, supra note 15.

33. *Canadian Charter*, supra note 3, section 7.

34. Ibid., section 15.

35. Ibid., section 7.

36. Expert Panel of the Royal Society of Canada: *End-of-Life Decision Making* (Ottawa: Royal Society of Canada, 2011) (Chair: Udo Schuklenk).

37. Tom Koch, "End of Life, Year after Year after Year," *Canadian Medical Association Journal* 181, no. 11 (2009): 868.

38. Susan Sontag, *Illness as Metaphor and AIDS and Its Metaphors* (New York: Anchor books/Doubleday, 1978), 3.

39. P. D. James, *The Children of Men* (Canada: Knopf Canada, 1992), chap. 9, 68–79.

40. T. Koch, *Thieves of Virtue: When Bioethics Stole Medicine* (Cambridge, MA: MIT Press, 1990), chap. 3.

41. Daniel Callahan, *Setting Limits: Medical Goals in an Aging* Society (New York: Simon and Schuster, 1987).

42. I am indebted to Canadian bioethicist, Dr. Tom Koch, for this formulation of the issue.

43. *Rodriguez* case, supra note 31.

44. Expert Panel of the Royal Society of Canada, supra note 36.

45. Report of the Select Committee of the Assemblée Nationale of Québec on "Dying with Dignity, *Mourir dans la Dignité* (March 2012) (Chair: Maryse Gaudreault).

46. Alberto Giubilini and Francesca Minerva, "After-Birth Abortion: Why Should the Baby Live?" *J Med Ethics* 39, no. 5 (2013): 261–263.

47. Supra note 36.

48. Supra note 45.

49. In this section, in using the word *euthanasia*, I intend it to include physician-assisted suicide.

50. Margaret Somerville, "Euthanasia by Confusion," *University of New South Wales Law Journal* 20, no. 3 (1997): 550–575. Also published in *Death Talk*, supra note 6, 119–143.

51. Jocelyn Downie, *Dying Justice: A Case for Decriminalizing Euthanasia and Assisted Suicide in Canada* (Toronto: University of Toronto Press, 2004).

52. Lauren Vogel, "Line between Acts and Omissions Blurred, Euthanasia Critics Argue," *Canadian Medical Association Journal* 184, no. 1 (2012): E19–E20.

53. Supra pp. 207–208, 211–212, 216, 220.

54. *Fleming v. Ireland & Ors*, [2013] IEHC 2. The Supreme Court of Ireland affirmed the High Court's judgment, *Fleming v Ireland & ors.*, [2013] IESC 19

55. See http://www.ibtimes.com/deaf-twins-euthanized-belgian-brothers-marc-eddy-verbessem-wanted-die-because-they-were-going-blind, accessed March 11, 2014.

56. Johan Bilsen et al., "Medical End-of-Life Practices under the Euthanasia Law in Belgium," *New England Journal of Medicine* 361, no. 11 (2009): 1119–1121, accessed March 11, 2014, <http://www.nejm.org/doi/pdf/10.1056/NEJMc0904292>.

57. See Margaret Somerville, "Is Dignity a Useful, Useless or Dangerous Concept?", unpublished manuscript, Montreal, 2009.

58. This question is fully explored in J. Donald Boudreau and Margaret A. Somerville, "Euthanasia Is Not Medical Treatment," *British Medical Bulletin* 106 (2013): 45–66.

59. Supra note 45.

60. See R. M. Sade and M. F. Marshall, "Legistrothanatory: A New Specialty for Assisting in Death," *Perspectives in Biology and Medicine* 1996;39, no. 4 (1996): 547–549.

61. As noted already, the High Court of Ireland found the opposite, see the *Fleming* case supra note 26.

62. Margaret Somerville, *The Ethical Imagination: Journeys of the Human Spirit* (Toronto: House of Anansi Press, 2006), 28–31, 62–72.

63. Leonie Welberg, "The Moral Brain," *Nature Reviews Neuroscience*, accessed March 11, 2014, http://www.nature.com/nrn/journal/v8/n5/full/nrn2141.html.

64. Supra note 62, 28–31, 53–93.

65. Margaret Somerville, "Legalizing Euthanasia: Why Now?", in *Death Talk*, supra note 6, 105–118.

66. *Death Talk*, ibid., 218–232.

PART FOUR

Religious Perspectives on Suffering and Medicine

11

Suffering: A Catholic Theological-Ethical View

Lisa Sowle Cahill

The first thing to be said about "suffering" in an ethical context is that the world bears "a barbarous excess of suffering," whose depth, pervasiveness, and horror are obvious without any philosophical or religious analysis whatsoever. In the words of feminist theologian Elizabeth Johnson,

> These centuries have witnessed millions of people gassed, burned, tortured, bombed and shot out of existence. Millions more continue to have the life ground out of them by the misery of poverty.... Everywhere is the suffering of illness, aging and death... a history of suffering weaves in and out of every moment so profoundly that suffering can be called the "red thread" that connects all living things in history. There is suffering, in other words, that does not simply punish or test or educate or work a greater good. Instead, it destroys.[1]

Humanly caused suffering of the sorts that involve dire health consequences afflicts the majority of people on this planet. While all destructive suffering should be avoided and ameliorated, the suffering caused by racism, sexism, economic inequality, war, and civil conflict calls most acutely for a moral response because it is caused by human agency and is in principle under human control. More than one billion people live on less than one dollar a day, with more than 2.7 billion surviving on less than two dollars. More than 800 million people go to bed hungry every night. Every year, more than six million children die from preventable causes like malaria, diarrhea, pneumonia, and malnutrition. More than fifty percent of Africans suffer from water-borne diseases like cholera.

Every minute, a woman somewhere dies in pregnancy or childbirth. But women in North America bear only a 1 in 3,700 risk of meeting this fate, whereas for an African woman, the risk is 1 in 16.[2] Women also face devastating forms of sexual violence. Between 100,000 and 250,000 women were raped in Rwanda during the three months of genocide in 1994. According to United Nations estimates, "more than 60,000 women were raped during the civil war in Sierra Leone (1991–2002), more than 40,000 in Liberia (1989–2003), up to 60,000 in the former Yugoslavia

(1992–1995), and at least 200,000 in the Democratic Republic of the Congo during the past 12 years of war."[3]

In the United States, health care professionals and ethical consultants may debate whether to provide emergency resuscitation, artificial nutrition and hydration, respirators, neonatal intensive care, experimental drugs, last-ditch surgery, terminal sedation, or physician-assisted suicide. In India, a doctor is faced with a shortage of neonatal ventilators. Not only that, this doctor's patient may well have been born into a destitute family that does not grasp the magnitude of the lifelong burdens to be incurred by caring for a critically ill or disabled child. The doctor asks, "My job is to keep him alive, but what about his brother and sister?"[4] In the Philippines, a seventeen-year-old boy from a very poor family is told that he permanently will need a respirator to survive after a car accident. Such an expense is completely out of the reach of his family, and to sustain it even short-term would devastate them. "Mr. C. looks sad. After a few days, he requests that the respirator be removed."[5] Situations like these caution first-world bioethicists of the moral blindness involved in considering health-related suffering only from the standpoint of the modern Western medical facility. Even in the United States, at this writing, more than forty-eight million people still lack health insurance, despite the beginning implementation of the 2010 Affordable Care Act.[6] The Institutes of Medicine reported in 2002 that eighteen thousand adults die every year because of lack of coverage, and in 2006, the Urban Institute raised that number to twenty-two thousand.[7]

In the face of such realities, extended philosophical rehearsals of the reasons that "we have a prima facie duty to relieve suffering because suffering is bad and ought not to occur," or that this duty is proportionate to "the intensity or duration of suffering,"[8] seem pedantic, otiose, and even self-indulgent. The author of the cited phrases rightly concludes that more fortunate individuals, with relative ease, should and "can prevent an enormous amount of suffering," suffering that is indubitable and egregious; "failure to do this is unjustifiable." A concluding "Author's Note" hammers home the worldwide differential in causes of suffering by advising readers that the book's royalties will go to Amnesty International, Doctors without Borders, and Oxfam.[9]

Religious and theological voices have also been raised in support of justice in health care access, among them Roman Catholic popes, bishops, and theologians. In 2003, John Paul II, mentioning AIDS and "dire epidemics," spoke of "*the very serious and unacceptable gap* that separates the developing world from the developed" in terms of health resources. He called for "justice and international solidarity" in order to redress the balance.[10] In his 2009 World Day of Peace Message, Benedict XVI laid out the "moral implications" of poverty, including children's lack of access to "vaccines, medical care and drinking water," and "*pandemic diseases*, such as malaria, tuberculosis and AIDS."[11] In late 2012, Benedict reiterated to a congress of health care providers that, in a time of economic crisis and scarcity of funds, it is crucial that health care facilities and structures better reflect the status of health as "a universal good" not to be "subjected to the laws of the market, hence accessible to the few." To work toward this end is a responsibility of health professionals themselves, beyond the immediate patients who enjoy access to their services.[12]

The U.S. Catholic bishops have repeatedly addressed the importance of health care justice in the domestic context. In 1993, during the Clinton administration's reform efforts, the United States Conference of Catholic Bishops (USCCB) issued a "Resolution on Health Care Reform" that called health care a basic human right.[13] The *Ethical and Religious Directives for Catholic Health Care Facilities* introduces its practical ethical guidelines by tying the Church's mission to the sick to the ministry of Jesus, whom the Gospels portray as healing not only "physical affliction" but also mental and spiritual distress and social isolation. The relief of human suffering is at the core of Catholic health care and informs the attention it gives to pastoral as well as physical support. Pastoral care includes "a listening presence, help in dealing with powerlessness, pain and alienation; and assistance in recognizing and responding to God's will with greater joy and peace."[14]

Human suffering in the biomedical context obviously results from multiple causes, and these can interact in complex ways, making the generation, intensity, duration, and resolution or relief of human suffering an equally complex and individual matter. This is true whether or not one experiences the primordial suffering of lack of food, shelter, or physical safety, but it is easier to see why suffering occurs when basic needs go unmet, and more difficult when suffering is caused by relatively idiosyncratic factors. Eric Cassell offers several poignant cases from his own experience as a doctor in the U.S. health care system.[15] In these cases, patient suffering does not seem to correlate closely with type or severity of disease, with physical pain, or with life expectancy. Other life factors, physical and nonphysical, can coalesce to intensify suffering. The emphasis of Catholic health services on pastoral care is a way of recognizing that although alleviating suffering is a major motivator of medical caregivers, not all suffering should be "medicalized." Medical and nonmedical forms of suffering intersect and magnify each other. The expertise of medical professionals does not extend to all equally. In addition, "patient autonomy" is an inadequate moral guide because suffering and vulnerability call for relationships of care and solidarity, nested in strong social supports.

Thus, medical, psychological, social, and pastoral services must work interdependently with patients and with patients' support networks. Patients' frequent sense of diminishment, of loss of self-image and dignity, of lack of control over their own lives and futures, of loneliness and fear can and should be addressed in creative and supportive ways that may well surpass the physician's competence. From a Catholic perspective, medical professionals should not ignore, suppress, or abandon the human needs and suffering of their patients. Yet they should have the humility and wisdom to recognize the human implications of disease and mortality, to acknowledge their own limits, and to call upon allied services to address complex suffering related to illness and death.

Catholic health care ethics recognizes that good care that keeps suffering to a minimum requires a multilayered social and institutional, as well as a personal, "bedside," response. Care at the bedside assumes a bed and a caregiver. Some ill or elderly persons have no access to a bed in a system of consistent professional care. In other cases, the bed is at home, and the primary caregivers are family members and informal networks, whose resources are often strained to the breaking point. Suffering and its alleviation extend beyond the purview of the directly medical context, and medical caregiving should interface creatively with other professional services, with families, and with social policy. Catholic social teaching brings such concepts as dignity of the person, common good, participation, and subsidiarity to bear on the social, economic, and legal causes and solutions to suffering.[16]

Mentioning the parable of the Good Samaritan (Luke 10:25–37), the *Directives* notes that the Christian vocation to heal suffering has taken social, organizational shape in the past and present through hospices for travelers and the ill, homes for children and the elderly, and hospitals, health care systems, and school or community clinics.[17] Catholic health care is especially committed to serve

> [t]hose people whose social condition puts them at the margins of our society and makes them particularly vulnerable to discrimination: the poor and uninsured; children and the unborn; single parents; the elderly; those with incurable diseases and chemical dependencies; racial minorities; immigrants and refugees. . . . [and] the person with mental or physical disabilities. . . . (Directive 3)[18]

Beyond faith-based charitable services, Catholic health care advocates for social protection of all marginalized groups, the poor, the uninsured and underinsured. It partners with other groups in civil society and government to seek access to basic decent health care for all as necessary to the "common good" of society.[19]

In 2007, the USCCB published *Forming Consciences for Faithful Citizenship,* a voting guide that termed health care reform "an urgent national priority," and reissued the guide for the 2012 national elections.[20] *Faithful Citizenship* repeats many of the themes of earlier statements: "**Affordable and accessible health** care is an essential safeguard of human life and a fundamental human right."[21] It adds a note of "global solidarity" in the face of undeniable forms of suffering worldwide that should inform the perspective of health care ethics. "The United States should take a leading role in helping to **alleviate global poverty** through substantially increased development aid for the poorest countries, more equitable trade policies, and continuing efforts to relieve the crushing burdens of debt and disease."[22]

Lamentably, health care reform did not become a practical political priority for most of the bishops or their national organization during the 2008 and 2012 presidential campaigns. Instead the more vocal bishops and the USCCB leadership focused on turning back a provision of the Affordable Care Act mandating that insurers cover free contraception as a form of basic preventative care.[23] However, the website of Catholic Relief Services, an international aid organization that comes under the authority of the USCCB, does feature many examples of advocacy and action for diminishment of human suffering in areas related to health. These include AIDS care, sustainable gardening, mosquito nets, and the strengthening of local health care systems globally.[24]

Although for Catholic bioethics, the mandate to alleviate human suffering applies first and most of all to the unjust suffering of those deprived of basic human goods that meet essential needs, Catholic ethics is also concerned with the morality of specific measures to restore health or end suffering, as these might be used in a particular health care setting. A general point about the Catholic approach to the use of medical treatments and technologies is that while the main goal is ending human suffering by restoring the person to healthy functioning insofar as is possible, the use of means to attain that goal is limited by their potential violation of other values related to human dignity and the common good. So, for example, the *Directives* caution, "While we rejoice in the potential for good inherent in many of these [new reproductive] technologies, we cannot assume that what is technically possible is always morally right."[25]

Judgments about what is morally wrong may be backed by Scripture or authoritative ecclesial pronouncements, but the more fundamental basis for the determination is an assessment of dignity, purposes, and goods, as pertaining to the individual person or to the common good. In the sphere of reproduction, infertility is seen as a dysfunction that can cause suffering. Yet any technologies that separate sex from conception (in vitro fertilization) or involve third parties (gamete donors and surrogacy) are viewed as violating the "natural" goods of sex, love, and procreation, whose authentically human meaning and fulfillment require their unity in each instance of conception. The human goods to be considered include the common good and justice. Commercialized surrogacy "denigrates the dignity of women, especially the poor."[26] Moreover, the suffering around a physical abnormality such as infertility may be partly socially caused. Possible solutions may likewise go beyond the medical, such as the forging of generous and life-giving relationships within the extended family and community, or adoption.

Many debates can be and are had, both within and about Catholicism, regarding whether in the case of reproductive technologies or in other instances, the determinations of the nature and relation of the goods at stake are correct. The main point here is that while human suffering makes a moral claim on medical expertise and resources, the fact that medical attention can relieve suffering is not the only consideration relevant to the morality of an intervention. If the intervention directly harms human goods that have equal or greater priority, then that means is ruled out. Moreover, adequate attention should be given to nonmedical ways to address suffering, such as more equitable distribution of health care resources, and social responses to physical dysfunction or to the psychological, emotional, and spiritual suffering associated with it.

The remainder of this essay will focus on care for those who are severely ill or dying, to allow development of the Catholic perspective on some of the most grievous occasions of human suffering in the spheres of health, illness, and mortality. It is generally agreed that even when the pain caused by illness or its treatment is severe, pain and suffering should not be equated. "Suffering" denotes a subjective state of affliction that can include isolation, desperation, hopelessness, bewilderment, and the dissolution of the self. Such affliction can originate either in human agency—in the form of war, poverty, and domestic or sexual abuse, for example—or in so-called natural causes, such as famines, floods, and disease. When such affliction is experienced as excessive and unjust, religious believers are forced to confront the contradiction between their situation and the existence of a God who is good and righteous, and who so orders the universe. Why does God permit this? Why did God so create the world? Where is God for me in the midst of such evil? These interrogations can produce an intense anguish better captured in biblical depictions of protest and lament than in any logical attempt to justify the ways of God in human terms ("theodicy"[27]).

The biblical story of Job attests both that the righteous are inexplicably afflicted and that their suffering runs deep. Job cries out:

> I loathe my life;
> I will give free utterance to my complaint;
> I will speak in the bitterness of my soul.
> I will say to God, Do not condemn me;
> let me know why you contend against me. . . .
> although you know that I am not guilty
> and there is no one to deliver out of your hand?
> (Job 10:1–2, 7–8)

Similar notes are sounded in psalms of affliction and lament.

> Hear my prayer, O Lord;
> Let my cry come to you.
> Do not hide your face from me
> In the day of my distress. . . .
> All day long my enemies taunt me. . . .
> I wither away like grass.
> (Psalm 102)

In the words of African American theologian Bryan Massingale, "Laments are cries of anguish and outrage, groans of deep pain and grief, utterances of profound protest and righteous indignation over injustice, wails of mourning and sorrow in the face of unbearable suffering. . . . Laments . . . are uncivil, strident, harsh, and heart-rending."[28] Dying almost abandoned on the cross, Jesus laments in the words of Psalm 22: "My God, my God, why have you forsaken me?" (Mark 15:34).

Can deep suffering—the sense of radical undeserved affliction—be given meaning within a monotheistic framework centered on a benevolent creator, redeemer, and sustainer? Catholic theology attempts to answer this question in the affirmative. Within the medical context, the question is most pressing and the answer displayed most frequently in the face of terminal illness or old age and the dying process.

Concisely stated, the contemporary Catholic approach is to exhort caregivers to relieve suffering, even at the expense of indirectly shortening life; yet try to give meaning to unavoidable suffering primarily by assuring patients of God's presence with them, revealed most of all by Christ's suffering on the Cross. Yet it is also stated that suffering can have a redemptive meaning, even though patients are not encouraged to suffer. This redemptive meaning derives from the patient's sharing in the salvific work of Christ. The idea that suffering (either that of Christ or that of a human being united with Christ) may have a meaning in itself, however, goes back to traditional interpretations of salvation through Christ's death on the Cross as "penal substitution" that have been problematized in modern theology. The motivation to reconceive cross theology lies in its questionable implications both for the human understanding of the divine nature and dispositions and for the ethical and political consequences that might follow. Revisioning theologians object to interpretations of Christ's suffering and death that seem to make God demand punishment or retribution as a precondition of forgiveness of sins and reconciliation of humanity and God, and that portray God as pleased by or even causing the death of an innocent man.

Rather than seeing the cross as a punishment for sin that Christ accepted on behalf of humans, these theologians tend to see the cross as the consequence of the way Christ lived his life, challenging the powers that be and reaching out to the excluded; or as necessitated by the fact that in Christ (who is both human and divine), God is "incarnate" and enters fully into the human condition. In such readings, the purpose of Christ's life is not as such to die or to suffer, but rather to embody the ministry of the inclusive "reign of God" (Mark 1:14) no matter what the consequences, or to redemptively unite all human sufferings to the divine nature, thus transforming them.[29]

On these or similar readings, the point of "redemptive suffering with Christ" drops out of the theological-ethical picture, and the cross becomes rather a symbol of divine solidarity with human suffering, and in no way an encouragement to take on suffering that is pointless or unnecessary. Suffering is justified or meaningful in pursuit of a higher end or cause. When human suffering does not serve such a cause yet is unavoidable, God in Christ is in solidarity with that suffering, without desiring its prolongation. Recent Catholic documents on suffering do not in fact repeat the traditional construal of the cross as a penalty for human sinfulness. They further undermine any idea that human suffering can have a redemptive effect by affirming that Christ's death is sufficient for the salvation of all people.[30]

Another area of development in Catholic thinking about suffering concerns the attitude religious believers ought to take to the inescapability of suffering. Traditionally and today, Catholic theology reminds us that suffering is an inevitable human reality, indeed a reality for all living things. Premodern thinkers, however, accepted that most human suffering cannot be changed and in fact might derive from an individual's station or lot in life. The worldwide emergence in the Enlightenment of movements for democracy and human rights brought changes in religious sensibilities, including the development of modern papal social teaching at the end of the nineteenth century, and in the twentieth, liberation theology.

According to current teaching, there is a moral and religious obligation to condemn and resist unjust or unnecessary human suffering, especially of the kinds discussed previously in the treatment of national and global inequalities and their impact on health. At the individual level, similarly, suffering is no longer seen as a concomitant of a sinful and broken world to which we must be resigned, or which we should see as penance to be borne now, in the hope of avoiding punishment after death.

This shift accounts for a much more activist stance toward pain and suffering in the modern medical setting. While Catholic teaching still holds out hope of eternal life with God, historical existence is no longer seen simply as a "vale of tears," as it is termed in the medieval hymn "Salve Regina," in contrast to the longed-for joy of heaven. "Salve Regina" is a good illustration of the connections traditionally drawn among sin, suffering, and deliverance after death. The lyrics depict the "poor banished children of Eve" beseeching Mary the Mother of Jesus to intercede with her son so that "we may be delivered from present evils and from everlasting death."[31] In current bioethical documents on care for the sick, suffering is said potentially to have a "redemptive" meaning, but sin and punishment are rarely if ever mentioned. The focus is on eliminating pain as far as possible and making human life and relationships satisfying, even in one's declining years or hours. Holistic, humane care and companionship at the end of life are seen as the best route to a meaningful and peaceful death and are a responsibility both of direct caregivers and families and of medical, social, and legal institutions, policies, and practices.

The multiple and ambiguous dimensions of the Catholic theology of suffering will be discussed in relation to three teaching documents, then examined for their implications for the ethics of care for severely ill or dying persons. These three are the Vatican *Declaration on Euthanasia* (1980),[32] the papal letter *Salvifici Dolores* (1984),[33] and the *Ethical and Religious Directives for Catholic Health Care Services*.

The *Declaration on Euthanasia* was composed at a time when "death with dignity" movements in Western Europe and the United States were gaining traction; the Dutch Supreme Court legalized euthanasia in 1984. The document aims to respond, with a certain amount of empathy, to the argument that direct killing represents a merciful action for, or even a right of, a person who is anxious about death or actively suffering. Sometimes, euthanasia is requested or performed "in good faith." Yet "the pleas of gravely ill people" should be interpreted as "an anguished plea for help and love," not for death.[34]

From the Christian perspective, suffering as death nears "has a special place in God's saving plan," and "is in fact a sharing in Christ's passion and a union with the redeeming sacrifice which he offered in obedience to the Father's will." Therefore, patients might even choose to moderate their use of painkillers to consciously share in the sufferings of Christ. "Nevertheless it would be imprudent to impose a heroic way of acting as a general rule. On the contrary, human and Christian prudence suggest for the majority of sick people the use of medicines capable of alleviating or suppressing pain," even "if one foresees that the use of narcotics will shorten life." In the latter instance, the intended purpose of the drugs would be to "relieve pain effectively," not to cause death, although death may be hastened as a secondary effect.[35] Although it is good to maintain consciousness to prepare for death in relationship with loved ones, diminished consciousness or lucidity maybe the necessary price to relieve pain and suffering.

Since this formulation of Catholic teaching on suffering was released, there has been, as mentioned before, a growing trend among both Catholic and Protestant Christian authors to rethink the meaning of the redemptive value of Christ's cross, and with it, the meaning of human suffering.[36]

The *Declaration on Euthanasia* seems to an extent caught between the old and the new interpretive frameworks. On the one hand, the more forceful and concluding message is that it is morally justified to avoid suffering by resorting to large doses of drugs, even if they hasten death, and to reject potentially life-prolonging treatments if they seem disproportionate to the benefit expected.[37] At the same time, redemptive suffering is mentioned, and patients are encouraged to share in it, even by foregoing pain relievers. This tension continues in John Paul II's much longer reflection on suffering, *Salvifici Dolores.*

This "apostolic letter" (considered to be of less authority than an encyclical) asserts that suffering poses "basic questions" that must be "dealt with, meditated upon, and conceived as an explicit problem."[38] The sufferer wants to know the cause of or rationale for suffering; these are difficult questions that must be answered cautiously.[39] The pope finds the key to the meaning of suffering in the mission of Christ. This mission is not described in the vocabulary of penal substitution, but rather as both the consequence of faithfully carrying out his ministry,[40] and as a way of overcoming sin, death, and suffering through divine solidarity with the human lot. "Christ drew close above all the world of human suffering through the fact of having taken this suffering upon his very self." The "saving power" of Christ's suffering derives from the fact that "he is *united to the Father in this love* with which he has loved the world and man in the world."[41] John Paul II grants that Christ's suffering *could* be termed "substitutive" but insists, "above all it is 'redemptive.'"[42] *Salvifici Dolores* alludes to the "Suffering Servant" of Isaiah 53:11 to stress that Christ's suffering was *voluntary* (in contrast to terminal patients) because his adherence to his role was voluntary. Still, his suffering on the cross was deep and intense, due most of all to his feeling of estrangement from God.[43]

Salvifici Dolores offers a clue to why the rubric of redemptive suffering has not entirely disappeared, even in an era in which the question of whether and how the cross saves is being rethought and in which patients and caregivers are being encouraged to take far-reaching measures to reduce suffering. The idea of redemptive suffering provides a way to see even unavoidable suffering as voluntary and purposeful. This is an interpretive framework with biblical roots.

Salvifici Dolores begins by citing a verse from Paul's New Testament letter to the Colossians: "I am now rejoicing in my sufferings for your sake, and in my flesh

I am completing what is lacking in Christ's affliction for the sake of his body, that is, the church" (1:24). As he traveled around the Mediterranean about twenty to thirty years after the death of Christ, founding new churches, Paul was attacked and rejected on several occasions, finally being imprisoned and executed by the Romans. It is speculated that he might have suffered a physical disability or illness because he mentions having a "thorn in the flesh" (2 Cor. 12:7), in which he seeks a divine purpose. Like Jesus, Paul suffers as a result of his fidelity to a mission. Like end-of-life patients, he does not seek out suffering, but it finds him. Paul is confronted with suffering that he cannot escape. He finds its meaning by seeing his own mission as a participation in that of Christ. His suffering is not meaningless, but purposeful. Suffering is not forced upon him; he embraces the good that it might bring.

As John Paul II sees it, Paul's words "have the value as it were of a final discovery, which is accompanied by joy. . . . The joy comes from the discovery of the meaning of suffering." Paul's discovery can help others to grasp "*the salvific meaning*" and therefore the purpose of suffering.[44] "A source of joy is found in the overcoming of the sense of the uselessness of suffering," the sense that one is "condemned" to be a burden to oneself and others. Instead even the most debilitated person can be assured that he or she has a mission of "special support for the powers of good."[45] People in the grip of uncontrollable pain, loss, or loneliness can regain dignity and a sense of self-determination by seeing that their suffering can be in a sense "chosen" for a higher purpose. Not only is Christ in solidarity with them, but they also are contributing to the work of Christ. Thus, suffering gains a "creative character."[46]

Notably, however, *Salvifici Dolores* culminates in an extended reflection on the parable of the Good Samaritan—not one who endured suffering courageously, but one who went out of his way to ameliorate the suffering of another. Belief in the salvific potential of suffering "*is in no way identified with an attitude of passivity.* Completely the reverse is true." Human suffering demands "sensitivity, compassion, and help." "At one and the same time Christ has taught man *to do good by his suffering and to do good to those that suffer*."[47]

The *Ethical and Religious Directives* take these issues back to the concrete dilemmas of providing and using health care. They concur in the ideas both that suffering can be a participation in Christ's mission and that healing and compassion are also continuations of that mission.[48] The *Directives* identify dependency, helplessness, and pain as the hardest parts of the dying process, and return to the centrality of relieving pain and suffering as definitive of Catholic health care ministry. "One of the primary purposes of medicine in caring for the dying is the relief of pain and the suffering caused by it. Effective management of pain in all its forms is critical in the appropriate care of the dying."[49]

The "suffer with Christ" strategy to deal with intense human suffering has the merit of restoring agency to the terminally ill and dying. Arguably, this strategy is not fully consistent theologically with the idea that Christ's suffering does not in and of itself redeem humanity, nor the tenet of "orthodox" Christian theology that redemption is accomplished by Christ alone. The conclusion might legitimately be drawn that the practical strategy of co-suffering with Christ should be dropped as a part of Catholic (or any Christian) pastoral care, and the emphasis should be placed solely on God's solidarity with human suffering, along with the ultimate purpose of God to end all suffering and restore all living things to fullness at the end of time. As one Catholic chaplain relates on the basis of his experience, there really are no "answers" to the question of why suffering and sorrow come one's way. Yet peace can be found in "the God of love," who knew the same "pain and hopelessness," and in knowing that just as God is accompanying us, so we can keep company with the suffering God. Suffering can be the occasion of greater openness to divine love and grace.[50]

It is important to listen and to learn from the personal and spiritual experiences of dying patients and others who have found redemptive co-suffering to be a freeing, consoling, and encouraging way to understand their reality in religious terms. God's ways with human beings will always contain an element of ineffable mystery that logic and theological theories may not approach as successfully as spirituality, prayer, biblical narratives, and community-defining rituals.

In addition to relief of pain, the care, companionship, and accompaniment of fellow human beings is an essential part of the Catholic Christian answer to suffering. To be in solidarity with those who suffer is a special vocation of religious communities. *Accompaniment* is a word used by staff of Jesuit Relief Services to denote their mission of "walking with" displaced persons, even when not much can be done to resolve their legal status or gain systemic recognition of their human rights. "Our accompaniment affirms that God is present in human history, even in its most tragic episodes. We experience this presence. God does not abandon us. As pastoral workers, we focus on this vision...."[51] Accompaniment and holistic care in the medical context fight back alienation and despair by locating the suffering patient in a compassionate community. The communal dimension of caregiving has a high profile in the Catholic approach and is particularly distinctive of pastoral care of the sick.

The Catholic approach to medical, psychosocial, and pastoral responses to suffering is set within a religious worldview, implicit in what has been argued thus far. The source and final destiny of all reality lies in the one God who creates, sustains, and redeems humanity and other creatures. On the one hand, historical human existence is not the whole human story: all human beings are offered unity with God in an existence that transcends and outlasts the world as we know it. For Christians, the hope of eternal life is focused on the presence of God in Jesus Christ, God incarnate in history, who sends his Spirit upon suffering creation and offers "resurrection life."

However, in Catholic perspective, the hope of life hereafter does not diminish the value of or responsibility to life in this world. Though life is not an "absolute" value, it is a very important one. The social teaching of the modern papal encyclicals stresses that each human being has dignity and that all are entitled to share in and are responsible to contribute to the common good. A priority is the inclusion of the most vulnerable members of society, whether racial-ethnic minorities, economically poor, immigrants and refugees, children and the elderly, or those made vulnerable by disability or illness. The Catholic liturgies of the "sacraments" celebrate the healing presence of God in human life by sacralizing common experiences of birth, meal sharing, repentance, growth to maturity, marriage, religious ministry, and preparation for death (the seven sacraments of baptism, Eucharist, penance, confirmation, marriage, ordination, and the anointing of the sick). In all of these, community, touch, language, and ritual celebrate God's action in the ordinary events of human lives. Trust in divine creative power and redeeming love can comfort and heal now.

In the Catholic worldview, a transcendent and personal Creator and Redeemer surrounds and sustains all life in the world and seeks its flourishing. Yet worldly life is not humanity's final end. Therefore, suffering that cannot be avoided or that is embraced in service of a higher good can be placed in the perspective of another dimension of reality in which "every tear shall be wiped away" (Rev. 21:4).

A holistic, communal approach to suffering attendant on illness and death is embodied in the Catholic sacrament of the anointing of the sick and in the contemporary reappropriation of the *ars moriendi* tradition. These religious enactments of communal presence, participation, and support are aimed at the most distressing aspect of human suffering, the experience of being abandoned or "forsaken" by God and other human beings. Among the seven sacraments of the Catholic Church, the Eucharist is undoubtedly the most central, and provisions normally are made for the reception of the Eucharist by the sick, even if they are hospitalized or unable to leave home.

While the Eucharist is a sacrament that binds the whole community, the anointing of the sick is especially conceived to enact the continuing membership of the severely ill or dying person in the faith community and to anticipate that person's coming union with God in an even more intimate way. The liturgy of the sacrament calls upon divine aid to succor the person, if possible to restore health, but above all to give hope. As the sick person is anointed with oil on the forehead and hands, the priest prays, "Through this holy anointing may the Lord in his love and mercy help you with the grace of the Holy Spirit" and "May the Lord who frees you from sin save you and raise you up."[52]

The tradition of *ars moriendi* ("art of dying") developed in Europe in the late Middle Ages as a response to the pervasive threat of death caused by the Black Plague.[53] The literature of the *ars moriendi* made available to the lay public the steps of preparation for death that in earlier eras had been reserved to clerical guidance. The dying are reassured that dying is the pathway to a better form of life; advised how to avoid temptations, including despair; and assured of the love of Christ and the importance of trusting in and imitating Christ. Family and others are instructed how to accompany the dying person and are given specific prayers to offer. While the cultivation of an "art of dying" may presume more control over the dying process than most people typically enjoy, its virtue lies in spiritual reassurance and in the expectation that at all times the dying person will be accompanied, encouraged, and consoled by loved ones who faithfully gather for that purpose.

As Christopher Vogt, a contemporary Catholic interpreter of this tradition, observes, while medieval tracts focused on patience, faith, and hope as virtues of the dying person, today's theologies and pastoral approaches give equal or more importance to what it means to be compassionate toward that person. A Christian approach recognizes that while pain relief must be a priority, not all existential suffering can be eliminated; and simply asserting patient "autonomy" in decisions about the dying process is not an adequate interpersonal or social response. [54] The suffering of the dying person calls for resources that go beyond the medical to the "communal and religious."

> Christian compassion can seek to instill patience and a sense of the dignity of the interrelatedness and receiving the love and care of others. For those in despair who are enveloped by their suffering, Christian compassion can bring hope by putting that suffering into a broader context—into a context where suffering can be understood sometimes to be redemptive or at least meaningful, and where that suffering is not the final word about one's life.[55]

In the practical context of biomedical decision making, suffering demands a holistic response, and part of that response still involves decisions to use, refuse, or discontinue means to prolong life or end pain, as well as whether to end life directly, as is now legally possible in the states of Oregon and Washington. This essay on suffering is not the place for a lengthy discussion of the ethics of end-of-life care.[56] However, the basic principles are stated concisely in the Vatican's *Declaration on Euthanasia* and the U.S. bishops' *Ethical and Religious Directives*.

Catholic tradition does not see physical life as an absolute value, but it draws the line at directly taking life.[57] "Dying patients who request euthanasia should receive loving care, psychological and spiritual support, and appropriate remedies for pain and other symptoms so that they can live with dignity until the time of natural death."[58] The legalization of euthanasia carries with it the danger of diminishing efforts to make the last period of life worthwhile despite limits and suffering; of medicalizing aspects of suffering that derive from the need to confront the reality of the human condition and of one's own disappointments and failures; and of validating patients' fears that their dependent, debilitated state renders them worthless and creates an undue burden on family and finances.

On the other side, no one wants to become a prisoner of medical technology that drags out the dying process without enhancing quality of life.[59] Patients are on good moral ground in refusing useless or burdensome treatments. The complexity of individual cases is acknowledged, and precise moral norms are eschewed in favor of the language of "proportionate and disproportionate" or "ordinary and extraordinary" means.[60] At its best, the Catholic tradition provides for nuanced medical decision making, with patient and family as primary decision makers, and puts the emphasis on humane and reasonable medical interventions, palliative care and hospice, over last-gasp tactics to eke out a few more days. A treatment may be discontinued or rejected if it carries a risk or is burdensome. Such a refusal is not the equivalent of suicide; on the contrary, it should be considered as an acceptance of the human condition, or a wish to avoid the application of a medical procedure disproportionate to the results that can be expected, or a desire not to impose excessive expense on the family or the community.[61]

One of the most difficult types of cases, however, are those in which patients suffer severe physical pain that is difficult to alleviate fully, disorientation, hallucinations, or a combination of these.[62] Situations in which the patient is truly in *extremis*, and virtually beyond the reach of the loving voice or touch, lead some Catholic theologians to question the absolute rule against direct killing as a form of compassionate care. Margaret Farley recounts her experience with a loved one dying of AIDS, then questions whether it is possible that "when death becomes inevitable and surrender to God is made in the face of it, then communal bonds can be preserved and not violated in an active as well as a passive dying-into-life?" "If it is possible that an individual can be in such dire straits that her very integrity as a self is threatened (by intractable pain, ravaging the spirit as well as the body), is it not justifiable in such circumstances to end one's life, to surrender it while it is still whole?"[63]

What is at stake here is the decisive weight Catholic tradition has given to the moral difference between directly and indirectly intending and causing an evil (the death of an innocent person). Suffering may be ended or avoided by removing or refusing life-prolonging treatments or by using large doses of painkillers, aimed specifically at ending pain; in such cases, death is only "indirectly" caused and intended. To take a drug "overdose" specifically to bring death about is seen as direct intention and causation of death and hence as a morally different matter. Farley is not disputing that there is a human difference between acting to cause an effect "directly" and allowing it to occur as a result of accomplishing some other purpose. She is not disputing that when the effect is an evil like death, indirect is morally preferable to direct causation. What she is suggesting, however, is that the difference between direct and indirect, while valid, is not decisive. Perhaps extreme, uneliminable suffering is enough to make direct killing morally acceptable in exceptional cases (whether or not it should be legalized).

A less radical alternative, and one arguably in line with Catholic teaching, is what is called "terminal sedation."[64] Terminal sedation involves putting the patient into a coma until the time of death and in addition foregoing the use of artificial nutrition and hydration, so that life in a comatose state is not prolonged. From the standpoint of Catholic moral theology, terminal sedation is acceptable only if enough drugs are administered to induce a coma, but without the intention of using the drugs to shorten life deliberately, and if the nonuse of artificial feeding is assessed as the refusal of a burdensome means of life support because it no longer can either enhance quality of life for the patient or meaningfully extend it, since the patient is already in the dying process.[65] In such cases, terminal sedation would fall under the approval that Catholic theology and official teaching have previously given to the use of heavy doses of analgesics that primarily control pain but secondarily shorten life.

In conclusion, the Catholic approach to suffering sees it as an inevitable part of life, but one that calls for empathy and a compassionate response. In a biomedical context, the first and most fundamental response is to strengthen or renew the patient's bonds of interpersonal, familial, religious, and community relationship because love and solidarity are life's most important meanings. A person may find consolation and hope in suffering by remembering that in Christ, God is in solidarity with human suffering and promises resurrection life. Although Catholic pastoral documents continue to portray human suffering as "redemptive," the suffering caused by illness should not be interpreted as a consequence of personal sin, sought out or encouraged. To the contrary, Catholic theology is emphatic about the bioethical responsibility to address the pain and suffering of ill and dying persons in as effective a manner as possible. While direct killing is excluded, patients or their representatives may refuse "disproportionate" life-saving means or choose methods of pain relief that might also shorten life.

Finally, however, the circumstance of health-related suffering that most calls for solidarity and concerted, compassionate action is the plight of millions globally who lack even the most basic means of sustenance or medical care.

Notes

1. Elizabeth A. Johnson, *She Who Is: The Mystery of God in Feminist Theological Discourse* (New York: Crossroad, 1992), 248–249.

2. "Fast Facts: The Faces of Poverty," U.N. Millennium Project, accessed March 12, 2014, http://www.unmillenniumproject.org/resources/fastfacts_e.htm.

3. "Background Information on Sexual Violence Used as a Tool of War," Outreach Programme on the Rwanda Genocide and the United Nations, accessed March 12, 2014, http://www.un.org/en/preventgenocide/rwanda/about/bgsexualviolence.shtml.

4. Ingrid Miljeteig and Ole Frithjof Norheim, "My Job Is to Keep Him Alive, but What about His Brother and Sister? How Indian Doctors Experience Ethical Dilemmas in Neonatal Medicine," *Developing World Bioethics* 6/1 (2006): 23–32.

5. Josephine M. Lumitao, "Death and Dying," in *Beyond a Western Bioethics: Voices from the Developing World*, ed. Angeles Tan Alora and Josephine M. Lumitao (Washington, DC: Georgetown University Press, 2002), 99.

6. Phil Galewitz, "Census: Uninsured Numbers Decline as More Young Adults Gain Coverage," Kaiser Health news, accessed March 12, 2014, http://www.kaiserhealthnews.org/stories/2012/september/12/census-number-of-uninsured-drops.aspx.

7. "Dying for Coverage," Families USA, accessed March 12 2014, http://www.familiesusa.org/issues/uninsured/publications/dying-for-coverage.html.

8. Jamie Meyerfeld, *Suffering and Moral Responsibility* (New York and Oxford, UK: Oxford University Press), 111, 113.

9. Ibid., 224–225.

10. John Paul II, "Address to the Members of the Pontifical Academy For Life," no. 6., February 24, 2003, Vatican, accessed March 12, 2014, http://www.vatican.va/holy_father/john_paul_ii/speeches/2003/february/documents/hf_jp-ii_spe_20030224_pont-acad-life_en.html.

11. Benedict XVI, "Message for the Celebration of the World Day of Peace," January 1, 2009, Vatican, accessed March 12, 2014, (http://www.vatican.va/holy_father/benedict_xvi/messages/peace/documents/hf_ben-xvi_mes_20081208_xlii-world-day-peace_en.html.

12. Benedict XVI, "Address to a Congress of Health Care Workers," November 17, 2012, Vatican, accessed March 12, 2014, http://www.vatican.va/holy_father/benedict_xvi/speeches/2012/november/documents/hf_ben-xvi_spe_20121117_hlthwork_en.html.

13. United States Conference of Catholic Bishops, "Resolution on Health Care Reform," *Origins* 23/7 (1993), accessed March 12, 2014, http://www.originsonline.com/index.html.

14. United States Conference of Catholic Bishops, *Ethical and Religious Directives for Catholic Health Care Services*, 5th ed. (Washington, DC: USCCB, 2009), 11–12.

15. Eric Cassell, *The Nature of Suffering and the Goals of Medicine* (New York: Oxford University Press, 2004), 29–30.

16. Meghan J. Clark, "Crisis in Care: Family, Society and the Need for Subsidiarity in Caregiving," *Journal of Catholic Social Thought* 7/1 (2010): 63–81.

17. *Directives*, supra note 14, 3–4, 7–8

18. Ibid., 8.

19. Ibid., 7.

20. United States Conference of Catholic Bishops, *Forming Consciences for Faithful Citizenship: A Call to Political Responsibility from the Catholic Bishops of the United States* (Washington, DC: USCCB, 2007).

21. Ibid., 23.

22. Ibid., 26.

23. See, for example, "USCCB: HHS Mandate for Contraceptive and Abortifacient Drugs Violates Conscience Rights," August 1, 2011, United States Conference of Catholic Bishops, accessed March 12, 2014, http://www.usccb.org/news/2011/11-154.cfm.

24. http://crs.org/search-results/?cx=010843626580803856021%3Akgdqn-okct8&cof=FORID%3A11&q=health&sa=Search, accessed March 12, 2014.

25. *Directives*, supra note 14, 21.

26. *Directives*, supra note 14, 30–42, quotation from no. 42; see also *Instruction on Respect for Human Life in Its Origin and on the Dignity of Procreation (Donum vitae)*, 1987, Congregation for the Doctrine of the Faith, accessed March 12, 2014, http://www.vatican.va/roman_curia/congregations/cfaith/documents/rc_con_cfaith_doc_19870222_respect-for-human-life_en.html.

27. *Theodicy* is the attempt to explain logically and rationally why a good and all-powerful God either causes or permits evil. I agree with Terrence Tilley that all theodicies ultimately fail. See Terrence W. Tilley, *The Evils of Theodicy* (Washington, DC: Georgetown University Press, 1991). For an attempted theodicy that deals better than most with the conundrums, see John E. Thiel, *God, Evil, and Innocent Suffering: A Theological Reflection* (New York: Crossroad, 2002). For historical examples, see Jeff Astley, David Brown, and Ann Loades, ed., *Problems in Theology 2: Evil* (London and New York: T&T Clark, 2005).

28. Bryan N. Massingale, *Racial Justice and the Catholic Church* (Maryknoll, NY: Orbis, 2010), 106.

29. For a much more detailed discussion of these problems, their history, and the contemporary alternatives, see Lisa Sowle Cahill, *Global Justice, Christology and Christian Ethics* (Cambridge, UK and New York: Cambridge University Press, 2013), chap. 6, "Cross," 204–246.

30. John Paul II, *Salvifici Dolores* (*the Christian Meaning of Human Suffering*), no. 24, 1984, Vatican, accessed March 12, 2014, http://www.vatican.va/holy_father/john_paul_ii/apost_letters/documents/hf_jp-ii_apl_11021984_salvifici-doloris_en.html.

31. The lyrics and history of this hymn may be found on Wikipedia, accessed March 12, 2014, http://en.wikipedia.org/wiki/Salve_Regina.

32. Sacred Congregation for the Doctrine of the Faith, *Declaration on Euthanasia*, 1980, Vatican, accessed March 12, 2014, http://www.vatican.va/roman_curia/congregations/cfaith/documents/rc_con_cfaith_doc_19800505_euthanasia_en.html

33. See supra note 50.

34. *Declaration on Euthanasia*, II.

35. Ibid., III.

36. See Marit Trelstad, ed., *Cross Examinations: Readings on the Meaning of the Cross Today* (Minneapolis: Fortress, 2006); and Robert J. Daly, S.J., "Images of God and the Imitation of God: Problems with Atonement," *Theological Studies* 68 (2007): 36–51.

37. *Declaration on Euthanasia*, IV.

38. *Salvifici Dolores*, no. 5.

39. Ibid., no. 9.

40. Ibid., no. 25.

41. Ibid., no. 16.

42. Ibid., 17.

43. Ibid., no. 18.

44. *Salvifici Dolores*, no. 1.

45. Ibid., no. 27.

46. Ibid., no. 24.

47. Ibid., no. 30.

48. *Directives*, supra note 14, 3.

49. Ibid., 25.

50. Andy Otto, "In the Garden: A Reflection on the Grace of Suffering," *America* (April 2, 2012): 23–24.

51. Bernard Arputhasamy, S.J., Regional Director of Jesuit Refugee Service—Asia Pacific, "The Core of JRS Is Accompaniment," Jesuit Relief Services, accessed March 12, 2014, http://jrsusa.org/accompaniment?LID=140.

52. See *Directives*, supra note 14, 14–16.

53. See Stefan Hartmann, "Ars Moriendi," in *The Brill Dictionary of Religion*, ed. Kocku von Stuckrad, Brill Online, accessed March 12, 2014, http://referenceworks.brillonline.com/entries/brill-dictionary-of-religion/ars-moriendi-SIM_00010; and Emily Rebekah Huber, "'Oh Death!': Death, Dying, and the Culture of the Macabre in the Late Middle Ages," in *Death, Dying, and the Culture of the Macabre in the Late Middle Ages* (Rochester, NY: Robbins Library, University of Rochester, 2012), accessed March 12, 2014, http://www.library.rochester.edu/robbins/home. The latter pictures the woodcuts from the original *ars moriendi* books.

54. Christopher P. Vogt, *Patience, Compassion, Hope, and the Christian Art of Dying Well* (Lanham, MD: Rowman & Littlefield, 2004), 53.

55. Ibid., 85.

56. For a more detailed treatment, see Lisa Sowle Cahill, *Theological Bioethics: Participation, Justice and Change* (Washington, DC: Georgetown University Press, 2005), 93–130.

57. *Declaration on Euthanasia*, II; Directive no. 60. See also Edmund Pellegrino, "Some Things Ought Never Be Done: Moral Absolutes in Clinical Ethics," *Theoretical Medicine and Bioethics* 26 (2005): 469–486.

58. Directive no. 60.

59. Richard A. McCormick, S.J., "Technology, the Consistent Ethic, and Assisted Suicide," *Origins* 25/27 (1995): 459–463.

60. See *Declaration on Euthanasia,* 11–12; and *Directives*, supra note 14, 55–59.

61. *Declaration on Euthanasia,* 12.

62. See Timothy E. Quill, "Physician-Assisted Suicide in the United States: Are the Existing 'Last Resorts' Enough?" *Hastings Center Report* (September-October 2008): 17–22.

63. Margaret A. Farley, "Issues in Contemporary Christian Ethics: The Choice of Death in a Medical Context," *The Santa Clara Lectures* 1/4 (1995): 14.

64. See James J. Walter, "Terminal Sedation: A Catholic Perspective," in *Contemporary Issues in Bioethics: A Catholic Perspective*, ed. James J. Walter and Thomas A. Shannon (Lanham, MD: Rowman & Littlefield,) 225–230.

65. Whether or not artificial feeding must be used in all cases, or at least when patients are unable to indicate their own wishes, has been hotly debated in Catholicism, ever since a March 2004 speech of John Paul II, in which he seemed to say that tube feeding is "natural" and should never be foregone. Yet in November of the same year, he reaffirmed the traditional teaching on ordinary and extraordinary means. The *Ethical and Religious Directives* (no. 58) prudently say that artificial hydration and nutrition must "in principle" be applied in all cases—which implies not in practice in every instance. See Thomas A. Shannon and James J. Walter, "The PVS Patient and the Forgoing/Withdrawing of Medical Nutrition and Hydration," and "Artificial Nutrition and Hydration: Assessing the Papal Statement," in *Contemporary Issues in Bioethics*, 231–268; and John J. Hardt, "Church Teaching and My Father's Choice," *America* (January 21, 2008), accessed March 12, 2014, http://www.americamagazine.org/content/article.cfm?article_id=10552.

12

The Orthodox Christian View of Suffering

H. Tristram Engelhardt Jr.

Any understanding of the Orthodox Christian appreciation of suffering is challenged by the differences in paradigm separating Western Christian and Orthodox Christian approaches to theology. In the early second millennium, Western Christian morality took a decisively scholarly and eventually academic turn through nesting its theology within a philosophical framework, while Orthodox theology in the strict sense remained noetic or mystical.[1] The Western Christian commitment to the dialectic of *fides et ratio*, faith and reason, made the discipline of philosophy the framing rationale for theology. This general approach, especially within Roman Catholicism, has been most recently underscored by Pope John Paul II in *Fides et Ratio*[2] and by Pope Benedict XVI.[3] Following this commitment, the West produced systematic intellectual examinations of major moral and theological themes such as suffering.[4] In contrast, Orthodox theology understands theology first and foremost to be a way of life, or more precisely a way of prayer, a relationship with God.[5] As Evagrios of Pontus (345–399) put it, the focus of theology is not writing about prayer, but engaging in prayer. "If you are a theologian, you will pray truly. And if you pray truly, you are a theologian."[6] As a result, Orthodox reflections on suffering generally have a more homiletic than scholarly or academic character. They are written to invite the reader into a proper way of appreciating and confronting tribulation, pain, suffering, and death. Dogma is to be lived and prayed. Thus, even the Nicean-Constantinopolitan Creed (A.D. 381) is approached as a prayer either recited or sung during liturgy.

The Ninth Ecumenical Council of the Orthodox Church (A.D. 1341, 1347, 1351), when it affirmed St. Gregory Palamas' (A.D. 1296–1351) position with regard to hesychastic theology[7] as the unbroken tradition of the Church, rejected an attempt to place a Scholastic, systematic theology at the core of Orthodox theology.[8] As Father John Romanides (1927–2001) glosses this position, "The Fathers do not say anything about God on the basis of philosophical reflection. They do not sit at their desks like the Scholastics in order to do theology because when the Church Fathers theologize, speculation or reflection is strictly forbidden."[9] Orthodox theology, as a result, also has an ahistorical character. It is written in a theological now in which there is no development of new doctrines, although there can be development of new expressions of old doctrines. As Metropolitan Hierotheos (1945–) puts it, "the scholastic theology of the West teaches that through the ages we have greater deepening in the dogmas of the faith and that they are still developing further. But this is not orthodox teaching."[10] The result is that what was written in the first centuries of Christianity carries the same theological weight today. For the issue of suffering and the use of medicine, this means a categorical exclusion of such interventions as physician-assisted suicide, euthanasia, and human embryo destruction. Medicine itself is recognized as a blessing to be engaged, so long as it does not distract from the pursuit of salvation.

For Orthodox Christianity, the theologian plays primarily an ascetically based, therapeutic role. The goal is not to think one's way to new articulations of the truth because the truth is not propositional but rather is the Persons of the Trinity. The goal is to turn, and to lead others to turn, from self-love to love of God and one's neighbor so that one can experience the Truth, God. Moreover, it is only in loving God rightly that we can love and turn to others rightly, even to ourselves. Thus, Nicholas Berdyaev (1874–1948) in commentary on Fyodor Dostoyevsky (1821–1881) observes, "Man's greatest duty is to love God: that is the first commandment. The second is to love his neighbour. And it is possible for two creatures to love one another only because God exists and is their common Father."[11] This requires breaking our habits of absorption in ourselves and in the distractions of the world. Suffering can be transformed into a means toward this end. It is because of this therapeutic focus that, as Metropolitan Hierotheos emphasizes, Orthodox theology works medicinally to cure us of sin. "The cure of the whole person, which is the essential aim of Orthodox spirituality, is effected by the sacraments of the Church and by the practice of the ascetic life. A break in the bond between sacraments and asceticism leads to pretentious moralizing or to total secularization."[12] Hence, the nonjuridical character of Orthodox Christianity's approach to sin is emphasized. The goal is on curing the penitent of sin, rather than punishing the penitent because of his sin. It is also for this reason that Orthodox theology and its understanding of suffering focus on spiritual therapy rather than on punishment.

The Orthodox Christian view of suffering and its account of the propriety of medical interventions in many ways contrast with those of Western Christianity. Before the Reformation, Western Christianity came to place suffering within an economy of sin, propitiatory punishment, and salvation, in which suffering plays a central role in paying off a penalty, namely, temporal punishment due to sin.[13] One's personal suffering, the suffering of another on one's behalf when offered up against the penalties of temporal punishment due for one's sins, or obtaining an indulgence from what Roman Catholicism holds to be the excess merits of the saints (*thesarum sanctificationem Christi et sanctorum*) could help pay off the penalty.[14] This view of suffering depends on a distinction the West draws between the guilt due to sin and the penalty or punishment merited by sin. This view conveys a special worth to suffering, in that suffering could help release souls from their punishment in purgatory. This view of suffering, when combined with the view that the penance a priest imposed in confession serves as a punishment merited by the temporal punishment due to sin, created an all-encompassing background spiritual currency in which the penalties of sin could be set aside by current tribulation, pain, and suffering. Suffering when patiently borne created merit that could be balanced against the temporal punishment due to sin. None of this exists in Orthodox Christianity. The absolution of the Orthodox priest at the end of confession absolves the penitent of the sins confessed so as to make pain and suffering to avoid purgatory beside the point.[15] Any penance imposed is to be imposed with a therapeutic goal focused on the particular needs of the penitent. The Orthodox view is that, by bearing tribulation, pain, and suffering in humility, one can cure the effects of sin through discipline. However, even when tribulation, pain, and suffering are a punishment due to sin (e.g., syphilis contracted after visiting prostitutes), suffering does not serve to discharge a debt of temporal punishment owed due to the sin Instead, the punishment offers an opportunity, causally connected with the sin, for recognition of the reality of one's sin, for healing, in particular for erasing the habits of sin.

In summary, tribulations, pain, suffering, death, and Christ's redemptive death are recognized as efficacious in setting aside the results of the death and suffering brought by Adam's sin and the sins of others.[16] All this having been said, there is a strong affirmation of not just the propriety of using, but the obligation to engage medicine for the amelioration of suffering and the treatment of disease.

Putting Tribulation, Pain, Suffering, and Death in Their Place

The Orthodox Church recognizes that tribulation, pain, suffering, and death, as well as our proper response to them, must be understood within a cosmic account of sin and salvation. On the one hand, pain, suffering, and death are the result of sin, the sins of individual humans and the sin of Adam. On the other hand, all suffering can help overcome sinful habits and sinful orientation. The Orthodox Church appreciates that the origin of all suffering is sin, although not all of suffering is punishment (i.e., in the sense of being causally connected with our pain and suffering). Again, strictly speaking, suffering does not cancel out a debt of punishment due to sin, although all suffering can be an occasion for repentance and salvation. Even where the suffering may be only the result of Adam's sin, it can help us to break our pride, to "wake us up" so that we reassess our situation and focus our lives away from sin.

First and foremost, suffering has its origin in the sin of Adam. Here, Orthodox Christianity affirms Genesis.

> To Adam He said, "Because you listened to your wife and ate from the tree about which I commanded you, 'You must not eat of it,' cursed is the ground because of you; through painful toil you will eat of it all the days of your life.

> It will produce thorns and thistles for you, and you will eat the plants of the field. By the sweat of your brow you will eat your food until you return to the ground, since from it you were taken; for dust you are and to dust you will return" (Genesis 3:17–19).

In his Commentary on Genesis, St. John Chrysostom (347–407) does not interpret God's curse punitively. Instead, St. John Chrysostom underscores the therapeutic force of the curse, of how suffering can be used to overcome the results of Adam's sin.

> Then, so that you may learn what "accursed" means, he added, "In pain may you eat from it all the days of your life." See how each punishment is extended for a lifetime, so that not only may they [Adam and Eve and their children] personally be the better off for it, but that those destined to follow in future may learn from these very events whence the source of this punishment derived in their case: "In pain," he says, "may you eat from it all the days of your life." Then, to teach us more precisely the kind of curse and the cause of the pain, he added, "Thorns and thistles let it yield you." Behold the reminders of the curse: thorns it will bring forth, he says, and thistles so as to give rise to great labor and discomfort, and I will ensure you pass the whole time with pain so that this experience may prove a brake on your getting ideas above your station and you may instead have a thought to your own make-up and never again bear to be deceived in these matters.[17]

The point is that all those who share Adam's nature and live in the world broken by Adam's sin, as well as by the sins of others, by virtue of this common fallen humanity and our fallen common world, are involved in the tribulation, pain, suffering, and death that result from that brokenness.

Suffering is often not a punishment (although it may be causally due to Adam's sin and the sins of others) or given as a direct intervention of God.

> Not all sicknesses for whose treatment we observe medicine to be occasionally beneficial arise from natural causes, whether from faulty diet or from any other physical origin. Illness is often a punishment for sin imposed for our conversion; 'For whom the Lord loveth,' says the Scripture, 'he chastiseth'.... [18]

In all cases, although suffering can be instructive and can be therapeutic, it is never imposed in order to strike out a temporal punishment owed because of sin, but always to help cure the soul.

Although pain, suffering, and death are the result of sin, they have been co-opted into the pursuit of salvation, the cure of sin, both through Christ's redemptive death and through the patient submission of individual humans to the will of God. Since Adam, the sin of each man has further contributed to the broken character of the world and the suffering that being in this fallen world involves. This is the point St. Paul makes in his Letter to the Romans. "Therefore, just as sin entered the world through one man, and death through sin, in this way death came to all men, because all sinned" (Romans 5:12). The central matter is that "the wages of sin is death" (Romans 6:23). Again, because all humans share in the fallen human nature of their father Adam, innocent persons can suffer because of the sins of others, just as a child can be born infected with HIV because his father frequented prostitutes and infected his wife, the child's mother, although the mother and child were innocent. Concerning the passage in Romans, St. John Chrysostom asks:

> "Through the sin of one." But what means, "for that all have sinned" [Rom. 5:12]? This; he having once fallen, even they that had not eaten of the tree did from him, all of them, become mortal.[19]

Given Adam's sin and the consequent sins of others, the whole world and the lives of humans in the world are defined by tribulation, pain, suffering, and death. St. Paul's statement in Romans 5:12 regarding the consequences of Adam's sin should therefore be read as clarifying that the guilt due to Adam's sin has not been passed on to his descendents as an inherited guilt, but only that the suffering and death due to Adam's sin have been passed on to his descendants.

Turning Through Suffering toward Salvation

This world broken by sin, full of tribulation, suffering, pain, and death, is ripe for being grasped as an opportunity to turn wholeheartedly to God. Tribulation, if borne with submission and humility, can benefit us in our struggle for virtue, as St. John Chrysostom observes:

> [T]ribulation maketh those who are troubled more approved; "For tribulation worketh patience; and patience, probation; and probation, hope; and hope maketh not ashamed" (Rom. V.3–5). Do you see that the probation, which comes of tribulation, fixes in us the hope of the good things to come, and that the abiding in trials causes us to have a good hope of the future? So that I did not say rashly, that these tribulations themselves mark out to us hopes of a resurrection, and make those who are tried the better; for, he saith, "as gold is tried in a furnace, so an acceptable man in the furnace of humiliation" (Ecclus. II.3).[20]

Again, it is not through one's own works that one has merited salvation, but only through one's turning fully to God to be united with his grace. Through accepting tribulation, pain, suffering, and death as God's will, one unites oneself ever more closely to the will of God and to his saving grace. In that turn to God, one's faith can grow stronger. As Mark the Ascetic (sixth century) taught, "The mercy of God is hidden in sufferings not of our choice; and if we accept such sufferings patiently, they bring us to repentance and deliver us from everlasting punishment" (i.e., by orienting us to God).[21] It is for this reason that "Affliction then is a great thing, beloved, for it accomplishes two great things; it wipes out sins, and it makes men strong."[22] In all of this, afflictions play an instrumental role in our spiritual self-discipline but are not in themselves valuable.

The reading is crucial, in that the first sin was that of pride, the pride of Adam wishing to go to heaven (achieve *theosis*[23]) on his own terms. Orthodox Christianity understands that in our coming to terms with suffering, it is not what we do, but what God does. That is, even our role in achieving the benefits of suffering must be put in its place by being balanced by humility, the acceptance of God's will. It is, to take the cardinal example, through the submission of the Theotokos to the will of God that Mary became the second Eve who gave birth to the second Adam, Jesus Christ, who finally offered all to the Father so that all those united with him through baptism may effectively set sin and its results aside through suffering properly accepted (Romans 6:3-7).

The deep fabric of the universe is recognized as broken by man's sin in such an encompassing fashion that it is only after the Second Coming of Christ with the resurrection and the restoration of all things that pain, suffering, and death are fully overcome once and for all. "I saw the Holy City, the new Jerusalem, coming down out of heaven from God, prepared as a bride beautifully dressed for her husband. And I heard a loud voice from the throne saying, 'Now the dwelling of God is with men, and he will live with them. They will be his people, and God himself will be with them and be their God. He will wipe every tear from their eyes. There will be no more death or mourning or crying or pain, for the old order of things has passed away'" (Revelation 21:2–4). This eschatological focus, which is central, underscores the importance of the seventh article of the Nicean-Constantinopolitan Creed: "And He shall come again with glory to judge the quick and the dead, Whose kingdom shall have no end." It is only after the Final Judgment through God's power that all is restored, free of the effects of sin.

Why Suffering Offers a Benefit

The answer to the question as to what can be gained from suffering is thus complex. The general point is that suffering can waken us out of an absorption in our selves and in the affairs of the world. That awakening out of the ordinary preoccupations of life can offer an opportunity, if taken, of turning anew, indeed wholeheartedly, to God. As Jean-Claude Larchet in *The Theology of Illness* recognizes: "That, of course, is never easy. Illness normally plunges us into unfamiliar territory, where the conditions of our life are significantly modified and where our relationships with those around us are disturbed and often weakened by imposed isolation."[24] Suffering also challenges our pride by bringing our confidence in ourselves and in our own capacities into question. Chrysostom underscores this: "God permits them to suffer evil, that they may not too easily be exalted into presumption, by the greatness of their good works."[25] If one takes advantage of this opportunity, then suffering has given one a chance to grow in virtue, disposing us to turn in response to God.

At this point, the significance of suffering can be radically re-valorized from a negative experience to one that is paradoxically positive.

> [5.] And let us therefore, when we suffer aught for Christ's sake, not merely bear it nobly but also rejoice. If we fast, let us leap for joy as if enjoying luxury; if we be insulted, let us dance as if praised; if we spend, let us feel as if gaining; if we bestow on the poor, let us count ourselves to receive: for he that gives not thus will not give readily.[26]

Examples of the transforming power of suffering when humbly accepted are afforded in particular in the accounts of the martyrs and confessors. The following short vignette from the reflections of the Romanian priest Fr. George Calciu (1925–2006), imprisoned under the Romanian communists, is illustrative.[27] The passage is from an interview after the fall of the Romanian communist regime and concerns Fr. George's time in Jilava Prison.

> ...we had a kind of nostalgia about the prison.... How could you miss prison? Because in prison we had the most spiritual life. We reached levels that we are not able to reach in this world. Isolated, anchored in Jesus Christ, we had joys and illuminations that this world cannot offer us. There are no words to express exactly the feeling we had there. Those who have not had our spiritual experience cannot understand that we could be happy in prison.... Can you imagine: we were in a cell without windows, without air, humid, filthy—yes, we had moments of happiness that we never reached in freedom. I cannot explain it. *Everything is stripped away, and God becomes real. He is not a theoretical God anymore.*[28]

Of course, this joy of which St. John Chrysostom and Fr. George speak is possible only for those who in full humility submit to their suffering.

The Obligation to Treat Disease and Ameliorate Suffering

Although the Orthodox Church recognizes the inevitability of pain, suffering, and death, it sees nothing intrinsically good in this state of affairs. Indeed, once in every Vespers, once in every Matins, and twice in every Liturgy, there is a petition for "A Christian ending to our life, painless, blameless, peaceful; and a good defense before the fearful judgment seat of Christ."[29] It is in this context that one finds Orthodox Christianity's strong affirmation of medicine. Although, if pain and suffering cannot be remedied, we are to accept with humility whatever God sends us, the medical treatment of pain and even difficulty in sleeping is endorsed. St. Basil says: "... with mandrake doctors give us sleep; with opium they lull violent pain."[30]

The use of medical interventions to prevent and cure disease, as well as to alleviate suffering, is strongly approved and in general considered to be obligatory. "And, when we were commanded to return to the earth whence we had been taken and were united with the pain-ridden flesh doomed to destruction because of sin and, for the same reason, also subject to disease, the medical art was given to us to relieve the sick, in some degree at least."[31] After all, pain and suffering can become an occasion for despair and temptation to sin (i.e., to use forbidden practices such as physician-assisted suicide and euthanasia). This endorsement of medicine and surgery was made in the face of the absence of anesthesia, recognizing that treatment itself can involve considerable pain and suffering.

> ...we must take great care to employ this medical art, if it should be necessary...[though] in using the medical art we submit to cutting, burning, and the taking of bitter medicines for the cure of the body...Right reason dictates...that we demure neither at cutting nor at burning, nor at the pains caused by bitter and disagreeable medicines, nor at abstinence from food, nor at a strict regimen....[32]

Medicine in Constantinople, it should be noted, was the best in Europe until the Fourth Crusade (A.D. 1204) and the pillage of the City.

This obligation to accept medical treatment is set within the constraint that it should not distract us from the pursuit of salvation. We should avoid any medical intervention that, context considered, would distract us from the pursuit of salvation. St. Basil enjoined us that "Whatever requires an undue amount of thought or trouble or involves a large expenditure of effort and causes our whole life to revolve, as it were, around solicitude for the flesh must be avoided by Christians."[33] This limitation is subtly but importantly different from the Roman Catholic doctrine regarding ordinary versus extraordinary, proportionate versus disproportionate cases. For the Roman Catholics, the duty to treat is proportionate to the benefits and inversely proportionate to the costs, which costs can be interpreted in quite secular terms, including financial costs.[34] For Orthodox, the duty to receive treatment is set aside whenever, all things considered, the treatment constitutes a distraction from the pursuit of salvation. The Orthodox concern thus remains explicitly Christocentric.

A Brief Summary

Orthodox Christian concerns regarding suffering are robustly theocentric without the envelope of philosophical systematicity and analytic focus found in most Western Christianities. Moreover, because all important Orthodox reflections regarding suffering are equal in their weight, the literature does not have the developmental character that one might expect from Western Christian reflections. The sources, instead, are laid out in a theological "now" that may be alien to some readers. The message is clear and central, namely, that suffering does not reflect a vengeful punishment from God, even when the punishment is causally connected to our sins or sent explicitly by God as punishment.

The appreciation of suffering always has a central spiritual therapeutic focus, as shown by the blessing for the sick.

> O Almighty Master, Physician of souls and bodies, Who humbleth and raiseth up, Who chasteneth and again healeth: As Thou art merciful, do Thou visit our brother, *N*., who is sick. Stretch forth Thine arm, full of healing and cures, and heal him, raising him up from his bed and illness.... And if there be imputed unto him iniquity or transgression, do Thou loose, remit and forgive him, out of Thy love for mankind.[35]

Consider also the prayers to be used by those who are ill.

> O Lord Jesus Christ, our Saviour, Physician of souls and bodies, Who didst become man and suffer death on the Cross for our salvation, and through Thy tender love and compassion didst heal all manner of sickness and affliction; do Thou, O Lord, visit me in my suffering, and grant me grace and strength to bear this sickness with which I am afflicted, with Christian patience and submission to Thy will... I know, O Lord, that I justly deserve any punishment Thou mayest inflict upon me for I have so often offended Thee and sinned against Thee.... Therefore, I humbly pray Thee, look upon my weakness, and deal not with me after my sins, but according to the multitude of Thy mercies. Have compassion on me, and let mercy and justice meet; and deliver me from this sickness and suffering.... Grant that my sickness may be the means of my true repentance and amendment of my life according to Thy will, that I may spend the rest of my days in Thy love and fear.... [36]

In all of this, it must be underscored that suffering has no intrinsic value. Therefore, we are encouraged to pray that we not suffer and to engage medicine for the prevention, cure, or at least remediation of pain and suffering, although we are in humility to accept what God sends. It remains in our hands to turn the evil of tribulation, pain, suffering, and death to means for the pursuit of virtue and salvation.

Notes

1. H. T. Engelhardt Jr., "Critical Reflections on Theology's Handmaid: Why the Role of Philosophy in Orthodox Christianity Is So Different," *Philosophy & Theology* 18, no. 1 (2006): 53–75.

2. Pope John Paul II, *Fides et Ratio* (Vatican City: Libreria Editrice Vaticana, 1998).

3. Just before becoming pope, Joseph Cardinal Ratzinger underscored the Roman Catholic commitment to philosophy in arguing, for example, "that ultimately the only weapon is the soundness of the arguments set forth in the political arena and in the struggle to shape

public opinion. This is why it is so crucial to develop a philosophical ethics that, while being in harmony with the ethic of faith, must however have its own space and its own logical rigor. The rationality of the argument should close the gap between secular ethics and religious ethics and found an ethics of reason that goes beyond such distinctions." Joseph Ratzinger and Marcello Pera, *Without Roots*, trans. Michael Moore (New York: Basic Books, 2006), 130–131.

4. See, for example,Peter J. Colosi, "John Paul II and Max Scheler on the Meaning of Suffering," *Logos* 12, no. 3 (Summer 2009): 17–32;J. L. A. Garcia, "Sin and Suffering in a Catholic Understanding of Medical Ethics," *Christian Bioethics* 12 (2006): 165–186; Thomas Aquinas, *Summa Theologiae*, 1st Part of the 2nd Part, Question 81, Article 5, Reply to Objection 3; Aquinas, *Summa Theologiae*, 2nd Part of the 2nd Part, Question and Aquinas, *Summa Theologiae*, 3rd., Question 46, Article 5.

5. H. T. Engelhardt Jr., *The Foundations of Christian Bioethics* (Salem, MA: Scrivener, 2000).

6. Evagrios of Pontus, "On Prayer," in *The Philokalia*, ed. Sts. Nikodimos and Makarios, trans. G. E. H. Palmer, Philip Sherrard, and Kallistos Ware (Boston: Faber and Faber, 1988), 1.62.

7. Hesychasm (from hesychia, "stillness, rest, quiet, silence") follows Christ's injunction: "when thou prayest, enter into thy closet, and when thou hast shut thy door, pray" (Matthew 6:6), so that in prayer (especially through the Jesus Prayer: Lord Jesus Christ, Son of God, have mercy on me, a sinner), one turns away from the world and the senses to experience God (theoria). Hesychasm is the process of retiring within oneself in order that through prayer, one ceases to regard the senses, so that one may be granted an experiential knowledge of God.

8. Metropolitan Hierotheos gives a useful summary of the position taken by the Ninth Ecumenical Council of the Orthodox Church (when John V Palaiologos [reigned 1341–1376] was emperor) and its condemnation of philosophy, of which Scholasticism was at the time the prime examplar.

"In the whole text of the 'Synodikon of Orthodoxy,' it is seen clearly that philosophy is condemned. Both the way in which philosophy refers to and presents God and the conclusions to which it comes are condemned. And of course, in speaking of philosophy, we mean metaphysics as it was developed by Plato, Aristotle, and other, later philosophers. . . .

"Yet it is not these [particular] works of the philosophers that are anathematized, but the fact that the teachings of the philosophers are preferred to the Faith, and that philosophy is used to distort the truth of the Church. It is not forbidden to study the works of the ancient Greeks, that is, of the pagans, but those Christians are reproached who follow and accept their futile theories. Anathema is pronounced 'on those who accept the Greek teachings, not on those who only cultivate them for culture, but on those who also follow these futile doctrines of theirs.' And as we said, before, those are censured who prefer 'the foolish so-called wisdom of the profane philosophers' to the orthodox teaching."

Metropolitan of Nafpaktos Hierotheos [Vlachos],*The Mind of the Orthodox Church*, trans. Esther Williams (Levadia, Greece: Birth of the Theotokos Monastery, 1998), 226–227.

9. John S. Romanides, *Patristic Theology*, trans. Hieromonk Alexis (Trader) (Dalles, OR: Uncut Mountain, 2008), 85.

10. Hierotheos, *The Mind of the Orthodox Church*, 58.

11. Nicholas Berdyaev, *Dostoevsky*, trans. Donald Attwater (New York: Living Age Books, 1957), 131.

12. Bishop of Nafpaktos Hierotheos [Vlachos], *Orthodox Spirituality*, trans. Effie Mavromichali (Levadia, Greece: Birth of the Theotokos Monastery, 1994), 98–99.

13. On November 25, 1551, during the 14th session, the Council of Trent published the following canons concerning the doctrine of the temporal punishment due to sin:

> "12. If anyone says that the entire punishment is always remitted by God along with the sin, and that the satisfaction made by penitents is nothing else but the faith by which they grasp that Christ has made satisfaction on their behalf: let him be anathema.
>
> "13. If anyone says that, for temporal punishment for sins, no satisfaction at all is made to God, through the merits of Christ, by the sufferings imposed by God and patiently borne; or by the penances enjoined by a priest; or, further, by those voluntarily undertaken such as fasts, prayers, almsgiving or other additional works of devotion; and consequently that the best penance is only a new life: let him be anathema. . . .
>
> "15. If anyone says that the keys have been given to the church only for loosing and not also for binding; and that, consequently, when priests impose penalties on those who confess, they are acting contrary to the purpose of the keys and to the institution of Christ; . . . : let him be anathema."
>
> Norman P. Tanner (ed.), *Decrees of the Ecumenical Councils* (Washington, DC: Georgetown University Press, 1990), 2:713.

14. The recent *Catechism of the Catholic Church* gives the following account of indulgences: "1478 An indulgence is obtained through the Church who, by virtue of the power of binding and loosing granted her by Christ Jesus, intervenes in favor of individual Christians and opens for them the treasury of the merits of Christ and the saints to obtain from the Father of mercies the remission of the temporal punishments due for their sins. Thus the Church does not want simply to come to the aid of these Christians, but also to spur them to works of devotion, penance, and charity." *Catechism of the Catholic Church* (San Francisco: Ignatius Press, 1994), no. 981, 371.

15. A widely employed Orthodox Christian prayer of absolution reads:

"Whatsoever thou hast said to my most humble self, and whatsoever thou hast not succeeded in saying, either through ignorance, or through forgetfulness, whatever it may be: God forgive thee in this present world, and in that which is to come. . . . God it was who forgave David through Nathan the Prophet, when he confessed his sins, and Peter weeping bitterly for his denial, and the sinful woman in tears at his feet, and the Publican, and the Prodigal Son: May that same God forgive thee all things, through me a sinner, both in this present world, and in that which is to come, and set thee uncondemned before his dread Judgment Seat. And now, having no further care for the sins which thou hast declared, depart in peace." *Pocket Prayer Book* (Englewood, NJ: Antiochian Orthodox Christian Archdiocese, 1956), 44–45.

16. The background Orthodox theology regarding the Redemption is summarized in the Anaphora of the Liturgy of St. Basil the Great:

> "But when he disobeyed thee, the true God, who had created him and was led astray by the guile of the serpent and rendered subject to death through his own transgressions,

thou didst banish him, in thy righteous judgment, O God, from paradise into this world, and didst turn him again to the earth from which he was taken, providing for him the salvation of regeneration, which is in thy Christ himself.... For as by man sin entered into the world, and by sin death, so it seemed good unto thine only-begotten Son, who is in the bosom of thee, the God and Father, to be born of a woman, the holy Theotokos and ever-virgin Mary; to be born under the Law, that he might condemn sin in his flesh, that they who were dead in Adam might be made alive in him thy Christ.... [H]aving sanctified us by the Holy Spirit, he gave himself a ransom to death, whereby we were held, sold into bondage under sin. And having descended into hades through the cross, that he might fill all things with himself, he loosed the pains of death and rose again on the third day, making a way for all flesh unto the resurrection from the dead, for it was not possible that the Author of life should be held by corruption, that he might be the First-fruits of those who have fallen asleep, the First-born from the dead, that he might be in all things the first among all."*The Liturgikon* (Englewood, NJ: Antiochian Orthodox Christian Archdiocese, 1989), 287–289.

17. St. John Chrysostom, *Homilies on Genesis 1–17*, trans. Robert C. Hill (Washington, DC: Catholic University of America Press, 1986), no. 39, 243.

18. St. Basil, *Ascetical Works*, trans. Sr. M. Monica Wagner (Washington, DC: Catholic University of America Press, 1962), "The Long Rules," 334.

19. St. John Chrysostom, *Homilies on the Acts of the Apostles*, in *Nicene and Post-Nicene Fathers*, First Series, ed. Philip Schaff (Peabody, MA: Hendrickson, 1994), "Homily X on Rom. V.12," 11.401.

20. St. John Chrysostom, *On the Priesthood, Ascetic Treatises, Select Homilies and Letters, Homilies on the Statues*, in *Nicene and Post-Nicene Fathers*, First Series, ed. Philip Schaff (Peabody, MA: Hendrickson, 1994), "Homily I concerning the Statues to the People of Antioch," no. 24, 9.340.

21. Mark the Ascetic, "On Those Who Think that They Are Made Righteous by Works," in *The Philokalia*, ed. Sts. Nikodimos and Makarios, trans. G. E. H. Palmer, Philip Sherrard, and Kallistos Ware (Boston: Faber and Faber, 1979), no. 139, 1.136.

22. St. John Chrysostom, *Homilies on the Gospel of Saint John and the Epistle to the Hebrews*, in *Nicene and Post-Nicene Fathers*, First Series, ed. Philip Schaff (Peabody, MA: Hendrickson, 1994), "Homily XXVIII on Hebrews XI.37, 38," 14.494.

23. Theosis refers to the transforming effect on us of the uncreated energies of God (i.e., the grace of God), so as to restore our likeness with God and lead to union with him.

24. Jean-Claude Larchet, *The Theology of Illness*, trans. John and Michael Breck (Crestwood, NY: St. Vladimir's Seminary Press, 2002), 10.

25. St. John Chrysostom, *On the Priesthood, Ascetic Treatises, Select Homilies and Letters, Homilies on the Statues*, in *Nicene and Post-Nicene Fathers*, First Series, ed. Philip Schaff (Peabody, MA: Hendrickson, 1994), "Homily I concerning the Statues," no. 14, 9.336.

26. St. John Chrysostom, *Homilies on the Epistles of Paul to the Corinthians*, in *Nicene and Post-Nicene Fathers*, First Series, ed. Philip Schaff (Peabody, MA: Hendrickson, 1994), "Homily XII on 2 Cor. VI.1–2," no. 5, 12.340.

27. For a literal "picture" of what it was like in these prisons, see the sketches made by one of the prisoners in Radu Bercea, *Images from the Romanian Gulag* (Brasov: Pastel Publishing House, 2010).

28. George Calciu, *Father George Calciu*, ed. St. Herman of Alaska Brotherhood (Platina, CA: St. Herman of Alaska Brotherhood, 2010), 131–132 (italics in original).

29. *The Liturgikon*, 28, 149, 281, 299.

30. St. Basil, "The Hexaemeron," in *Nicene and Post-Nicene Fathers*, Second Series, ed. Philip Schaff and Henry Wace (Peabody, MA: Hendrickson, 1994), Homily 5, §4, 8.78.

31. St. Basil, *Ascetical Works*, "The Long Rules," no. 55, 331.

32. Ibid., 331–332, 334.

33. Ibid., 331–332.

34. Daniel Cronin, "The Moral Law in Regard to the Ordinary and Extraordinary Means of Conserving Life" (dissertation for Pontifical Gregorian University, Rome, 1958); H. T. Engelhardt Jr. and Thomas J. Bole III, "Entwicklungen der medizinischen Ethik in den USA: die Verführung durch die Technik und der Irrtum einer Lebenserhaltung um jeden Preis," *Arzt und Christ* 36 (1990): 113–121.

35. St. Tikhon's Monastery, trans., *The Great Book of Needs* (South Canaan, PA: St. Tikhon's Seminary Press, 1999), 3.3.

36. *Pocket Prayer Book*, 22–23.

13

Redemptive Suffering Redeemed: A Protestant View of Suffering

Karen Lebacqz

Lawyer and noted Episcopal layman William Stringfellow moved to Block Island in the fall of 1967. He was already ill, but little did he know what he was about to endure.[1] That winter, he lost nearly 60 pounds in 7 short weeks and was dying of malnutrition. As doctors struggled to understand what was happening, Stringfellow was wracked with pain. The pain became "incessant, unremitting, and, as it seemed to me, insatiable." It matured into "a kind of possession of not only my body but my person, so that the facility of concentration was crippled" and "sanity itself" was at issue.[2] The comforts and distractions that he had once known were "neutralized" by the pain. Medical examinations and tests were "tortures." Every movement became an ordeal. He was unable to write or to practice law, he lost his income and went heavily into debt, and he was not expected to live. With missed diagnoses and failed treatments, finding a physician he could trust was itself a trial. To add insult to injury, he experienced rejection from one important person who, "upon beholding my disease, abhorred me rather than the disease. . . . "[3]

Stringfellow writes primarily about physical pain. Like other commentators, I do not equate pain with suffering.[4] The root of suffering lies in a disruption of identity or a challenge to self and world.[5] One can certainly experience pain without suffering, and one can experience suffering without pain. Still, Eric Cassell reminds us that "physical pain remains a major cause of human suffering."[6] This is particularly true when the pain is severe, prolonged, and seemingly intractable, as was Stringfellow's. But in addition to pain, it is clear that Stringfellow suffered challenges to his sense of self and world on a number of levels: to lose one's ability to work and hence to lose one's income and face an uncertain future, to be rejected by a loved one, and to lose faith in the medical profession that is supposed to help one is surely to suffer in many ways.[7] Stringfellow suffered on physical, mental, emotional, social, and structural levels.[8]

What is a Protestant to make of such suffering? Throughout history, suffering has variously been considered to be a punishment for sin; an enemy to be overcome;

an evil to be resisted; a chastisement for our correction; a representation of Christ on earth and, hence, a means of communion with God (God suffers with us); a vehicle for purifying the soul or strengthening faith and, hence, a divine blessing (admittedly, in disguise); a means to deeper faith or commitment; a mark of moral piety; a prod to resist oppression or to envision reality differently; and/or a path to humility or perseverance or hope.[9] Protestants at different times have embraced all of these understandings of suffering. Suffering can be seen as ennobling, transformative, redemptive, and mysterious. Most contemporary Protestants would agree that Christians are called to stand by and with those who suffer, to alleviate suffering where possible, and to attempt to find transformative meaning in suffering when it cannot be eliminated. All of us know people whose inordinate suffering has transformed their lives—sometimes for worse, sometimes for better.[10] That suffering can be transformative is thus absolutely unquestionable. But is it also *redemptive*?

Of course, much depends on how redemption is understood. The history of theories of atonement and theologies of redemption goes far beyond the scope of this essay. For our purposes, I will begin with a simple definition of redemption as the act of rescuing from sin by "paying a price."[11] I will argue here that, from a Protestant perspective, only certain suffering is redemptive, and that applying the concept of redemptive suffering to the situation of a dying or very ill patient eviscerates the true meaning of redemptive suffering. Transformation and redemption are not the same. In making this argument, it will be clear that I am dependent upon some Protestant views and sources more than others: I write as a feminist theologian informed by liberation theology. Since liberation theology "is a theology that formally addresses the question of suffering caused by injustice,"[12] it should come as no surprise that I will argue that true redemptive suffering takes place only in the social and political arenas where justice is at stake.

This position stands in contrast to classical Roman Catholic theology. In his examination of *Health and Medicine in the Catholic Tradition,* Richard A. McCormick comments that "without glorifying suffering, Catholic Christianity has always viewed it within a larger perspective—that of the redemptive process."[13] Grave illness can be seen in this perspective as "an intensifying conformity to Christ." The notion that the suffering of a gravely ill patient conforms to the suffering of Christ leads to the notion that such suffering is redemptive. It brings the sufferer closer to Jesus and to God; it is therefore redemptive because it mirrors or participates in the suffering of Jesus, which was redemptive for humankind.[14] In Wikipedia, one finds redemptive suffering *defined* as "the Roman Catholic belief that human suffering, when accepted and offered up in union with the Passion of Jesus, can remit the just punishment for one's sins or for the sins of another."[15] While I hope to show that any definition limiting redemptive suffering to Roman Catholic beliefs is inadequate, it is noteworthy that Roman Catholics have a sufficiently strong doctrine of redemptive suffering for the author in Wikipedia to consider it definitive, and that within that Roman Catholic doctrine, the suffering of a patient can be redemptive.[16]

Do Protestants share such a perspective? As a Protestant, is it part of my own understanding? To these questions, I must answer both yes and no. On the one hand, Protestants worship a God who suffered and died for our sake. Indeed, the symbol of Christ on the cross is, as David Smith puts it, "the characteristically Christian datum in the debate about suffering."[17] As Sharon Thornton avers, the cross is the central symbol of Christian faith.[18] We may not know much about God, but in a Protestant Christian view, we know at least this much: God suffered and died on the cross. Hence, the suffering person is in some way "in the likeness of God."[19] Suffering can be a means to drawing closer to God and so can be transformative for the individual.

Indeed, some would go so far as to say that Christians should not shun suffering, but rather should embrace it as a discipline that can purify the soul and ennoble the person.[20] Lutherans in particular tend to emphasize a "theology of the cross," in which the suffering of Jesus on the cross shows us that God is among us precisely in suffering and that therefore when we suffer, God is very much with us, and we are with God. In language strikingly similar to that used by McCormick, Luther embraced the notion that suffering "conforms" us to Christ. To be a Christian is to accept suffering; to refuse to suffer is to deny Christ.[21] We must bear our cross, as Jesus bore his. Suffering can be seen as a gift given to us by a God who loves us enough to consider us worthy of such a visitation.[22] Jesus is a savior who can sympathize with our suffering because of his own; this permits Christians to bear their suffering because they know that God understands and has compassion—God "suffers with" them. Barbara Brown Taylor opines: "...we need a God who knows about pain." And she adds that sometimes the mere knowledge that God (or Jesus) is "with" us in our suffering "becomes dearer...than the hope of recovery."[23]

Notwithstanding these traditional views of the possible value of suffering, most Protestants pray each week, "deliver us from evil." Protestants desire suffering to cease. Still, suffering that comes as a by-product of a life devoted to Christ can have deep meaning and is not always to be avoided.[24] Thus, John Wesley, founder of the Methodist tradition, did not advocate a simple resignation to suffering, but he did opine that suffering can benefit the human spirit by drawing our hearts away from the world and toward piety, yielding a form of happiness far greater than any worldly pleasures.[25] Suffering was, for Wesley, an enemy, yet an enemy that could be a great teacher for those who took it seriously and saw in it a meaning beyond itself.[26] To this extent, then, Protestants would agree that suffering *can* be transformative. But is this the same thing as saying that it is redemptive?

I think not. Although Luther sees our suffering as "conforming" us to Christ, he does not see our suffering as "redeeming" us. For Luther, redemption has already been accomplished by Christ. Dietrich Bonhoeffer continues this tradition, claiming that Christ suffered vicariously for the whole world and that "his is the only suffering which has redemptive efficacy."[27] Indeed, Bonhoeffer considered asceticism dangerous because it tempted people to choose suffering and to think that by imitating the sufferings of Christ, we would be undertaking the work of redemption.[28] Christ fulfilled all the suffering necessary for redemption. When we suffer on earth as Christians, we are suffering in a representative capacity "for" the church, which is the body of Christ, but we are not effecting redemption.[29]

Stringfellow himself never viewed his ordeal of pain as redemptive.[30] Indeed, quite the opposite. To believe that enduring pain brings redemption is, for Stringfellow, a form of "justification by works," wherein bearing pain substitutes for doing good deeds. The idea that we can pursue our own justification or redemption by enduring pain is, therefore, for Stringfellow, a "vanity" of the first order. "[T]o view pain as a means of justification . . . is an especially pathetic ridicule of God. . . . [T]he victim becomes an idolator of his own pain."[31] Further, Stringfellow writes that, as his pain progressed, it became his work. We usually understand work either in terms of a job or in terms of something that requires effort. This was certainly true for Stringfellow: "Pain commandeered, engaged and exhausted all my faculties, energies, and talents; pain tested all my weaknesses and shortcomings; pain filled most of the time and dictated the use of all of the time. . . ."[32] The recognition that pain was his work, however, means something additional for Stringfellow. From a biblical perspective, work is a reality of *fallen* existence—it is a sign of our disorientation, a premonition of death. "[P]ain is a specific instance and endurance of that . . . fallenness," and hence, "pain is work."[33] Far from being a part of redemption, then, Stringfellow seems to signal that enduring pain is simply and exquisitely a sign of our *fallen* existence. We cannot transcend that fallenness or obviate the burden of our brokenness. We must face and accept the brutality of death's vigor in our lives. Only when we accept that life is an incredible gift do we transcend in some way the power of death. To the extent that pain might force us to accept the vigor of death and to see life as the incredible gift that it is, pain might be a teacher for us, but it is never, itself, a form of redemption.

Similarly, Bradley Hanson writes regarding his own experience of illness and incredible pain that one of the hardest of the Pauline lessons for him was trying to see how his suffering could be said to be a sharing in Christ's suffering: ". . . I felt that my own affliction from pain did not qualify as suffering that shares in the suffering of Christ."[34] Christ suffered political persecution and unjust crucifixion. Following Christ, Paul suffered from persecution, from imprisonment, from being beaten and lashed, and from the dangers he encountered as a traveling missionary. None of these, suggests Hanson, are equivalent to the suffering caused by illness, even extreme illness and pain. Thus, at least prima facie, suffering from illness and even from great pain would not be, for Hanson, redemptive.

Bonhoeffer, too, argued that not all suffering is a sign of discipleship. Rather, for Bonhoeffer, suffering *and rejection* signal that one is a disciple of Christ. "Suffering and rejection sum up the whole cross of Jesus."[35] Christian suffering is not just *any* suffering, "not the sort of suffering which is inseparable from this mortal life," but rather, "the suffering which is an essential part of the specifically Christian life."[36] For Bonhoeffer, therefore, the natural ills of the body do not constitute redemptive suffering, nor are they a sign of discipleship. Only the suffering and rejection that come at the hands of men can be considered a form of discipleship.

It is in this vein, I believe, that Martin Luther King Jr. declared that "unearned suffering is redemptive."[37] Crucial to understanding Martin Luther King Jr.'s view of redemptive suffering is to begin with the understanding that the Negro in America suffered greatly from oppression. Segregation was a reality. Black people in America were treated as second-class citizens—forced to sit in the back of the bus, denied access to public places or required to use separate entrances, living often in extreme poverty, and expected to endure being belittled, assaulted, intimidated, and shunned. Oppression and exclusion caused enormous suffering. Such suffering is unearned but it is *not* redemptive. As Barbara Brown Taylor puts it, "there is nothing redemptive about famine, genocide, or incest...and no one should have to endure them."[38] Redemptive suffering is a more specific category.

Redemptive suffering, for King, is the suffering that comes as a consequence of struggling for justice within an unjust system. In seeking to defeat an unjust system, "suffering can be a most creative and powerful social force."[39] When his own home and the homes of other members of the freedom movement were bombed, King urged his followers not to return violence for violence. "We must somehow believe that unearned suffering is redemptive," he declared.[40] Thus, King introduces the notion of redemptive suffering in connection with the violence and suffering imposed on those who were struggling for justice. The unearned suffering that becomes redemptive is neither the "natural" suffering of disease nor the unjust suffering of oppression; rather, it is the suffering voluntarily undertaken by those who struggle against oppression and injustice. It is *this* kind of suffering that is redemptive in King's view. I concur.

Martin Luther King Jr. suffered often yet spoke little of his own sufferings. Finally, on invitation from the *Christian Century*, he wrote briefly, enumerating as follows: "I have been arrested five times....My home has been bombed twice. A day seldom passes that my family and I are not the recipients of threats of death. I have been the victim of a near-fatal stabbing. So in a real sense I have been battered by the storms of persecution."[41] These personal trials, he writes, taught him "the value of unmerited suffering." "Recognizing the necessity for suffering I have tried to make of it a virtue. If only to save myself from bitterness, I have attempted to see my personal ordeals as an opportunity to transform myself and heal the people involved in the tragic situation which now obtains. I have lived these last few years with the conviction that unearned suffering is redemptive."[42] What makes unearned suffering redemptive is not the suffering itself, but the hope that it will lead to social transformation.

It should therefore be noted that the redemptive suffering King proclaims is not primarily individual. It is primarily social. To be sure, unearned suffering may result in the reformation of people's views and attitudes, and in that way can be transformative on an individual level. For King, unearned suffering would come through following the way of nonviolent resistance to violence—or of nonresistance. Chilton argues that nonresistance is not the same as acquiescence, and that it is a deliberate social tactic to undermine injustice: "The injustice that is done is never accepted as if it were just. The acts of turning the other cheek, giving the garment... are all designed to be excessive, so that the fact of the injustice of what is demanded is underlined."[43] For Chilton, such nonresistance becomes a policy of "exemplary response." It is the only authentically Christian response to suffering in the present: to accept the pains of injustice without retaliation is to model Christ.[44]

As King puts it, the way of nonviolent resistance "first does something to the hearts and souls of those committed to it. It gives them new self-respect; it calls up resources of strength and courage that they did not know they had."[45] To this extent, unearned suffering could be transformative for the soul of the sufferer. But more important were its effects on the outside world. Unearned suffering in the struggle for justice, King believed, would finally reach the opponent "and so stir his conscience that reconciliation becomes a reality."[46] "We will soon wear you down by our capacity to suffer," he insisted.[47] In this way, unearned suffering is redemptive because it moves the social system toward more justice. The struggle for justice of necessity will cause suffering: every step toward justice requires sacrifice, suffering, and struggle. King summed it up dramatically: "The way of nonviolence... may even mean physical death. But if physical death is the price that a man must pay to free his children and his white brethren from a permanent death of the spirit, then nothing could be more redemptive."[48] Thus, the ordeals of his generation were "the opportunity to transfigure... American society."[49] Unearned suffering in a righteous cause can be redemptive.

In short, the suffering that is redemptive—or creative, as King often calls it—is not every and all suffering, but rather the suffering that comes from practicing civil disobedience in ways that are geared to bring attention to injustice and to bring about more justice. Martin Luther King Jr. rarely links this suffering directly to Jesus.[50] Perhaps the closest he comes is when he says that the nonviolent demonstrator "sees the misery of his people so clearly that he volunteers to suffer in their behalf and put an end to their plight."[51] Suffering "in behalf of" someone is what Jesus did, and in this way, redemptive suffering today might be said to reflect or mirror the suffering of Jesus. Ultimately, this kind of redemptive suffering is based on hope—on the conviction that "even though the arc of the moral universe is long, it bends toward justice."[52]

A view similar to King's emerges in the work of contemporary pastoral theologian Sharon Thornton. "This is a book about suffering" begins her work on pastoral theology and the cross.[53] Thornton does believe that there is a kind of suffering that is redemptive. But she is quick to clarify that she does not suggest that suffering in and of itself is redemptive: "On the contrary and emphatically, no!"[54] Drawing on numerous theologians, Thornton decries the habit of seeing all suffering as "taking up your cross." Jesus did not simply suffer and die. He was crucified under Pontius Pilate, an official of the Roman government.[55] Early interpretations of his death never suggested that a messiah would substitute for others or die "for" the world.[56] Rather, his suffering was because he did not give up the way of love and justice even when injustice was done to him. Hence, "on the cross, historically imposed suffering exposes the structures of violence, the inhumane way people treat one another."[57] The cross, then, argues Thornton, should not be interpreted in an individualistic, internalized manner. The cross is very explicitly a *political* symbol, pointing us to the historical injustices under which Jesus suffered and died. "The political cross illumines the social contours of suffering."[58]

For Thornton—and for Dorothee Soelle, on whom Thornton draws extensively—love must necessarily act to undo injustice. As it does so, love will inevitably suffer because the world is full of forces that resist the movement toward more justice. Hence, those who act to bring about justice in the world must expect to suffer. In this way, their work continues the suffering of Jesus. But Thornton is careful to clarify: "The purpose of carrying out an act of suffering is not for the sake of suffering itself. . . . Carrying out the act of suffering is aimed at making those who are suffering visible and the causes of their suffering known."[59] It is in exposing the social and political causes of suffering that we might participate in redemptive suffering.

Some important nuances are evident in this discussion. First, there is no single "Protestant view" of suffering. Second, there is a sense in which Protestant commentators want to walk a fine line. On the one hand, neither I nor most Protestants quoted here believe that the physical suffering that attends disease or its treatment is redemptive. Only certain suffering qualifies as redemptive: not the suffering that comes from the natural order of human disease, not the suffering that comes from oppression and injustice in the world, but only the suffering that is incurred in the struggle for justice, dignity, and human fulfillment. When Jesus said, "he must suffer for my name" (Acts 9:16), he was talking not about suffering from illness but rather about suffering from persecution experienced in the struggle for the kingdom of God.

On the other hand, all interpretations of the meaning of suffering will draw on cultural constructs. As Mohrmann puts it, the work of finding sense in pain is perilous, and we always begin with some conceptual framework.[60] If believing that suffering brings one closer to God or participates in Jesus' redeeming work helps a patient to reconstruct meaning and hope, I would be loath to diminish that hope or take away a conceptual framework that helps that patient to restructure a shattered life.[61] Having endured breast cancer and the pains and indignities of its treatment, I understand how crucial it is for patients to find meaning in the midst of chaos. Bradley Hanson eventually did come to see his illness and suffering as a form of participation in the suffering of Christ. For Christians, he urges, "suffering is not alien to their relationship to Christ, but an integral part of it."[62] To the extent that Jesus suffered extreme pain on the cross, any person who suffers extreme physical pain, as both Hanson and Stringfellow did during their illnesses, may apprehend what Jesus suffered and be drawn closer to the mystery of his sacrifice. Dorothee Soelle stresses the importance of seeing our suffering as a continuation of Jesus' work in the world. While I do not believe that the suffering that patients endure is itself redemptive from a Protestant perspective, I want to honor the depths of *meaning* that emerge for some sufferers. Suffering certainly can evoke resistance to all the powers of death that operate in human life. Nonetheless, because Jesus' suffering was not from illness but from political injustice, and his physical pain and suffering were the result of such injustice, I argue that redemptive suffering per se comes only in the political context and is redemptive for the social order. I want to "redeem" redemptive suffering from its role as a salve to the sick and restore it to its proper place, which is social and political, not biomedical.

What are the implications of this view for bioethics?

First, because suffering from disease is *not* redemptive, there is no reason to value such suffering. In general, therefore, we have a mandate to remove or reduce that suffering to the extent possible, even though patients can and do find meaning in it.[63] Protestants turn to Scripture as a source of authority, and in Scripture we find Jesus *healing* the sick and suffering (Mark 1:32–34). Protestant churches have founded many hospitals and other places dedicated to healing the sick. Christians who, out of compassion, risk their lives by exposing themselves to contagion in an effort to heal others could be said to be modeling Christ's compassion. While the moral obligation to relieve suffering is not distinctively Christian, it is certainly central to Christian belief. Others share this sense of obligation; for example, Iris Marion Young argues that "there is a moral imperative to minimize suffering, wherever it occurs."[64] Here, the Protestant view coheres with general obligations of beneficence and nonmaleficence and with a wide range of literature in the field of bioethics.[65]

At the same time, Protestant Christians do not expect to be healed by God of all illness; the letters of the New Testament speak frequently of the illnesses suffered by those who were following Christ (1 Tim. 5:23; 2 Tim. 4:20; Phil. 2:27; Gal. 4:13). Suffering is part of human life, and there will always be disease and deterioration that present challenges to Christians as to others. While Protestants affirm the sovereignty of God, this does not translate to an expectation that God will remove all pain or suffering from human life, even from the lives of those who love God. There can therefore be limits to the obligation to remove suffering: we are not mandated to expend all resources in an effort to overcome the sufferings of illness and disability. When suffering cannot be removed, it is the task of Christians to "suffer with"—to have compassion, and to attempt to help the sufferers to find meaning in their illness. "[S]uffering waits for sympathy," says Portmann. "Hell is a place where people do not, cannot, console one another."[66] In Reformed Protestantism, where I place myself, social support—the offering of community—is essential. There is much that we can do to relieve suffering by standing in solidarity with those who suffer.[67] As philosopher Iris Marion Young notes, solidarity need not connote homogeneity or unity of a group; rather, it refers to a relationship among separate and even dissimilar actors who decide to stand together and be "for" one another.[68] Solidarity with the sick and suffering is the second implication of a Protestant view of suffering.

Third, some of the suffering experienced in illness is the result of "natural" evil, while some is either the result of "moral" evil—of what humans have done to each other—or is exacerbated by moral evil.[69] Thus, we have a mandate to look behind the physical or emotional suffering of the ill to the possible social causes of that suffering. In North America, says Margaret Lock, efforts to reduce suffering tend to focus on control and repair of individual bodies while ignoring the social origins of suffering and distress, including poverty and discrimination[70]—the very factors that King fought so ardently. Paul Farmer points to the hidden causes of disease—the social policies and political decisions that often determine the course of illness. In Haiti, for example, the construction of a new dam flooded a fertile plain, causing many families to flee to less fertile hillsides. To survive, those families had to carry their meager crops to sell in distant villages; their daughters were sometimes raped and other times seduced on the road, and some contracted and died of AIDS.[71] Farmer concludes: "The social and economic forces that dictate life choices in Haiti's Central Plateau affects many millions of individuals, and it is in the context of these global forces that the suffering of individuals receives its appropriate context of interpretation."[72] To this, I would only add the clarification that those "global forces" must include both social structures and cultural constructions. Our love of automobiles may be responsible for more than 125,000 cases of cancer each year in the United States.[73] If we make the connections, as feminists stress,[74] between the personal and the political, we will probably find that sources of suffering—including much illness—are seldom divorced from the actions of those with power. Where illness results from abuse of power or injustice in the world, we have a duty to struggle for justice.

Fourth, there is always a spiritual dimension to suffering. Because suffering is an assault on the self and the world that sustains that self, suffering challenges our sense of self and world. Faith traditions attempt to address that dimension partly by offering social support to the sufferer and partly by offering structures of meaning. Thus, we encounter the theodicy question: Does God *will* our suffering?[75] How can there be a good God and still be so much suffering in the world? This perennially troubling question goes beyond the scope of this essay, though hints of possible answers are couched herein. Christians will always struggle with the meaning and place of suffering in a world created and sustained by a loving God. Part of the importance of chaplaincy in a hospital is precisely to help sufferers find answers to such mysteries. Perhaps most important, however, is to reshape the questions and not permit the theodicy question to distract us from addressing the very real injustices and oppressions that cause so much suffering around the world. It is in the struggle to eliminate those injustices that we encounter the possibility of genuinely redemptive suffering.

Notes

1. William Stringfellow, *A Second Birthday: A Personal Confrontation with Illness, Pain, and Death* (Eugene, OR: Wipf and Stock, 1970).
2. Ibid., 46.
3. Ibid., 196.

4. See, for example, Daniel P. Sulmasy, "Finitude, Freedom, and Suffering," in 92; Mark J. Hanson, "Bioethics and the Challenge of Theodicy," in ibid., 176.; David H. Smith, "Suffering, Medicine, and Christian Theology," in *On Moral Medicine: Theological Perspectives in Medical Ethics*, ed. Stephen E. Lammers and Allen Verhey (Grand Rapids: William B. Eerdmans, 1987), 255. Simmons distinguishes them bluntly: "pain is physical; suffering is psychic and emotional." Paul D. Simmons, *Faith and Health: Religion, Science, and Public Policy* (Macon, GA: Mercer University Press, 2008), 24. However, Portmann would challenge this, reminding us that Mark Zborowski's classic study of pain showed that the experience of pain is influenced by culture; hence, pain is not *simply* physical. John Portmann, *When Bad Things Happen to Other People* (New York: Routledge, 2000), 49. To suffer is not merely to endure a misfortune, but to feel distress at that misfortune. See Jamie Mayerfeld, *Suffering and Moral Responsibility* (New York: Oxford, 1999). Although pain and suffering are generally distinguished today, it should also be noted that when philosophers such as Sidgwick, Bentham, or Brandt use the term *pain,* they may be referring to what we would today call *suffering*. See Mayerfeld, chap. 2. It is also noteworthy that *The Merriam-Webster Dictionary* (Springfield, MA: Merriam-Webster, 2004, 715) offers "to feel or endure pain" as the first definition of "suffer."

5. See, for example, Eric Cassell's classic description of suffering; also Per Anderson, "To Change and To Accept in a Technological Society," in *Pain Seeking Understanding: Suffering, Medicine, and Faith*, ed. Margaret E. Mohrmann and Mark J. Hanson (Cleveland, OH: Pilgrim, 1999), 141.

6. Eric J. Cassell, *The Nature of Suffering and the Goals of Medicine*, 2nd ed. (2004), 31. Cassell points out (35) that pain generally involves suffering when the pain is (1) severe, (2) uncontrolled, and (3) apparently endless. All three were true for Stringfellow. In *The Body in Pain: The Making and Unmaking of the World* (New York: Oxford, 1985), Elaine Scarry notes how pain shatters language. This shattering of language cuts the one in pain off from communication and hence from community, causing more suffering.

7. In her study of seventeenth-century texts on suffering, Ann Thompson notes that these early authors focused largely on external afflictions or painful events in the life of the sufferer. The effect of these afflictions on the sufferer's state of mind, however, was the true source of suffering. Such inner distress needed to be alleviated so that the suffering was made bearable. Suffering, then, became an "art"—we must learn how to use our suffering so that it yields spiritual fruits. Ann Thompson, *The Art of Suffering and the Impact of Seventeenth-Century Anti-Providential Thought* (Burlington, VT: Ashgate, 2003), 2f.

8. I say "structural" here because of Stringfellow's struggle to find adequate health care despite being well educated and well situated. Indeed, he acknowledges—with some anger—that he would probably have died if he had been poor and black rather than white and well situated.

9. For a listing of Bible verses associated with many of these interpretations, see Joni Eareckson Tada and Steven Estes, *When God Weeps: Why Our Sufferings Matter to the Almighty* (Grand Rapids: Zondervan,1997), appendix B.

10. A fascinating study of three people whose sufferings bore fruit in incredible creativity is John Piper's *Tested by Fire: The fruit of Suffering in the Lives of John Bunyan, William Cowper and David Brainerd* (Leicester, UK: Inter-Varsity Press, 2001).

11. Merriam-Webster, *The Merriam-Webster Dictionary* (Springfield, MA: Merriam-Webster, 2004), 605.

12. Lucien Richard, O.M.I., *What Are They Saying about the Theology of Suffering?* (New York: Paulist Press, 1992), 91.

13. Richard A. McCormick, *Health and Medicine in the Catholic Tradition* (New York: Crossroad, 1984), 116. Similarly, Henry C. Simmons, C.P., speaks of a "bond" between our suffering and Christ's. *Valuing Suffering as a Christian: Some Psychological Perspectives* (Chicago: Franciscan Herald Press, 1976), 9.

14. On Wikipedia, redemptive suffering is described as a Roman Catholic doctrine, but that is not correct and is far too limited.

15. http://en.wikipedia.org/wiki/Redemptive_suffering, accessed March 12, 2014. This entry was updated January 30, 2014.

16. In one of those difficult paradoxes of faith, one must also note that if suffering brings one closer to God, then in one sense suffering must yield joy because closeness to God is the goal of the Christian life. Hence, as Cassell notes, there is a sense in which the Christian's suffering would not be considered suffering at all. Cassell, supra note 6, 44.

17. David H. Smith, "Suffering, Medicine, and Christian Theology," in Stephen E. Lammers and Allen Verhey, *On Moral Medicine: Theological Perspectives in Medical Ethics* (Grand Rapids: William B. Eerdmans, 1987), 259.

18. Sharon G. Thornton, *Broken Yet Beloved: A Pastoral Theology of the Cross* (St. Louis: Chalice Press, 2002), 65. Dr. Thornton's careful reading of a first draft has helped this project immensely.

19. Martin E. Marty, *Health and Medicine in the Lutheran Tradition* (NewYork: Crossroad, 1983), 60.

20. Marty, 55, 59.

21. Blair Kasfeldt, "Martin Luther on Suffering and Theodicy for the Christian," http://suite101.com/article/martin-luther-on-suffering-and-theodicy-for-the-christian-a3498, accessed October 2, 2012.

22. Amanda Drury, "Luther on True Christian Suffering," www.drurywriting.com/amanda/Luther%20on%20Suffering.doc, accessed October 2012.

23. Barbara Brown Taylor, *God in Pain: Teaching Sermons on Suffering* (Nashville: Abingdon Press, 1998), 12.

24. Ibid., 64.

25. E. Brooks Holifield, *Health and Medicine in the Methodist Tradition* (New York: Crossroad, 1986), 63.

26. Ibid., 65.

27. Dietrich Bonhoeffer, *The Cost of Discipleship* (New York: MacMillan, 1974), 102.

28. Ibid., 190.

29. Ibid., 273.

30. Because Stringfellow writes as an Episcopalian, some might not consider him a Protestant thinker. I believe, however, that his views on this subject cohere with the Protestant approach that I take.

31. Stringfellow, supra note 1, 53.

32. Ibid., 55.

33. Ibid., 65; 97.

34. Bradley Hanson, "School of Suffering," in Stephen E. Lammers and Allen Verhey, *On Moral Medicine: Theological Perspectives in Medical Ethics* (Grand Rapids: William B. Eerdmans, 1987), 251.

35. Bonhoeffer, supra note 27, 96.

36. Ibid., 98.

37. Martin Luther King Jr., *A Testament of Hope*, 219. I am grateful to Dr. Randall Miller of Pacific School of Religion for his careful and critical reading of my interpretation of Martin Luther King Jr.

38. Barbara Brown Taylor, supra note 23, 63.

39. Martin Luther King Jr., supra note 37, 47.

40. Ibid., 466.

41. Ibid., 41.

42. Ibid.

43. Bruce Chilton, "Christianity," in *Evil and Suffering*, ed. Jacob Neusner (Cleveland: Pilgrim, 1998), 84f.

44. Ibid., 88.

45. Martin Luther King Jr., supra note 37, 487.

46. Ibid., 487.

47. Ibid., 485.

48. Ibid., 485.

49. Ibid., 487. At some points in his ministry, at least, King clearly believed that it worked—for example, he enumerates the many forms of violence perpetrated against the freedom movement and notes that every attempt to end the protest by intimidation or force or violence simply further "cemented the Negro community and brought sympathy for our cause from men of good will all over the world." Ibid., 79.

50. He did say, however, that the early Christians "were willing to face all kinds of suffering in order to stand up for what they knew was right...." So should we be. Ibid., 50.

51. Ibid., 57.

52. Ibid., 52. This famous quote from King also demonstrates what many Protestants would hold: that suffering in a righteous cause is sustained by the hope of justice, and thus that suffering and hope are inextricably bound.

53. Thornton, supra note 18, 1.

54. Ibid., 24.

55. Ibid., 68.

56. Ibid., 73.

57. Ibid., 79.

58. Ibid., 117.

59. Ibid., 157.

60. Margaret Mohrmann, "Someone Is Always Playing Job," in Mohrmann and Hanson, supra note 5, 65. See also J. W. Bowker, "Religions, Society, and Suffering," in Arthur Kleinman, Veena Das, and Margaret Lock, ed., *Social Suffering* (Berkeley: University of California, 1997), 363: "no matter how true it is that there must be an individual *locus* of suffering, the meaning of suffering arises out of the relations of individuals together in society...." supra note 70.

61. I venture to suggest that Thornton would agree because she offers an example of a patient who found comfort in thinking that Jesus suffered as she was suffering: "If Jesus could stand the cross, I can live with this," she told Thornton. Thornton, supra note 18, 10.

62. Hanson, supra note 34, 253.

63. Roman Catholics would agree with this. "The attitude of the good Samaritan, to reach out in compassion...to relive the pain of neighbors, is the posture toward suffering that we must remember," writes Bernard J. Bush, S.J. See Bush "All Creation Groans,"

in Richard J. Gilmartin, ed., *Suffering: Issues of Emotional Living in an Age of Stress for Clergy and Religious* (Whitinsville, MA: Affirmation Books, 1984), 32.

64. Iris Marion Young, *Responsibility for Justice* (New York: Oxford University Press, 2011).

65. See, for example, Erich Loewy, *Suffering and the Beneficent Community: Beyond Libertarianism* (Albany, NY: State University of New York Press, 1991); Tom L. Beauchamp and James F. Childress, *Principles of Biomedical Ethics* (New York: Oxford University Press, 2001). The obligation to relieve suffering is not exclusive Christian, but it is widely shared in human community and religious traditions. "Because suffering ought not to occur, we have a prima facie obligation to prevent it," declares Mayerfeld, op. cit.112.

66. Portmann, supra note 4, 52.

67. Whether we should always attempt to relieve suffering is a challenging ethical question, addressed by Portmann in his study of Schadenfreude, which he defines roughly as pleasure in the suffering of others when we think that suffering is *deserved.* Thus, there are strong connections between the emotions caused by suffering and our sense of justice. Without an appeal to justice, pleasure in the suffering of another seems to amount to perversity, cruelty, or both. Ironically, of course, when we suffer, then, we must acknowledge that others probably assume that we 'deserve' to, and this knowledge may increase our suffering. Portmann, op. cit., passim.

68. Young, op. cit., 120.

69. For a definition of natural and moral evil as they cause suffering, see Paul D. Simmons, *Faith and Health: Religion, Science, and Public Policy* (Macon, GA: Mercer university Press, 2008), 21–23.

70. Margaret Lock, "Displacing Suffering: The Reconstruction of Death in North America and Japan," in Arthur Kleinman, Veena Das, and Margaret Lock, ed., *Social Suffering* (Berkeley: University of California, 1997), 210.

71. Paul Farmer, "On Suffering and Structural Violence," in Kleinman et.al., 264ff.

72. Farmer, 273.

73. James B. Martin-Schramm, *Climate Justice: Ethics, Energy, and Public Policy* (Minneapolis: Fortress Press, 2010), 7.

74. Beverly Wildung Harrison, *Making the Connections*, ed. Carol S. Robb (Boston: Beacon Press, 1985).

75. See, for instance, Tada and Estes, *When God Weeps,* 57ff. We are not promised healing from all our diseases, they argue; when Jesus says, "I will do whatever you ask in my name" (John 14:13), it does not mean that we can ask for healing and receive it. Rather, it means that we should ask for the things that Jesus himself requested: the spread of the kingdom of God, forgiveness, and sustenance for the day. 61 Thus, they argue that God's plan for Christians can include suffering. They caution that we tend to see God in miracles of healing, but not in trials of suffering. 91 It is worth mentioning that one of the authors of this book—Joni Tada—broke her neck as a teenager and coauthored this book some 30 years later when she was, as she puts it, constantly suffering and weary from battling the encroaching limitations of her paralysis. 13.

14

Suffering: Reflections from the Jewish Tradition

Laurie Zoloth

> R. Johanan once fell ill and R. Hanina went in to visit him. He said to him: Are your sufferings welcome to you? He replied: Neither they nor their reward. He said to him: Give me your hand. He gave him his hand and he raised him. Why could not R. Johanan raise himself?—They replied: The prisoner cannot free himself from jail.
>
> Talmud Bavli, Barochot, 5b[1]

In a long passage in the Babylonian Talmud, the rabbinic authorities debate the matter of suffering and its meaning. Is there value in suffering? Can suffering act as atonement for sinful behavior? Can the suffering one, at the least, understand this agony as an expatiation? The answer in the text is a long and complex argument, in which the protagonists, experiencing terrible loss and illness, repeat to one another: "Are your sufferings welcome to you? And reply: Neither they nor their reward."

We will return to this text in some detail. Such a text notes the complexities of tradition, raises questions within the narrative, telling us, the readers, that suffering in normative rabbinic Judaism is not here welcomed as a meaningful or pedagogical experience, nor as a preliminary threshold to a postmortem reward, nor as an exchange of goodness for grace, nor as the Event that shapes our humanity. How unlike, one is immediately moved to consider, this view of suffering from other religious traditions, how unlike many normative constructions of faith within contemporary American discourse, most especially, the discourse of bioethics. For on the personal level, in such a text, pain, grief, illness, and befallenness are understood as chaos, as disorder, which is largely without spiritual value—is "useless"—and is not linked to a spiritual journey or a holy transformation. This essay will address a core difference in religious text and tradition, which, I will argue, have come to define and delineate one of the most salient issues in American bioethics, for example, the way that human suffering and its tragic or redemptive nature is at stake in debates as varied as stem cell research, end-of-life care, or reproductive policy. But bioethics is not the only venue in which the view of suffering animates the policy discussion—it is a quiet and steady presence behind much political and social discourse.

Behind the passion of these debates and the logic of their argumentation live core belief structures animated by substantially different religious traditions. Perhaps nowhere are these differences as deeply shaped into policy as in medicine and medical research, but it can be argued that the entire public debate about worth, harms, or entitlements rests on the fulcrum of the meaning of suffering in human life and our responsibility to the suffering of the other. In this essay, I will briefly sketch some outlines for how the view of suffering in Jewish thought is developed and debated, show how one rabbinic text structures a response, and end with some suggestions for how to appreciate the different voice that Judaism brings to ethics because of its different evaluation of suffering.

There is another, critical difference about suffering that is carried by Jewish tradition, perhaps most especially as a reality by all of post-Shoah (Holocaust) Jewish thought. Jews have both an individual and a corporate body, an individual and a collective fate. The question of suffering is always about the ontological, individual Jew who lives in a particular place, time, and narrative and the suffering of the Jewish People as a whole, for whom place and time are both diachronic and synchronic. For while it has been a question since the destruction of the Second Temple, the issue of why the Jewish people suffer is intensified to blinding after the Second World War, in which the entire project of European Jewry, the elegant and intricate life of six million men, women, and children, from the voices rising in the Grand Synagogue to the small breath of a waiting boy in a village kitchen, was utterly and irrevocable obliterated. Suffering, for the Jewish ethicist, always has a first-person and a third-person grammar, a single tone and multiple register.

Let me state the obvious: the Christian narrative is based on a cluster of traditions in which the individual person exists in a world that has been redeemed and forgiven by the central sacrifice of Jesus, who is crucified as atonement of collective human sin. The link between embodied corporal suffering and atonement for sin offers a strong mimetic for an individual Christian in physical pain. Texts of Christian bioethics often stress this link, suggesting that it our capacity for suffering that makes us both most fully human and capable of transcendence. But if the Cross is at the center of history for Christians, the problem of human suffering is a central issue for most religions. Thus, while my claim that suffering does not have the centrality that it has within many classic Christian texts found within bioethics, the consideration of its meaning surely has a place in Jewish thought. Jewish devotional liturgy addresses suffering; one prays, as a Jew three times daily, prayers that include petitions for healing, to avoid suffering, and to have the strength to endure disaster when it inevitably occurs. It is true, of course, that this particular world, in this particular religious cosmology, is created in such a way that tragic events will happen, and the rabbinic editor that links the textual accounts of debates about suffering writes under conditions of serious collective suffering, during Roman Imperial power and, later, the long night of Diasporic exile. But suffering does not purify or redeem the world. Suffering, in these texts, creates a crisis, an injustice, a rupture, and the possibility of repair, and if it cannot be righted, but only witnessed by another, it is an occasion of tragedy. Most important, one is not elevated by the suffering of the other. Jewish understanding of healing therefore runs counter to a Christian understanding—toward protest, toward healing, toward repair.

Thus, suffering, within most normative Jewish texts, is not a problem of being, it is a problem of ethics and of response: first, because of the way that the moral gesture of medicine as the primary response to personal human suffering is enriched by a narrative approach that is rooted in the aggadic as well as the halachic tradition; second, because the primary act of healing involves not only the direct encounter with the other on both the physical embodied level but also a direct encounter with the other at the moral and existential level, meaning that to be a healer is to be willing to participate in the act of moral repair and reciprocity; third, because the long tradition of lived experience of the Jewish people is replete with suffering on a collective as well as individual level, thus the question of meaning has a social as well as psychological dimension. Finally, it is the entire moral argument behind this Jewish view of suffering that the social welfare, charity, medicine, and science needed to respond to suffering are acts of justice, the response of the human, the argument of the human hand, against an unjust and as yet unredeemed and darkened world.

Suffering in the Classic Traditions and Texts: A Brief Historical Account

The view of suffering and its role in the medical process is one way that Jewish texts take account of a core problem in religion: Why would a powerful, compassionate, and just God allow innocents to suffer? Judaism argues for several answers. First, some philosophic texts suggest that suffering is merely a characteristic of physical existence,[2] or that individual suffering can only be understood as alienation or privation of the good, a "turning away," in the Buberian sense,[3] or a "refusal" of the ethical command, a command that is made by every suffering person, for Levinas.[4] What is stressed in such texts is that while physical pain is part of the mere physicality of creaturely existence, suffering occurs when pain does not evoke a response from fellow humans—in this sense, it is a result of simple human failure. Every suffering person creates an interruption and thus a chance for the enactment of a duty.

The tension between the idea that sin results in suffering and that suffering is independent of sin but is linked to human behavior only as a condition of response arises in the classical texts of Jewish tradition. In two key Biblical texts (Abraham's bargaining for the salvation of Sodom and the debate with friends who want to make a facile link between sin and suffering in Job), the idea of connection between sin and suffering is raised, and left unresolved. Further, in rabbinic texts like the one from the Gemora, as cited earlier, in which the idea that suffering is "an affliction of love," is presented, then strongly debated, then strongly refuted.

The inclusion in the Hebrew Bible of the Book of Job creates deep and remarkably more open questions about suffering. The book ends with a complex move that is both opening and closure, submission and speech—"I will withdraw myself to ashes and to dust," says Job (42:6)—then narratively filling the empty space from which he has withdrawn with prayer on behalf of others, his friends whose formal and standard pieties have been rejected. Such a debate is made vivid by the refusal of many Jewish texts to resolve the problem of suffering by recourse to the sort of heaven populated with angels so clearly drawn in contemporary medieval Christian texts. When some commentators suggest this, they are queried promptly by others even within the narrative, as we will see in the passage we explore in the next section of this essay. While it is true that Rabbinical narratives cover a wide range of views on suffering, the tension about its meaning is unresolved. For philosopher Moshe Habertal, commenting on these texts, rabbinic narratives struggle with the meaning of individual suffering:

> "The midrash, quoting a second century source, designates affliction as a preferable alternative to sacrifice."... When suffering is not mere retribution but instead serves as atonement, it is a different kind of substitute."

However, the Talmud shifts and debates with this argument, as we will see in the final section of this essay.

As the Christian accounts of suffering as redemption became more elaborated in the medieval and early modern construction of the problem, Jewish thought diverged, in part as a method of differentiation. Maimonides, medieval philosopher and physician, is particularly opposed to a fully developed concept of a literal afterlife, for like most within the Jewish tradition, the "world to come" is understood as a collective, messianic redemption, not as a personal domain in which suffering is given meaning or reward. Later commentators reflect on the problem as well. In this next section, we turn to three representative writers of European modernity: Nachman of Brezlov, Franz Rosenzweig and Emmanuel Levinas. Each man struggled with enormous personal tragedy. (Nacham struggled with depression and the loss of a child; Rosenzweig with the devastating disease amyotrophic lateral sclerosis (ALS); and Levinas with the murder of his entire family and village by the Nazis, the imprisonment and the betrayal of his beloved mentor.)

Rabbi Nachman of Brezlov (April 4, 1772–October 16, 1810) lived within a circle of devotees, the great-grandson of the Baal Shem Tov, the founder of modern Hassidism. He traveled widely in the Jewish Pale of Settlement and in Israel, returning to Brezlov, in the Ukraine, where he settled and established a large set of followers. In a sense, his work bridges the period in which Jews emerged from completely contained settlements to engage with the wider world. Beset with both personal tragedy, and in a time when attacks on long established villages were on the rise, Nachman developed a response to suffering that emphasized a personal capacity to withdraw from pain into a personal meditative experience he call *bitul*. This deep inner focus would allow one to "focus on the true goal, which is entirely Good"

(Garden of the Souls 48). In this retreat—eyes closed, fierce concentrated brow furrowed—the suffering one could find the capacity to entreat God through prayer.

> This is why we have to narrow our eyes to see a distant object. We have to limit our vision so that other things should not interfere and we have to focus on the desired object to strengthen our vision... so it is when we want to look at the ultimate goal, which is all good, all unity. (Garden of the Souls, 48)

Returning, as one must always return, to the world, did not ease the suffering. In fact, Nachman realized that to live in the world was difficult; the burden was lessoned by the realization that some deeper order could be revealed, that prayer and mediation allowed a return to that state of peace.

After a series of personal losses, and after the painful death of both his wife and his infant son, Nachman gave an hours-long sermon about the meaning of suffering: suffering was endured by the Jew, and most intensely by the Jewish *tzaddik* or "righteous one, because of the reality that "each Jew is responsible for one another" and thus the sinfulness of each becomes the burden of the leaders of the community. But he refused the direct, cause-and-effect notion of suffering as a consequence of sin—rather, it was a reality of the time, place, and body of the person. It could be addressed by doctors and medication, and it could be made more or less intense by participation in a community of Torah study, daily *bitul* as a practice and the deep and lifelong struggle to understand the ultimate purpose of God to be beneficent, albeit unfathomably difficult to understand.

> Whatever evil and suffering you go through, God forbid, if you will just look at the ultimate goal—God's purpose—you will not experience it as suffering at all. The deepest truth is that there is no evil in the world, everything is good.... Then why do we feel pain when we suffer? The pain... is only because their *da-at* (divine understanding) is taken from them and they are unable to focus on the ultimate purpose, which is entirely good. (Garden of the Souls, 59)

This teaching, the "Garden of the Souls," was collected and published as a part of his corpus and widely read and studied in thousands of Eastern European Jewish communities. The idea that life is supposed to be free of suffering was an illusion, Nachman insisted, and it was surely reflected in the deepening oppression of the nineteenth century.

> Whether you are rich or poor, you cannot avoid pain. The world is filled with pain and suffering and there is no escape.... No matter who you are, you will find that the world abounds with real suffering and pain... [T]here is no escape, except in Torah. (Garden of the Soul, "Other Teachings" 76)[5]

Here, is it important to note that while pious Jews understood suffering as inevitable, it was not welcomed, nor in any sense was one passive when suffering was encountered. Doctors were sought after, and when cures proved beyond their skill, a deliberate and intellectual resistance was necessary.

For Franz Rosenzweig (1886–1929), suffering is not a distinctive experience to be theorized apart from the essential human condition—his condition and the condition of every son who loses his father. Writing after his father's death, he speaks of the inherent and essential place of suffering.

> It is true that every loss makes us more familiar with our own death, but none can bring me closer to it, none has the power to turn me out of the house of life. In spite of all losses, I still retain myself, with the unfathomable and continually surprising store of tasks that each new day brings. And each loss, by making me more familiar with death, makes me more ready for life. The less I fear death, indeed the more I love it, the more freely I can live. That is to say, the more I cease to expect happiness on this earth... if you should feel the despair of having nothing more to lose, remember what I just told you: it is only then that perfect life commences, the perfect freedom to do and suffer anything.[6]

Writing of his own physical condition, as he lies slowly and terribly dying of ALS, he notes the same "ordinariness" of suffering. Replying to a letter of sympathy from a follower, he notes:

> The words pain and suffering which you use seem quite odd to me. A condition into which one has slithered gradually, and consequently gotten used to, is not suffering but simply—a condition. A condition that leaves room for joy and suffering like any other. A Homeric god might see human life only in terms of pain and suffering. This notion is... false.... What must appear suffering when seen from outside, is actually only a sum of great difficulties that have to be overcome.[7]

And again, reflecting on his fate, he rejects the event of physical decline as a lesson or gift: "the sufferer alone is permitted to praise God in his works. But all men suffer" (163). Since suffering is essential, and ordinary, it is part, for Rosenzweig, of the "Godliness" of ordinary life. Suffering, for Rosensweig, is a part of his Jewish theological structure of wholeness:

> Everything created has a double function: first, it is simply there, it has its own being, and its own purpose. But it is also there for the sake of something else, in the final analysis for the sake of everything else. Insofar as it is itself and its own purpose, it experiences the near God. For the remote God is the God of the world, which is always a whole.... While the near God is the God of the heart, the heart which is never as much itself, and nothing but itself, as when it suffers.[8]

Suffering is a problem and a puzzle not only personally but also in a corporate sense. In a note to a poem by Judah Ha-Levi, Rosenzweig considers the problem of suffering of the Jews as a people, something he argues can best be understood as prayer or poetry. Note here how similar are themes and responses in the Nachman texts we reviewed. Rosenzweig ties individual suffering to the large narrative of peoplehood:

> He has elected his people, but elected it to visit upon them all their iniquities.... and the strands of suffering and guilt, of love and judgment, of sin and atonement, are so inextricably twisted that human hands cannot untangle them[9]

And in considering the larger problem, he notes, again, stressing prayer, like Job, as the only human response:

> .... The question as to how the Jewish people has survived all its sufferings has often been put and there have been many more or less clever... answers. The true reason... emerges in this poem. It begins with a cry from the abyss of suffering.... And in the very act of crying out... the eye still recognizes that He to whom the cry mounts is circled with stars. The unburdened mouth professes the power of Him who commands the hosts of heaven, the heart drowns in the ecstasy of beholding the glory of God—and all suffering is forgotten."[10]

John Bowker argues that Rosenzweig's view is consistent with the long tradition of complex views on suffering within Jewish thought. Bowker notes that the Hebrew Bible's concern is "not on the existence of suffering, but on the distribution of suffering." Thus, it is the problem of justice, not the existence of suffering (which, as Rosenzweig notes is the fate of all) to which the Biblical narratives turn. The rabbinic narratives cover a wide range of possible responses, as we will see in the next section of this essay.

For Emmanuel Levinas (1906–1995), the issues of suffering and its meaning are key to understanding why Judaism is " a religion for adults." In two essays about the tragic blunder that links human suffering to God's judgment, he reflects on the horror of the Shoah.

Levinas begins his essay ("Loving Torah More than God") by alluding to an essay, "purporting to be" a letter written in the last flames of the Warsaw Ghetto, by a desperate Yossel ben Yossel Rakover, a resistance fighter who has lost his entire family—wife and six children—as well as all of his friends, including, just before the letter was written, a 5-year-old boy who lies beside him as he writes. The letter is a fiction, which Levinas knows but understands as presenting an honest fictive account of actual events. ("in which everyone who has survived recognizes his own life in astonishment"). Yossel ben Yossel, after his account of his losses, still "believes in the Torah of God," in the law, justice and duties commanded be a God who is entirely absent who may even be "the God of the Nazi's."

How should a Jew reflect on this narrative, Levinas asks the reader. For Levinas, the correct way to understand the suffering described is to precisely and starkly begin the decoupling of meaning, of cause and effect, of the illusion of control from the experience of suffering:

> What is the meaning of the suffering of the innocent? Does it not bear witness to a world which is without God, to a land where man alone measures Good and Evil? The simplest and most common response to this question would lead

> to atheism. This is no doubt the sanest reaction for all those for whom up until then a God, conceived a bit primitively, distributed prizes, inflicted sanctions or pardoned faults, and in His kindness treated men as eternal children. But with what narrow-minded demons, with what strange magicians have you thus populated your sky, you who nowadays declare it to be a desert?[11]

The God of an adult, argues Levinas, manifests himself precisely in the emptiness—the noncausality—of the sky. There is no simple answer to the suffering of innocent ones, surely not that is deserved, or an expiation. Indeed, perceiving the existential absence of a "God-in-the-Sky" who allows "prizes" and "sanctions" is the first step in a fully adult religious faith.

> A God who conceals his face: I think this is neither a theologian's abstraction nor a poetic image. It is the hour when the just person has nowhere to go in the outside world: when no institution affords him protection; when even the comforting sense of the divine presence, experienced in a childlike person's piety, is withdrawn; when the only victory available to the individual lies in his conscience, which necessarily means, in suffering. This is the specifically Jewish meaning of suffering—one that never takes on the quality of a mystical expiation for the sins of the world. The condition in which victims find themselves in a disordered world, that is to say, in a world where goodness does not succeed in being victorious, is suffering. Suffering reveals a God who, while refusing to manifest Himself in any way as help, directs His appeal to the full maturity of the integrally responsible person." ("Loving Torah More than God," 3)[12]

Levinas recalls for us that the link between suffering and justice is only met by a "lived" "concrete" Jewish life. Like Nachman, Levinas asserts that living as a Jew means understanding the ultimate task of communal response—that everyone is responsible for everyone, that one's fate is tied to the fates of every soul in the garden.

"The suffering of the just for a justice which is without triumph is lived concretely as Judaism..."[13]

A key part of such a life is the continual story of the paradoxical texts themselves. God is not incarnate, and suffering is not the key to meaning.

> The characteristic features of Judaism; the relationship between God and the human person is not an emotional communion within the context of the love of an incarnate God, but a relationship between minds that is mediated by teaching, by the Torah. The guarantee that there is a living God in our midst is precisely a word of God that is not incarnate. Trust in a God who does not reveal Himself through any worldly authority can rest only on inner clarity and on the quality of a teaching[14]

Note again this theme—put forth both by Nachman and Rosenzweig—that while God is unrevealed, the Torah is revealed. The capacity for study, teaching, and performance of the Law is the response that is possible—for adults.

In other work, Levinas returns to the theme of suffering. Suffering is "useless" in that it refuses meaning and rational order—it is inchoateness itself. The suffering itself is "for nothing," and theodicy that attempts "to prove God innocent" is "a scandal." He plays on the word in French—the world for suffering and evil is the same. There is no meaning in suffering, nor does it perform any worthy task. It is entirely evil. But the world, as in Nachman, does allow a response beyond "uselessness"—the response of "use" or duty.

If theodicy is "a scandal," especially after the "malignancy of the 20th century," and we might add, the losses of the twenty-first century, then what can be said about the religious ethics and the discourse of suffering from a Jewish perspective? Levinas believes we can/must carry on the responsibility of Jewish life as teachers of Torah, whose laws and whose justice are plain, healing where we can, and answering as witness when we cannot.

Suffering and Substitution: Creating a Jewish View of Suffering for Contemporary Bioethics

We live a generation later, still in the long shadow of Jewish History. The tradition within Jewish thought allows us to understand how different theologies and histories lead to different responses to suffering in contemporary medical decision making. But how would this work in clinical practice? Let us return to the story with which we began: Talmud Bavli, Barochot, 5b.

> It has been taught: R. Simeon b. Yohai says: The Holy One, blessed be He, gave Israel three precious gifts, and all of them were given only through sufferings. These are: The Torah, the Land of Israel and the world to come. Whence do we know this of the Torah?—Because it is said: Happy is the man whom Thou chastenest, O Lord, and teachest him out of Thy law. (Ps. XCIV) Whence of the Land of Israel?—Because it is written: As a man chasteneth his son, so the Lord thy God chasteneth thee, (Deut. XXVIII) and after that it is written: For the Lord thy God bringeth thee into a good land. (Duet. XXVIII) Whence of the world to come?—Because it is written: For the commandment is a lamp, and the teaching is light, and reproofs of sufferings are the way of life. (Prov. VI:23)
>
> A Tanna recited before R. Johanan the following: If a man busies himself in the study of the Torah and in acts of charity and [nonetheless] buries his children, all his sins are forgiven him. R. Johanan said to him: I grant you Torah and acts of charity, for it is written: By mercy and truth iniquity is expiated. 'Mercy' is acts of charity, for it is said: He that followeth after righteousness and mercy findeth life, prosperity and honour. 'Truth' is Torah, for it is said: Buy the truth and sell it not. But how do you know [what you say about] the one who buries his children?—A certain Elder [thereupon] recited to him in

the name of R. Simeon b. Yohai: It is concluded from the analogy in the use of the word 'iniquity'. Here it is written: By mercy and truth iniquity is expiated. And elsewhere it is written: And who recompenseth the iniquity of the fathers into the bosom of their children.

R. Johanan says: Leprosy and [the lack of] children are not chastisements of love. But is leprosy not a chastisement of love? Is it not taught: If a man has one of these four symptoms of leprosy, it is nothing else but an altar of atonement?—They are an altar of atonement, but they are not chastisements of love.

If you like, I can say:—This [teaching of the Baraitha] is ours [in Babylonian], and that [saying of R. Johanan] is theirs [in Palestine]. If you like, I can say: This [teaching of the Baraitha] refers to hidden [leprosy], that [saying of R. Johanan] refers to a case of visible [leprosy]. But is [the lack of] children not a chastisement of love? How is this to be understood? Shall I say that he had children and they died? Did not R. Johanan himself say: This is the bone of my tenth son?—Rather [say then] that the former saying refers to one who never had children, the latter to one who had children and lost them.

R. Hiyya b. Abba fell ill and R. Johanan went in to visit him. He said to him: Are your sufferings welcome to you? He replied: Neither they nor their reward. He said to him: Give me your hand. He gave him his hand and he raised him.

R. Johanan once fell ill and R. Hanina went in to visit him. He said to him: Are your sufferings welcome to you? He replied: Neither they nor their reward. He said to him: Give me your hand. He gave him his hand and he raised him. Why could not R. Johanan raise himself?—They replied: The prisoner cannot free himself from jail.

R. Eleazar fell ill and R. Johanan went in to visit him. He noticed that he was lying in a dark room, and he bared his arm and light radiated from it. Thereupon he noticed that R. Eleazar was weeping, and he said to him: Why do you weep? Is it because you did not study enough Torah? Surely we learnt: The one who sacrifices much and the one who sacrifices little have the same merit, provided that the heart is directed to heaven. Is it perhaps lack of sustenance? Not everybody has the privilege to enjoy two tables. Is it perhaps because of [the lack of] children? This is the bone of my tenth son!—He replied to him: I am weeping on account of this beauty that is going to rot in the earth. He said to him: On that account you surely have a reason to weep; and they both wept. In the meanwhile he said to him: Are your sufferings welcome to you?—He replied: Neither they nor their reward. He said to him: Give me your hand, and he gave him his hand and he raised him.[15]

What is happening in this long complex midrash?

We are introduced to an unnamed teacher, a Tanna, which means an authority of the teaching of the Mishneh. We are in Tiberias, Palestine, in the Roman

Empire, and the culture of Rome is everywhere as dominant and oppressive as the punishing heat of the Jordan Valley. The talk has turned, in the House of Study, the Beit Midrash as described in the Talmud, to the relationship between suffering and meaning. The claim is made that the three most critical and enduring veracities in a Jew's life, amid the chaos of Roman occupation, the Torah, the land, and the world to come, are related to each other because they are given only after punishments. In the word play that is the serious business of the Talmud, they make that point by finding three times that the word "chastisements" is used in linkage with these three things. The Tanna leading the discussion makes an assured statement: If a man studies Torah, and if he does acts of charity, his sins are forgiven him. Even if the mans' sins have been so great, he implies, that his children have died as a result of them.

The text insinuates that this is Rabbi Eleazer's meaning—at least Rabbi Johanan, his student, takes it this way. Enter Johanan, who will become a central figure in rabbinic texts,[16] the compiler of the Jerusalem Talmud, and the intellectual leader of the Jerusalem community.[17] He is noted to be always unbearded, and is the most perfectly beautiful man in the rabbinic imagination, and it is a tender beauty, a famously womanly beauty, so striking that once, bathing naked in the Jordan, he is perused by Resh Lakish, who perhaps takes him for, as a woman, a sexual conquest. His beauty is compared to a freshly minted silver vase, filled with red roses, the sun striking the silver, shadows playing across the flowers—a rich, gorgeous image of female beauty. (Think here of Georgia O'Keefe!) Johanan is a student of the Tanna and, we are told, a particularly obedient student, a particularly careful one. He is an orphan, raised by his grandfather, and taken to the Beit Midrash as a child. He states in another section of the Talmud, that every word of the Mishneh is absolute, with the status of the Mosaic law. Not here. He has here the "text" of his own life that he (literally, it will turn out) wears on his body.

He has had ten sons, and they have all died—he has buried every single one.

Johanan answers steadily to his teacher: How do you know anything about the father who digs the hole in the earth and, shovel by shovel, buries his children there? How can you know this? Another unnamed older teacher replies: but here is the proof text, the parallel of language is the same! And the *Tanna Kamma* (the Elder) shows that this trick of the word game binds the literal moral universe together.

But Johanan, this time, still steadily objects: illness, and the loss of children—these are not "the chastisements of love." It is a flat statement.

The elders argue back: (one thinks of Job's friends here,) but it has been taught, in the *text*! The mark of illness is an "alter of atonement," meaning that the bearer of illness is marked by his suffering and his redemption, his pain and his penance.

Perhaps his own illness is, replies Johanan, perhaps it is that the ill body is this "alter of atonement," the place of sacrifice and of amends. But the illness, that is not a condemnation of a loving God.

Then the argument seems to shift to an attempt to use language to resolve the tension that has built up steadily in the scene. The Elder, or perhaps another voice, argues: let me put it this way, if you like. He offers to compromise. The teaching of the Mishneh will hold in the exiled community of Babylonia, but in Palestine, in the Beit Midrash of those who know Johanan (and his personal tragedy), his opinion holds, and we will not challenge it. Or, if you like, we can say, continues the other voice, another compromiser, we can say that the Mishnah refers to hidden illness, and Johanan is referring to the horrific catastrophe of visible illness.

But what about the *children*, what will you say about that, persists another voice in the text, perhaps the *stam*, or editor.

The text insists that we cannot turn away from the original problem. How can the death of children possibly be understood as having anything to do with a reprimand of love from God? Can it be even said neutrally, without moral resonance? That "he had children and that they just died?" And someone speaks up, An Amora, teacher in a later generation years after the original argument in historical time, but the debate is not finished: "Remember our teacher, himself, saying: this is the bone of my tenth son?"

And that stops the debate, the image of the Rabbi Johanan, with the bones of his last, lost baby son carried in his pocket, held in his hands as he argues the law of healing. Here, the narrative abruptly breaks off, and suddenly we are in the midst of the actions of healing that have occurred long before.

We are in a sick room, and we "see" Johanan at work as a healer. He is at the bedside of Rabbi Hiyya b. Abba, one of his old teachers, perhaps the unnamed one who had argued with him in the earlier passage. Johanan asks his patient about the meaning of his sufferings: are they welcome? It seems to be a kind of informed consent negotiation—do you want my intervention, or would you prefer that I do not touch you? And the sick man is clear that he would want the intervention, that the illness is not bearable, nor is he learning anything of spiritual value. No, not the illness, not the suffering, and not any possible spiritual reward for my bearing of them. At that, Johanan "gives" him his hand, and raises him from the bed, presumably having cured him.

But then the scene shifts again, and this time we have Johanan in bed, ill and vulnerable, and another teacher and great friend, the healer Hanina is there to visit. What is not said is also important: Hanina and Johanan have had a dispute so profound that Johanan has left the Sepphoris, where he studied as Hanina's pupil, to found an academy in Tiberias. And, later in the story of this deep and complex friendship, things will reverse again, and Hanina will die just as Johanan hurries to his bedside, and he will mourn his teacher as a son mourns a father, tearing his clothes, all the "thirteen that he wore."[18] But first this story of Johanan, the ill healer, and Hanina, the one to heal.

The exact question is asked: Tell me, is there meaning, goodness, welcome in illness? And the answer is exactly the same as well. No, and the act of hand-to-hand healing is accomplished.

But a voice interrupts—but wait a minute! Isn't this the great healer? Didn't he just heal the other guy? And the answer is given: but now he is imprisoned by the illness, and he cannot free himself without this help, without both the question of meaning and the human gesture of friendship, embodied connection, and tangible response.

There is more. Now another scene: Rabbi Eleazar is now in the bed. He is a student of both Hanina, and of Johanan, and Eleazar is one who has disappointed Johanan in the past. He is now ill, Johanan now well, the healer again. The room is dark, and it is a bleak time. There is terrible tragedy for the society, they are driven from Yavnah by Roman oppression, and in Babylon the Zoroastrians have seized power. The lighting of fires, including the kindling of the Sabbath candles, is forbidden and must be done secretly. It is a dark time for Johanan as well. He is a failed healer.

And in this darkness, Johanan lifts his arm from his scholar's cloak, from his thirteen garments, and holds it up, and it fills the darkness with light. And when the younger man sees this, he begins to cry. Johanan, the healer, asks why: Is it regret, that you have not studied enough, is it poverty, or is it that you have had few children? He attempts to comfort him—what matters is intention, not quantity, wealth is not important, many are poor. And finally, startlingly, he takes that shining hand from the air and puts it into his pocket and takes out that last bone from his last dead son, his youngest son, the trump card of loss itself. Some translate this bone as the tooth of his son, perhaps the bone imagery is too stark, or perhaps they do mean the tooth, and I, the feminist scholar, imagine this, that he carries the baby tooth of his last baby boy.

But Eleazar is not crying for himself, he is crying for the whole tragic journey of mortality itself. He is struck by the understanding that he, the lost children, and finally even the beautiful, sad, gifted teacher, the very image of rabbinic power, the wounded healer, filled with the light of faith in the midst of darkness, even that, will be lost. (And here a modern reader is powerfully reminded of the Catholic poet and priest, Gerald Manley Hopkins, "It is Margaret that I mourn for.")

I am weeping, he says, on your account, on the account of all that beauty that is going to rot in the earth. And we are back to burial, to the red clay of the Galilee piled shovel by shovel over the graves that have been theorized at the beginning of the section. For this, Johanan tells his patient, for mortality itself, for seeing the fate of us both, you surely have a reason for existential grief, beyond that which I can talk you out of.

And the healer and his patient sit in the room, and they weep together, the reversal of self and other, healer and patient fully accomplished. After a while, the ritualized question and the ritualized response, I find no meaning in this, and I want rescue, and the healer, not with incantations, and not with potions, though both are fully available as textual strategies (and both are used by Hanina and other rabbinic healers, for example, in other texts of healing). He gives him his hand, which is to say, gives him the relationship of one embodied mortal self to another, hand to hand, body to body, substitution, for you, doctor, could be you, patient, and Jewish thought reminds us of this. It seems the story is completed.

But we, as readers of the story in the section of the Talmud on Blessings, know more about the characters from another section of the Talmud, Baba Metzia, in which these same characters appear. We know that the healer Johanan has once famously refused to heal, and it was a terrible turning away. Johanan's dearest friend, the man who had surprised him in the river, Resh Lakish, becomes trained by Johanan, marries his sister, and challenges him in the language games of study. But suddenly there is a disputation, and Johanan mocking refers to Lakish's past as a warrior, and perhaps a corrupt one. Lakish never speaks to him again and becomes mysteriously ill. As he lies dying, Lakish's wife, who is, of course, Johanan's sister, comes to beg him to visit him, to see him, to heal him with both the gifts and light for which he is famous, and to engage him in the study of Torah which heals. But despite her pleas—"Look at me!" "See my face!"—Johanan will not see her, nor will he look at the face of his friend. And when his friend dies, Johanan steadily loses his mind and wanders lost. His colleagues bring him Eleazar to study with, but Eleazar is not Lakish and cannot comfort nor heal him (which is to say, cannot argue with him cogently enough) (Baba Metzia). He takes to standing at the gates of the city, calling out, "Son of Lakish! Where are you!" He becomes so hysterical, so lost, that the rabbis pray for his death, and he does die. And that is the tragic end of Johanan in that narrative. Note how it is existential loneliness that is fatal, and note how in our other text, it is the capacity for companionship in suffering (even irredeemable suffering) that allows healing to occur and pain to be mitigated. Reading the two stories together—as one can assume Jews have done since the Talmud was codified, presents a meta-argument over the textual argument, as if several people crowded into the room of the tale: memory and community entering the narrative.

But even the logic of the text looks odd—the tale is repeated three times, perhaps there has been some mistake? Since the same story is told in different ways, it suggests that perhaps the writer of the text had got it wrong, didn't know which was the real story, and just left all the versions in the last draft. But that is not my understanding. In fact, I think that the whole point of the story is the exactness of the odd retelling of the same scene and the peculiarities of the way that the figure in the bed switches from being the person of Johanan to the persons of his teacher and student. The reversal then not only teaches us about the nature of mortality, that haunting question that Eleazar will raise in the last bit of story, but also serves as a commentary on the first premise, the relationship between suffering and meaning, and one's just deserts.

Through it all, the healer-teacher carries his bone, the tangible symbol of loss itself. We are introduced to this bone, which is to say, the body, the blood, and the sacrifice, in the first paragraph, and we see it reemerge at the end. Hence, for the entire narrative, that bone grounds us in the physicality of the grief. And it is this sense that allows Johanan his point, that it is not illness, nor loss, that allows for redemption, but the responsive act of healing that allows for it.

It is not reading too much into the language, I think, to make this claim. The story has been left "open," the rabbinic discussion is interrupted by the action itself.

Here we see the struggle to decide what is the meaning of the words left to us by the academy. But unlike the Greek symposium, the conversation, while important, must be interrupted—stopped by an action, the moral gesture of healing, which is, of course, for the rabbis of the Talmud, primarily another sort of conversation, the talk with the ill person.

Here, the text seems to be saying: "do you want to know the meaning and the moral value of suffering, the weight of the mark of leprosy? Ask the one at the center of the issue, the patient himself."[19] Starting with this idea of asking the patient the moral value of suffering centers the problem of healing on the other, not the self, and it allows for more—it means that the ill one, who in the first part of the conversation in the house of study only appears as the object of the gaze—the visible sign of atonement—becomes the subject of the talk, and importantly the one whose words will guide your actions. It is to this that we can draw our first conclusion of what is being asked and answered by the healing gesture. The meaning of healing is first, then, conversive, as in the sense of being a participant in a conversation about value, and in this, it is the patient's value that is determinative (something, I might add, that modern American medicine finds difficult). Let me note here that it is clearly not that the healer has nothing to offer, so that he might as well play a secondary role; it is that not that he is merely attending to the ill person, because he would have every reason for simply coming in, giving his hand, and doing that which works every time, raising the patient up to heal. There is something required of the healer in the exchange, more than this as remedy.

Something else, the text argues, might be required at this juncture, and it is clearly consent, even to a question that the healer knows the answer—or, perhaps, this is what we are being told—this is why Johanan does know the answer! And it is the responsible action—the response-able action that is the gesture of healing. In the ritual that is repeated each time, the healer must give his hand—not place his upon the head of the patient, like a superior to an inferior, but *give up his hand into the hand of the other.* The hand of the healer is taken by the patient as opposed to the other way around. And only then, when the classic trust gesture of equality and friendship is made, only then can the healing "work."

The next story in our section of the Talmudic passage pulls us deeper into the problem, for here, suddenly, the hero of our story until now is himself ill, marked by atonement, suffering. It is in this sense also that healing is conversive, as in reversed, as in having to be "turned around" (which is to say, in Hebrew, to do *teshuvah,* to change course). This time, Johanan is answering the questions that he has asked and will ask of the other. He is the object of the healing ritual—he is given to, and he takes. It is this ability to reverse that lies at the heart of the healing act. Unlike a medical dictum that teaches that the ill are different from us, to be pitied, to bear some complex burden for us, or to be object in our moral world, the ill are us, we; each of us is a participant, and we are interrupted ourselves by illness and suffering, the humanness that we share, that is the essential part of healing.

And finally, in case that point is not fully made, there will be one more story, the dark room of illness entered one more time, the story interrupted yet again by another story. Here we have Johanan enter, well again, as healer, to the bedside of the man that will be later sent to heal him (in the part of the story not mentioned here, but that you, reader, must remember.[20]) But the talk is far more detailed and starker. Because the sick room is full of such darkness (of despair? of death?) that he cannot see the face of his patient, and one must, clearly see the face of the partner in the conversation, and sees the body of the ill one. He first raises his arm, naked. It radiates light to fill the room—the act of healing has a power to change the world. But this act, a display of beauty and potency, of the tools of healing, perhaps a kind of arrogance—will not be what is needed, in fact, it seems to make it all worse, and the patient breaks down. Then Johanan seems annoyed, trying first to argue him out of his sobbing and, finally, tries to tell him his suffering is not fully warranted compared with the broken healer's own heart, to his own broken life. Here, words fail—he shows him the relic itself, and it flashes white in the dark room, held in that golden radiant hand, a man carrying the death around. "I, too," says this part of the conversation that stops even the language of conversation, "I, too" am horribly marked, and there is no alter of atonement on which to place the body of my son, not the alter, not the temple, not the rock of the Akedah (Genesis 22) beneath the temple, an image that floods beneath the text (and beneath all sacrifice at that place) at this moment.

But this is precisely the point—it is the recognition that the human is limited and is mortal, that even the beauty, and even the power, fleeting, that is the truest thing that can be said between them, spoken, again by the patient, that allows the patient and the healer to reverse most powerfully. As we are in the dark box of the room, we are in the dark box of our own mortality, and in the dark of the earth itself we will return.

But the rabbis are not entirely existential, they are practical prophets after all, and the text has a way of going on: it is the action of healing. After a time in tears, the work of a commanded life must go on—the mitzvot (commandments) are as clear to them as they are to our contemporaries—that healing is mandated. And, finally, this is the answer to the suffering—healing is the answer. And it is this that is the *altar of atonement* in this place, the Palestinian world in which the pragmatism of Johanan will be decisive—it is not the theory, but the practice of healing the actual person in pain. Truthful telling, seeing the tragedy of limits, is what then allows for the phroneses (the practical wisdom) of healing.

As Emmanuel Levinas notes for us, truth telling is the first act of ethics:

> To hear a voice speaking to you is *ipso facto* to accept obligation toward the one speaking. Intelligibility does not begin in self-certainty, in the coincidence with one's self from which one can give oneself time and a provisional morality, trying everything, and letting oneself be tempted by everything. Intelligibility is a fidelity to the true; it is incorruptible and prior to any human enterprise.[21]

Hearing always, and telling truthfully, and fully (these are the bones of my dead) begins the act of healing. Note, here, the connection between truthfulness to the other and truthfulness about obligation, an obligation taken on fully, and taken on faith.

But truth is only the first act of healing. Let us return to the problem of expiation. Here, the rabbis of the Talmud struggled with a real crisis, perhaps most critically the rabbis most involved in the act of healing. For in the period of the Second Temple and before, the disease, especially the leprosy alluded to in the original argument, had clear biblical therapeutic interventions. The leper was required to bring animal sacrifices to the real Altar of Atonement, and the blood of the slain animals was used to cleanse the affected place of leprosy. The healers, the priests, had elaborate interventions and rituals for a practice of the healing. The Jews controlled the state then, so the entire civic-religious system could function for quarantine, for reentry, and for the explanation of illness. But in the darkness of the Roman rule, where the Jews were unarmed—or rather that they had nothing but their own bright arms, their own hands—the entire system of healing was disrupted, the narrative flow of Biblical edict, physical act, and spiritual redemption, destroyed.

What will be done? If the priests cannot come sweeping into your house, hands full of birds, and the cedar-wood, and hyssop and scarlet, and light them into a sweet bright fire, and clean the walls with the blood, and wipe the wings of the birds with blood, and set them free out of the windows and the doors, as is described in Leviticus, what exactly can the healer do? If the healing priests cannot slaughter the goat, and place his hands in its blood, and wipe the blood on your right ear, your right hand and your right foot, and then drip the healing oil on your right ear, your right hand and your right foot, what can be done instead? If you cannot strip off your blood-soaked garments, all of you at the ritual, and if the healed one and the healer cannot go to the Great Baths, and then to the Temple again, with noise and gladness and the songs of the Levites, the gold of the gates in the mountain sun, what can possibly replace this?

And these quiet healer texts tell us: you must come into a dark and desperate room, and you must sit, and you must listen to the voice of the other in need. And when the other asks for the truth about death, you must tell him, and in this act, you must seek justice. What you are obliged to be is the one who can hear the voice of the one who is vulnerable, and if you can, then the loss of might and State power will not disrupt that which is central to the world, the intimate and daily acts of justice upon which the world depends.

For it is justice—*tzedakah*—which has the dual meaning in Hebrew of both social justice and of charitable acts. The other is not an event for you, a commodity for you, nor a job for you. It is a challenge—the other, *as you, after all*, are the one who demands that the sickened world, and the sickness of alienation, and the dark room of the unfair and incomprehensible fate of illness be lit up with your presence your very body, in all of its limits and all of its light. The texts of justice cannot be unhitched from the rabbinic understanding of healing. "For the commandment is a lamp, and the teaching is light, and reproofs of sufferings are the way of life" (Prov. VI:23).

If the commandments are the lamp, and if teaching the commandments is the light that radiates from it, and suffering is the way of the world, then in this story, in the life without the Temple, the human healer who enacts the commandment literally becomes a lamp, his body filled with light, transformed, thus linking the continuous text together as one whole. As David Hartman explains, healing stands in for the entire enterprise of human responsibility.[22]. In an unjust world, then, and certainly now, in which a great deal of what reads as illness and suffering is caused by indifference, greed, and injustice—in an unjust world, the gesture of medicine and of healing might be the essential gesture of justice itself. How do we answer the darkness of leprosy, which in the Biblical period clearly meant the illness of the soul, the illness of the society? We answer, now, with ritual of a far different sort, the hand in the hand of another, the light of sheer beauty transformed into the warm of the hand at the end of the story. And the blood that is streaked everywhere is the blood of the healer, the sacrifice of the animal, transformed into the sacrifice of the self to the other, and in this case, also the way that being a father and a teacher has meant loss of son, student, and brother.

For Levinas, the utter chaos of the world is mirrored by the utter enormity of our responsibility. Reading Levinas, I think of our dilemmas in modern bioethics: Should the healer stand outside the case, should she not use everything in her power to alleviate suffering? Can she be overwhelmed by the context, the tragedy, or the helplessness that "leaves not a corner" of the sensible world intact? Is she not to be marked, and not to think of her body and the body of the patient as, in a way, fundamentally interchangeable?

Johanan the healer is as marked by blood as the lost altar of the temple. It is the healer, and not the ill one, that is the "altar of atonement," and it is the act of healing, in physical, tangible ways, that restores order and justice to the world. And we are, hence, restored to the first claim that Johanan has made: that it is acts of *tzedakah* that heal the world, justice that will stand in for the system of sacrifice and return.

I (will) grant you (that) Torah and acts of charity (can absolve sin,) for it is written: By mercy and truth iniquity is expiated. "Mercy" is acts of charity, for it is said: He that followeth after righteousness and mercy findeth life, prosperity, and honor.

In the Yom Kippur liturgy, three things both replace the Temple sacrifice and mediate the harsh sentences of the year to come: *teshuvah,* which usually means repentance, but for this account, let us say "reversal into the other"; *tzedakah*, charity and hence justice; and *tefillah*, prayer. Healing at its heart is reversal and justice, *teshuvah, tzedakah*, and for the rabbis, perhaps prayer is that which allows us to hear first the cry of the one in need. For the Jewish tradition that argues that evil is not inherent, nor sin an inevitable fate, nor sufferings the punishment for frail and flawed human choices, the problem is largely about what to do next, and next, what to do to repair the rupture of the communal memory, how to pass on the truthful talk. In this essay, I have argued that the turn to Torah, duty, and healing is the correct response to suffering. I have made the claim that whenever the point is made that links the suffering of innocents to sin, or to redemption, there is another voice that refutes that idea. That not only is true in the Talmudic passage but also is embedded in the Biblical tradition, when the idea that sin leads to suffering is put into the mouths of Job's foolish friends; in the rabbinic tradition; and in the texts of medieval and modern Jewish thought, from Hassidic masters and academic philosophers alike.

Suffering, argues this voice within Jewish tradition, needs not to be explained in terms of God's plan, nor offered up as mimetic action, nor celebrated, nor sought. It is to be opposed. The correct response is to ask how to find life in the middle of death, healing in the dark room of death, to raise again from the dark understanding that mortality cannot be defeated by even by the best medicine, but must be risen from all the same. It is about what to do and how to carry on in the face of this knowledge. In this text, the suggestion is made by the structure of the story itself and by the simple gestures across a bed, 2000 years ago and rivers and oceans away, remembered and carried, like the beloved's white bone. We only understand the healer after we have seen him at work, after we have "heard" him and allowed him to hear the ones he is healing, after the discursive universe, and thus the moral world is set right by simple acts of goodness.

Conclusion

It is my claim that the relationship between the healer and the ill can be extrapolated and theorized here as a fruitful way to understand the role that suffering plays in the twenty-first century, when we, as readers of the historical textual tradition, come to differ with our Christian, Buddhist, and Hindu colleagues, for example, about the centrality of suffering.

I am going to suggest a few things about suffering and Jewish ethics, and in particular, for the discourse of modern bioethics. Why this is critical is obvious: in the past decade, the differences about the meaning of suffering have dominated debates about both end-of-life care and advances in new scientific research such as stem cell science. The claim has been made that support for such research and support for the discontinuation of intensive care are wrong because they suggest that we have as a goal the elimination of human suffering. For Christians, this is a disturbing idea. But for Jewish bioethicist, for whom suffering plays no redemptive role, it seems like a very good idea indeed.

The first point is methodological. Let me first argue that reading texts in which the narratives of suffering are debated allows an important voice within Jewish tradition to be heard. This method of writing about Jewish texts and their mobilization to support the moral gesture of medicine can be enriched by a narrative approach that is rooted in the aggadic (storytelling) as well as the halachic (legal) tradition because, in most cases, as Wimpfhiemer and other argue, the two occur together.[23] Reading texts in this way is different from reading secondary sources that codify law, and it expresses the complexities and shifting positions of the texts.

The second point is a claim about the content of a Jewish response to suffering. The primary act of healing involves not only the direct encounter with the other, on both the physical embodied level, but also a direct encounter with the other at the moral and existential level, meaning that to be a healer is to be willing to participate in the act of moral reversal and reciprocity.

And finally, I would argue that the entire moral argument behind this Jewish view of healing is that medicine is an act of justice, the response of the human, the argument of the human hand, against an unjust and as yet unredeemed and darkened world. This claim lies clearly within the tradition as expressed by Nachman, Rosenzweig, and Levinas—that suffering requires a correspondent response. Medicine, and the research science that pushes medicine forward, is a gift, it is never opposed or denied. The right to medical care is an act of basic justice. It may not be sufficient, and the essay notes that the need for witness in the face of suffering, indeed, a capacity for empathy so profound that it allows imaginative reversal, is part of what the healer is expected to provide.

Jewish thought, I would claim in this chapter, argues the that arc of Jewish theology and philosophy can be directed to serious policy decisions informed by the view that human suffering can be—and must be—elevated by all our efforts. It is not our capacity for suffering that makes us human. It is our capacity for response.

Jewish thought, argues this text, and I would claim in this essay, argues the arc of Jewish philosophy, is directed to clinical contexts and the pursuit of emerging research, and is expressed in the policies of states that drive ahead, relentlessly, to fund quests to alleviate, address, and yes, to seek to eliminate suffering—all this can be understood as the best possible pursuit in Jewish thought.

This is dramatically different from many traditions within religious ethics. There is little anxiety in our tradition about whether a world with less suffering would be less spiritual or less moral. There is a long tradition that rejects the experience of suffering of individuals or of the Jewish people as a sign of judgment in the tradition of modern Jewish thought. Instead, there exists a deep understanding that the brokenness of the world, the groaning of the world, the inexplicable tragedies of human existence say little about the nature of God and much about the work before us. Suffering's existence in our befallen creaturely lives creates primary duties of one to another, and the small responses: study, abundant generosity, the careful attention to a Law that exists when the law of state has fallen and the "order of the city" has failed are all that is available, and all that is required. The steady working within history to repair history's catastrophe and the steady acts of healing, of person and place, the living for justice in a time of injustice—these are the workings of theology and ethics of a suffering world.

Notes

1. Barochot, 5b, *Soncino Talmud* (CD ROM) (Davka Publications, 1998).
2. Maimonides, "Guide of the Perplexed" 3, 8–25.

3. Buber, "Martin, Good and Evil" (1952).

4. Emmanuel Levinas, "To the Other" (1985).

5. Nachman, Garden of the Souls, op. cit. 76.

6. Franz Rosenzweig, *Franz Rosenzweig, His Life and Work, edited and collected by Nachum N. Glazer*. (New York: Shocken Books, 1961), 66

7. Ibid, 142.

8. Ibid, 281.

9. Ibid., 305.

10. Ibid., 349.

11. Emmanuel Levinas, "Loving Torah More than God," in *Difficult Freedom: Essays on Judaism*, ed. Sean Hand (London: Athlone, 1991), 145.

12. Ibid., 146.

13. Ibid., 148.

14. Ibid., 148.

15. Barochot, 5b, op. cit.

16. Daniel Boyarin, "Rabbis and Their Pals," in *Unheroic Conduct: the Rise of Heterosexuality and the Invention of the Jewish Man* (Berkeley: University of California Press, 1997), 127–151.

17. Gersom Bader, *The Encyclopedia of Talmudic Sages*, trans. Solomon Katz. (Northvale, NJ: Jason Aronson, 1988), 481.

18. Ibid., 530.

19. Taking "him" to mean the actual men that the rabbis were nearly always thinking about.

20. For this to work, one must imagine the world of the Talmud, in which this occurred—the story, remember, is being told years later by the students, as a flashback memory after Johanan has died. But having Eleazar here in this text functions neatly in the scheme of reversal.

21. Emmanuel Levinas, *Nine Talmudic Readings* (Bloomington: Indiana University Press, 1993), 45; R. Nachman, *Gardens of the Soul: Rebe Nachman on Suffering*, from Likutey Moharan, trans./ed. Avraham Greenbaum (Jerusalem: Breslov Research Institute, 1990).

22. David Hartman, *The Living Covenant: The Innovative Spirit in Traditional Judaism* (New York, Free Press, 1985), 229–230. I was lead to this work by Noam Zohar in his book, *Alternatives in Jewish Bioethics* (Albany: State University of New York Press, 1997); Emmanuel Levinas, "Useless Suffering" and "Loving the Torah More than God," op. cit.; Franz Rosenzweig, *Collected Writings*, op. cit.

23. Barry Wimpfhiemer, *Narrating the Law* (Philadelphia: University of Pennsylvania Press, 2011).

15

Human Suffering through Illness in the Context of Islamic Bioethics

Abdulaziz Sachedina

As an Abrahamic religion, Islam is a theocentric tradition in which the all-powerful God exercises limitless power in managing all aspects of creation, including wellness and illness, whether individual or collective. Suffering through illness can occur through natural causes over which humans have no control; or, it may occur as a result of bad habits. Naturally caused physical evil functions as a grim reminder of human fragility and mortality, whether the source of misfortune is an external power like God or the internal agency of human fallibility. In Islam, the suffering that attends such natural or physical evil, combining personal culpability with circumstances beyond human control, is often regarded as some sort of divinely sanctioned evil inflicted to teach humanity in general a lesson in humility. By contrast, the guilt and suffering that attend the evil perpetrated by a free human agent are often viewed as the just deserts of the wrongdoer. Accordingly, it is possible to draw correlations between the freely committed evil and the personal suffering endured by the human author of the evil. What is clear, though, is that the foundational sources of Islamic teachings, Qur'an and the tradition, prescribe maintaining good health as a duty. Physical and psychological health cannot be taken for granted—they are a divine benefaction that depends on human moderation in food and drink and regular physical activities, including swimming and horse riding, as the founder of Islam, Prophet Muhammad instructed his followers. However, there are people who suffer from illnesses that are genetically transmitted, in which case they have exercised no choice whatsoever. Who is the author of this suffering? Is it God's determination? Or do human choices somehow play a role?

These troublesome questions constitute a major challenge to the belief in God's justice and goodness. Muslims, like other peoples of faith, have struggled to reconcile God's omnipotence with the persistent evils of the world, including the pain and suffering that attend illness. I do not wish to treat the problem of suffering beyond the context of Islamic biomedical ethics. My objective in raising the issue of suffering in this chapter is to demonstrate the importance of understanding religious and cultural attitudes among Muslims that influence their choices in health care and medical treatment. The principle of "No harm, no harassment"—which means there shall be no harming, injuring, or hurting of one human by another, in the first instance, nor in return, or requital, as taught by the Prophet—has become the major source of bioethical decisions in the Muslim community and obliges an active response to unparalleled medical advancements in prolonging the life span of terminally ill patients.

The predominant theological belief among the majority of Muslims is in predestination, and yet, it is refreshing to observe a transformation from thoroughgoing fatalism to choice-oriented human action in modern times. This shift to activist theology is subtle yet noticeable in the areas of biomedical ethics and protection of human rights. The classical theological notions of resignation and submission in the face of death and suffering have yielded to a growing awareness of the possibilities offered by modern medicine. In addition, modern education, with its assertive operational agnostic culture, has minimized the influence of superstitious beliefs about the human body and its ailments; yet even today, the perceived impact of hidden maleficent powers still plagues large sectors of Muslim rural populations that lack access to adequate health care facilities.

Religion and Culture in Muslim Attitudes toward Medical Treatment

Given the diversity in Muslim cultures, different ethnic groups that make up this diversity are not a monolithic population when it comes to understanding illness and wellness. Muslims with different cultural backgrounds approach suffering with a wide range of deeply entrenched traditional and religious attitudes about its causes and consequences. Sometimes, these attitudes undermine the efficacy of treatments that require the patient to summon the will to fight the disease. A holistic medical approach, which treats both psychosomatic and physical conditions, obliges clinicians to be aware of the patient's emotional condition and cultural background in order to formulate an accurate diagnosis and successful treatment plan. It is important, therefore, to promote sensitivity to the patient's religious and traditional presuppositions about the nature of suffering.[1]

Promoting such sensitivity to the patient's presuppositions requires an investigation of illness viewed as a form of evil. Such an inquiry should seek to furnish objective criteria by which serious medical conditions are perceived as evil. Such criteria will enable health care providers and ethicists to understand, articulate, and address preconceptions that foster despair and loss of confidence in the fight against life-threatening diseases. Generally, a situation that is negatively described as evil refers to an objective state of affairs ("It is unbearable!") as well as a subjective response ("It is harmful for the patient!") of a judging individual. In other words, assessing suffering as a form of evil, either objectively or subjectively, requires a recognition of the agent, the act of suffering, and any potential harm, all of which can influence a positive or a privative understanding of evil. When both subjective and objective elements are present in an illness, the resulting suffering is sometimes deemed to be undesirable and maleficent. Both physically and morally, such judgments posit an objective standard that most people would judge as tragically harmful to the agent, without any reference to any ontology or complex metaphysical or theological explanation.

This is the point at which physical dimensions of medical care come to terms with human condition and limitations of human endeavors to alleviate suffering. Whereas the Qur'an teaches humility and reveals human limitations in comprehending the ways of the powerful and yet compassionate God, who gives and takes life, medicine, taking the responsibility for removing the evil of pain and suffering, seeks a cure or at least a prolongation of life, irrespective of the wishes or intentions of any divine agency. The Islamic approach to illness inculcates faith in God's goodness and an acceptance of suffering as part of the overall divine plan for humanity's spiritual and moral development. Whereas medicine takes the entire responsibility for determining a patient's life span through technological intervention, the Qur'an emphasizes human finitude and reminds humanity not to defy God's will to take life at a predetermined time known to God alone. In the Muslim view, when the time comes for the person to depart, then she has to leave everything behind: family, wealth, and status: "All that dwells upon the earth shall perish; except the face of thy Lord, majestic and splendid" (Q. 55:26).

To be sure, medical practice seeks to cure or lessen the illnesses that cause pain and suffering. The relief of human suffering through curing and healing is the main justification for investing large sums of money in health care institutions in the world. Because all humans will experience illness at some point in their lives, both physicians and nurses are obliged to approach suffering with the requisite cultural-religious sensitivity. Modern bioethics, deeply rooted in the dominant secular culture marked by a radical reduction of the religious to the moral, tends to ignore theological questions connected with understanding of the evil of human suffering, whether divinely ordained or humanly acquired. By contrast, religion-based bioethics emphasizes the divine will and nurtures hope and trust in God in the face of incurable illness. Hence, understanding suffering is central to Islamic bioethics.[2] In the context of health care, the idea of God's omnipotence has enormous implications, breeding a quietism that discourages the ill from prying into God's unfathomable ways and encourages resignation to suffering. With modern medicine's enormous strides in healing the sick and alleviating suffering, the inexorability of God's decrees provides little comfort to those who want to see an end to agonies of incurable diseases.

Muslim theologians have striven to comprehend the rationale of suffering, for instance, of children and even animals. Whereas, explaining the causes of suffering of bad people, even though unconvincing, has been easier because of the causal link drawn between sins and suffering by majority of Muslim theologians, what sins can one count for the suffering of the innocent children?

Suffering of the innocent is liable to make people doubt God's goodness, even if such suffering turns out to be the cause of some greater good. In a similar vein, the promise of the future reward of the righteous in the hereafter does little to placate the fear of earthly misery and suffering. The idea of predetermined suffering implicates God in the authorship of an act that seems to cause both physical and moral evil. More critically, the problem of undeserved physical evil generates a struggle between hope and despair—an inner conflict that arises often in the face of the grim reality of inherited diseases like cancer. In their endeavor to absolve God from any blame of concocting physical evil, Muslim theologians defended God's goodness, asserting that whatever happens "happens for the best." They devoted a great deal more attention to God's omnipotence than to human freedom, pushing the problem of evil deep into the realm of theology, thereby pushing the ethics and psychology aside. Ironically, the more they conflated the problem of evil with God's absolute will, the more they absolved human beings from assuming responsibility for the moral evil. The ethical dimension of evil with moral culpability was important in acquitting God for non-natural evil, which occurred as a consequence of human free will, with each person fully responsible for the choices he or she made. The neglect of psychological dimension of evil had ramifications in the field of education where human behavior is scrutinized in terms of human intention and capacity to execute the plan to perform an action, good or bad. In both these dimensions, some Muslim thinkers undertook to explain the ethical and psychological dimensions of human action and individual responsibility for moral evil.[3]

In the recent case of inoculation against polio in Nigeria, the religious authorities discouraged Muslims from getting inoculated because, as they contended, there was a Western conspiracy in such an encouragement that was designed to make Muslims sterile, and that in turn was against the will of God, who had determined that the Muslim community will be the most numerous in comparison with other faith communities. It is not uncommon to observe such conspiracy theories in third-world countries, Africa, and the Middle East that, at their worst, generate passivity and resignation among the people living under the most unacceptable conditions of poverty and inflicted with incurable diseases. The increase in the number of AIDS sufferers in African countries has been blamed on the religious attitudes that perpetrate deterministic quietist theology based on the sin-suffering doctrine.[4]

The Qur'an, regards the world—that which exists—as being equivalent to good. Everything is inherently good; if it is evil, it is so only in a relative, privative sense. The mosquito that causes malaria is not evil in itself. It is evil because it is harmful to humans and causes disease. In other words, that which is created is a thing in and of itself, and hence a true existence; contingent existence has no place in the order of being and is not real. That which is real must derive its being from the Creator. Only those things and attributes are real that exist outside the mind. Relative attributes are created by the mind and have no existence outside it.

Accordingly, it is not the act in itself that is evil. In fact, it is almost neutral. It receives its classification only through the divine command, which in its turn correlates to the objective nature of good. However, this objective good is good because God has created it as such. It is subject neither to rational thinking nor questioning. It is God's will alone that determines its value. There are no criteria that can in any way limit or determine God's absolute will. So evil in the Qur'an is not defined by any reference to an objective criterion in itself but is reduced to that which, if performed, transgresses the limits set by God's command. This is, then, a religious ethics of obedience to divine command.[5]

Suffering Caused by Illness or Loss of Good Health

Just as the Qur'an treats evil and human afflictions as the part of the overall plan for human spiritual and moral growth, so the traditions ascribed to the Prophet elaborate on the ramifications of the belief in God's omnipotence and omniscience and its impact upon human well-being. In general, the treatment of suffering caused by illness or loss of good health appears to have been taken up in the light of certain theological positions maintained about the divine will and human will. Hence, there are traditions that speak of illness as a form of divinely ordained suffering based on the belief that God is the author of all that befalls human beings. In fact, such traditions have been the major source of quietism and an attitude of resignation toward seeking medical treatment in some quarters of Muslim society because God is regarded as the only healer, who, if he willed, could cure the illness and eliminate suffering. A true believer in these traditions should put her trust in God and depend on him and none other for deliverance from pain and suffering. Some of these traditions speak about the temporary nature of all forms of suffering, including illness; they persist only for a "fixed period" in God's decree, after which relief is guaranteed either through complete cure or death. Furthermore, in some traditions, illness is evaluated as a form of divine mercy to expiate a believer's sins. According to a well-known tradition, the Prophet is reported to have said: "No fatigue, nor disease, nor sorrow, nor sadness, nor hurt, nor distress befalls a Muslim, even if it were the prick he received from a thorn, but that God expiates some of his sins for that."

In contrast, there are traditions that contradict this attitude of passivity in the face of suffering. These traditions hold that because God is just, he cannot cause gratuitous pain to his creatures. In fact, there is a strong emphasis on God's goodness, a belief that he wills only beneficence. Reconciling God's benevolence and absolute goodness with the suffering of the innocent, as discussed earlier, has not been easy in any religious tradition. Even when the general trend in Muslim piety is to hold human beings accountable for their own suffering and to recommend righteous acts to rid the world of suffering, the suffering of infants and animals has presented an interpretive challenge. Some Muslim scholars have tried to explain the suffering of an infant as an admonition for adults; children's suffering is viewed as a response to the parents' sins. Rarely have these scholars paid attention to the suffering of the animals. But when they have, they explained away the suffering of animals in terms of a hierarchy of existence, in which the creatures of lower rank, like animals, serve the purposes of the higher, like human beings. They argue that because all God's acts are purposeful, nothing can be in vain, including the suffering of the children and other beings. In most theological discussions, suffering was construed with reference only to human beings. Since moral evil referred merely to human actions perpetrated upon or afflicting human beings, other instances of being were not included. In that sense, the suffering of children, and not that of animals, served as a divine sign and warning.[6]

This view raises a serious question: Is human suffering the only form of evil worth considering in the light of divine justice and benevolence? If only human suffering is regarded as evil, then other earthly creatures are relegated to a lower status. This relegation seems to conceive a unique moral status for human suffering in light of human capacity for willing and executing evil acts. If moral evil is the main source of human suffering, then the suffering experienced by lower forms of life are devoid of moral implications. According to this view, the desecration or destruction of the natural environment or cruelty to animals would constitute a lower order of evil than the destruction of human life. Such a doctrine has serious implications for the use of animals in medical research. In the literature examined for the present work, there are rarely rulings prohibiting the use of animals for human ends, although one can find numerous traditions that treat cruelty toward animals as a sin against God, punishable by him in the hereafter.

There are numerous traditions that provide religious incentives for the care and curing of the sick. Some function as prophetic directives about the proper etiquette for dealing with illness or visiting the sick and bereaved. One tradition cites a paradigm case for the community to emulate. According to this tradition, it was the Prophet's custom, when he visited the sick, to say, "Don't worry. It is a purification, if God wills"—and he said to him, "Don't worry. It is a purification." On one occasion, the Prophet entered into the home of an ailing desert Arab and said to him, "It is a purification, if God wills." The man replied, "Never! Rather it is a fever boiling on an old man, which will send him on a visit to the grave!" The Prophet replied, "Very well, then be it so." In another tradition, it is related that when a person fell ill, the Prophet used to rub him with his right hand and then pray to God, saying: "O Lord of the people, grant him health, heal him, for Thou art a great healer."[7]

Other traditions recognize a religious purpose for illness, as for other forms of suffering, as a cleansing challenge and trial decreed by God. Hence, in one tradition, the Prophet says that the patient evolves spiritually because of these trials and can attain the rank of a true believer. "When God intends to do good to somebody, he afflicts him with trials."

Aṣābahu bi-maraḍin: He (i.e., God) afflicted him with disease; or rendered him diseased), like its converse, *aṣābahu bi-ṣiḥatin* (He rendered him healthy), is a common expression of God's activity in everyday human situations in Muslim cultures. In a Muslim thanksgiving prayer, besides praising and thanking God for all the blessings, a believer affirms: "To You [O God] belongs praise for all the good affliction (*balā'in ḥasanin*) with which you have inured me."

The characterization of affliction as "good" in the previous prayer indicates that suffering as such does not create a theoretical problem in Islam. Rather, it is treated in direct terms as part of the divine plan for humanity. When it occurs, it is identified, and its impact is reversed by education and discipline in a true affirmation and submission to the will of God (*islām*). The Qur'an and the traditions provide an uncommon interpretation of suffering as a concrete human experience, an unavoidable condition of human existence. They do not always regard suffering from natural causes as an evil and hence a problem that needs to be explained or vindicated because its author is the good God.

Suffering and Bioethical Decisions

To recapitulate, two distinct explanations for the purpose of suffering emerge in Islamic teachings. First, suffering is part of natural evil within God's plan for the betterment of humanity; all forms of suffering, including illness, serve two purposes: they are a form of punishment that expiates a sin, and they are a test or trial to confirm or reinforce a believer's spiritual status. Second, suffering is part of moral evil caused by human free will in choosing to disbelieve and face the consequences of this choice. Disbelief, then, is treated as the source of human misconduct that results in suffering. Suffering in this situation serves an educational function, helping to reveal the consequences of disbelief and its attendant afflictions. However, when the righteous suffer affliction, it is seen as an agent of purification and attainment of higher spiritual station.

However, an important dimension to the question of suffering through illness brings us face to face with cultural and religious attitudes regarding human existence and the control over life and death decisions, more particularly when an individual is overcome by suffering. Furthermore, it underscores the view that the human being has only the stewardship, not the ownership, of his body and thus is not free to do with it whatever he pleases. He is merely the caretaker, the real owner being God, the creator. As a caretaker, it is a human's duty to take all necessary steps to preserve himself in a manner that would assist him in seeking the good of both this world and the next. To seek the good of this world requires Muslims to pay attention to their health by maintaining a balanced diet and exercise. They have an obligation to maintain their own health. If, despite such precautions, a person falls prey to pain or illness, the tradition instructs the believer to understand that suffering is a form of a test or trial to confirm a believer's spiritual station (Q.

2:153–57). Suffering in this situation is a divinely ordained trial, a way of revealing that humanity belongs to and will return to God. Accordingly, suffering cannot be regarded as evil at all. Human travail and suffering should not lead to despair and lack of faith in divine mercy.

This religious and spiritual valuation of suffering does not answer the critical question: Should one take upon oneself to alleviate suffering where possible and endure it otherwise? This question is critical to the present-day discussion, namely, the patient's right to die. In Islam, this question cannot be negotiated because, in the first place, life is a divine trust and cannot be terminated by any form of active human intervention; and, in the second, its term has been fixed by the unalterable divine decree.

The belief in God's unalterable decree is also revealed in the Muslim ethics, where not only is the right to die not recognized, but also the right to be assisted in dying, whether through "passive" or "active" means, is ruled out. It is important to clarify here that because decisions about life and death are through divine decree, Islamic religious law—the Shari'a—refuses to recognize an individual's right in those matters. However, with its emphasis on the principle of promoting or seeking what is in the best interest of all concerned (*istiṣlāḥ*), Muslim jurists have recognized the possibility of arriving at a collective decision through consultation (*shūra*) by those involved in providing health care, including the attending physician and the family. Besides the principle of promoting the best interest, it is the ethical principle affirmed in the most unequivocal terms by the Prophet that has been evoked when matters concerning critical care have been under consideration. This is the principle of "No harm, no harassment." It lays down the justificatory force of the ruling to avoid causing harm or harassment to the patient. It also allows for important distinctions and rules about life-sustaining treatments in terminally ill patients. The distinctions upon which ethical decisions are made include the distinction between "mercy killing" (active euthanasia) and "letting die" (passive euthanasia). The killing–letting die distinction often underlies distinctions between suicide and forgoing treatment or between homicide and natural death. The rule of "no harm" in some ways functions like the principle of nonmaleficence. But it goes beyond preventing harm. It raises a critical moral question about the intention of the health care providers in forgoing life-sustaining treatment: whether such a decision can be regarded as a form of killing, and if so, whether it is assisted suicide or homicide. There is no immunity is Islamic law for the physician who unilaterally and actively decides to assist a patient to die.

There are, however, two situations in the treatment that could be interpreted as "passive" assistance in allowing a terminally ill patient to die. Pain relief treatment that could shorten life, but that is administered to relieve physical pain and psychological distress and not to kill, is permitted in Islamic law simply because the motive is regarded as a sufficient justification, protecting the physician against criminal or other liability in such circumstances. As long as the situation does not involve an intention to cause death, a medical intervention to provide necessary treatment for the relief of pain or other symptoms of serious physical distress is not regarded as criminal.

Similarly, in withdrawing treatment, whether pursuant to a refusal of death-delaying treatment or through mutual and informed decision making by patient, physician, and other parties involved in providing care for the patient, although there is an intention to allow the person to die when it is certain that death will result from its omission, Islamic law regards it as a nonculpable act. The reason is that delaying the inevitable death of a patient through life-sustaining treatment is regarded as being against the benefit of the patient. Moreover, the principle of juristic preference protects the physician by authorizing departure from the already established ruling about the prohibition of allowing death in order to avoid any rigidity and unfairness in recognizing the incurable pre-existing conditions of the patient. Furthermore, by authorizing the removal of life-sustaining treatment in cases in which it results merely in a death-delaying procedure, the juristic preference serves the ideals of justice and the public in a better way. Notwithstanding a fine line between having and not having an intention to cause death in such omissions, Islamic law does not forbid withdrawal of futile and disproportional treatment on the basis of the consent of immediate family members who act upon the professional advice of the physician in charge of the case. Some Muslim jurists have recognized the validity of a competent patient's informed refusal of treatment or "a living will," which allows the person to die under circumstances in which there is no medical reason to continue treatment. However, even in such rare instances of recognition of the patient's autonomy in Muslim culture, the law actually takes into consideration the patient's long-term treatment relationship with a physician whose opinion, in the final analysis, serves, for example, as the grounds for turning off the respirator. In this case, the death is regarded as having been caused by the person's underlying disease rather than the intentional act of turning off the respirator.

The moral principle that is operative in this ruling is that intention alone does not make an act culpable. The person's death is actually caused by the preexisting disease when the withdrawal of the treatment becomes justified through the expert medical opinion. In other words, the Shari'a would not consider withdrawal of the treatment as the cause of the person's death. This can be contrasted to the death that occurs by giving a person a lethal injection. The injection is the sole cause of the person's death and is clearly regarded as the cause of this in fact and in law by Muslim jurists and hence is forbidden.

To recapitulate the Islamic legal-ethical perspective on the end-of-life decision of a terminally ill patient without any hope of getting better, it is important to restate that the justificatory force of the rulings on "allowing to die" by withdrawal of life-sustaining treatments is contingent upon a well-informed consultation with the physician and other parties involved in the patient's treatment. More important, because Islamic legal deliberations contain and ground morality as part of the spiritual response to God in interhuman relationships, the patient's own determination and the physician assisting him to terminate life are both held accountable for acts of disobedience against God. Pain relief treatment or withholding or withdrawing of life-support treatment, in which there is an intention of allowing the person to die when it is certain that the disease is causing untreatable suffering, are permissible as long as the structures of consultation between all parties are in place. In final analysis, besides the exceptions noted in the two situations, in Islam there are no grounds for the justifiable ending a terminally ill person's life, whether through voluntary active euthanasia or physician-assisted suicide.

Concluding Remarks

Should one take upon herself to alleviate suffering when possible or just endure it? Two responses are offered in the light of two previously mentioned positions, which have negative and positive implications for medical treatment, respectively:

1. A passive response based on the belief that because God is testing human faith, one must endure suffering. A corollary of this belief is that, as reported in the words of Abraham in the Qur'an, God is the only Healer on whom a believer should depend:

"... Lord of all Being who created me, and Himself gives me to eat and drink, and, whenever I am sick, heals me, who makes me die, then gives me life...." (Q. 26:80).

The statement "whenever I am sick, heals me," became a source for a skeptical attitude toward medical treatment. This skeptical attitude is not limited to any particular school of thought in Islam. Rather, it is commonly held in the culture without sometimes any reference to the aforementioned belief in God's sole power of healing.

2. An active response based on the belief that because the human being is the cause of his own suffering, he should undertake to do righteous acts to rid the world of suffering. Good works negate suffering. Obviously, the latter belief generates a positive attitude to medical treatment, and it derives its strength from the oft-quoted Prophet Muhammad's advice to his followers:

"O servants of God, seek the cure, because God did not create a disease without creating its cure, except for one disease... senility."

Theological-ethical debates on these two responses are based on the two forms of Islamic theodicy: the determinist and free-will theodicies, based on the concepts of the divine omnipotence and the divine justice.

Ethical decisions in alleviating suffering through illness take medical treatment in the sense of an active response to human suffering based on traditions that relate the following:

a. Health is preferable to sickness.
b. "A powerful believer is preferred and better liked by God than a weak believer."
c. Seeking cure does not contradict the trust in God and submission to God's decision about humanity.

As for the place of life-sustaining treatment in Islamic bioethics, the fundamental criteria include the following:

a. There is an absolute obligation to save human life. In the case of a patient in the vegetative state, ethical deliberations in Islam are not only concerned with determining the value of the patient's life. The principle of public good (*maṣlaḥa*) demands that an individual's life must be weighed in the scale of general well estate of those who are related to the patient. End-of-life decisions require taking into consideration an individual's interpersonal relationship with her own family and society in general. If active medical intervention in the case of a severely brain-damaged patient leads to further suffering of the patient and those related to her in society, then the ethical judgment cannot ignore the ensuing general harm, including the rising cost of prolonging such life for the entire society. In keeping with the principle of "no harm," there is no obligation to prolong the life of a patient in a persistent vegetative state through intensive care technology. In this latter case, Islamic jurisprudence views aggressive medical treatment as a source of harm and obstruction of nature's course toward terminating human suffering through death. Moreover, necessity renders the prohibited permissible, which in this case will make it permissible to discontinue the life-sustaining equipment.
b. Availability of affordable resources, both human and technological, to sustain a terminally ill patient's life must be assessed in terms of collective social needs.
c. Benefits of active medical intervention must be open to all.

Principles of "justice" and "utility," as known in the secular bioethics, would be hard to implement in the case of inclusiveness and the community-oriented nature of the Islamic ethics of medical treatment. Moral problems connected with the allocation of scarce resources in the majority of Muslim societies in the third world remain unaddressed because of the authoritarian and paternalistic nature of health care in these countries. However, the requirement to adhere to the principle of equal worth of human life as a mere fact of being human suggests that no human life can be treated lightly when it comes to the distribution of limited medical resources.

As for physician-assisted suicide and euthanasia in Islam, it is important to keep in mind that illness as a form of divinely ordained suffering serves two purposes:

First, as a form of punishment to expiate a sin;

Second, as a form of a test or trial to confirm a believer's spiritual station.

Suffering is, thus, instrumental in revealing God's purposes for humanity. Should one take it upon himself to alleviate suffering where possible? Obviously, the Qur'anic directives make it clear that death cannot be negotiated because life is a divine trust and cannot be terminated by any form of human intervention. Hence, the rulings are as follows:

a. "Mercy killing" or "physician-assisted aid in dying" of terminally ill patients is prohibited.
b. Withdrawing or withholding necessary-to-life interventions is construed as murder because a physician is responsible to maintain the process of life, not of deciding death. However, there is no obligation to continue these interventions if these simply prolong the imminent death of a terminally ill patient.
c. If a patient determines that death is a better outcome and a physician assists her to terminate life, both are committing an offense against God.
d. "Killing" and "letting die" carry equal moral consequences even if the person to be killed is competent to determine that death is a better outcome.

In final analysis, there are no grounds for justifiable killing whether through voluntary active euthanasia or physician-assisted suicide in Islam.

Notes

1. Peter Antes, "Medicine and the Living Tradition of Islam," in *Healing and Restoring: Health and Medicine in the World's Religious Traditions*, ed. Lawrence E. Sullivan (New York: Macmillan, 1989), 173–208, discusses the problem of assessment and diagnosis of culturally diverse individuals in Germany and underscores the importance of understanding Muslim patients' religious and cultural backgrounds for a successful diagnosis and treatment.

2. A number of traditions to this effect have been cited in George F. Hourani, "Ibn Sina's 'Essay on the Secret of Destiny,'" in *Bulletin of School of Oriental and African Studies* (London: University of London, 1966) 25–48.

3. Although the bases in the Qur'an for these assertions would require another paper to develop, there are some key texts supporting the existence of evil in the world. Its positive or negative estimation among Muslims has depended upon the way pertinent scriptural texts are interpreted by various scholars representing different schools of thought. But it is also the cryptic nature of some of the scriptural language about God's role in creating or "permitting" evil in the world that lends itself to the problems of justifying the purpose of evil. Moreover, one can detect some kind of an unofficial state theology at work in furthering unquestioning submission to the all-powerful God, reaching almost psychological numbness in dealing with evil in the society in general, which actually led to quietism and acceptance of adverse social and political conditions without holding the authorities responsible for their unjust behavior.

4. For a sample of Sunni creed on this subject and its theological discussion, see A. J. Wensinck, *The Muslim Creed* (London, 1965), 188–190; for relevant traditions, see *Ṣaḥīḥ al-Bukhīrī, Kitāb al-marḍa,* Vol. 7 (Chicago: Kazi Publications, 1979) 371–372, Ḥadīth 545.

5. Theodicy in the Qur'an remains marginal. It is not a major concern of the Qur'an to show that good God does not commit evil; rather, the concern is to generate faith in God's wisdom and power over everything God has created. Neither does the Qur'an impute evil on God. In the final analysis, the existence of evil is squarely ascribed to human arrogance and disbelief in the final day.

6. Eric L. Ormsby, *Theodicy in Islamic Thought: The Dispute over Al-Ghazali's "Best of All Possible Worlds"* (Princeton, NJ: Princeton University Press, 1984), 241–245, discusses various views held by Muslim theologians regarding the suffering of children and animals in the context of God's "doing the best for His creatures."

7. *Ṣaḥīḥ al-Bukhārī, Kitāb al-marḍa*, Ḥadīth 566.

16

Endure, Adapt, or Overcome? The Concept of "Suffering" in Buddhist Bioethics

Jens Schlieter

> Most people either dread death as the greatest of suffering
> or long for death as a relief from suffering.
> One who is wise neither deprecates life, nor fears not living.
>
> Epicurus, *Letter to Menoeceus*

The central position of "suffering" in its fundamental doctrines is, without doubt, a characteristic of Buddhism.[1] Accordingly, its core teachings, conveyed by the historical Buddha in a succinctly worded formula, the "Four Noble Truths," are all related to "suffering." The first "Noble Truth" states the existence of "suffering" (Sanskrit: *duḥkha*, Pali: *dukkha*); the second, the "Origin of Suffering"; the third, the "Cessation of Suffering" (*duḥkha-nirodha*); and, finally, the fourth discloses the "Path Leading to the Cessation of Suffering," which is the "Noble Eightfold Path." The latter, a "training guide" to reach the end of suffering, comprises elements of wisdom, ethical self-cultivation, and mental development (such as concentration and meditation).

Even though the "negative" diagnosis of unrestricted "suffering" of the first "Noble Truth" is obviously put into perspective and "neutralized" by the "positive" third and fourth "Noble Truths," which emphatically claim that there is (a way to) "cessation of suffering," early Western scholars of Buddhism were nevertheless repelled by the weight of the allegedly single negative truth of suffering in Buddhist doctrine. As a result of this centrality of suffering, Buddhism seemed to comprise for them—in combination with the abstract goal of "Nirvāna" as an end to suffering—a kind of "pessimism," "nihilism," or "cult of nothingness." Recent publications trace this interpretation to the early apprehension of Buddhism by Jesuit missionaries and other Christian apologetics,[2] but it remains influential and still constitutes a popular criticism of Buddhism. Therefore, it is important to discuss suffering in relation to the overall positive claim that Buddhists make, namely, that there is a way to overcome suffering. But what constitutes suffering in a Buddhist context?

A stock phrase, to be found in discourses of the Buddha transmitted in Pāli, explains: "And what, monks, is the Noble Truth of Suffering? Birth is suffering, ageing is suffering, death is suffering; sorrow, lamentation, pain, sadness, and distress are suffering. Being attached to the unloved is suffering, being separated from the loved is suffering, not getting what one wants is suffering."[3] Here, the concept of "suffering" includes a wide spectrum of heterogeneous characteristics ranging from the fundamental anthropological situation of "being human" (birth, ageing, sickness, morbidity) to physical, emotional, and mental states and attitudes. Other texts portray the social side of human suffering: loneliness, depression, never-ending stress.[4] Therefore, "the Buddhist concept of duhkha, often translated as 'suffering,' is not simply an unpleasant feeling. Rather, it refers most deeply to a basic vulnerability to suffering and pain due to misapprehending the nature of reality."[5]

The translation of the technical term for "suffering" in early Buddhist texts, Skt. *duḥkha*, poses some difficulties: No single English term captures the full range of this crucial concept. Renderings, depending on the context, include "despair," "fear," "pain," and "vulnerability," but also "stress," "frustration," "aversion," "longing," "uncertainty," and "boredom."[6] Some scholars of Buddhism have proposed to render it primarily as either "unease," "uneasiness," or "unsatisfactoriness"—in order to cover the larger range of its meaning.[7] Therefore, it seems to be both necessary and useful to distinguish between different Buddhist concepts of "suffering": Suffering as a feeling (e.g., pain), suffering as an emotion, and also purely "cognitive" suffering as an outcome of "false views" (mental attitudes), such as suffering as a result of the belief one will undergo unpleasant states in the future.[8]

According to early texts and later commentaries, suffering has its origin in "desire," "thirst," or "craving" (Skt. *tṛṣṇā*, P. *taṇhā*); in the attachment to one's own body and clinging to a concept of an "adamantine personhood"; and, finally, in the cycle of unpleasant rebirths. Already in canonical texts, however, there appears a distinction of "three kinds of suffering": "suffering due to pain," "suffering caused by conditioning," and "suffering caused by change."[9]

Yet, one might ask whether or not these different kinds of suffering may be subsumed under the category of "suffering" as understood in recent Western psychology and academic discourse. By way of clarification, we might take a short look at some recent Western approaches to define "suffering": according to the influential view of Eric J. Cassell, suffering "can be defined as the state of severe distress associated with events that threaten the intactness of the person."[10] Without question, the first criterion of "distress" plays an important role in the Buddhist definition of suffering. Already, early Buddhist texts offer a "psychological" view on suffering. There, the Buddha is portrayed to explain that human beings have "contact" to the world by way of sense perception. With "contact as condition," he proceeds, "there is feeling. What one feels, that one perceives. What one perceives, that one thinks about. What one thinks about, that one mentally proliferates."[11] "Distress" is, therefore, a conditioned mental reaction triggered by unpleasant sense perceptions (e.g., pain, but also hurtful words of others). The second criterion, however, the threat to the "intactness of the person," seems to be less fitting: Although "ageing" and "death" figure prominently in the Buddhist concept of suffering, they are not understood as suffering because the "intactness of the person" is in danger.[12] Quite to the contrary: According to the Buddhist concept of personhood, the very idea of a substantial "self" is a prominent source for suffering: "Whether we use the term self, or ego, or personal identity, for Buddhists it is precisely the notion of an enduring entity that is the root cause of suffering. The mutable nature of phenomena comes into conflict with the hope that our self will endure."[13] Moreover, at least in early Buddhist discourse, the concept of human suffering is part of the general suffering all "sentient beings" (Sanskrit: *sattva*) share; to tie suffering per definition to "persons" seems to presuppose a certain Western "speciecism," which many Buddhists reject quite emphatically.[14]

The different apprehension of suffering in Buddhist (as well as other Indian) and in Western traditions can be shown in a telling example. In the view of Western traditions, the life of the embryo and fetus in the mother's womb has been conceptualized as very pleasant, secure, carefree, and guarded—thus, far from being considered as suffering. As it seems, this depiction emerged already in the Jewish-Christian tradition: In Isaiah (44:2), we read of the Lord, "who made you, who formed you in the womb, and who will help you." The embryo, in short, is cared for already in the womb. Sigmund Freud diagnosed some patients as being affected by nothing less than the desire to return to the mother's womb. Not coincidentally, for Freud and other psychoanalysts, the womb is a mythical, archaic, and even "holy" space free from suffering—an "intrauterine paradise."[15] In contrast, in the Buddhist tradition, the "embryo/fetus" had, according to the karma-and-rebirth doctrine, already lived previous lives and is, therefore, not a "blank sheet" ("tabula rasa") and hence bound to suffering.[16] In Buddhaghosa's important manual of Buddhist doctrine (fifth century C.E.), we read: "When this being is born in the mother's womb, he is... born... like a worm in rotting fish, rotting dough, cesspools, etc., he is born in the belly in a position that is below the receptacle for undigested food (stomach), above the receptacle for digested food (rectum), between the belly-lining and the backbone, which is very cramped, quite dark..... And on being reborn there, for ten months he undergoes excessive suffering, being cooked like a pudding in a bag by the heat produced in the mother's womb, and steamed like a dumpling of dough, with no bending, stretching, and so on. So this, firstly, is the suffering rooted in the descent into the womb."[17] Another text on the "Descent of the Embryo," the *Garbhāvakrāntyavadāna*, explains that a fetus has to suffer—because of its negative karma—from that moment onward, when it is "equipped with the consciousness of [experiencing] suffering" (Skt.: *duḥkhasaṃjñā-prapanna*).[18] The assumption of prenatal-fetal stress, in Western medicine a rather recent discovery,[19] has likely influenced the critical stance of Buddhist scholars in regard to abortion, too. Again Buddhaghosa: "When the mother has an abortion, the pain that arises in him through the cutting and rending in the place where the pain arises that is not fit to be seen even by friends and intimates and companions—this is the suffering rooted in abortion."[20]

To return to the discussion of "Western" concepts of suffering, a definition that seems to be more in line with Buddhist accounts of suffering is the "intuitive" definition of Edwards: "The first is that suffering must involve a phenomenological element. This may include pain but need not. Second, pain is neither a necessary nor a sufficient condition of suffering. Third, suffering has to have a significant duration. This is in clear contrast to pain. Fourth, for a state to count as suffering, it must have a fairly central place in the mental life of the subject."[21]

This definition converges with the "emic" Buddhist concept of suffering in several respects: the "centrality" of suffering, the difference to "pain," the temporal extension, and the "nonpersonalist" approach. These characteristics lend themselves to the argument that not only other sentient beings, such as animals, suffer, but also fetuses, babies, and human beings in "nonrational" mental circumstances (e.g., individuals with dementia). Nevertheless, applying such a definition, Buddhists may not necessarily conclude that all these cases of suffering are equal in regard to quality or intensity. Concerning the animals' suffering, however, early texts explicate—which may astonish only at the first glance—that for them hunger, thirst, heat, abuse, cruelty, struggle, and so forth, will be even more agonizing than for human beings.[22]

But what about those humans that seek to suffer deliberately (as radical ascetics do), or those who will sometimes—if perhaps only in certain situations—find "joy" in their suffering? According to textual sources of early Buddhism, it seems to be clear that there is no religious justification for practices of extreme mortification for the historical Buddha. His teaching of the "middle way" implies to steer clear from any indulgence of sense-pleasures on the one hand, and self-mortification on the other, which is judged as either a finite pleasure or a painful and unprofitable undertaking.[23] There is, indeed, no appreciation of self-afflicted suffering in early Buddhist sources. Any religious indulgence in suffering and likewise any pleasure in suffering (e.g., masochism, unnecessary endurance, or unmet desires) are altogether counted as suffering to be overcome. Clifford Geertz's depiction that, as a religious problem, "the problem of suffering is, paradoxically, not how to avoid suffering but how to suffer, how to make of physical pain, personal loss . . . something bearable, supportable—something, as we say, sufferable,"[24] is, therefore, only partly true with respect to Buddhist attitudes. Most Buddhists distinguish between "pain" and "suffering," claiming the former to be unavoidable, while regarding the latter to be completely overcome by the spiritually advanced practitioner. The anthropological—or, probably better, the "theriological"—basis of Buddhist views on suffering lies in the capacity of sentient beings to recoil if they experience aversion (e.g., pain, violence) and seek situations in which they are secure, happy, and at ease. This is already stated in verses of the canonical *Dhammapada*: "All tremble at violence, to all life is dear. Comparing (others) with oneself, one should not kill or cause to kill. When a man considers this, he does not kill or cause to kill. Whoever injures with violence creatures desiring happiness, seeking his own happiness he does not gain happiness when he has passed away. Whoever does not injure with violence creatures desiring happiness, seeking his own happiness he gains happiness when he has passed away."[25] This feature is to be found in later texts of the Mahāyāna tradition, too, such as Śāntideva's "Guide to the Buddhist Path to Awakening" (seventh century C.E.), which states that "happiness is liked by me and others equally," whereas "fear and suffering are disliked by me and others equally."[26] And the current Dalai Lama, Tenzin Gyatso, explained: "In your personal view, is a bacterium a sentient being? The question is important in the Buddhist context because when you take the life of a sentient being, that constitutes a wrong deed. So is it wrong to kill an amoeba? Buddhists would say that if the amoeba feels pleasure and pain, wishes to be happy and free of suffering, then it is wrong to kill it, and otherwise it is not wrong."[27]

In the Dalai Lama's definition, it seems to be of ethical relevance if a being is endowed with the capacity of feeling pleasure or pain. There is, however, to my knowledge no classical text that explicates how the victim's capacity to feel pain should guide ethical decision making in regard to human beings. Again, this may be illustrated with the Buddhist notion of fetal development: as stated previously, there are several texts in which the fetus is depicted as being bound to suffering; she is—at a certain advanced stage of fetal development—equipped with the "consciousness [or: clear knowledge] of suffering" (Skt. *duḥkhasaṃjñā*).[28] In premodern Buddhist tradition, an exact date (as a "terminus ante quem") for the initial development of the fetus's capacity to feel pain or pleasurable feelings does not seem to be of ethical importance.[29] Remarkably, though, some Vinaya traditions distinguish between a "human being" (Skt. *manuṣya*, Tibetan *mi*) and a being "that possesses a humanlike form [or body]" (Skt. *manuṣyavigraha*, Tib. *mir chags pa*).[30] According to some texts, the "humanlike" phase spans over the first forty-nine days,[31] which would more or less comprise the Western definition of "embryonic development." However, even killing an embryo in "humanlike form" is explicitly forbidden—yet, it might, according to some Vinaya texts relevant to Buddhist traditions in East Asia, be interpreted as comparably less serious.[32] Nonetheless, Tibetan embryological texts stress the homogeneous continuity of the development with the fact that the karmic "consciousness principle" may even "experience" entering the womb.[33]

To summarize, the acceptance of the fact that human beings suffer is seen as an essential prerequisite for Buddhist practice—essential, because it is the ultimate motivation to pursue the goal of overcoming one's own suffering as well as to help others who suffer. Suffering has, therefore, also "a positive side. It makes us aware of the vulnerability of life."[34] The latter is especially emphasized in the Mahāyāna tradition, that is, those schools that focus on the spiritual ideal of the Bodhisattva. A Bodhisattva generates—out of compassion—the wish to attain Buddhahood for the benefit of all suffering beings. And again, in the words of Sharon Salzberg, "the first step in developing true compassion is being able to recognize, to open to, and to acknowledge that pain and sorrow (suffering) exists."[35]

The relevance of these ideas and motivations in concrete bioethical decision making will be discussed later; here, however, a more general remark may be in place: claiming the existence of suffering, Buddhist texts emphasize that the overall, long-term goal can be neither to mitigate nor to endure (or adapt to) suffering, but instead to accept it—in order to enter the path of Buddhist practice, which is intended to fully overcome suffering. Pursuing strategies to prevent a priori any kind of *anticipated* suffering for sentient beings would—assuming that these strategies would work—preclude the motivation to search for efficient ways out of the "ocean of suffering."[36]

The Japanese philosopher Masahiro Morioka has coined a brilliant term for this enterprise, namely to follow the ideal of a "painless civilization": such a civilization, he says, "is one in which the mechanism of preventive reduction of pain spreads throughout its society";[37] a development that, he holds, actually already takes place in highly industrialized nations with advanced biomedicine. For example, he asks "why many people choose to abort when a congenital disability, such as Down syndrome, is found in the fetus." For him, "there are various reasons for that decision. Some would say that a severe disability will bring great suffering to the child itself in the future.... However, I believe that one of the strongest reasons for choosing selective abortion is... that parents tend to think that having a disabled baby may cause great pain and suffering to the parents themselves, both economically and psychologically.... They try to avoid pain and suffering that may fall upon them in the future, and usually this avoidance is accomplished in a preventive way. I have called this kind of act... 'preventive elimination of pain.'"[38]

Buddhist ethicists may subscribe to Morioka's view in a crucial aspect—in Buddhism, ethics pertain first and foremost to the first-person perspective: "Each person must monitor his or her own life."[39] This attitude, which is substantiated with the theory of karma, may be called a "perpetrator"-centered view of ethics—instead of a "victim"-centered approach. Practices of selective abortion and the use of preimplantation genetic diagnostics are not related to real pain and suffering of affected individuals—simply because they will not be born. Their expected suffering remains, therefore, still a sheer possibility. At the time of the decision making, the emotional stress of the expecting is much more manifest.

Answers on How to Alleviate or Overcome Suffering

Overall, Buddhist texts stress that pain and suffering are central to the mental life of human beings. Nevertheless, they likewise express the optimistic idea that all people are—in the long run—able to overcome suffering. Because "craving" is considered one of the fundamental origins of suffering, strategies that aim to abandon desire will have to eliminate craving as the root cause. "Craving" (Skt. *tṛṣṇā*; P. *taṇhā*), literally "thirst," is defined as the intensive desire to experience sensual pleasures and as longing either for the "eternal existence" of the individual self or the soul or for "non-existence" or total "annihilation" after death. Another important theoretical doctrine, which can already be found in early Buddhist sources, the "dependent origination" (Skt. *pratītyasamutpāda*), explicates the origination and cessation of suffering by a conditional nexus: "by the cessation of craving clinging ceases; by the cessation of clinging becoming ceases; by the cessation of becoming birth ceases; by the cessation of birth ageing and death, sorrow, lamentation, pain, grief and distress cease. And thus this whole mass of suffering ceases."[40]

More generally, "suffering"—with "craving" as its root cause—leads to a process called "clinging" or "attachment" (P./Skt. *upādāna*) to the world and a person's own self. "Attachment" can become manifest in various ways: attachment to pleasures, emotions, material possessions, or to the very own identity of the "self." The latter seems to be the most crucial yet, at the same time, the most difficult moment of the Buddhist explanation of the coming into existence of "suffering." In later Buddhist thought, such as Buddhaghosa's *Visuddhimagga* (and elsewhere), it is the highest sense (ultimate truth) that there is no "person" that feels, no "experiencer": "For there is suffering, but none who suffers; 'doing' exists although there is no doer."[41]

Thus, ultimately, any therapy for "suffering" has to succeed with the abandonment of any strong notion of a "substantial" self. This is emphasized in most schools of Mahāyāna Buddhism, too: "As a result of misapprehending the self as independent, there arises a strong sense of the absolute separation of self and other. Then, craving naturally arises for the 'I' and for what is mine, and repulsion arises toward the other. The erroneous belief in the absolute distinction of self and other thus acts as the basis for the derivative mental afflictions of craving, hatred, jealousy, and arrogance. Such toxins of the mind are regarded, in Buddhism, as the sources of all mental suffering."[42] In a famous and influential work of Mahāyāna Buddhism, the philosopher Śāntideva argues that focusing on one's own suffering cannot to be justified if the claim of "selflessness" is taken seriously: "Without exception, no sufferings belong to anyone. They are to be warded off simply because they are suffering. Why is any limitation put on this?"[43] It is therefore the ideal of the Bodhisattva, his "regulative idea," if I may allude to Kant here, to champion the benefit of all sentient beings by directing his compassion to them, and furthermore, to work indirectly toward alleviating their suffering by guiding them in their Buddhist practice.[44] Especially, Mahāyāna Buddhist texts emphasize that the Bodhisattva is obliged to pursue a greater benefit even if it may cause some small amount of harm: "The Bodhisattva makes an effort . . . with all the forces of body, word and mind for assuaging all bodily and mental pain, both present and future, for all beings, and for producing bodily and mental happiness present and to come. But if he does not search for the complicated causes leading to all this, nor strive for the remedy of obstacles in its way; if he does not engender a little pain and grief in himself which becomes the remedy of much grief in others; nor relinquishes a little wealth for the sake of great prosperity, yea, if he overlook[s] these duties for even a moment, then he is guilty of sin."[45]

As is well known, the Buddhist tradition developed techniques of concentration and meditation, which are instrumental in the alleviation of suffering.

Notwithstanding that other philosophical traditions—such as the Greek-Roman Stoa, namely Epictetus or Marcus Aurelius—have developed certain techniques for dealing with suffering, it is a quite remarkable, if not distinct, feature of the Buddhist tradition that these techniques have been elaborated into some kind of systematic training. The Stoics, for example, developed some basic exercises how one should refrain from hasty judgments. One should observe one's own state of mind in a neutral and disengaged manner—the famous stoic "mental unperturbedness"—and should, moreover, enjoy this passionless state of mind as the most happy to achieve.[46] Likewise, one should "premeditate" (Latin: *praemeditatio*) possible painful experiences to come and one's own process of dying and death in order to stay calm and peaceful when the time has come. Someone who is trained in precise observation of negative feelings, such as aggression, self-hate, or jealousy, will henceforth be probably less governed by these.

This is exactly what the core of Buddhist training (in a more systematic manner) seems to consist of: to gain knowledge of these feelings and emotions in their most sublime initial stage. Buddhist practitioners who are able to refine their sensitivity in this respect are hoped to cut off conditioned modes of reactions (e.g., certain automatized, aversive responses to pain). Paramount in this context is the "mindfulness" meditation. Already, early Buddhist texts declare that there is "one path" (or, a "unified path") "which purifies beings, surmounts grief and fear, eliminates suffering and distress, abandons crying and weeping...—namely the four establishments of mindfulness."[47] Directing attention to the process of breathing marks the beginning of mindfulness meditation. Subsequently, the mind is trained to concentrate on body postures, movements, and the impermanence of the body; feelings and emotions; thoughts and cognitive states; and finally, central Buddhist teachings, such as the "four truths." The overall goal of mindfulness training, which has in modern Theravāda Buddhism been systematized as "[realization through] direct insight" (P. *vipassanā-bhāvanā*), is equanimity, peace of mind, and liberation from craving and attachment. Buddhist teachers explain that a systematic training in attention, concentration, and equanimity will lead to their mutual reinforcement: one who is able to strengthen his concentration will be able to deepen his equanimity; and one who is tranquil will be able to raise his level of concentration and attention.

A more concrete case of Buddhist views and attitudes with regard to the alleviation of suffering can be drawn from the popularization of meditation techniques as a means to understand—and deal with—stress and chronic pain. The still growing clinical application of "mindfulness-based stress reduction" (MBSR) may serve as an example here. This technique, developed by Jon Kabat-Zinn as a clinical or therapeutic group program for alleviating pain and dealing with depression, stress, and anxiety,[48] is devoted to the training of mindfulness in nonreligious settings. "Mindfulness," as understood in this technique, "is characterized by dispassionate, non-evaluative and sustained moment-to-moment awareness of perceptible mental states and processes."[49] While designed for individual self-practice, MBSR presupposes participation in weekly group sessions for eight to ten weeks, where patients not only learn a basic form of mindfulness meditation but also are introduced to yoga and current scientific knowledge of the psychophysiology of stress and pain. Over the course of four decades, MBSR has developed into a widely used program.[50] Whereas some of its teachers claim the Buddhist background of the technique to be of minor importance, the founder, Kabat-Zinn, has reinforced a Buddhist foundation of the therapy in several important aspects, such as in his implementation of Buddhist "loving-kindness" as a means to foster self-acceptance[51] and his conviction that suffering is essentially a reaction to expected pain, which can be overcome.[52]

Restricted space precludes me from discussing the MBSR approach in detail here. It may suffice for our purpose to employ it as an example how traditional Buddhist meditation techniques are regarded as relevant for the treatment of pain and suffering in therapeutic settings. Compared with traditional formulas of mindfulness meditation, practices such as MBSR[53] represent in certain respects the approach of "Buddhist modernism." They focus essentially on those elements of Buddhist teachings and practices that seem to provide helpful action-guides for coping with the predominant ways of suffering in modern society, whereas other strands of Buddhist explanations of suffering, such as the karmic roots of suffering, are no longer appealing.[54] Moreover, modern mindfulness meditation contains insights from humanistic psychotherapy, namely, "strong" concepts of self-acceptance, "self-efficacy,"[55] and self-esteem, whereas in early Indian Buddhism (and sometimes in monastic Buddhism even today), an important exercise of mindfulness meditation was to disassociate with the embodied self by rather drastic means (e.g., contemplation of one's future fate as a corpse in various stages of decay).[56] This practice is meant to reveal "the repulsive nature of the body . . . during the stages of its decay, and the fact that death is the inescapable destiny of all living beings."[57] These practices, intimately tied to a certain negative image of the body in early Buddhist India, seem to be less fitting to modern Western representations of a generally neutral, if not positive, image of embodiment and hence one's own body.

Exploring the possibility of whether the Buddhist understanding of suffering might serve as a public notion of suffering within a modern pluralistic society, it seems that modernized Buddhist conceptions of suffering share a common ground with other major therapeutic approaches in two respects. First, suffering is defined on an "empirical," "phenomenological," and "psychological" basis. Second, both share the conviction that a successful treatment of suffering can be achieved by "innerworldly" means: through forms of cognitive training, which are in principle thought to be open to every human being, provided they are endowed with a certain level of cognitive abilities. Nevertheless, these similarities do not pertain to Buddhism in general but rather to Buddhist modernism only. Most important, it is the nonempirical doctrine of karma that has to be discounted, if not suspended, which has been done in some Western philosophical reconstructions of Buddhist ethics[58] or in a straightforward "Buddhism without beliefs."[59]

To summarize, from early on, Buddhist texts and teachers have suggested meditation as a technique to overcome suffering. This kind of training should enable an experienced meditator to sustain a tranquil but attentive state of mind, which allows the practitioner to realize the ephemeral and transient quality of any intense feeling (such as pain). It follows that persistent states of suffering may not arise—for those who are able to unmask a certain interpretation of pain, namely, to identify with a "strong" notion of "one's own self bound to suffer." Moreover, this kind of "self-help" attitude averts those "unwholesome" thoughts that consist of attempts to blame others to be accountable for one's own suffering. From this perspective, any effective therapy of suffering is, therefore, mainly a cognitive undertaking, which aims not to enhance capacities to endure or adapt to suffering but to eliminate suffering.

This being said, Buddhist perspectives seem to converge largely with the (neo-Buddhist) Schopenhauerian "cognitive" definition that "all happiness rests solely upon the relation between our demands and that which we receive…and likewise, that all suffering actually emerges from the discrepancy between what we demand and expect and what happens to us—a discrepancy that apparently lies only in knowledge and could, through better insight, be fully dissolved" (Schopenhauer 1818 [my translation]).[60]

Suffering: Implications for Buddhist Bioethical Decision Making

Considering recent Buddhist discourse on suffering in bioethical decision making, it is important to acknowledge the diversity of opinions voiced in the field. As my own empirical research on Buddhist bioethics suggests,[61] Buddhist discourse on bioethics seems in fact to be as complex as the respective discourses in the Jewish, Christian, or Muslim traditions.

Before discussing concrete examples, an overall question must be addressed, namely the relationship between Buddhist ethics and suffering. It is a remarkable fact that there are no direct equivalents that correspond with Western "ethics" in the various premodern Buddhist traditions—neither as a term nor as a discipline. In a way, ethical reasoning on Buddhist grounds was initiated and systematized by Western scholars—for example, in the field of bioethics, by Damien Keown.

Nevertheless, from early on, ethical reasoning and morality have formed an essential part of Buddhist discipline and philosophy. Of utmost importance is the goal to refrain from intentionally harming sentient beings ("nonviolence," Skt. *ahiṃsā*). Ethical reasoning, furthermore, implies the analysis of an intended action with regard to whether it is "skillful" or "unskillful" for all parties involved. This ethical reasoning—illustrated with the mirror metaphor for ethical "reflection"—has been portrayed by the Buddha with the following words: "What do you think, Rāhula? What is the purpose of a mirror?" "For the purpose of reflection, venerable sir." "So too, Rāhula, an action with the body should be done after repeated reflection; an action by speech should be done after repeated reflection; an action by mind should be done after repeated reflection. Rāhula, when you wish to do an action with the body you should reflect upon that same bodily action thus: 'would this action that I wish to do with the body lead to my own affliction, or to the affliction of others, or to the affliction of both? Is it an unwholesome bodily action with painful consequences, with painful results?' When you reflect, if you know: 'This action that I wish to do with the body would lead to my own affliction, or to the affliction of others, or to the affliction of both; it is an unwholesome bodily action with painful consequences, with painful results,' then you definitely should not do such an action with the body."[62] The Buddha advises Rāhula and his other followers to reflect in the same manner on verbal and mental actions—and not only to do so before any bodily, verbal, or mental action but also to continue to reflect while acting, and even after the deed is done. For some Western scholars but also some Theravāda Buddhist scholars, this and other similar passages provide "powerful evidence" for a "consequentialist interpretation of early Buddhist ethics."[63]

There is, however, also a strong emphasis on the intention behind an action.[64] With an intention to kill or harm a living being, any action is thereby rendered unwholesome because motives, greed, fanaticism, and delusions all have the same unwholesome effect. In this respect, Buddhist ethics have thus been called "intentionalist" ethics. Yet, this is not to be confused with a pure evaluation of the mind's intentions only. Already, classical commentarial texts of the Vinaya (regulation of moral conduct of monks and nuns) define explicitly that an intention (Skt., P.: *cetanā*) can only be a morally relevant intention if the intended action is executed. Interestingly, however, there are only few Buddhist texts of the Mahāyāna tradition that argue ethically by balancing and weighing harms and benefits for all parties concerned. This obvious lack of casuistry (leaving casuistry concerning the application on Vinaya rules aside, which is in most cases ethically not relevant) makes a strong case for Buddhist ethical reasoning having an intentionalist core.

Buddhist ethics include a reflection of the consequences that actions have for others, but still the main focus is on the consequences for the offender or perpetrator: "Ultimately decision-making power rests with the agent of the action, since it is that person who will reap the fruits of the action."[65] Every ethically relevant action is believed to have an effect on the perpetrator's next life; unwholesome actions will lead to bad karma and will therefore imply an increase of personal suffering in the next rebirth. I have proposed to denote this kind of perspective on ethics as "offender centered"—in contrast to "victim centered" ethics, which focus on the dignity and inviolability of other affected individuals.[66]

However, Buddhist ethics have also been conceptualized as contextual ("situation ethics"), or "virtue ethics" (e.g., by Damien Keown). Finally, another important facet of Buddhist ethics is the notion of a self-transformative enterprise, which looks at individual moral practice from a salvific point of view (in line with the "offender centrism" mentioned previously). A Sri Lankan professor of Buddhist philosophy,

P. Don Premasiri, has acknowledged this transformative quality of "morality" (*sīla*) with the following words: "If the entire spiritual training is understood as an attempt to transform the moral nature of man, sīla can be considered as the beginning of this conscious and deliberate process of self-transformation."[67] To conclude, the best (Western) way to describe the different aspects of Buddhist ethics seem to be some kind of "polythetic" approach: Buddhist ethics combine certain elements of utilitarian consequentialism, intentionalist ethics, situation ethics, and virtue ethics.

To provide some insights into current Buddhist discourse with regard to the alleviation of suffering in bioethical decision making, I will now examine concrete cases of Buddhist evaluations within three ethical domains: (1) prenatal genetic diagnostics and abortion; (2) end-of-life issues—palliative care and euthanasia; and (3) alleviation of suffering through psychotropic drugs.

Prenatal Genetic Diagnostics and Abortion

To evaluate suffering in bioethical decision making with respect to the beginning of individual human life, I will start with some general remarks concerning traditional Buddhist notions of conception and prenatal life. According to early Buddhist texts of various traditions, life is inaugurated by the convergence of three factors: the fertile substances of father and mother, the fertile period of the mother, and a "consciousness-principle" (Skt. *vijñāna*, P. *viññāṇa*).[68] The "consciousness-principle," which is said to descend into the mother's womb at the time of sexual intercourse, is propelled by karmic forces and destined to take rebirth in a new worldly existence. The traditional attitude might therefore be called "conceptionalism" because it identifies the appearance of a new being with conception. This new life, addressed as "embryo" (Skt. *garbha*) or "being" (Skt. *sattva*), is further qualified by terms such as "mind" (Skt./P. *citta*), or, again, "consciousness." In texts on monastic discipline (Vinaya), we read the definition: "*Human being* means: from the mind's first arising, from (the time of) consciousness becoming manifest in a mother's womb until the time of death, here meanwhile he is called a *human being*."[69] An important aspect of this being is its possession of (or, sometimes, identification with) a "vital force" or "life-faculty" (P./Skt. *jivitīndriya*). The ethical relevance of these definitions becomes visible in the evaluation of abortion: for monks and nuns, it is clearly forbidden to engage in practices of abortion[70]—abortion is regarded as taking the life of a human being. Whereas this quite strict position is most clearly expressed for monks and nuns, it should pertain to lay Buddhists as well. They should likewise practice the training rule to abstain from "killing."[71] For L. P. N. Perera, it is "the Buddhist view that the right to life commences at the very first embryonic stage of a being, since *maitrī* or love, according to the *Mettasutta* (Sn vv. 143–152) should be extended even to the embryo or 'one seeking birth'– *sambhavesī* (Sn v. 147)."[72] For some Buddhists, even the embryo is entitled to a "right to self-determination," equated with the idea of karma, "which puts total responsibility on the individual for his life."[73]

Moving to the recent Buddhist discussion on prenatal diagnostics, I will not be able to present the ethical discussion (e.g., on abortion of a defective embryo or fetus) thoroughly. Instead, I will try to highlight some aspects related to the question of suffering. Prenatal (in vivo) diagnostics of severe genetic diseases (e.g., Down syndrome, cystic fibrosis, Duchenne muscle dystrophy, beta-thalassemia) raise the probing question of whether—and if so, in which cases—abortion might be justifiable.

Buddhists may approach this issue from various angles.

First, there is the question of whether prenatal diagnosis of such defects can establish any secure knowledge about the amount of suffering the "nasciturus," or human-to-be, will be confronted with. Are there—for Buddhists—any criteria to estimate the suffering of challenged individuals? Would the situation improve if the respective life were terminated? Nevertheless, such a judgment should be based on criteria that allow for a conclusive deliberation over whether no longer being alive would be better than living an impaired life.

Intricate questions already arise with the *interpretation* of prenatal test results: What does it mean, for example, to be confronted with a probability of 1in 280 that the child-to-be will be affected with trisomy 21? Far from being able to predict the grade of the individual occurrence of every single genetic disease, even for medical specialists, it is sometimes difficult not to confuse population statistics with the prediction of the individual's medical fate.[74]

Furthermore, it will not count as evidence here to rely on the testimony of individuals who judge from *their* life that *for them* it was not worth living. This kind of circular reasoning is splendidly portrayed in the paradoxical words of a Yiddish joke: Two rabbis are musing about life. One of them sighs and says to the other, "How hard is life. So much suffering! In fact, sometimes I think it's better not to have been born at all." "True," says his friend. "But how many are that lucky? Not one in a million!"[75] For Buddhists, however, karma is the force that propels the cycle of rebirths. Therefore, "[not] to be born" is not perceived as an act of divine creation, which transforms into pure contingence, if there is no longer (knowledge of) a divine will. For Buddhists, "to be born" as a human is, nevertheless, a very valuable achievement, regulated by the "natural law" of karma (P. *kammaniyama*).[76] There are, to my knowledge, no classical Buddhist sources arguing that termination of a living being may be a justifiable means to prevent further suffering of the affected victim. "The fact that we are suffering now does not make us immune from future harm if we do harm to someone else. We cannot, in the long run, get out of suffering by causing more suffering."[77]

Again—in classical texts, and for those Buddhist scholars who adhere to the traditional "conceptionalist view"[78]—the focus on the doer of deeds will be of importance here. To terminate a form of life implies suffering not only for the life that gets terminated (and will likely be reborn) but also for the decision-making perpetrators because it is they who will suffer from the negative karma they took as burden through their action.[79] Furthermore, some more traditional Buddhists may argue that the diagnosed genetic disease of the embryo or fetus is a karmic force that will only be reduced by exhausting itself.[80] By any third-party interruption of this process, negative karma will still be there, influencing the next life to come. Altogether, the expected suffering of a being not yet born seems for many Buddhists in itself no argument for aborting a positively tested embryo—even if with high probability it will be hindered to live a normal life (in terms of the amount of suffering to be expected, even a normal life is merely an abstract statistical illusion).

Although classical texts do not discuss these aspects because modern diagnostic technologies were not within their reach, one might nevertheless argue that for Buddhists, these new diagnostic-prognostic technologies open up a new dilemmatic situation, too. In this situation, which in certain aspects is similar to the ethical reflection on the legitimacy of euthanasia (discussed later), the expected amount of suffering could indeed matter. Let us assume as a premise (1) the conviction of many intellectual Buddhists that in principle every practitioner is capable of generating potent mental strategies for alleviating her suffering. Assuming, moreover, (2) that many Buddhists hold the opinion that practitioners will need, for an efficient use of these potentials, some basic cognitive capacities at their free disposal. If, now, (3) a certain person has been born with such a genetic disease that typically includes a severe degree of intellectual disability, such as Down or Tay-Sachs-syndrome, she will most likely not be able to learn the Buddhist cognitive strategies (such as meditation) in order to alleviate her suffering. So, in other words, she will not be able to develop sufficient means to ward off pain and suffering. Some Buddhist ethicists fell into a pondering silence or admitted the intricacy of the problem when questioned regarding this matter.[81] But again, the main criterion is the question of the status of the embryo. Obviously, it is less problematic for Buddhist bioethicists to divert from a conceptionalist view and argue instead that the descent of the "consciousness principle" takes place later—for example, when the primitive streak and the nervous system develop[82] —than to declare that "killing" might be justified with the hypothetical prevention of the affected individual's future suffering.[83]

Second, there is the pressing question of whether the suffering of other parties, such as the parents-to-be, or effects to society at large[84] should also be taken into consideration. Especially in poor countries and circumstances, considerable economic and social costs accompany parents with disabled children. According to the Buddha's advice for Rāhula, the doer should reflect not only if harm is done to others but also if harm is done to himself (e.g., by generating unwholesome thoughts)—and this reflection should take place before, during, and after his action. Actually, reformulating Morioka's argument given previously, the embryo's suffering in the future is usually the decision maker's own suffering—the latter being troubled by scenarios of the affected embryo's as well as his own future. Thereby, the decision maker dismisses not only the embryo's actual situation but also his own because the anticipated negative scenario may not actually come to pass. With regard to the intentionalist vein of Buddhist ethics, a Buddhist evaluation could therefore also begin with the motives of parents who decide that having a child with a severe inherited disease means an unbearable burden to them. Apart from a critical evaluation of the motives (compassion, convenience, or egoism?),

Buddhist ethicists might also consider the long-term effects on society: "The parents' desire for their offspring to have the most desirable genetic makeup is everyone's dream. But should science develop to meet this desire? The concern with the welfare of the yet-to-be-born is good intention. However, it could lead to an eugenic movement.... If this happens, genes will become the determining factor for discrimination,"[85] resulting, in an extreme scenario, in a society in which people with undesirable genes will—in one way or other—be forced not to have offspring (an extreme case of what Michel Foucault called "biopolitics").[86] Buddhists stress here, again, the perpetrator's intention: whether or not the doer believes or could notice the embryo to be a living being (or, inversely, just an agglomeration of cells) is decisive because the action will—in terms of negative karma—be even more harmful if the intention is a conscious act of killing.

End-of-Life Issues: Palliative Care and Euthanasia

With regard to suffering in the final stage of dying, a critical aspect for Buddhists is in which state of mind the person actually dies. If this state is "wholesome" (Skt. *kuśala*), it is expected to have positive effects on the next rebirth; if it is unwholesome, the effect will be accordingly.[87] Thus, scholars of Theravāda and Mahāyāna Buddhist traditions declare unanimously that retaining a clear and "present" state of mind when dying is of utmost importance. The dying person should be able to develop skillful, wholesome mental attitudes—such as being content, tranquil, and focused, and not being angry, jealous, regretful, or aggressive.

The aim to retain a clear consciousness and a focused mind is an essential part of several meditation techniques, which focus on the "recollection of death" (P. *maraṇasati*). The importance of the very last moment of consciousness (P. *cuti viññāṇa*) has been already stressed in early texts; Sugunasiri could bring the Buddha's advice to the point by speaking of an "exit mind."[88] Of special importance, too, is the dying person's state of mind in most schools of the Tibetan tradition, in which a comprehensive teaching and ritual, the reading of the *Tibetan Book of the Dead*[89] (and other texts) has been developed for escorting the dying person or, more precisely, the departing consciousness.

Many Buddhists explain that even the intention or wish to commit suicide is usually[90] governed by the intention to kill. For them, the suicidal person may likely be motivated by some kind of hidden self-hate—which is, of course, an unwholesome mindset. Generally, there is a more depreciative attitude toward suicide as a means to end physical pain or suffering in this life: "Because a human lifetime is an ideal opportunity for achieving liberation, the practice of euthanasia or assisted suicide is antithetical to Buddhist thinking. Even a life of suffering and hardship is counted as a valuable opportunity for realization and spiritual evolution."[91] Hence, for those Buddhists, who believe in the negative quality of the intention to kill, direct euthanasia or assisted suicide will be no plausible way to end pain, suffering, and despair because they will fear the negative karmic effect on future lives: instead of ending or reducing suffering, suffering is actually expanded.

Moreover, a palliative therapy, which uses strong analgesics, might likewise not be adequate if, as a side effect, the consciousness and mental presence of the patient become blurred or disturbed. Some Buddhist scholars argue, however, that a person's fear of the pain becoming unbearable may also disturb the process of focusing the mind—and, accordingly, vote for a more permissive attitude with respect to medical pain treatment.[92] The majority of Buddhist ethicists regard any form of active euthanasia as intended killing and consequently recommend abstaining from it. With respect to passive or indirect euthanasia, however, there are a significant number of Buddhist scholars opting for more permissive options on a case-by-case basis (e.g., in regard to the withdrawal of life support).[93] As a matter of fact, even the current XIV Dalai Lama offers liberal opinions. In an interview regarding human beings in "hopeless" irreversible states (being, as we may say, beyond "the point of no return"[94]), he took not only into consideration the amount of suffering these futile treatments might cause to the family but also financial aspects: "From the point of view of a Buddhist, any pain has to be faced, if not in this lifetime, then some other lifetime. One can use this chance to eliminate the pain by meditating or thinking about compassion.... This is a very complicated issue and has to be individually assessed on a case-to-case basis. If the person cannot think because of too much pain, or is in a coma with no hope of recovery, then the family will also eventually suffer. In the meantime, this is costly in resources, so then euthanasia may be considered."[95]

If dying persons proclaim their wish that their pain shall be eased by strong analgesics, doctors and relatives will presumably decide in their favor—even if Buddhist specialists would argue that doing so poses a greater challenge to realize the "exit mind" for the dying person.

As noted previously, Buddhist ethics are, especially for lay persons, a matter of training precepts, which should be cultivated as persistently as personal abilities allow. More difficult are those cases in which someone is no longer able to articulate her preferences. In many Asian countries with a significant Buddhist population (Japan being an exception here), a more pragmatic attitude with regard to irreversible states such as brain death seems to prevail. Accordingly, also financial constraints of the family, and the quite often limited resources in intensive care facilities are taken into consideration.

Pharmacological Mood-Lifting: Alleviation of Suffering through Psychotropic Drugs

Western biomedicine established over time a distinction between clinical forms of depression, mood disorders, and so forth, and milder, nonclinical forms of depressive moods and episodes (e.g., as a reaction to loss). It would be interesting, however, to discuss how this psychiatric differentiation of clinical from nonclinical forms might converge with traditional Buddhist perspectives on suffering. An intriguing aspect here is the—in comparison with the United States—hesitant use of fluoxetine (Prozac) and other antidepressants in Japan, a fact that has been connected to cultural differences in labeling depression—that is, to more "positive" evaluations of moods of melancholy, sadness, and grief, as well as of impermanence and loss, in Japan.[96] In the following discussion, I examine some Buddhist positions regarding pharmaceutical treatment of the latter, of healthy persons. As is well known, antidepressants such as fluoxetine have been extensively used in nonmedical contexts, bringing the topic of "pharmacological" alleviation of suffering to the forefront.

The example of emotional and cognitive enhancement may provide an interesting test case for Buddhist ethicists. On the one hand, it might be construed as a competing "therapy" for suffering. On the other hand, it is not tied to the decisive ethical question of how to evaluate certain states of human life, such as embryonic life or aphasic, persistent vegetative, or brain-dead states, in which the affected are not yet—or are no longer—able to articulate how much they actually suffer.

First, I will summarize some arguments that were put forth by Buddhist ethicists relating to pharmaceutical emotional enhancement. For Karma Lekshe Tsomo, the use of these new generations of pharmaceuticals "may alleviate suffering temporarily, but may also result in a loss of perspective and/or personal agency, create unhealthy dependencies, and lead to even greater suffering."[97] Accordingly, her central argument revolves around whether these pharmacological treatments will lower or better the appreciation of one's own personal agency. For her, the Buddhist model of mental cultivation is indeed an efficient method to alter one's own consciousness (the latter not being just an epiphenomenon of brain functions). Therefore, meditation is held to be a superior method for the alleviation of nonclinical forms of depression because for Tibetan Mahāyāna Buddhists, there is "a subtle form of mental consciousness" that "is not fully dependent on the brain."[98]

Let us assume as a thought experiment, that, for a certain practitioner, the result of Buddhist mental cultivation and pharmaceutical enhancement is experienced as absence of suffering, as happiness, or even as bliss. But because pharmaceuticals do not reach to the origins of suffering according to a Buddhist framework (e.g., impermanence, ego-centeredness, clinging), they will be efficient as a treatment only of symptoms and not of causes. Enjoying some kind of transient relief of suffering—something that is, in Buddhist cosmology, a characteristic of gods in their respective realms—the practitioner may simply delay the pursuit for a permanent way out of suffering.[99]

Even though, for Buddhists, ultimate reality is beyond suffering, there is an intricate, if not dialectical, relation between suffering as experience and the motivation to practice the Buddhist way to get out of suffering. Not to acknowledge the reality of suffering—mythologically speaking, the failure of gods absorbed in pleasure, power, and longevity—will prolong suffering because no efforts are made to end transmigration.[100] Seen from this perspective, the permanent use of mood-lifting pharmaceuticals as the only means of therapy in nonclinical circumstances might for some work as a "clutch" for decoupling certain aspects of reality. The undesirability of enthusiastic feelings that do not correspond to sufficient cause has been demonstrated by Robert Nozick's philosophical thought experiment of an "experience machine."[101]

Leaving the topic of antidepressants behind, I will move to the recent discussion of whether a more general pharmaceutical cognitive enhancement of humans, which might enable a more efficient cognitive handling of suffering, should be considered administrable.

Presenting Buddhist thoughts on neuroethics, philosopher Andrew Fenton takes a quite permissive stand, focusing, however, on pharmaceutical enhancement of cognitive abilities. If a consequence of pharmaceuticals is to achieve "further insight into our self-nature or the reduction or alleviation of *duḥkha*,"[102] they should, according to Fenton, not be opposed from a Buddhist point of view. Arguing that the supposed ends of pharmaceutical enhancements—"greater skill in concentration or a more exact perception of events or changes of processes in one's environment"[103]—are quite similar to the ends meditation and self-cultivation aim for, there should be no principle objections in regard to the overall goals. Using these substances as "helpers" for cognitive or affective enhancement will equally contribute to boosting the ability to focus on compassion, thereby accumulating good karma, which in turn may help to alleviate suffering. If objections arise, Fenton argues, they must therefore address obviously unwholesome effects of the pharmaceutical means used. Such effects might include a certain false conception of "self" (e.g., self-aggrandizement, attachment to social reputation, or engagement in social competition) or adherence to a dualist framework of upper and inferior mental qualities. Yet, all these possible dangers, Fenton concludes, are not causally connected to these pharmaceutics; they are, therefore, not intrinsic arguments for a rejection.

Assessing this position with traditional Buddhist descriptions of suffering in mind, one might be skeptical with regard to Fenton's claim that the "ends" of enhancement—pharmaceutical enhancement and self-cultivated cognitive enhancement—are really the same. Should a "pharmaceutically enhanced mind" be regarded as an end in itself, or a means for the reduction of suffering—a means that nevertheless might be claimed applicable by Buddhist modernists in the future?[104] The most important difference between nonmedical use of antidepressants and pharmaceuticals for cognitive enhancement seems to be the possible effects on the motivation to start with, and maintain, Buddhist practices: namely, if they will prevent practice through avoidance of a certain psychological strain (which is definitely more present in the application of antidepressants). In consequence, it may discourage personal efforts necessary for coming to terms with suffering in the long run.

Summary and Discussion

Do Buddhist scholars of ethics advise individuals mainly to endure, or to mitigate, or to adapt, or to (try to) overcome suffering regarding bioethical decisions? A pivotal aspect of the Buddhist discourse on suffering seems to be—as we could see regarding the end of life—that there is no "higher" justification for suffering that people "have to endure" in these situations. Suffering, albeit an important aspect of human life, has no "natural quality" of "fate," "retribution," or the like. In Buddhism, there is no blueprint of "good" suffering. Instead, the final goal is to cultivate capacities in order to overcome—and not to endure, nor to mitigate—suffering. This has to be done individually, motivated by one's own conscious intentions, and as persistently as the individual abilities permit. This "first-person view" on suffering implies that, for Buddhist ethicists, it is important to stress the individual's capacity to overcome suffering through mental strategies such as meditation. Accordingly, for Buddhist specialists, these long-term strategies of overcoming attachment, craving, and so forth are more valuable than any method of transient relief of suffering. Moreover, Buddhists scholars emphasize that it is "never too late to exercise"—for example, in their recommendation that dying persons should try to retain a clear consciousness and mental presence.

An important regulative idea of Buddhism in regard to one's own suffering appears in the form of certain self-critical questions. Tackling, for example, the problem of genetic enhancement, Yao characterizes the "the Buddhist approach" quite aptly: "we are required to think first about why we want to do genetic enhancement since all forms of genetic enhancement are our cravings."[105] This "first-person," or "offender-centered" approach is also of influence for decisions in regard to the suffering of others. A substantial criterion is the ideal of not harming or killing sentient life (including oneself); if taken literally, it implies some confinements in regard to Prenatal-Diagnosis-cum-abortion (see note 79) or "mercy killing." On the other hand, Buddhist texts do not offer criteria to estimate (future) suffering of others. The amount of suffering to be expected is, for that reason, no important ethical action-guide—notwithstanding, that to generate "compassion" for all beings that suffer is a very important Buddhist virtue.

Interestingly, there is in regard to the central place of the actor's "no injury" maxim in Buddhist ethics some similarity with Karl Popper's proposal to replace the traditional utilitarian principle of "maximizing pleasure" with "minimizing pain": "I believe that there is, from the ethical point of view, no symmetry between suffering and happiness, or between pain and pleasure.... In my opinion... human suffering makes a direct moral appeal, namely, the appeal for help, while there is no similar call to increase the happiness of a man who is doing well anyway.... Instead of the greatest happiness for the greatest number, one should demand, more modestly, the least amount of avoidable suffering for all."[106] Yet, the Bodhisattva should also work for the happiness of others (as Śāntideva declared previously). Another difference between Popper's "negative utilitarianism" (Ninian Smart) and Buddhist attitudes toward suffering is, however, that the latter do not conceptualize ethics primarily from the victim's point of view but rather, as I pointed out earlier, from the perpetrator' point of view. Even though the Buddhist idea of "compassion" is intimately tied to the aim of alleviating suffering, it has traditionally not been defined by certain "therapeutic" obligations in a practical manner. The Bodhisattva's "compassion" may, for example, consist of his "energetic empathy" directed toward the sufferer; or the Bodhisattva may offer, motivated by compassion, instructions on how to cope with suffering. With other words, "compassion" in Buddhism is—in contrast to the Christian conception of active "charity" (*caritas*)—much less defined in terms of concrete actions of healing, curing, or other ways of restoring a former "good condition" of others.

Going through the different cases presented, one might finally ask if there are, in regard to the suffering of others, any clear-cut Buddhist ethical imperatives for medical professionals. Are there any first principles that rule Buddhist Bioethical decision making? For modern Buddhists, the ideal of "compassion" should also be an action-guide for medical professionals. For Pinit Ratanakul, "compassion" figures as a "prima facie duty" of Buddhist medical ethics—along with veracity, noninjury to life, and justice.[107] Other scholars of ethics, however, came to the conclusion that Buddhist ethics—in the form it has been presented so far—are not very helpful for pressing ethical dilemmas. Approaches of Western ethics (and bioethics, respectively), it has been remarked, possess a considerable strength in supplying a hierarchy of ethical principles, in offering hermeneutics of concrete cases and so forth, whereas, in contrast, Buddhist ethics sometimes lack clear guidelines "besides 'caution,' which is too vague to be of any practical value."[108] Indeed, Buddhist ethics do not seem to offer—at least in their premodern types—in-depth studies of ethical dilemmas in regard to the suffering of others. Instead, Buddhist ethics offer rather unwieldy (and sometimes uncomfortable) instructions for "not killing" and "not harming," and for the primacy on the actor's motivation and self-cultivation, which is for others exactly the strength of Buddhist ethics. Quite tellingly, only very few early or classical Buddhist texts discuss situations in which an actor is forced to sacrifice a precept (e.g., the abstention of killing) in order to mitigate a greater mass of suffering. It seems that Buddhist specialists are largely agreeing that "not to act at all" (or even to act intuitively) is in most dilemmatic situations a legitimate option. Here, credit may again be given to the theory of karma, which regulates the final outcome of deeds for the perpetrator, while the victim's perspective is left aside. Already, early texts (such as the *Dhammapada* verses 130–132 quoted earlier) had explained that generally everybody seeks to be happy. This seems not to be meant as a moral obligation—nevertheless, being without greed, hate, or fear is, without doubt, held to be an important precondition for acting morally wholesome.

Notes

1. Here, *Buddhism* is used generically and should be understood as a cover term, despite the diversity of different traditions, both past and present. Abbreviations for Pāli texts follow the editions and translations of the Pali Text Society.

2. Cf. Urs App, *The Cult of Emptiness: The Western Discovery of Buddhist Thought and the Invention of Oriental Philosophy* (Tokyo: University Media, 2012); Roger-Pol Droit, *The Cult of Nothingness: The Philosophers and the Buddha* (Chapel Hill: University of North Carolina Press, 2003).

3. *Mahāsatipaṭṭhāna Sutta*, D II.306–307, in *The Long Discourses of the Buddha: A Translation of the Digha Nikāya*, trans. Maurice Walshe (Boston: Wisdom, 1995), 344.

4. Asanga Tilakaratne, "Suffering and Liberation in Theravāda Buddhism," *International Journal of Buddhist Thought and Culture* 10 (2008): 87–103, 101–102.

5. Paul Ekman, Richard J. Davidson, Matthieu Ricard, and B. Alan Wallace, "Buddhist and Psychological Perspectives on Emotions and Well-Being," *Current Directions in Psychological Science* 14, no. 2 (2005): 59–63, 60.

6. Cp. Narendra Kumar Dash, ed., *Concept of Suffering in Buddhism* (New Delhi, Kaveri Books, 2005).

7. Cf. Damien Keown, *Buddhism and Bioethics*, 2nd ed. (London, New York: St. Martin's Press, 2001), 2; Bhikkhu Ñāṇamoli, *The Path of Purification (Visuddhimagga)*, by Bhadantācariya Buddhaghosa (Kandy, Sri Lanka: Buddhist Publication Society, 2010), XVI.34, note 8.

8. The latter concept of suffering might be termed the "metaphysical" understanding of suffering: because it has its roots in the individual's production of "negative karma," the strategy of overcoming this kind of suffering is connected to moral behavior, i.e., ethical training. Asian Buddhist cultures, however, admittedly still use some more traditional means of coping with suffering: safeguarding amulets and formulas, sacrifices, healing rituals, etc.

9. P. *dukkha-dukkhatā, saṅkhāra-dukkhatā, vipariṇāma-dukkhatā* (D III. 216); trans. Walshe, supra note 3, 484; in the later Mahāyāna tradition, e.g. in Asaṅga's compendium of "philosophical systematization" (Skt. *abhidharma*), the threefold scheme is explained by an eightfold typology: the sufferings of birth (1), aging (2), disease (3), and death (4) and suffering associated with what is unpleasant (5) are "sufferings due to pain" (Skt. *duḥkha-duḥkhatā*). The five aggregates of attachment (8) are "suffering caused by conditioning"; whereas the suffering of separation from what is pleasant (6) and the suffering caused by not obtaining what one desires (7) are "suffering caused by change" (cf. *Abhidharmasamuccaya: The Compendium of the Higher Teaching (Philosophy)*, by Asaṅga, trans. Walpola Rahula and Sara Boin-Webb (Freemont, CA: Asian Humanities Press, 2001), 84-85.

10. Eric J. Cassell, *The Nature of Suffering* (Oxford: Oxford University Press, 1991), 33. Here, I discuss Cassell's classical definition of the 1990s; for Cassell's current thoughts on "suffering," the reader is advised to consult his contribution in this book (see chapter 1). Additionally, the reader may consult David DeGrazia's contribution (see chapter 7) for a discussion on the relationship of distress and suffering.

11. M I.111–112; *The Middle Length Discourses of the Buddha: A Translation of the Majjhima Nikaya*, trans. Bhikkhu Bodhi with Bhikkhu Nanamoli (Boston: Wisdom, 1995), 203.

12. "Death is the greatest suffering of all, because it is the ultimate threat to our self-identity and self-interest. As long as we cling to ourselves or our loved ones, death brings great suffering. But when we analyze the notion of self and try to identify an independently existing self, we cannot find one. The notion that dying is a tragedy is therefore based on a false premise," as Karma Lekshe Tsomo, *Into the Jaws of Yama: Buddhism, Bioethics, and Death* (Albany, NY: State University of New York Press, 2006), 34, explains.

13. Ibid., 34. The concept of "selflessness" is, moreover, closely tied to the "compassion"—Pinit Ratanakul, "Buddhism and Human Genome Research," in *GenEthics and Religion*, ed. Georg Pfleiderer, Gabriella Brahier, Klaus Lindpaintner (Basel: Karger, 2010), 138–150, 140: "Compassion in Buddhism is the quality of the heart and is not an ephemeral

sentiment. It is a sublime emotion arising from the knowledge of suffering inherent in all sentient beings, and also from the realization of their unsubstantial nature (anattā) and inter-relatedness (paticcasamuppada)."

14. Cf. Lambert Schmithausen and Mudagamuwe Maithrimurthi, "Tier und Mensch im Buddhismus," in *Tiere und Menschen: Geschichte eines prekären Verhältnisses*, ed. Paul Münch, Rainer Walz (Paderborn: Ferdinand Schönigh, 1998), 179–223.

15. Cf. Carola Bindt, A. Huber, and K. Hecher, "Vorgeburtliche Entwicklung," in *Entwicklungspsychiatrie: Biopsychologische Grundlagen und die Entwicklung psychischer Störungen*, ed. Herpertz-Dahlmann, Beate, Franz Resch, et al. (Stuttgart: Schattauer, 2007), 89–117, 95.

16. Because of this existence of prenatal suffering, some embryological texts of the Tibetan tradition argue that the fetus may in fact be able to "practice Buddhism," e.g., to meditate—cf. Frances Garrett, *Embryology in the History of Tibetan Medicine: Becoming Human* (New York and London: Routledge, 2008), 103-105.

17. Vism 500; Ñāṇamoli, supra note 7, 512.

18. Michael Hahn, "Kṣemendras Garbhāvakrāntyavadāna (Sanskrittexte aus dem tibetischen Tanjur II)," *Journal of the European Ayurvedic Society* 5 (1997): 82–112, 89.

19. Cf. K. O'Donnell and V. Glover, "New Insights into Prenatal Stress: Immediate and Long-Term Effects on the Fetus and Their Timing," in *Neonatal Pain: Suffering, Pain and Risk of Brain Damage in the Fetus and Newborn*, ed. G. Buonocore and C. V. Bellieni (Milan: Springer, 2008), 57–64.

20. Vism 500; Ñāṇamoli, supra note 7, 512; cf. Garrett, supra note 16, 108.

21. Steven Edwards, "Three Concepts of Suffering," *Medicine, Health Care and Philosophy* 6 (2003): 59–66, 65.

22. Cf. Schmithausen and Maithrimurthi, supra note 14, 208–211.

23. E.g. in S V.420; trans. in Bhikkhu Bodhi, *The Connected Discourses of the Buddha: A Translation of the Saṃyutta Nikāya* (Somerville, MA: Wisdom, 2000), 1843–1844.

24. Clifford Geertz, *The Interpretation of Cultures: Selected Essays* (London: Fontana Press, 1993), 103.

25. Dhp 130–132; Kenneth Roy Norman, *The Word of the Doctrine. Dhammapada*, translated with an introduction and notes (Oxford: Pali Text Society, 2000), 20.

26. Bca VIII.95–96; trans. in Kate Crosby and Andrew Skilton, *Śāntideva. The Bodhicaryāvatāra: A Guide to the Buddhist Path to Awakening*, 2nd ed. (Birmingham, UK: Windhorse, 2002), 128.

27. XIV Dalai Lama, in Jeremy L Hayward and Francisco Varela, ed., *Gentle Bridges: Conversations with the Dalai Lama* (London, Boston: Random House, 1992), 67; cf. Dalai Lama XIV (His Holiness Tenzin Gyatso), *Kindness, Clarity, and Insight*, Jeffrey Hopkins, trans. and ed.; Elizabeth Napper, co-ed. (Ithaca, NY: Snow Lion, 2006 [1984]), 75. XIV Dalai Lama explained his basic approach like this: "My approach—and you can call it a leap of faith—is based on two premises. One is that life is precious. The second is that at the core of human nature there is a need to seek happiness.... These are the first principles. Everything else is based on them" (Richard J. Davidson, Anne Harrington, ed., *Visions of Compassion: Western Scientists and Tibetan Buddhists Examine Human Nature* [Oxford, New York: Oxford University Press, 2002], 216).

28. Cf. Hahn, supra note 18, 89.

29. Relevant embryological texts of the Mahāyāna tradition usually adhere to descriptions found in the most prominent texts of Indian Āyurveda medicine, which assume

that consciousness of feelings or mental activity will spring forth between the third and fifth month of fetal development. According to Vāgbhaṭa's medical compendium, the *Aṣṭāṅgahṛdayasaṃhitā* (ca. seventh century C.E.), "conscious knowledge of pleasure and pain" (Skt. *jñānaṃ ca sukhaduḥkhayoḥ*; Ah Śā II.55) starts in the third month. In the *Suśrutasaṃhitā* (second or seventh century C.E.) "mental activity" (*cetanā*) starts in the fourth month (SuS Śā III.18); according to Vāgbhaṭa in the fifth (Ah Śā II.57b; cf. Rahul Peter Das and R. E. Emmerick, ed. "A Machine-Readable Transcription of the Aṣṭāṅgahṛdaya by Vāgbhaṭa," accessed March 15, 2014, http://gretil.sub.uni-goettingen.de/gretil/1_sanskr/6_sastra/7_ayur/vagaah_u.htm.

30. Prātimokṣa-Sūtra (Tib. *so sor thar pa'i mdo*) of the Mūlasarvāstivādin (Derge Kanjur, 'dul ba, ca, 1b1–20b7); quoted according to Mahāmahopādhyāya S. C. Vidyabhusana, "Sor-sor-thar-pa; or, a Code of Buddhist Monastic Laws. Being the Tibetan Version of Prātimokṣa of the Mūla-sarvāstivāda School," *Journal and Proceedings of the Asiatic Society of Bengal*, New Series, XI (1915): 29–139, 79.

31. Cf. Huimin Bhikkhu, "Buddhist Bioethics: The Case of Human Cloning and Embryo Stem Cell Research," *Chung-Hwa Buddhist Journal* 15 (2002): 457–470.

32. Cf. Giulio Agostini, "Buddhist Sources on Feticide as Distinct from Homicide," *Journal of the International Association of Buddhist Studies* 27, no. 1 (2004): 63–95, p. 73.

33. Cf. Garrett, supra note 16.

34. Ratanakul, supra note 13, 146.

35. Sharon Salzberg, *Loving Kindness: The Revolutionary Art of Happiness* (Boston: Shambhala, 1995), p. 104.

36. In Buddhist mythology, this is the fate of the gods (devas), who, although virtually free from pain and sorrow, are not able to experience full liberation and are still subject to migration after their good karma is consumed.

37. Masahiro Morioka, "Painless Civilization and Fundamental Sense of Security: A Philosophical Challenge in the Age of Human Biotechnology," *polylog: Forum for Intercultural Philosophy* 6 (2005): 17, accessed March 15, 2014, http://them.polylog.org/6/fmm-en.htm.

38. Ibid.

39. Somparn Promta, "Buddhism and Human Genetic Research," in *Genomics and Bioethics: Interdisciplinary Perspectives, Technologies, and Advancements*, ed. Soraj Hongladarom (Hershey, NY: IGI Global/Medical Information Science Reference, 2011), 1–14, 11.

40. D II.35; trans. Walshe, supra note 3, 212. The Thai Buddhist bioethicist Pinit Ratanakul holds that the "Buddhist perspective on life, suffering and death can never be truly understood apart from the Buddhist law of conditionality (*paṭiccasamuppāda*)," which he, as many other Theravāda Buddhists, regards as a "natural law" (Pinit Ratanakul, *Bioethics and Buddhism* [Bangkok: Mahidol University, 2004], 299; cf. Promta, supra note 39, 6.

41. Vism 513; Ñāṇamoli, supra note 7, 529.

42. Ekman et al., supra note 5, 61.

43. Bca VIII.102; trans. Crosby and Skilton, supra note 26, 129.

44. Buddhist bioethicists emphasize that generating compassion is not merely a religious goal—it is of concrete help in decision making: "Compassion . . . involves both beneficence and non-maleficence. With compassion as motivation, science and technology will

be steered towards the optimum relief of human suffering.... This needed compassion and conscience are already inherent in our hearts and minds, but in a slumber-like state because of our egoism" (Ratanakul, supra note 13, 149). The importance of "compassion" in Buddhist bioethics—as the Bodhisattva's guiding therapeutic attitude toward the suffering of others, e.g., as a justification of genetic intervention—is stressed by Fuchuan Yao, *An Ethical Study of Genetic Intervention based on Rawlsian Justice and on Buddhism*, dissertation thesis (Norman, OK: University of Oklahoma, 2006).

45. *Śikṣā Samuccaya: A Compendium of Buddhist Doctrine. Compiled by Śāntideva Chiefly form Earlier Mahāyāna Sūtras*, trans. Cecil Bendall and W. H. D. Rouse (Delhi: Motilal Banarsidass, 1999 [1922]), 16.

46. Cf. Martha C. Nussbaum, *The Therapy of Desire: Theory and Practice in Hellenistic Ethics* (Princeton, NJ: Princeton University Press, 1996), 316–318; Dougal Blyth, "Suffering and Ancient Therapy: Plato to Cicero," in *Perspectives on Human Suffering*, ed. Jeff Malpas and Norelle Nickiss (Dordrecht, Heidelberg, etc.: Springer, 2012): 131–154, 144–146.

47. T 1, 582b, trans. Tse-Fu Kuan, *Mindfulness in Early Buddhism: New Approaches through Psychology and Textual Analysis of Pali, Chinese and Sanskrit Sources* (Abington, Oxon/New York: Routledge, 2008), 146; cf. M I.55, trans. Ven. Anālayo, *Satipaṭṭhāna: The Direct Path to Realization* (Birmingham, UK: Windhorse, 2007), 3.

48. Cf. Jon Kabat-Zinn, *Full Catastrophe Living: Using the Wisdom of Your Body and Mind to Face Stress, Pain and Illness*, 15th ed. (New York: Bantam Dell, 2005 [1990]).

49. Paul Grossman, Ludger Niemann, Stefan Schmidt, and Harald Walach, "Mindfulness-Based Stress Reduction and Health Benefits: A Meta-Analysis," *Journal of Psychosomatic Research* 57 (2004): 35–43, 36.

50. For the historical background of this approach, see W. Dryden and A. Still, "Historical Aspects of Mindfulness and Self-Acceptance in Psychotherapy," *Journal of Rational-Emotive & Cognitive-Behavior Therapy* 24 (2006): 3–28.

51. Kabat-Zinn (supra note 48, 185) advised this Buddhist practice in its literal form: "'May I be free from anger, may I be free from hatred; may I be filled with compassion, may I feel kindness toward myself.' Then we can go on to invoke someone else, perhaps a particular person we care about. We can visualize that person in our mind's eye or hold the feeling of the person in our heart as we wish that person well: 'May he or she be happy, may he (she) be free from pain and suffering, may he (she) experience love and joy'."

52. "Aversion to pain is really a misplaced aversion to suffering. Ordinarily, we do not make a distinction between pain and suffering, but there are very important differences between them. Pain is a natural part of the experience of life. Suffering is one of many possible responses to pain.... It involves our thoughts and emotions and how they frame the meaning of our experiences. Suffering, too, is perfectly natural.... But it is important to remember that suffering is only one response to the experience of pain. Even a small pain can produce great suffering in us if we fear that it means we have a tumor or some other frightening condition.... So it is not always the pain but the way we see it and react to it that determines the degree of suffering we will experience. And it is the suffering that we fear most, not the pain" (ibid., 285–286).

53. For a critical review of studies claiming evidence for the effectiveness of MBSR, see S. R. Bishop, "What Do We Really Know about Mindfulness-Based Stress Reduction?" *Psychosomatic Medicine* 64, no. 1 (2002): 71–83 (e.g., the problem of operationalizing constructs of "mindfulness"; dismantling the core effects of mindfulness in regard to other aspects of MBSR, such as psychosocial group expectations; or other methodological problems).

54. The role of karma as an explanation of suffering has been a disputed topic in Buddhist traditions. Some Theravāda Buddhist texts convey the Buddha's statement that karma is only one cause among several others, whereas some Buddhists, especially of Tibetan Mahāyāna, argue that karma is the origin of all forms of "suffering." Patrul Rinpoche (1808–1887), an influential teacher of the Tibetan Nyingmapa school, explains: "In all their inconceivable variety, the pleasures and miseries that each individual experiences—from the summit of existence down to the very lowest depth of hell—arise from the positive and negative actions [i.e., wholesome and unwholesome karma, J. S.] that each has amassed in the past" (Patrul Rinpoche [O rgyan 'jigs med chos kyi dbang po Dpal sprul], *The Words of My Perfect Teacher: Kunzang lama'i shelung. A Complete Translation of a Classic Introduction to Tibetan Buddhism*, trans. the Padmakara Translation Group [New Delhi: HarperCollins India, 1998], 118). The same argument can be found in Karma Lekshe Tsomo's work on bioethics from a Tibetan Buddhist view: "Coming face-to-face with death and impermanence, suffering, and the immanent dissolution of the illusory self are all opportunities for gaining insight into these basic Buddhist truths. Sufferings can be understood as the result of one's own actions in the past, rather than some inexplicable injustice. Through the experience of suffering of illness and approaching death, this negative karma is expiated, and it is possible to achieve profound realizations" (Tsomo, supra note 11, 188).

55. Kabat-Zinn, supra note 31, 201–203.

56. Cf. M I.58, trans. Anālayo, supra note 47, 6, 152–155.

57. Ibid., 153.

58. Cf. Mark Siderits, *Buddhism as Philosophy* (Cambridge, UK: Hackett, 2007); ibid., "Buddhist Reductionism and the Structure of Buddhist Ethics," in *Indian Ethics: Classical Traditions and Contemporary Challenges*, Vol. 1, ed. P. Bilimoria, J. Prabhu, and R. Sharma (Burlington, VT: Ashgate, 2007), 283–296.

59. E.g., Stephen Batchelor, *Buddhism without Beliefs* (New York: Riverhead Books, 1998); ibid., *Confession of a Buddhist Atheist* (New York, Spiegel & Grau/Random House, 2010).

60. In Schopenhauer's own words: "[dass] alles Glück nur auf dem Verhältniß beruht zwischen unsern Ansprüchen und dem, was wir erhalten...: und eben so, daß alles Leiden eigentlich hervorgeht aus dem Misverhältniss dessen, was wir fordern und erwarten, mit dem, was uns wird, welches Misverhältniss aber offenbar nur in der Erkenntniss liegt, und durch bessere Einsicht völlig gehoben werden könnte." Arthur Schopenhauer, *Die Welt als Wille und Vorstellung*, Vol. I., 1: § 16 (Zurich: Haffmans, 1999 [1813]), 137–138.

61. Interviews on matters of bioethics were conducted with Buddhist scholars, monastics, and decision makers (e.g., members of bioethics committees) in Sri Lanka and Thailand (Theravāda), and with Tibetan Buddhists in India (Mahāyāna), as well as with members of both traditions in Western countries. The results are due to be published soon (*Bioethics in Buddhist Traditions: Doctrinal Background and Global Discourse* [habilitation thesis]).

62. M I. 416; trans. Bhikkhu Bodhi with Bhikkhu Nanamoli, supra note 11, 524.

63. Charles Goodman, *Consequences of Compassion: An Interpretation and Defense of Buddhist Ethics* (Oxford: Oxford University Press, 2009), 48; cf. P. D. Premasiri, "Place of Ethics in Buddhism," in *Encyclopedia of Buddhism*, Vol. 5., ed. G.P. Malasekera and W.G. Weeraratne (Colombo: Government of Sri Lanka, 1990), 144–165.

64. For Karma Lekshe Tsomo, "Compassion, Ethics, and Neuroscience: Neuroethics through Buddhist Eyes," *Science and Engineering Ethics* 18, 3 (2012): 529–537, 532,

Buddhist ethical decision making "is guided by three general considerations: the law of cause and effect (karma), the intention that motivates an action, and compassion."

65. Tsomo, supra note 12, 207.

66. Cf. Jens Schlieter, "Some Observations on Buddhist Thoughts on Human Cloning," in *Cross-Cultural Issues in Bioethics—The Example of Human Cloning*, ed. Heiner Roetz (Amsterdam: Rodopi, 2005): 179–202.

67. Premasiri, supra note 63, 150.

68. E.g., in M I.265–266; cf. Peter Harvey, *An Introduction to Buddhist Ethics: Foundations, Values and Issues* (Cambridge, UK: Cambridge University Press, 2000), 312.

69. Vin III.73; quoted in ibid., 313.

70. cf. Keown, supra note 7, 93–96.

71. cf. Suwanda H. J. Sugunasiri, *Embryo as Person. Buddhism, Bioethics and Society* (Toronto: Nalanda College of Buddhist Studies, 2005), 7–9, 24–27; and generally Damien Keown, ed., *Buddhism and Abortion* (Honolulu: University of Hawaii Press, 1998).

72. L. P. N. Perera, *Buddhism and Human Rights: A Buddhist Commentary on the Universal Declaration of Human Rights* (Colombo: Karunaratne & Sons, 1991), 30.

73. Ratanakul, supra note 13, 144.

74. Cf. the contributions in Georg Pfleiderer, Edouard M. Battegay, and Klaus Lindpaintner, ed., *Knowing One's Medical Fate in Advance: Challenges for Diagnosis and Treatment, Philosophy, Ethics and Religion* (Basel: Karger, 2012). Simpson points out that in some respect the "genetic forecast" and its notions of predeterminism and susceptibility correspond with traditional astrology and its schema of causality and fate (cf. Bob Simpson, "Negotiating the Therapeutic Gap: Prenatal Diagnostics and Termination of Pregnancy in Sri Lanka," *Journal of Bioethical Inquiry* 4, no. 3 [2007]: 207–215, 213).

75. Cf. Robert Nozick, *Anarchy, State, and Utopia* (Oxford, UK, and Cambridge, MA: Blackwell, 1999 [1974]), 38–39, 338.

76. Cf. Ratanakul, supra note 13, 144.

77. Nyanasobhano, *A Buddhist View of Abortion*, Bodhi Leaf Booklet no. 117 (Kandy, Sri Lanka: Buddhist Publication Society, 1989), 19; cf. Ratanakul, supra note 13, 147. In the words of Karma Lekshe Tsomo (supra note 11, 188): "To cut short a life prematurely merely perpetuates the suffering; it simply postpones the suffering to another time, when it might be even more unbearable, and it sows the seeds of further, even greater sufferings through the non-virtue of taking life."

78. Those Buddhist ethicists that argue for a more permissive attitude toward a termination of pregnancy in case of positively tested embryos usually do not argue with the amount of expected suffering but instead argue that if the intention of lay Buddhists is not governed by greed, hate, or delusion, they may opt for a termination—taking, however, into consideration the karmic consequences their actions may have. Rather liberal attitudes with regard to selective abortion in cases of detected genetic defects have been reported from countries with a significant Buddhist population such as Sri Lanka (cf. Bob Simpson, V. H. W. Dissanayake, and R. W. Jayasekera, "Contemplating Choice: Attitudes towards Intervening in Reproduction in Sri Lanka," *New Genetics and Society* 24, no. 1 [2005]: 99–118; Simpson, supra note 74, 210–212) and Thailand (cf. Robert Florida, "Abortion in Buddhist Thailand," in *Buddhism and Abortion*. ed. Damien Keown [Basingstoke, UK: Macmillan, 1998], 11–30).

79. In general, the same holds true for embryo research and preimplantation diagnostics, cf. Keown, supra note 7, 119–121; Harvey, supra note 68, 319; Ratanakul, supra note 13, 143–144; yet, Buddhist ethicists voiced generally much more "permissive" positions in regard to the justification of research on superfluous and "orphaned" extracorporal embryos than on Prenatal-Diagnosis/Preimplantation-Diagnosis-cum-subsequent-abortion, cf. Schlieter, supra note 66; Keown, supra note 7, 97–100, 118–122.

80. Cf. Pinit Ratanakul, "Socio-Medical Aspects of Abortion in Thailand," in *Buddhism and Abortion,* ed. Damien Keown (Basingstoke, UK: Macmillan, 1998), 53–65, 59.

81. E.g., an interview with P. D. Premasiri on October 4, 2012 (conducted with Dr. E. Guhe, Fudan University, Shanghai). Contrarily, one may pose the question of whether a truly severe intellectual impairment will prevent the affected person to experience all forms of "suffering" (as per Buddhist definition).

82. Cf. Simpson, Dissanayake, and Jayasekera, supra note 78; Simpson, supra note 78.

83. These observations could be made in interviews conducted with Buddhist ethicists Somparn Promta, Mano Laohavanich (Bhikkhu Mettānando), P. D. Premasiri, Sumana Ratnayake, and others.

84. Promta, supra note 39, 11–14.

85. Ratanakul, supra note 13, 145.

86. Foucault is mainly interested in practices of power and neoliberal governmentality—the transition of a classical system in which a sovereign executes power over life and death to a modern nation state with the power to install eugenics and other forms of managing "life" itself (cf. Michel Foucault, *The Birth of Biopolitics: Lectures at the Collège de France, 1978–1979*, trans. Graham Burchell (New York: Palgrave MacMillan, 2008).

87. Ratanakul, supra note 40, 319–322.

88. Sugunasiri, supra note 71, 78, 80.

89. The best translation of these Tibetan teachings, which became increasingly popular in Western hospice care, can be found in *The Tibetan Book of the Dead: The Great Liberation of Hearing in the Intermediate States*, trans. Gyurme Dorje (London: Penguin Books, 2005).

90. It is necessary to note here that some Buddhist texts portray examples of ethically justified self-induced death: some spiritually advanced practitioners ("arhats") were able to develop wholesome thoughts even in such moments (cf. Bhikkhu Dhammavihari, "Euthanasia: A Study in Relation to Original Theravada Buddhist Thinking" (1996), accessed March 15, 2014. http://www.metta.lk/english/euthanasia.htm; Padmasiri de Silva, *Buddhism, Ethics, and Society: The Conflicts and Dilemmas of Our Times* (Clayton, Victoria, Australia: Monash Asia Institute, 2002), 81–96; Martin Delhey, "Views on Suicide in Buddhism: Some Remarks," in *Buddhism and Violence*, ed. Michael Zimmermann (Lumbini, Nepal: Liri, 2006), 25–63.

91. Tsomo, supra note 12, 177.

92. Cf. Dhammavihari, supra note 90; Keown, supra note 7, 184–185.

93. Cf. Ratanakul, supra note 40, 322–325.

94. Cf. Jens Schlieter, "Karma, Contingency, and the 'Point of No Return': Predictive Medicine and Buddhist Perspectives," in *Knowing One's Medical Fate in Advance: Challenges for Diagnosis and Treatment, Philosophy, Ethics and Religion*, ed. Georg Pfleiderer et al. (Basel: Karger, 2012), 106–120.

95. XIV Dalai Lama, in Wendy Bainbridge and Elizabeth Baines, "Insight into Palliative Care: An Audience with the Dalai Lama," *European Journal of Palliative Care* 8, no. 2 (2001): 66–69, 67.

96. Laurence J. Kirmayer, "The Sound of One Hand Clapping: Listening to Prozac in Japan," in *Prozac as a Way of Life*, ed. Carl Elliott, Tod Chambers (Chapel Hill: University of North Carolina Press, 2004), 164–193, 174.

97. Tsomo, supra note 64, 533.

98. Ibid. This argument, however, should not be confused with the argument of authenticity, which uses concepts of a normatively loaded "naturalness" and "enduring personal identity," which are both problematic for Buddhists (cf. James J. Hughes, "Using Neurotechnologies to Develop Virtues: A Buddhist Approach to Cognitive Enhancement" (three parts, 2012), accessed March 15, 2014. http://ieet.org/index.php/IEET/more/hughes20121016.

99. Cf. ibid.

100. Cf. Susanne Mrozik, *Virtuous Bodies: The Physical Dimensions of Morality in Buddhist Ethics* (Oxford: Oxford University Press, 2007), 67.

101. Nozick, supra note 75, 42–43. In the summary of Thomas Metzinger, *The Ego-Tunnel* (New York: Basic Books, 2009), 198, the relevance of Nozick's thought experiment for the question of treating suffering through pharmaceutical means (or other external stimulants) becomes immediately clear: "You have the option of being hooked up to an 'Experience Machine' that keeps you in a state of permanent happiness. Would you do it? Interestingly, Nozick found that most people would not opt to spend the rest of their lives hooked up to such a machine. The reason is that most of us do not value bliss as such, but want it grounded in truth, virtue, artistic achievement, or some sort of higher good." Actually, we do not want to be "deluded Bliss Machines but conscious subjects who are happy for a reason.... We want an extraordinary insight into reality, into moral value or beauty as objective facts. Nozick took this reaction to be a defeat of hedonism."

102. Andrew Fenton, "Buddhism and Neuroethics: The Ethics of Pharmaceutical Cognitive Enhancement," *Developing World Bioethics* 9, no. 2 (2009): 47–56, 47.

103. Ibid., 51.

104. Surprisingly, Fenton himself argues with the cognitive enhanced mind as a means—as it shall be used, like meditation, for "deepening the insight into the nature of the self and world and the gradual elimination of *duḥkha*" (ibid., 53).

105. Yao, supra note 44, 214.

106. Karl Popper, *The Open Society and Its Enemies. Volume 1: The Spell of Plato* (London: Routledge, 2002), 284–285.

107. Pinit Ratanakul, "Bioethics in Thailand: The Struggle for Buddhist Solutions," *Journal of Medicine and Philosophy* 13 (1988): 301–312, 301–302; this approach of four principles has been modeled in reaction to Tom L. Beauchamp; James F. Childress, *Principles of Biomedical Ethics*,5th ed. (Oxford: Oxford University Press, 2001), 12–13: "autonomy, beneficence, non-maleficence, justice."

108. Yao, supra note 44, 214.

17

Human Suffering and the Limits of Secular Bioethics

Mark J. Cherry

Medicine has long been the focus of marked human passion. It extends the hope of remedying the perceived deficiencies of human nature, the reduction of suffering, and the postponement of death. As a result, medicine fascinates, commanding moral and political attention, and evoking a set of expectations that often have a momentum of their own. For example, in the United States, more than one out of every seven dollars is spent on some form of health care. In 2011, such expenditure amounted to approximately 17.7 percent of the entire gross domestic product: roughly $8,507.60 for every man, woman, and child. Health care expenditures in Canada, Germany, and the United Kingdom in 2010 represented 11.2, 11.3, and 9.4 percent, respectively, of each country's gross domestic product, or approximately $4,521.60, $4,494.70, and $3,405.50 per capita.[1] Technologically advanced medicine dedicated to extending life plays a significant role in such expenditures. In the United States, between 17.4 and 39 percent of all hospital costs are expended on critical care medicine, representing as much as 11.2 percent of all health care spending in the country.[2] This increasingly consequential consumption of personal and social resources is driven by very real concerns to ameliorate the physiological collapse and human suffering brought on by age, accident, injury, and disease.

Yet, even from the time of Plato (427–347 B.C.), medicine has been associated with an appropriation of authority that threatened to undermine proper virtue (see *The Republic* 405a–410a).[3] Plato understood that medicine can be a source of temptation to hubris: an excessive pride, a passion to control life and death. Plato, for example, explored the ways in which medicine could be utilized to cleave unhealthy and diseased subjects from the state. He cites approvingly:

> ...the remedies... were enough to heal any man who was healthy and sound.... But they would have nothing to do with unhealthy and intemperate subjects, whose lives were of no use either to themselves or others; the art of medicine was not designed for their good, and though they were as rich as Midas, the sons of Asclepius would have declined to attend them.[4]

As Plato appreciated, because all medical choices must be made in the face of human finitude, they encourage existential questions regarding the attributes of the good life and the good death. Insofar as one is honestly to face the challenges of human suffering in an age of life-sustaining therapy, one must come to terms with the limits of human knowledge and resources, even when confronted with the collapse of human abilities, suffering, and death.

The challenge, however, is that this is a core set of existential questions to which secular bioethics can, in principle, give no unequivocal response. Indeed, the international, secular ethical and bioethical debate routinely fails adequately to appreciate the depth of the difficulties of providing such answers. To provide a definitive response to such existential concerns, to make unequivocal moral judgments in response to suffering requires a canonical morality, a binding moral standpoint from which to know truly the nature of the right, the good, and the virtuous. As I argue, secular ethics, and thus secular bioethics, possesses no such definitive moral point of view. Consequently, all attempts by secular bioethics to grasp the meaning of human life and human suffering so as authoritatively to guide medical decision making and public policy are inevitably no more than socially and culturally conditioned preferences regarding lifestyles and death styles.

Privileged Secular Assumptions: Autonomous Choice and Egalitarian Social Justice

The dominant secular approaches to bioethics and health care law in the United States and Western Europe tend to support an unqualified affirmation of persons as the source of authority over themselves. Persons appear as atomic individuals, outside of families or other social structures, and endowed with a right to determine their own future.[5] Cardinal moral value is assigned to liberty as individual autonomous choice and an egalitarian understanding of social justice. Persons as rational moral beings are appreciated as autonomous and self-determining individuals, who are to shape their moral values and perceptions of the good life and the good death for themselves. Individual autonomy is highlighted as integral to human good and human flourishing. As a result, Western health care law and public policy are generally framed in terms of individual-oriented consent, reflecting the centrality of the individual for medical decision making, and ensuring adequate opportunity for persons to free themselves from familial relationships[6] or traditional religious perspectives that are perceived as too restrictive of personal choice.[7] The focal point of the moral life is assumed to reside in autonomous self-determination, where liberty as the celebration of free individualistic choice is accented as integral to the good life for persons. Each person is understood as possessing an equal liberty-based entitlement to realize his own understandings of the good life and the good death, unhampered by the choices of others or the constraints of nature.

This conceptual point regarding the equal liberty of persons must be underscored. Here, liberty functions as a value, rather than a side constraint.[8] So conceived, liberty frames inequalities as social injustices because some persons are less able to realize their own understandings of the good life. In turn, there is a presumption that such injustices ought to be redressed through regulatory state action. Natural talents and abilities are, as John Rawls urges, to be appreciated as arbitrary from a moral point of view[9] and as common assets for the creation of social benefit.[10] Insofar as all do not have an equal chance at realizing their own appreciation of the good, justice is perceived as requiring state action to mitigate the influences of social contingencies and natural fortune.[11] Such concerns are usually encapsulated as the need to sustain more than the conditions of formal liberty, as freedom from constraint, but to guarantee material liberty, as expressed in fair equality of outcomes.[12] The underlying concern is for equal worth of personal and political liberty, especially concerning the material and social conditions necessary to eliminate natural and social disadvantages so that each may enjoy fair equality of outcome in terms of the freedom to fulfill their potential, however defined.

Within such a political framework, access to the full range of health care possibilities receives special attention because medicine is assumed to be a key instrumental good, which is integral to the protection and realization of other interests and opportunities.[13] Entitlements to health and health care, for example, are often captured under the general rubric of basic "human rights." Consider, for example, the United Nations Educational, Scientific and Cultural Organization (UNESCO) Universal Declaration on Bioethics and Human Rights (issued October 19, 2005), which simply announced a significant array of "human rights" as welfare entitlements. Article 14 asserted rights to personal health and health care, medicine, nutrition, water, improved living conditions, environmental protection, and so forth—as well as corresponding governmental duties to promote and provide for such public health measures:

1. The promotion of health and social development for their people is a central purpose of governments that all sectors of society share.
2. Taking into account that the enjoyment of the highest attainable standard of health is one of the fundamental rights of every human being without distinction of race, religion, political belief, economic or social condition, progress in science and technology should advance.
   (a) Access to quality health care and essential medicines, especially for the health of women and children, because health is essential to life itself and must be considered to be a social and human good.... [14]

Not only is "...the highest attainable standard of health.. " judged to be a fundamental human right, but the claim that "...promotion of health and social development for their people is a central purpose of government that all sectors of society share" rhetorically places such expansive regulatory powers under the rubric of legitimate political authority.[15]

Here, UNESCO is drawing on the popular idea that health as a fundamental human right is essential to achieving equal worth of individual liberty. The state is envisaged as a liberal morally pluralistic democracy, framing economic, institutional, and social structures that guarantee equal access to the basic goods of society (health care and other welfare entitlements) so as to sustain progressive notions of fair equality of opportunity and outcome. Advocates who defend human rights as basic welfare entitlements usually attempt to justify such entitlements as essential to the "equal consideration for all persons":

> We suggest instead that human rights should be understood as moral claims grounded in *basic human interests*. These are interests that are universally shared by all (or nearly all) human beings, and they are the kinds of interests that justify assigning obligations to others, or to society generally, to secure or protect those interests... health care is a human right because being healthy is a universal interest, common to all people, that grounds duties in others. The basic human interest in health grounds negative duties—duties not to make anyone sick—and, especially for government, positive duties—duties to protect and/or to promote the health of others.... Ultimately, what grounds human rights, including corresponding obligations, is something fundamental to morality: equal consideration for all persons.[16]

Because health care helps guarantee the chance to enjoy the normal range of human opportunities, access to health care as a basic entitlement, without income, gender, religious, or other barriers, is accented as foundational to preserving individual liberty and fair equality of opportunity.[17] Preserving personal capacities for forming, revising, and achieving one's own goals and objectives, for defining individual meaning and self-satisfaction requires removing, as much as possible, the physical, mental, and social handicaps of illness, disease, and disability. Unless personally chosen and valued, all mental, emotional, or physical suffering is to be set aside.

Moreover, because the focal point of the moral life is assumed to be autonomous self-determination, limits on the expression of one's autonomy are assessed as unjust. Further accent is, therefore, given to health care services that are judged integral to the realization of important lifestyle projects so as to avoid the mental, emotional, or physical suffering resulting from their frustration. Such services include easy access to reproductive technologies and abortion services, as well as to control over one's death style, such as access to euthanasia services to avoid suffering at the end of life.

Activists, for example, have come to appreciate access to abortion without restriction as central to social and political justice for women.[18]

> Lack of access to abortion is arguably the most important barrier to economic and social equality for women in the United States. Legal access to abortion ensures that women will not be forced to continue pregnancies against their will, which is necessary if women are to enjoy a level of human rights equal to those afforded men.[19]

Access to abortion is assumed to be important so that women can avoid the "...mandatory dungeon of motherhood."[20] The United Nations statement, "HIV/AIDS and Human Rights" (1996) specifically calls for easy access to contraception and abortion as the means for liberating women from traditional biological and social constraints on their freedom: "Laws should also be enacted to ensure women's reproductive and secular rights, including the right of...means of contraception, including safe and legal abortion and the freedom to choose among these, the right to determine the number and spacing of children...."[21] The United Nations Convention on the Elimination of All Forms of Discrimination against Women prohibits policies that "...require women seeking health services to obtain authorization from their husbands, or that criminalize medical procedures that only women need, such as abortion."[22] Abortion is interpreted as giving women personal control over their reproductive lives,[23] freeing them from the burdens of pregnancy and child care, and, therefore, as essential to preserving their individual liberty.

Since individuals are perceived as choosing life values and moral content for themselves, even medical killing with consent and assistance in self-killing have been placed within a context of permissible autonomous choices. Voluntary euthanasia and physician-assisted suicide are encapsulated as no more than personal choices regarding death style. The shift in accent is again toward individual authority in medical decision making.[24] Many bioethicists conclude, for example, that physician-assisted suicide is an appropriate exercise of autonomy to avoid further unwanted suffering; however, such "suffering" is personally defined. Consider, for example, the recent case of the deaf adult male twins in Belgium, who chose to be euthanized after they discovered that they were going blind. According to published reports, the twins were neither terminally ill nor in any real physical pain. Instead, they choose to be medically "put down" so as to avoid the "suffering" of slowly going blind and never seeing each other again.[25] To many commentators, the autonomy-based argument for voluntary euthanasia and physician-assisted suicide appears to be an obvious and appropriate response to human suffering. Assisted suicide is affirmed as preserving oneself from unnecessary pain and suffering, while fulfilling one's last act of self-determination. Such deaths are presented as alleviating the physical pain and mental anguish of those beyond effective therapy. Adversity can drain a person's life of meaning, and from such a perspective, individuals appear to have a right of self-determination to judge when to end their own lives. It is not wrong painlessly to kill someone who wishes to die, it is argued, because they are not thereby deprived of anything they value.[26] Insofar as the individual sufficiently substantiates the wish to die, the value of personal autonomy, it is claimed, is straightforwardly affirmed.

In short, contemporary medicine evokes a technological imperative; that is, a moral assumption that any health care technology that promises to satisfy human desire or to relieve suffering ought to be available for utilization at the patient's request. The very existence of such high-technology medical interventions for many demands its use. For many, any possibility to relieve human mental or physical suffering appears permissible, if not obligatory. Suffering is only appreciated as surd. Health care, as a result, is assessed primarily in terms of its ability to satisfy personal choice. Physicians and other health care professionals have been reconceptualized as technicians, whose public role it is to help fulfill the autonomous lifestyle and death-style preferences of their patients/clients. Such assumptions offer real temptations to spend significant sums of money in pursuit of self-fulfillment (e.g., cosmetic surgery) and marginal chances incrementally to postpone death (e.g., the use of very expensive intensive care unit resources for nonsalvageable patients[27]), as well as to satisfy lifestyle choices (e.g., abortion, gender reassignment surgery, and treatments for erectile dysfunction) and death-style preferences (e.g., voluntary euthanasia, physician-assisted suicide).

Coming to Terms with Moral Pluralism

What is necessary, but has not been forthcoming, is a definitive general secular moral standard to guide medical decision making. As a field of inquiry, bioethics rarely pays adequate attention to the significant challenges that religious, cultural, and secular moral diversity presents to decision making. Compassing persons from disparate and more or less intact moral communities with varying moral intuitions, taken-for-granted moral norms and commitments, as well as diverse understandings of the common good, the national and international moral landscape is highly complex. Western culture routinely confronts a deep fragmentation of moral visions regarding human goods and human flourishing. Secular reason has been unable definitively to secure a uniquely authoritative account of the right, the good, and the virtuous to guide medical decision making and health care policy. Moral pluralism is empirically real and very substantial. One need only consider the bitter bioethical debates concerning abortion, human embryo research, health care allocation, stem cell research, and euthanasia to note that this fragmentation is significant. The contrast among divergent moral viewpoints and morally licit approaches for addressing human suffering is often stark and intractable.

In this regard, human embryo experimentation is heuristic. The often acrimonious debates regarding human embryonic stem cell research involve deliberation regarding the moral status of the embryo and the aspired to goods of medical research to address human suffering. On the one hand, human embryonic research has been heralded as the key for unlocking future treatments for diabetes, Parkinson's disease, immunodeficiencies, cancer, metabolic and genetic disorders, and a variety of birth defects, as well as for discovering new methods for generating tissues and organs.[28] On the other hand, many argue that the killing of the embryo is the moral equivalent of murder.[29] Deliberation regarding the moral status of human embryo experimentation typically concerns at what moment the child possesses a soul, or at what point the embryo crosses the development and moral threshold to be protected as a person. It has become commonplace in secular bioethics to hold that biological development is gradual, with no clear moment between conception and birth to draw a moral dividing line between person and nonperson. As a result, there is fairly broad agreement among secular bioethicists that moral responsibility for killing embryonic life probably does not begin at the early blastocyst stage, and thus that it is unreasonable to conclude as a matter of public policy that it is wrong to utilize embryos for experimentation. Proponents of embryonic stem cell research routinely motivate public opinion with a vision of the future in which innovative medical technologies extend human life, cure disease, or otherwise relieve suffering. If human suffering is at stake, how can we fail to act? Yet, such secular judgments reflect just one particular moral perspective among many.

By way of contrast, a statement from the Holy Synod of Bishops of the Orthodox Church in America reaffirmed the traditional Christian unambiguous conclusion of the spiritual implications of the destruction of human embryos: it possesses the moral and spiritual impact equivalent to murder. The *Didache,* which dates from the first century A.D. states, "Do not murder a child by abortion, nor, again, destroy that which is born."[30] Canon 91 of the Quinisext Council, A.D. 691, reads: "Those who give drugs for procuring abortion, and those who receive poisons to kill the fetus, are subjected to the penalty of murder."[31] Moreover, as Saint Basil (A.D. 329–379) makes clear, neither an account of ensoulment nor of the state of the formation of the fetus is relevant to this traditional Christian understanding. "The woman who purposely destroys her unborn child is guilty of murder. With us there is no nice enquiry as to its being formed or unformed."[32] St. Basil recognized that even early embryocide possesses the same spiritual effects as murder, without committing himself to understanding the embryo as already possessing a soul or to any particular view regarding the states of embryonic development. As the Holy Synod of Bishops of the Orthodox Church in America notes, to appreciate the destruction of embryos rightly, we must understand this practice in terms of its full spiritual implications.[33]

Here, the conceptual point is that as the underlying metaphysical, theological, and epistemological assumptions for how to approach reality change, so also do our understandings of responsible human choice and permissible action. Whose understanding of the deep nature of reality should be taken as definitive to set permissible limits on medical research aimed at the reduction of human suffering and the extension of life? Whose understanding of morally responsible action should guide such innovation in high technology medicine: the fully secular or the traditionally Christian, among the many possibilities? The decision is not neutral. Making such choices will guide the crafting of public policy for the use of life-sustaining therapy and thereby affirm one out of the many possible social and moral realities.

Even appealing to "justice" will not suffice because one must provide definitive content to give substance to one's account of justice. To privilege any one account of justice over others (e.g., utilitarian, Rawlsian, Marxist, egalitarian) requires granting a particular moral theory of the good, a specific view of moral rationality or assessment of the morally reasonable. John Rawls's arguments in service of his theory of "justice as fairness" are in this respect heuristic. Although Rawls is often taken as having provided a straightforward defense of a universally binding account of justice, the particularity of his thin theory of the good[34] and of the lexical ordering of his principles of justice indicate otherwise.[35] Rawls, in the end, articulated only one very specific secular account of justice, driven by a lexical prioritizing of values in which he ordered liberty first and fair equality of opportunity second; concern for the maximization of resources is affirmed only insofar as it rebounds to the benefit of the worst-off members of society and is prioritized third. As others have noted, this ranking leads to counterintuitive consequences.[36] Among other puzzles, given his lexical ordering, no amount of gain in the maximization of resources is permitted to offset losses in political liberty. One is not permitted to trade off great advantages in economic prosperity for losses in equal voting rights, for example. His theory implies, all things considered, that it is more rational and socially just to maintain a poor society, while politically sustaining an equal right to vote, than to give up one's voting rights in favor of wealth maximization. Those who care more about advantaging themselves, or those whom they love, economically, than they do about casting their one vote among millions of other votes are easily left asking why it is that anyone should affirm Rawls's specific ranking of primary goods that constitute his particular principles of justice.

Even in 1971, with the original publication of *A Theory of Justice*, Rawls recognized that his exploration constituted only one particular, rather than a supposedly universally binding, theory of justice that governed outside of context and history. At times, Rawls indicated his own awareness that he could not offer an account of justice outside of a particular sociohistorically conditioned circumstance. He acknowledged, for example:

> For while some moral principles may seem natural and even obvious, there are great obstacles to maintaining that they are necessarily true, or even to explaining what is meant by this. Indeed, I have held that these principles are contingent in the sense that they are chosen in the original position in the light of general facts. More likely candidates for necessary moral truths are the conditions imposed on the adoption of principles; but actually it seems best to regard these conditions simply as reasonable stipulations to be assessed eventually by the whole theory to which they belong. There is no set of conditions or first principles that can be plausibly claimed to be necessary or definitive or morality and thereby especially suited to carry the burden of justification.[37]

> It may be said that the agreement in considered convictions is constantly changing and varies between one society, or part thereof, and another.[38]

In these passages, Rawls steps away from a strong Kantian reading of his position. Here, even the early Rawls at least implicitly recognized that all secular moral viewpoints are sociohistorically conditioned. As a result, what has been taken by many to be an account advanced by Rawls as the morally rational can at best be defended as only one among a plurality of very particular accounts of the politically reasonable.

By 1985, Rawls acknowledged the particularity of his position. In "Justice as Fairness: Political not Metaphysical," Rawls clearly stepped back from the claim that his position could be understood as a universally true account of justice.[39] Rawls acknowledged that his project is ultimately fundamentally limited: "Whether justice as fairness can be extended to a general political conception for different kinds of societies existing under different historical and social conditions, or whether it can be extended to a general moral conception, or a significant part thereof, are altogether separate questions."[40] Rawls had come to the conclusion that his position is simply the framework as he saw it of the political commitments central to the Western liberal social-democratic constitutional state.[41] He had come to acknowledge that the position he was advancing was that of a particular sociopolitical agenda. He had come to advance the position that his account compassed only that which he took to be involved in framing justice as the politically reasonable with regard to sociodemocratic constitutional states. "Thus, political liberalism looks for a political conception of justice that we hope can gain the support of an overlapping consensus of reasonable religious, philosophical, and moral doctrines in a society regulated by it."[42] He had gathered together a cluster of more or less reflective and interconnected moral and political intuitions supported by no more than a particular moral political narrative.

As Rawls came publicly to acknowledge, his account of political liberalism is not grounded in anything other than the political conception itself. "Political liberalism, then, aims for a political conception of justice as a freestanding view. It offers no specific metaphysical or epistemological doctrine beyond what is implied by the political conception itself."[43] The viewpoint Rawls embraces, as he acknowledges, is a political vision that possesses no particular moral necessity; indeed, the moral view is only a contingently persuasive socially conditioned freestanding view of liberty, equality, and social justice. Nor can Rawls's account be appreciated as properly structuring the primary goods and basic social institutions of a just society as such without simply assuming the truth of his theory. Rawls's account of justice as fairness and their applications to health care policy are without final foundations. As a freestanding moral political viewpoint, Rawls's theory of justice can be met by other, albeit contrasting, freestanding moral political viewpoints. There exist no independent, secular, noncontingent grounds for preferring Rawls's account of social justice over other competing accounts of justice and the politically reasonable. In the end, Rawls's arguments exist as no more than intellectual support in service of a very specific socio-political agenda.

More generally, any particular secular account of the right, the good, the virtuous, or the just can, in principle, only advance one viewpoint among a plurality of accounts of morality and social justice to direct medical choice in the face of human suffering. Rather than being guided by a canonical moral vision anchored in being-as-such, secular bioethics is situated within currently popular socially and culturally conditioned preferences. As a result, it can demonstrate neither a definitive connection between its particular ideological commitments and the deep nature of reality, nor why following such precepts would necessarily be politically reasonable or particularly rational. Rather than providing an objective moral viewpoint, for example, Rawls presents just one, idiosyncratic, understanding of social justice, among a plurality of alternative accounts, grounded in one out of a plurality of moral viewpoints, embodying at best a very particular normative content and social ethos, whose proponents seek to establish at law.

In similar fashion, international pronouncements on egalitarian justice and individual liberty, such as the Convention on the Elimination of All Forms of Discrimination against Women, encapsulate only one particular set of secular moral intuitions. Nor has any sound rational argument successfully been advanced to establish the various political declarations, such as UNESCO's Universal Declaration on Bioethics and Human Rights, which continue to give political and institutional expression to the Enlightenment hope that ethics "... should liberate from unjustified customs and constraints, those contrary to the demands of universal moral reason."[44] Any particular account of secular bioethics inevitably expresses an ideological viewpoint that is at best a cluster of moral intuitions held together by one narrative chosen from among a plurality of moral narratives that can only present itself as a freestanding moral view without foundations. Secular bioethics is thus starkly limited in its ability adequately to respond to human suffering in the face of human finitude, in that it cannot express a unique, universally binding, moral point of view.

As a result, we are left with significant questions regarding how public policy should be crafted adequately to address suffering in an age devoted to the medical manipulation of the human condition and the control of death. Should public policy simply acquiesce to the deep moral intuitions of academic bioethicists, to current bioethical convention, or to whatever policy seems best able to produce innovative medical therapy? Or, should society seek moral content to guide public policy through appeal to intuitions, consequences, casuistry, the notion of unbiased choice, game theory, or middle-level principles? All such attempts, as Engelhardt has argued, confront insurmountable obstacles. Particular moral content must already be presupposed in order to choose among intuitions, rank consequences, evaluate exemplary cases, or mediate among various principles; otherwise, no rational choice at all will be possible. Even if one merely ranks cardinal moral concerns differently, such as liberty, equality, justice, and security, one will thereby affirm different moral visions, divergent understandings of the good life, varying senses of what it is to act appropriately. Each attempt straightforwardly assumes the moral rationality of its own particular moral content. Each account affirms its own particular understanding of the politically reasonable. Each viewpoint reconstructs a particular socially, historically, and culturally conditioned perspective. In general secular terms, it is impossible to break through the seemingly interminable bioethical debates to definitive truth.[45] Secular morality, and thus secular bioethics, is without definitive foundations; it is ultimately ambiguous.

Conclusion

Secular bioethics offers at best a deflated plurality of moral perspectives. Matters that had once been held to have cardinal significance (e.g., birth, copulation, suffering, and death) have been recast as no more than socially and culturally conditioned personal preferences regarding legitimate lifestyle and death-style choices. Without a canonical point of view, a binding standpoint that is not already conditioned by a particular society, culture, or point in history, all accounts of morality are necessarily contingent. Secular morality possesses no ultimate binding significance; at best, its import is contingent upon individual judgments regarding personal prudential interests and potentially idiosyncratic desires.[46] Without definitive foundation in being-in-itself, morality shatters into numerous incommensurable perspectives; its hold on us becomes fragmented and contingent[47]; and it becomes impossible, even in principle, to secure a definitive moral understanding of human suffering or of the proper limits on high-technology medicine. This is why secular morality, and thus secular bioethics, is inherently ambiguous and irreducibility plural. There exists no standpoint outside of particular cultural sociohistorically conditioned perspectives from which to communicate any deeper perspective of morality, suffering, or life-sustaining therapy that such a perspective would secure.

Despite such lack of definitive foundations, particular ideological worldviews may falsely claim to establish how one ought in secular terms to act *sub specie aeternitatis*. Secular worldviews (e.g., human rights discourse) and particular secular philosophers (e.g., John Rawls) often rhetorically give the impression that their views bind moral agents as such. However, such robust claims regarding the capacities of secular reason are unjustifiable. General secular reason cannot secure a single authoritative account of the characteristics of the appropriately flourishing human life, that is, of basic human goods, true integral human fulfillment, or proper approaches to suffering. Instead, contemporary society, much like the ancient world, discloses a significant plurality of moral visions. Our contemporary moral discussions are embedded in what Alasdair MacIntyre has characterized as a cosmopolitan culture articulated in the international language of secular modernity, that is, a morality isolated from traditional cultures and religions and devoid of a shared ethics to provide a common moral compass.[48]

What ranking of potential human goods or proposed moral principles should one adopt? Whose appreciation of harms versus benefits or account of human flourishing should guide our approach to human suffering? Which social goals should frame the public health care policy challenges for addressing such concerns? Which of the competing accounts of the right, the good, and the virtuous should guide appreciation of the politically reasonable or the morally rational such that we would know when and how to address suffering? The deep tensions among various possible, competing and incommensurable moral perspectives are irresolvable. There are as many moral understandings as there are different religions and secular moral worldviews.[49] Secular morality exists as no more than the various narratives we tell each other. Even our deepest moral intuitions about human suffering are no more than particular human emotions or political creations floating on current social and cultural fashion. Secular bioethics is irreconcilably plural.

Secular bioethics is unable to provide a definitive meaningful account of pain and suffering, disability, and death, beyond a descriptive account of the firing of synapses, the collapse of human abilities, and the end of life. It cannot provide definitive canonical moral guidance for proper medical choice. This is why contemporary Western bioethics is remarkably thin. Populated with the rhetoric of personal autonomy, equality, and social justice, secular bioethics encourages the expansion of choice and the elimination of suffering so as to satisfy lifestyle and death-style preferences, but it is utterly unable authoritatively to determine which choices to make, which kinds of physical, mental, or emotional suffering to ameliorate, or whose deaths to postpone. Given different taken-for-granted background starting points, underlying assumptions, and personal values, one will be led to embrace varying accounts of proper medical choice. One will judge differently regarding the intrinsic or instrumental value of human suffering and will come to varying conclusions regarding which types of human suffering to embrace, ignore, or eliminate. Moreover, all such considerations affect our understandings of the appropriate allocation of medical resources to address human suffering and the proper use of life-sustaining therapy.

Having begun with the privileged presumption of the sovereignty of the individual, who judges physical and mental suffering for himself, secular bioethics can provide no particular meaning to suffering. Instead, the definition of suffering and its proper appreciation are left up to individual, potentially idiosyncratic, choice. Suffering may be instrumentally useful, helping to identify a physical ailment (e.g., gallstones) or psychological interest (e.g., gender reassignment) that medicine may have the capacity to address. Suffering may be embraced in the pursuit of other instrumental goods (e.g., "no pain, no gain") or rejected as hampering one's lifestyle choices (e.g., prescription medication to address erectile dysfunction in HIV-positive men). All suffering and death, and thus all medical choice, are set fully within the particular interests of particular persons. As a result, despite the lack of firm foundations in sound rational argument, secular bioethics routinely sanctions access to nearly any means to satisfy individual lifestyle and death-style choices so as to avoid emotional, mental, or physical suffering, as at least morally permissible, if not obligatory. Moreover, secular bioethics seeks state-based authority to create and regulate access to health care because it judges such "entitlements" as necessary to secure the equal liberty of persons. In short, contemporary circumstances are much as Plato described: modern medicine and contemporary secular bioethics embody the potentially unconstrained human passion to control life and death.

Notes

1. Organisation for Economic Co-operation and Development, Health Data 2013 (last updated October 11, 2013), accessed March 27, 2014, www.oecd.org.

2. C. M. Coopersmith et al., "A Comparison of Critical Care Research Funding and the Financial Burden of Critical Illness in the United States," *Critical Care Medicine* 40, no. 4 (2012): 1072–1079.

3. Plato. *The Dialogues of Plato*, trans. B. Jowett (New York: Charles Scribner's Sons, 1892).

4. Ibid., 408a.

5. P. Applebaum, C. Lidz, and A. Meisel, *Informed Consent: Legal Theory and Clinical Practice* (New York: Oxford University Press, 1987); President's Commission for the Study of Ethical Problems in Medicine and Biomedical and Behavioral Research. *Making Health Care Decisions* (3 vols.) (Washington, DC: U.S. Government Printing Office, 1982).

6. This view of individuals in medical decision making approaches patients as if they are not members of intact functioning families, unless there is good evidence to the contrary. Patients who wish to be treated as members of families, such as a mother who wishes to have her eldest son make medical decisions on her behalf, have usually been required explicitly to authorize the involvement of family members in the decision-making process. See, e.g., Ruth Faden and Tom Beauchamp, *A History and Theory of Informed Consent* (New York: Oxford University Press, 1986); Stephen Wear, *Informed Consent: Patient Autonomy and Physician Beneficence within Clinical Medicine* (Dordrecht: Kluwer Academic 1993). As H. Tristram Engelhardt Jr. marks this practice: "Those who regard autonomous individualism as the presumptively appropriate relation among persons would require any deviations to be established by explicit statement and agreement. For example, patients would be presumptively treated as autonomous individuals willing and committed to choosing on their own, unless they explicitly demanded to be regarded and treated within a traditional family structure." H. Tristram Engelhardt Jr., "Morality, Universality, and Particularity: Rethinking the Role of Community in the Foundations of Bioethics," in *Cross-Cultural Perspectives on the (Im) Possibility of Global Bioethics*, ed. J. Tao Lai Po-wah (Dordrecht: Kluwer Academic, 2002), 19–38, 24–25. It is the individual, rather than the family, who is appreciated as possessing decisional authority. See also Mark J. Cherry and H. Tristram Engelhardt Jr., "Informed Consent in Texas: Theory and Practice," *Journal of Medicine and Philosophy* 29, no. 2 (2004): 237–252.

7. Traditional religions and cultures are also appreciated within a hermeneutic of suspicion. Elements of the feminist movement, for example, adopted a highly critical stance against the traditional family precisely because they saw the family as an institution of unequal power relationships and female subordination. As Susan Okin rightly perceives, the traditional family embodies particular understandings of proper family structures, including appropriate gender roles. That is why, for example, she concludes that traditional religious groups should not be permitted to nurture and educate their children within the religion itself, decrying such pedagogy as indoctrination. Susan Okin, "'Mistresses of Their Own Destiny': Group Rights, Gender, and Realistic Rights of Exit," *Ethics* 112 (2002): 205–230, 218, 226.

Okin argues that "The liberal state . . . should not only not give special rights or exemptions to cultural and religious groups that discriminate against or oppress women. It should also enforce individual rights against such groups when the opportunity arises and encourage all groups within its borders to cease such practices" (Ibid., 229–230). Amy Gutmann argues similarly: "The basic principles of liberalism, those necessary to protect every person's basic liberties and opportunities, place substantial limits on social diversity. . . . The limits on racial and gender discrimination, for example, enable many people to pursue ways of life that would otherwise be closed to them by discriminatory practices at the same time as they undermine or at least impede some traditional ways of life." Amy Gutmann, "Civic Education and Social Diversity," *Ethics* 105 (1995): 557–579, 559.

8. See Robert Nozick, *Anarchy, State and Utopia* (New York: Basic Books, 1974).

9. John Rawls, *A Theory of Justice*, revised ed. (Cambridge, MA: Harvard University Press, 1999), 63–64.

10. Ibid., 87.

11. Ibid., 63.

12. As Kai Nielsen expressed this view: "If we want a world of moral equals, we also need a world in which people stand to each other in a rough equality of condition. To have a world in which a condition of equal respect and concern obtain, we need ... a rough equality of resources. If equality as a right is to be secure; that is, if that is a right that people can securely exercise, we must obtain the good of equality of condition." Kai Nielsen, *Equality and Liberty: A Defense of Radical Egalitarianism* (Totowa, NJ: Rowman & Allenheld, 1985), 10. See also Norman Daniels, "Equal Liberty and Unequal Worth of Liberty," in *Reading Rawls*, ed. Norman Daniels (New York: Basic Books, 1975), 253–281; Norman Daniels, *Justice and Justification* (Cambridge, UK: Cambridge University Press, 1996).

13. See, e.g., Norman Daniels. *Just Health Care* (Cambridge, UK: Cambridge University Press, 1985); Norman Daniels, *Just Health: Meeting Health Needs Fairly* (Cambridge, UK: Cambridge University Press, 2008); Allen Buchanan, *Justice and Health Care: Selected Essays* (New York: Oxford University Press, 2009).

14. United Nations Educational, Scientific and Cultural Organization (UNESCO). 2005 Universal Declaration on Bioethics and Human Rights. in *Records of the General Conference* (Geneva: UNESCO, 2005), accessed March 16, 2014, http://portal.unesco.org/en/ev.php-URL_ID=31058&URL_DO=DO_TOPIC&URL_SECTION=201.html.

15. In its "Aims," the Universal Declaration on Bioethics and Human Rights affirms that the intention is "to provide a universal framework of principles and procedures to guide States in the formulation of their legislation, policies or other instruments in the field of bioethics." Section 36 of the Resolutions of the October 2005 General Conference states: "*The General Conference* ... 1. *Adopts* the Universal Declaration on Bioethics and Human Rights, as annexed hereto; 2. *Calls upon* Member States: (a) to make every effort to adopt measures, whether of a legislative, administrative or other character, to give effect to the principles set out in the Declaration, in accordance with international human rights law; such measures should be supported by action in the sphere of education, training and public information ... " Ibid. The authors' purpose is to introduce new political obligations, statutory rights, welfare entitlements, and moral duties under the general rubric of "human rights," through the simple expedient of making the announcement. UNESCO's goal is to delineate a legislative, administrative, and educational agenda for state action.

16. Allen Buchanan, supra note 13, 213.

17. It is common in bioethics to decry market-based systems as advantaging the healthier and wealthier segments of society. For a positive account of the free market in medicine and the development of medical technologies, see Mark J. Cherry, "Scientific Excellence, Professional Virtue, and the Profit Motive: The Market and Health Care Reform," *Journal of Medicine and Philosophy* 28 (2003): 259–280; John Meadowcroft. "The British National Health Service: Lessons from the 'Socialist Calculation Debate,'" *Journal of Medicine and Philosophy* 28 (2003): 307–326.

18. Consider, for example, the centrality of access to contraception and abortion to President Obama's Patient Protection and Affordable Care Act. The law requires health insurance plans to cover contraception without copayments. As Health and Human Services Secretary Kathleen Sebelius argued: "President Obama is moving our country forward by giving women control over their health care.... This law puts women and their doctors, not insurance companies or the government, in charge of health care decisions."

Quoted in Caroline May, "Obamacare Contraception Mandate Takes Effect." *The Daily Caller,* August 01, 2012, accessed March 16, 2014, http://dailycaller.com/2012/08/01/obamacare-contraception-mandate-takes-effect/.

19. Ely E. Gretchen and Catherine N. Dulmus, "Abortion Policy and Vulnerable Women in the United States: A Call for Social Work Policy Practice," *Journal of Human Behavior in the Social Environment* 20 (2010): 658–671, 658.

20. S. Sella, "Maternal Indications," *Atrium: The Report of the Northwestern Medical Humanities and Bioethics Program* Summer (2010): 1–3, 3.

21. United Nations. *HIV/AIDS and Human Rights* (New York: United Nations, 1996). Consider also the *Protocol to the African Charter on Human and People's Rights on the Rights of Women in Africa,* which asserts that states must "...protect the reproductive rights of women by authorizing medical abortion in cases of sexual assault, rape, incest, and where the continued pregnancy endangers the mental and physical health of the mother or the life of the mother or the foetus." African Union, *Protocol to the African Charter on Human and People's Rights on the Rights of Women in Africa* (Maputo: African Union, 2003), article 14c.

22. United Nations, *Convention on the Elimination of All Forms of Discrimination Against Women,* accessed March 16, 2014, www.un.org/womenwatch/daw/csw/index.html. See also United Nations, *Beijing Platform for Action,* Fourth World Conference on Women, accessed March 16, 2014, www.un.org/womenwatch/daw/beijing/platform, which holds that the failure to provide for safe abortions is a violation of human rights; and Voravit Suwanvanichkij et al., "Gender and Sexual Health Rights: Burma," in *Public Health & Human Rights: Evidence Based Approaches*, ed. Chris Beyrer and H. F. Pizer (Baltimore: Johns Hopkins University Press, 2007), 391–418.

23. Abortion advocates urge that legal limits be placed on the ability of physicians and nurses to refuse to participate in such services. Julie D. Cantor argues, for example, that conscientious objections to medical treatments should be starkly limited so as to enhance the liberty interests of female patients: "Conscientious objection...is worrisome when professionals who freely choose their field parse care and withhold information that patients need.... Conscience is a burden that belongs to the individual professional; patients should not have to shoulder it." Julie D. Cantor, "Conscientious Objection Gone Awry: Restoring Selfless Professionalism in Medicine," *New England Journal of Medicine* 360, no. 15 (2009): 1484–1485. The moral concerns of physicians not to be involved in what they judge to be murder is cast as less important than the liberty interests of women, who might wish to terminate a pregnancy.

24. As Engelhardt argues, "At stake was a widespread change in who was accepted in the dominant culture as an authority for health care decisions. The authority of physicians, the clergy, the family, and traditional authority figures was displaced by the authority of autonomous, rights-bearing individuals. The result was the disestablishment of those who had traditionally been in authority for giving advice and direction with regard to health care, namely respected physicians, priests, rabbis, and ministers." H. Tristram Engelhardt Jr., "Introduction: Bioethics as a Global Phenomenon," in *Regional Perspectives in Bioethics*, ed. John F. Peppin and Mark J. Cherry (Lisse: Swets & Zeitlinger, 2003), viii–xxii, xviii.

25. James Rush and Damien Gayle. "Deaf Twins Who Discovered They Were Going Blind and Would Never See Each Other Again Are Euthanized in Belgium Hospital," *Daily Mail,* January 14, 2013, accessed March 16, 2014, http://www.dailymail.co.uk/news/article-2261985/Belgian-twin-brothers-killed-doctors-choosing-euthanasia-able-again.html. See also "Deaf Belgian Twins, 45, Helped to Die after Losing Sight," *Reuters*,

January 14, 2013, accessed March 16, 2014, http://www.reuters.com/article/2013/01/14/us-belgium-euthanasia-idUSBRE90D0W620130114.

26. As John Harris encapsulates this viewpoint: "The value of our lives is the value we give to our lives." John Harris, "Euthanasia and the Value of Life," in *Euthanasia Examined*, ed. J. Keown (Cambridge, UK: Cambridge University Press, 1995), 6–22, 11.

27. See, e.g., Michael Rie, "Respect for Human Life in the World of Intensive Care Units: Secular and Reform Jewish Reflections on the Roman Catholic View," in *Allocating Scarce Medical Resources: Roman Catholic Perspectives*, ed. H. Tristram Engelhardt Jr. and Mark J. Cherry (Washington, DC: Georgetown University Press, 2002); Paulina Taboada, "What Is Appropriate Intensive Care? A Roman Catholic Perspective," in *Allocating Scarce Medical Resources: Roman Catholic Perspectives*, ed. H. Tristram Engelhardt Jr. and Mark J. Cherry (Washington, DC: Georgetown University Press, 2002).

28. See, e.g., Suzan Holland, Karen Lebacqz, and Laurie Zoloth, ed. *The Human Embryonic Stem Cell Debate: Science, Ethics, and Public Policy* (Cambridge, MA: MIT Press, 2001).

29. See, e.g., Christopher Kaczor, *The Ethics of Abortion: Women's Rights, Human Life, and the Question of Justice* (New York: Routledge, 2010).

30. Jack N. Sparks ed., "The Didache" in *The Apostolic Fathers*, trans. R. Kraft (Minneapolis: Light and Life, 1978), 309.

31. P. Schaff and H. Wace, ed., "The Canons of the Council in Trullo (Often Called the Quinisext Council)," in *Nicene and Post-Nicene Fathers*, second series, Vol. XIV (Peabody, MA: Hendrickson, 1995), 404.

32. St. Basil, "Basil Letters and Selected Works: The Nine Homilies of the Hexaemeron and the Letters of Saint Basil the Great, Letter CLXXXVIII," in *Nicene and Post-Nicene Fathers*, second series, Vol. VIII (Peabody, MA: Hendrickson, 1995), 225.

33. Questions about the moral status of embryos created through in vitro fertilization are in certain facets complex. As Engelhardt summarizes: "To be a person is to be a being whose proper destiny is theosis. What of the zygote or early embryo before it is or would have been in the womb? What of the circumstance that, because of the high loss of zygotes and early embryos, human biological life at this stage may not be of the sort that inevitably leads to the life of a person?... On the one hand, one must be careful to follow the injunction of St. Basil not to split hairs as to when there is a soul, a person. Yet, on the other hand, while regarding the non-implantation of 'excess' zygotes and early embryos as a serious moral matter, it may be appropriate to consider the wrong as not fully equivalent to abortion, especially when no direct violence is done against these zygotes and early embryos." H. Tristram Engelhardt Jr., *The Foundations of Christian Bioethics* (Lisse: Swets & Zeitlinger, 2000), 255. (See generally the discussion on pages 254ff.) Experimentation on such zygotes and early embryos would constitute illicit and deeply sinful direct violence.

34. John Rawls, *A Theory of Justice* (Cambridge, MA: Belknap Press, 1971), § 46, 302–303.

35. Ibid., § 60, 395–399.

36. See, for example, H. Tristram Engelhardt Jr., *The Foundations of Bioethics*, 2nd ed. (New York: Oxford University Press, 1996), 50–53; Robert Nozick, *Anarchy, State and Utopia* (New York: Basic Books, 1974), 183ff.

37. John Rawls, supra note 34, § 87, 578.

38. John Rawls, supra note 34, § 87, 580.

39. Rawls begins by noting that his motivation for clarifying his conception of justice is "...because it may seem that this conception depends on philosophical claims I should like to avoid, for example, claims to universal truth, or claims about the essential nature and identity of persons." John Rawls, "Justice as Fairness: Political not Metaphysical," *Philosophy & Public* Affairs 14, no. 3 (1985): 223–251, 223.

40. Ibid., 225.

41. "In particular, justice as fairness is framed to apply to what I have called the 'basic structure' of a modern constitutional democracy." Ibid., 224. See also John Rawls, *Political Liberalism* (New York: Columbia University Press, 1993).

42. John Rawls, *Political Liberalism* (New York: Columbia University Press, 1993), 10.

43. Ibid.

44. H. Tristram Engelhardt Jr., "The Search for a Global Morality: Bioethics, the Culture Wars, and Moral Diversity," in *Global Bioethics: The Collapse of Consensus*, ed. H. Tristram Engelhardt Jr. (Salem: M&M Scrivener, 2006), 20.

45. H. Tristram Engelhardt Jr., *The Foundations of Bioethics*, 2nd ed. (New York: Oxford University Press, 1996).

46. As Alasdair MacIntyre summarizes a similar point: "There is no standing point, no place for enquiry, no way to engage in the practices of advancing, evaluating, accepting, and rejecting reasoned argument apart from that which is provided by some particular tradition or other." Alasdair MacIntyre, *Whose Justice? Which Rationality?* (Notre Dame, IN: University of Notre Dame Press, 1988). 350.

As G. E. M. Anscombe (1919–2001) once famously observed, with a variation on a Kantian insight, once God is removed from the understanding of morality, it is doubtful that moral claims will be compelling: it is "as if the notion 'criminal' were to remain when criminal law and criminal courts had been abolished and forgotten."G. E. M. Anscombe, "Modern Moral Philosophy," *Philosophy* 33 (1958): 1–19, 6. Or, as Jürgen Habermas critiqued: "...it is altogether a different matter to provide a motivating response to the question of why we should follow our moral insights or why we should be moral at all."Jürgen Habermas, *Religion and Rationality: Essays on Reason, God, and Modernity*, ed. Eduardo Mendieta (Cambridge, MA: MIT Press, 2002), 108.

Secular philosophy and secular bioethicists may offer their own moral insights, intuitions, and perspectives, but they cannot secure universal and unconditioned moral truth, much less unconditioned and unconditional reasons to act morally.

47. This is why Immanuel Kant, even though he was likely an atheist, concluded that "Without a God and without a world invisible to us now but hoped for, the glorious ideas of morality are indeed objects of approval and admiration, but not springs of purpose and action." Immanuel Kant, *Critique of Pure Reason*, trans. Norman Kemp Smith (London: Macmillan, 1964), 640, A813–B841.

48. Alasdair MacIntyre, supra note 46.

49. H. Tristram Engelhardt Jr., supra note 45, chaps. 1–4.

PART FIVE

Suffering in the Ethics of Contemporary Medicine and Biotechnology

18

Reproductive Technology in Suffering's Shadow

Paul Lauritzen

> There is an elemental moral requirement to respond to innocent suffering. If we were not to respond to it and its claim upon us, we would be without conscience and, in some basic sense, not completely human.[1]
>
> Precisely because of its value—social, medical, economic—medical research tempts us to invest too much hope in it as a way of relieving the human condition or leads us to excessively commercialize it, to cut moral corners in pursuit of therapies and cures, or with human research subjects, or to divert attention from the social and economic sources of sickness.[2]

In his magisterial work, *Victims and Values: A History and a Theory of Suffering*, Joseph Amato makes a persuasive case that responding to suffering is central to the moral life. Equally important, however, says Amato, is acknowledging that the universal imperative to ameliorate suffering does little "to settle the arguments about what types of suffering we should respond to, what grounds we should use to choose between the contradictory claims of different victims, and why and how to respond appropriately to victims."[3] Strange as it may seem, we need to ask whether some victims are "purer, nobler, and more deserving" than others[4]; stranger still, we need to confront the reality that the demand that suffering be relieved may be the shrill cry of the moral nihilist.

Nowhere is the moral complexity of the commitment to alleviate suffering more apparent than in the field of bioethics, and, as the chapters in this volume demonstrate, the range of bioethical issues that are fruitfully examined with a focus on suffering is broad. My task in this chapter is to turn that lens on issues of assisted reproduction. I will argue that debates about the moral significance of suffering and the appropriate limits of medical efforts to alleviate suffering have been central to bioethics discourse on reproductive technology. Close attention to the rhetoric of suffering in debates about assisted reproduction also highlights two serious dangers when suffering is the focus of moral inquiry. Following Amato, I will refer to these dangers as the medicalization of suffering and the banalization (or trivialization) of suffering.[5] Daniel Callahan has written about the dangers of treating suffering as a kind of trump card when considering the funding of medical research. He speaks of these dangers as the shadow side of suffering.[6] Borrowing from Daniel Callahan, I call the problems that emerge when the suffering of the infertile is medicalized and trivialized the *shadow side of suffering in assisted reproductive technology* (ART). I will conclude with some comments about the need to recover an understanding of professional responsibility that suggests resources for avoiding the problems raised by the medicalization and trivialization of suffering in treating infertility.

From the start of bioethics debates about ART, the issue of suffering was central. For example, one of the first sustained critiques of reproductive technology, the Vatican Instruction *Donum vitae*, acknowledged that its opposition to various forms of assisted reproduction, including artificial insemination and in vitro fertilization (IVF), might seem callous without a proper understanding of the role of suffering in human life. According to the Vatican, the suffering of infertile couples is real and substantial, but not ultimate. "Whatever its cause or prognosis," *Donum vitae* asserts, "sterility is certainly a difficult trial," and for that reason it is appropriate to support in their suffering those couples who are unsuccessful in their efforts to conceive.[7]

Whether one finds helpful the Vatican's suggestion that an infertile couple might seek comfort in a spiritual fruitfulness when material fruitfulness is not possible, there is no denying the centrality of the question *Donum vitae* raises: Must the suffering of the infertile be addressed through medical means? That this is an important question in discussions of assisted reproduction can be seen by the fact that the nature of infertility has been regularly debated since the first IVF child was born in 1978. Although the American Society for Reproductive Medicine (ASRM), the American College of Obstetricians and Gynecologists (ACOG), and the World Health Organization (WHO) all define infertility as a disease, critics of ARTs have often noted the peculiarity of treating infertility as a medical condition.

Consider, for example, one of the most common causes of male infertility, namely, a varicocele. A varicocele is the technical medical term for an enlarged vein in the testicle. Like a varicose vein in the leg, a varicocele allows for pooling of blood, in this case, in the veins of the scrotum. Because sperm production is sensitive to temperature variation, it can be affected by the rise in temperature caused by the pooled blood in the vein. According to the ASRM, about 15 percent of men have a varicocele, and 40 percent of men who have fertility problems have a varicocele.[8] For those men with both a varicocele and infertility, a surgical procedure can reroute blood flow by tying off the dilated veins. In two thirds of cases, semen parameters are improved by surgery.[9]

Given that surgery is minimally invasive, relatively inexpensive, and a reasonably good way to address one class of male infertility cases, what is the problem? The short answer, say critics, is that infertility is not a disease and a varicocele is not a medical condition. At best, infertility is a symptom of a physiological condition, which itself is not a disease. As the ASRM fact sheet on varicoceles makes clear,

15 percent of men have varicoceles, and many of these men will never know they have one. The reason is that a varicose vein in the testicle is not typically associated with any health-related problems.[10] The only reason the varicocele needs to be "repaired" is that the man wants to have child.

For this reason, ARTs are often compared with cosmetic surgery, and discussions of cosmetic surgery are in fact instructive. For example, Miller, Brody, and Chung have framed the concerns about cosmetic surgery in a way that illuminates reproductive medicine.[11] As they note, the critique of cosmetic surgery typically observes the highly unusual nature of this form of medical practice because it involves invasive procedures performed on healthy bodies for the sake of appearances.

Of course, the fact that cosmetic surgery appears to lie on the periphery of established medical terrain does not mean it is morally problematic. Breast enhancements, eyelid surgery, facelifts, and liposuction may be the bread and butter of most cosmetic surgery practices, but reconstructive surgeries to ameliorate the ravages of disease or injury or to correct gross physical abnormalities also falls to cosmetic surgeons, and few would question the appropriateness of these latter procedures. Why the difference?

The answer, say Miller, Brody, and Chung, is that while it is a proper goal of medicine to relieve pain and suffering, "it is not within the purview of physicians to attempt to relieve any and all pain and suffering that may afflict human beings."[12] What forms of suffering fall outside the purview of medicine? According to Miller, Brody, and Chung, the answer is that suffering unrelated to "maladies" is beyond the pale of legitimate medical practice. They illustrate this standard with a discussion of contraception and sterilization. Their account is worth quoting at some length.

> Although not a disease or a malady, pregnancy is a condition that in our society brings women under medical attention. Unwanted pregnancy can be understood as a disability, which interferes with the ability of women to function normally in social life. This suggests the conclusion that contraception promotes the health of women. The health promotion rationale for contraception or sterilization is stronger in the case of women who are likely to experience serious health risks from becoming pregnant, which would support including these procedures within the core of medicine in these circumstances.[13]

By contrast, male sterilization through vasectomy is, at best, on the periphery of legitimate medical practice. If it is undertaken to prevent unwanted pregnancy, they write, "the pregnancy it prevents belongs to another person, not to the one sterilized. Unwanted paternity, unlike unwanted pregnancy, does not qualify as a medical condition to be prevented."[14]

Miller, Brody, and Chung's attempt to distinguish access to contraception as a medical issue for women but not for men and their talk about pregnancy as a condition that interferes with a woman's ability to function "normally" in social life suggests how difficult it will be to specify criteria that identifies the sort of suffering to which medicine ought to respond. I will return to this point shortly, but for now it is enough simply to note that Miller, Brody, and Chung seek to do for medicine what Amato says we need to do generally, namely, prioritize the types of suffering to which we should respond, when we cannot respond to all types. They do not deny that individuals who seek enhancements through cosmetic surgery may be suffering; they simply deny that the suffering of those with a negative body image is the sort of suffering to which medicine should appropriately respond. One reason they are wary of "treating" this kind of suffering is that, too often, it is rooted in socially constructed desires that are themselves unhealthy.[15] But even apart from feminist concerns about the dangers of reinforcing sexist ideals of feminine beauty, Miller, Brody, and Chung insist that the suffering cosmetic surgery relieves is not an appropriate object of medical concern.

That the nature and the quality of the suffering involved is central to the legitimacy of cosmetic surgery can be seen from the fact that its supporters adamantly insist that they are responding to real and acute suffering. Even if cosmetic surgery does not typically treat a physical malady, psychological suffering is an appropriate area for medical concern, and the fact that many patients presenting for cosmetic surgery have formal psychiatric diagnoses may be cited as a reason to offer surgery. This fact could, of course, cut both ways, because it might be argued that a diagnosis of, say, body dysmorphic disorder should be grounds for ruling out cosmetic surgery. [16] Yet, at least one study suggests that surgeons do not always see it this way. Only 30 percent of surgeons in one survey reported that body dysmorphic disorder is always a contraindication for surgery. Presumably, the other 70 percent felt that at least in some cases a surgical procedure might help alleviate the marked distress with bodily appearance associated with this condition.

If we return at this juncture to consider ARTs, we see why critics cite parallels between ARTs and cosmetic surgery. In both cases, many treatments are offered to "patients" who have nothing medically wrong with them. In both cases, treatment frequently responds to suffering, not to sickness. Childlessness and a negative body image are thus said to be alike in that what is fundamentally not a medical condition gets conceptualized as a problem that requires or at least permits a medical intervention. This is not to say that infertility is never the result of a medical condition. The point is that childlessness itself is not.

The Medicalization of Suffering

Amato's history of suffering helps explain the larger point of this comparison. As he makes clear, in the nineteenth century, "all Western societies had launched attacks against the roots of human misery."[17] Improvements in personal hygiene, sewage disposal, and nutrition, combined with procedures for slowing the spread of contagious diseases, had led to significant progress against disease and illness. Cholera, diphtheria, and tuberculosis were all in retreat, and people began to believe that pain and suffering from disease and illness were avoidable. As Amato puts it:

> In unprecedented numbers, infirmaries and hospitals, armed with the new tools of anesthesia, antiseptics, and surgery, sprung up in the nineteenth century to meet the afflictions of growing urban populations. Qualified public health and administrative officials and professional medical associations of doctors and nurses and surgeons established themselves as society's experts on illness, disease, and pain. Supported by medical schools, a growing body of scientific materials, a new concern for medical records, and laws for certification, doctors and health officials launched a major offensive to take control of the kingdom of pain and suffering.[18]

Yet, conquest of the kingdom of suffering was not limited to the local counties and parishes of medicine, but expanded beyond medicine's traditional territorial limits. Medical sociologists refer to this process as medicalization, by which they mean "the extension of the conceptual and normative domain of medicine to problems, states, or processes not previously within the medical sphere, leading to medical management and treatment of them."[19] In broad terms, this process might be described as the medicalization of suffering.

The term *medicalization* is typically used pejoratively to suggest a kind of medical imperialism, but there is nothing intrinsically problematic about the effort to extend medical knowledge and expertise into domains where it might be used to alleviate suffering. I know from my own experience of infertility that the suffering of the involuntarily childless is real, and I see no reason in principle that physicians should not seek to help the infertile, even if a particular instance of infertility is not the result of a medical condition. Nevertheless, Amato is right to insist that we ask about the types of suffering to which we should respond. In the case of reproductive medicine, we need to ask whether every case of involuntary childlessness is one that merits a medical response. In other words, we need to ask whether the only check on what reproductive medicine provides should be the desire of a patient who is suffering, no matter the reason.

Unfortunately, the answer to this question is too frequently "yes." Once again, the work of Miller, Brody, and Chung is helpful because they recognize that medicine is degraded when it is regarded strictly as a fee-for-service business and not as a profession. Medicine, they say, is a professional practice that should be "governed by a moral framework consisting of goals proper to medicine, role-specific duties, and clinical virtues."[20] This is why they say that physicians should not be expected to relieve any and all suffering; the attempt to relieve some forms of suffering may simply be inconsistent with the goals that should define a physician's professional life. Miller, Brody, and Chung refer to the goals, duties, and virtues that should define a physician's professional life as the "internal morality of medicine."

It is beyond the scope of this chapter to explore the idea of an internal morality of medicine in any detail, but the core idea of this notion is that there is a regulative ideal that should govern the practice of physicians. Physicians are not, or at least should not be, "hired guns" that sell their expertise to the highest bidder or anyone prepared to pay for their services. A comparison to other professions may help illustrate this point. Consider, for example, the debate that has taken place in recent years within higher education about whether universities should be run more like businesses than they have been in the past.

In his book, *Universities in the Marketplace—the Commercialization of Higher Education,*[21] Derek Bok, a former president of Harvard University, asks whether the regulative ideals governing higher education are compatible with the logic of the marketplace. He begins the book by imagining various money-making schemes that might be considered for easing the constant pressure on college presidents to raise money. He wonders what the problem would be with turning Harvard's football program into a big-time college bowl contender, or auctioning off the last hundred spaces in every entering class to the highest bidder, or selling advertising space in Harvard syllabi, classrooms, and websites. Consider this last proposal. Should faculty members sell advertising space in their syllabi?

Almost every faculty member with whom I have discussed this has been adamantly opposed to the idea of having ads in syllabi. But why? Arguably, selling advertising space might benefit all parties involved. The university increases revenues, faculty members might receive increased remuneration, tuition might be lowered, and advertisers reach a target audience in new ways. Why, then, do faculty appear to be so opposed to the idea? The answer, I believe, is clear if we consider the idea of the regulative ideals governing the profession of education.

Particularly, if we focus on the ideals governing traditional liberal arts education, we see a commitment to the transfer of knowledge from previous to later generations with the assumption that the search for knowledge can be personally transformative. The regulative ideal of a professor in the liberal arts is that of a mentor and role model for students whereby one's relation to one's students is neither that of parent nor friend, but closer to that of a guide. If this is the regulative ideal governing teachers in higher education, then selling advertising space in a syllabus is something a virtuous educator simply would not do. Selling advertising space may not violate any provisions in a faculty handbook or contradict one's contractual obligations to a university, but doing so is incompatible with the regulative ideal of higher education.

The logic of the marketplace that would put a price on access to students in the classroom is corrosive of the ideal of a faculty–student relationship. I do not mean to deny that universities are a business or that, in one sense, classes are commodities for sale in the marketplace. Neither do I want to romanticize faculty–student interactions. There are certainly times when both teachers and students interact in fairly calculating ways. Still, most faculty members do not take a merely calculative interest in their students, and most understand their work of generating, preserving, and transmitting knowledge as part of a social commitment to shape habits of mind that are crucial to securing the common good. The idea of selling advertising space in a syllabus—with its accompanying vision of faculty–student interactions on the model of seller–buyer—is profoundly at odds with the regulative ideal of a professor concerned about students as individuals whose future is importantly shaped by the disinterested pursuit of knowledge, including the pursuit of self-knowledge.

If we return to the profession of medicine with this analogous regulative ideal drawn from education, we see why Miller, Brody, and Chung are right to insist that the internal morality of medicine rules out certain forms of professional practice. For example, if a physician's overriding goal in practicing medicine is to make money, he has betrayed the profession of medicine. This is not to say that the goal of making money is incompatible with the ethical practice of medicine. It is to say that a physician whose primary goal is making money is not a virtuous physician, and not merely because his greed is likely to lead to actions that violate codes of professional conduct. He has simply not internalized the regulative ideals of medicine and thus is likely to betray those ideals in a variety of ways.

In *Virtue Ethics and Professional Roles,* Justin Oakley and Dean Cocking offer an example that resonates both with the case of a professor selling advertising space in his or her syllabus and with Miller, Brody, and Chung's concerns about cosmetic surgery. They cite an advertisement placed in an Australian newspaper by a cosmetic surgery practice. The ad reads: "World leading cosmetic surgery clinic [invites applications for a] Patient Advisor: Working closely with the principal surgeon and other team members, you will develop long term relationships with patients *to insure repeat business.*"[22] Oakley and Cocking are not condemning cosmetic surgery as a field of medicine; their point is that, by making repeat business the focus of this cosmetic surgery practice, the physicians associated with this practice violate the regulative ideals of medicine.

This is a point that Miller, Brody, and Chung make when they argue that governance by the internal morality of medicine is what distinguishes medicine from business. "Patient autonomy," they note, "is not the same as consumer sovereignty."[23] Patients may demand specific medical interventions, but physicians are under no obligation to meet those demands unless they are consistent with medical indications and professional judgment. Informational advertising may alert patients to possible medical problems, but advertising merely to create demand for services is morally suspect.

This is why Miller, Brody, and Chung believe that advertising associated with cosmetic surgery is problematic. In their words, advertising these services "puts physicians in the position of selling invasive procedures for which there is no medical need."[24] Worse, still, advertising cosmetic surgery sends a signal that these procedures are medically necessary and thus legitimates unnecessary surgical and other risky interventions.

The Trivialization of Suffering

If Miller, Brody, and Chung are correct in thinking that cosmetic surgery is worrisome, at least in part because it is an area in which patients are treated like mere consumers, then we ought to be troubled by the field of reproductive medicine as well. It is another area of medicine in which suffering appears to be commoditized and medicine is uncomfortably aligned with the market.

Consider, for example, a story the *New York Times* ran in October 2012 about a Long Island infertility clinic that was advertising for potential patients by sponsoring a contest in which infertile couples shared their stories through essays and videos in return for a chance to win a free cycle of micro-IVF at the clinic, a $3,900 value.[25] The ad copy for the contest says it all. "That's right . . . one lucky woman will win the ultimate chance at starting or building her family. All from the practice that brought Long Island its very first IVF baby, first cryo baby, and first donor egg baby! Imagine it." Contestants in the "Extreme Family-Building Makeover Contest" were required to mention Long Island IVF—at least once for essays and twice for videos—and they were encouraged to "be creative!"[26]

At the start of this chapter, I spoke about the twin dangers of the medicalization of suffering and the banalization (or trivialization) of suffering. Both are displayed dramatically in this contest. For example, a review of the essays submitted by contestants shows that, for many, infertility is only one of a series of life frustrations that a child is expected to redress. The following entry is fairly typical.

> Hi, I am L. H., and my wonderful husband is R. H. We would love to win an IVF cycle at Long Island IVF because our hearts ache not just for a baby, but to be a family. We have been married since February 2006, and spent our first years of wedded bliss getting all of our ducks in a row before trying to start our family. Well, it turns out that our ducks had other ideas. We endured R. H.'s job layoff and resulting loss of health insurance, four moves, me being unable to continue working, and the loss of our beloved 16 year old cats. We really didn't think things could get worse. Through the ups and downs we stuck together and had hope that the future would be brighter.[27]

Unfortunately, R. H. was diagnosed with Wegener's granulomatosis. Treatment with Cytoxan rendered R. H. infertile. The couple's narrative continues:

> IVF treatment (using R. H.'s frozen sample) is prohibitively expensive and not covered by our health insurance, so we first decided to try a lower-cost treatment at home using a donor. R. H. carefully performed an IUI (intra-uterine insemination), but it turned out to be unsuccessful. I spent an entire day in bed sobbing for the child that never was.[28]

This case highlights the ambiguous character of much of the field of reproductive medicine. On the one hand, R. H.'s infertility is directly related to a medical condition; indeed, it is an iatrogenic problem. Thus, the standard that Miller, Brody, and Chung set out, that treatment be related to a malady, is clearly met. On the other hand, as the use of artificial insemination with donor sperm suggests, the turn to medical professionals is not primarily about treating R. H.'s medically induced infertility, but rather is about meeting the couple's desire for a child. The failure to conceive a child is presented as one in a series of life setbacks that the couple has endured. Both L. H. and R. H. lost jobs; they have had to move four times in rapid succession early in their marriage; their beloved cats died.

Here we confront in acute form the problem I previously identified, namely: How do we identify criteria for distinguishing between desires to which it is appropriate for medicine to respond and those that it may responsibly ignore? In this case, given that R. H.'s infertility is medically induced, we might well conclude that his desire for a child is one to which medicine should respond. I certainly do not wish to dispute this conclusion; indeed, iatrogenically frustrated desires may be prime candidates for medical response. Nevertheless, most cases of infertility will not fall into this category of iatrogenically caused problems, and we need some way to distinguish appropriate from inappropriate medical interventions that respond to childlessness.

One possibility at this juncture would be to attempt to map appropriate medical interventions to cases in which medical treatment responds to suffering caused by disease. The problem with this strategy is that the definition of disease is highly contested. As Marc Ereshefsky argues, most positions in the literature on health and disease can be framed in terms of two distinct accounts of illness: naturalism and normativism.[29] Naturalists seek to define disease independently of value judgments by offering an account of species-typical functioning that provides a standard, the deviation from which defines illness and disease. By contrast, normativists argue that definitions of disease are inescapably value laden. As H. Tristram Engelhardt puts the point, "disease does not reflect a natural standard or norm, because nature does nothing—nature does not care for excellence, nor is it concerned with the fate of individuals qua individuals."[30] Even if we can clearly identify species-typical dysfunction, we have to evaluate the dysfunction negatively before it will be treated as disease or illness.

We can now see that, on either account of disease, there are difficulties using "disease-frustrated" desire as a norm for evaluating suffering. On a naturalist account of disease, the inability to reproduce might be thought to be the quintessential case of biological dysfunction. A varicocele that renders a man infertile would thus be a paradigm case of disease to which medicine should respond. The problem is that, unless the man wants to have children, this dysfunction is not medically relevant.

Yet, the normativist position also fails to generate useful criteria because although it captures the importance of evaluative judgment, it offers no explanation of the possibility of a negatively valued condition that is not a disease. As Ereshefsky points out, alcoholism is widely evaluated negatively, but there is no consensus on whether it is a disease.[31] In other words, the fact that a state like childlessness is devalued does not alone make it a candidate for medical intervention.

Some combination of a naturalist and normativist account of disease might help us to develop criteria for distinguishing suffering that is the appropriate object of medical attention from suffering that is not, but I will leave that for another time.[32] My point about the medicalization of suffering in relation to infertility is that the mere desire for children is not enough to turn the suffering of involuntary childlessness into a medical concern. In short, I am particularly worried about a normativist account of infertility as illness.

If we return to the case of L. H. and R. H., we see the danger of a normativist model that understands medicine as merely responding to desire. Let us suppose that R. H. was not rendered infertile by treatment with Cytoxan and that L. H. and R. H. have simply been unable to conceive. Their involuntary childlessness has been very painful for them, and their suffering is real and deserves our sympathy. But should the mere existence of a frustrated desire, however much suffering the frustration of the desire may have caused, lead us to conclude that a medical intervention is appropriate? If the answer to this question is "yes," then why should we resist—as I believe we would—the conclusion that preventing R. H.'s layoff or the death of the couple's cat is a medical concern?

Unfortunately, the frame of this couple's contest entry suggests that they understand infertility treatment as addressing all of their frustrated desires. The job losses, the moves, the insecurity of not having health insurance all can be made right if only they had a child, any child. As the couple says at the conclusion of their essay: "Winning a free Micro-IVF cycle from LIIVF would mean the world to us!"[33] Undoubtedly, conceiving a child would mean the world to this couple, but it is not the job of medicine to make dreams come true, and not all suffering should be treated as a problem medicine should seek to address.

Ironically, when suffering is treated as so significant that any and every one of its forms demands relief, it is trivialized. We also see this banalization of suffering at work in the Extreme Family-Building Makeover Contest. The process is especially striking in the video-entry category. Once again, the instructions from the IVF clinic set the tone. "For videos, you can use your regular selves, or consider make-up or costumes. Create a skit. Use family and friends as actors or to give testimonials on your behalf. Maybe use the kids in your life."[34] Judging from the video entries, the advice to consider a "straight-forward tear-jerker" in order to "make us feel something" was widely followed.

The winning YouTube entry, by "itshippychick," did indeed follow the strategy of emotional manipulation.[35] Entitled, "We'll never stop hoping," it offered a collage defined by the "hope/despair" trope that dominates discussions of infertility. A series of images of "itshippychick" giving herself injections, greeting a FedEx deliveryman, doing acupuncture, receiving the news of another failed cycle, and looking at ultrasound pictures of "a true miracle" are set to the music of Jodi Picoult and Ellen Wilber's song, "Sing You Home." The video ends with a barefoot "itshippychick" walking down a sidewalk where she steps on each word of the message: "To win an extreme family building makeover from LIIVF could give us an opportunity we'll never have again." To put the point gently, one might say that the video does not have high production values; nevertheless, it was apparently just what the doctor ordered for use in marketing his clinic. "Itshippychick" and her partner won the grand prize of a "free" cycle of IVF.

Again, the point is not to discount the suffering that infertility has caused this couple. Rather, the point is that there is something troubling about the couple's suffering being used as the currency by which they hope to purchase a round of IVF. Seeing "itshippychick" giving herself hormone injections and watching the quotidian detail of "itshippychick" brushing her teeth, wrapped in a towel as she prepares for artificial insemination, and then listening in on the phone conversation when she gets the bad news that she is not pregnant is just creepy. And it is a special kind of creepy; it's reality television for the infertile. "Itshippychick" is not Honey Boo Boo, but the difference is one of degree, not kind.

The Problem with Commoditizing and Trivializing Suffering

We have already discussed some of the general problems created when medicine is understood largely in market terms. At this point, it is useful to explore more fully the idea of commodification in order to understand just how problematic the commoditization and trivialization of suffering are. One of the best accounts of commodification in the bioethics literature is found in a focus issue of the *Journal of Medicine and Philosophy* edited by M. Cathleen Kaveny. In the introduction to the focus issue, Kaveny discusses features of commodification that are helpful to understanding how market logic works.[36] According to Kaveny, commodification is best defined by noting some common features of goods that are commodities, that is, goods that are "inserted into a stream of commerce." Three characteristics of commodities are crucial. Commodities have a price; they are typically interchangeable with other goods of a similar type and quality; and they are thought to have instrumental rather than intrinsic value.

Moreover, these core characteristics give rise to others. The fact that commodities have a price results in a tendency to reduce their worth to something measurable in terms of a single scale of (monetary) value. This value, in turn, is a function of what buyers are willing to pay for the commodity. Thus, although similar goods are in theory interchangeable without loss—that is, commodities are, in the technical language, fungible—their fungibility is not a function of any intrinsic property of the good, but is instead a function of the desires of consumers. In addition, the three core features of commodities are mutually reinforcing and contribute to a market logic in which the value of goods is largely instrumental and is essentially determined through a negotiation between buyers and sellers in which worth is reducible to price. In this regard, the logic of market transactions also diminishes any sense that the identities of the buyers or sellers are important or that the transaction itself might be valuable.

With this analysis in mind, think about how suffering is understood in market terms in the Extreme Family-Building Makeover contest. Contestants are encouraged to put their suffering on public display for a price. The price is theoretically $3,900, the estimated cost of one round of IVF at the clinic. But more than this, the relationship between the physician and patient is instrumentalized. The physicians who own the clinic are using the suffering of prospective and actual patients as a marketing tool, and patients, in turn, are selling their suffering, as if it were not exquisitely personal. To borrow Kaveny's language, suffering has entered the stream of commerce. Personal pain gets transmuted into a fungible commodity because, for marketing purposes, pain is pain. Whether it is the suffering of "itshippychick" or of "L. H." does not really matter, as long as its public offering brings the clinic customers. Nor does it really matter what the patient needs; what matters is what the customer wants. "L. H." had her husband perform donor insemination at home and, when that did not work, she went to the clinic to try IVF. But is there any reason to think that the clinic would not have performed donor insemination if she had gone to them first? As long as making money is the primary objective, a service is a service; never mind that there may be a moral difference between donor insemination and insemination with a husband's sperm. Eggs and sperm are fungible.

The further difficulty here is that when the market swallows up the personal and moral significance of individual pain and suffering, it becomes extremely difficult to evaluate and thus prioritize the sort of suffering that has a moral claim on us. The best illustration of this point in relation to reproductive technology is seen in how the increase in twins, triplets, and other multiple-gestation pregnancies associated with ARTs has been handled. Unfortunately, the pain and suffering caused by multiple-gestation pregnancies is too frequently ignored. By all accounts, multiple-gestation pregnancies increase both maternal morbidity and fetal and neonatal morbidity and mortality. Indeed, multiple-gestation pregnancies are one of the most serious problems confronting ART.[37] Preeclampsia, gestational diabetes, cholestasis, excess weight gain, anemia, chronic back pain, umbilical hernias, and postpartum laxity of the abdominal wall are all associated with multiple-gestation pregnancies. When we add to the maternal complications of multiple-gestation pregnancies the effects on children of such pregnancies, namely the numerous and potentially devastating consequences of preterm birth and low gestational weight at birth, the pain and suffering associated with ART can be considerable. Consider just a few of the many potential problems associated with preterm birth or low gestational weight at birth: cerebral palsy, retinopathy, bronchopulmonary dysplasia, polycythemia, hypoglycemia, necrotizing enterocolitis, and infant death.[38]

This is why both the ASRM and the Society of Assisted Reproductive Technology recommend transferring very few embryos as part of IVF treatment. Yet, as the Practice Committee Opinion of the ASRM points out, there are multiple factors that lead infertile couples and their physicians to ignore these practice guidelines. The absence of health care coverage or strict limits on the number of cycles of IVF covered by insurance leads many couples to seek superovulation followed by the transfer of multiple embryos with IVF or superovulation followed by artificial insemination with a partner's or donor's sperm when IVF is not used. As one study in *The Lancet* observed, "In a commercial environment in which IVF is mostly practiced at present, the customer usually decides about timing and choice of treatment."[39]

As the language of "customer" signals, patients are largely understood as consumers with a demand for a product. Yet, because infertility has been framed as a form of existential suffering, we tend to overlook the fact that ARTs are often used to "treat" infertility of unknown origin. Physicians do not necessarily know what is causing the infertility, but they are asked to provide infertility treatment, even when the health risks to both women and children are real and known. To echo *The Lancet* piece, we might say that in a commercial environment, we should remind patients of the time-honored advice to consumer, namely, *caveat emptor*: let the buyer beware.

Moving beyond a Consumer Model

How might the field of reproductive medicine take seriously the suffering of the infertile and not be consumed by it? To answer that question, we need briefly to explore the idea of professionalism in medicine. Unfortunately, there has been a profound shift in the social understanding of the professions over the past fifty years that makes the effort to resist patients' demands to end suffering difficult. The sociologist Steven Brint has captured the shift in paradigms of professionalism in terms of two models: first, the "social-trustee" model, which dominated roughly from the end of nineteenth century until the early 1960s; and second, an "expertise" professionalism model, which emerged in the 1960s and has become ascendant today.

Brint quotes R. H. Tawney's characterization of professions as an example of social-trustee professionalism. "[Professions uphold] as the criterion of success the end for which the profession, whatever it may be, is carried on, and [subordinate] the inclinations, appetites, and ambitions of individuals to the rules of an organization which has as its object to promote the performance of function."[40] One can hold a social-trustee model of professionalism without embracing such a high-minded conception of self-sacrifice in service of a social good, but the contours of a social-trustee model are clear in the passage. Professions have a higher purpose than promoting the avaricious desires of individuals or market interests in efficiency and productivity. Under this model, professions would have special status in the labor force premised on mastery of a complex knowledge base recognized through a system of credentialing that is state sanctioned in collaboration with professional associations, but the technical expertise of professionals and their control over labor markets is understood to be for the purpose of promoting the common good. This, alas, is not the case with expertise professionalism.

As Brint notes, the idea of professions as in some ways the guardians of the public good did not always sit easily with notions of populist democracy and business entrepreneurship, even when few questioned a social-trustee model. Yet, it was not until the early 1960s that this model came under serious assault. Many reasons have been offered for why this was the case, everything from explosive growth in the number of professionals—which in turn fueled concern for individual interests—to the erosion of trust in ruling elites. For our purposes, the causes of this assault are less important than the consequences. The fundamental result was that professions came to be defined almost exclusively in terms of expertise. Brint puts the point this way: "Over the last thirty years, the idea of professions as a status category has become increasingly disconnected from functions perceived to be central to the public welfare and more exclusively connected to the idea of 'expert knowledge.'"[41] Indeed, continues Brint, "powerful social and economic forces have brought the older idea of professionalism linking social purposes and knowledge-based authority close to an end."[42]

Brint's analysis that expertise professionalism has very nearly eclipsed social-trustee professionalism is indisputable, and no one has explored the consequences of this change for the professional lives of physicians better than Eliot Freidson. Although Freidson is much more focused than Brint on the social environments in which professional work takes place and how the work environment affects professional behavior, like Brint, he is profoundly concerned about the way in which professions have come to neglect service to the common good. Part of the problem is connected to the dynamic we have already described in which consumer demand is almost the sole determiner of what services the physician delivers.

To be sure, the traditional fee-for-service arrangement provided some degree of autonomy for a solo practitioner, but as Freidson point out, such an arrangement is inherently unstable and ultimately compromises autonomy by ceding control of medical decisions to patients or competing physicians.[43] Professionalism in medicine thus requires avoiding the dangers of both consumerist and managerial models. Here, we see one of the most serious threats that emerge from the medicalization of suffering. It obscures the consumerism in much of contemporary medicine. Although a free-market, consumerist ideology is widely accepted in our society, it would be recognized as unseemly in medicine, were it not for medicine's relation to suffering. If physicians were understood merely to be technical experts for hire, if they were understood to be mere purveyors of potions or devices, then certainly there would be little reason to treat medicine as a profession and provide physicians protection in the labor market through a system of licensing and credentialing.

But when medicine is understood to respond to medical need and not just desire, when it is understood to serve the suffering and not merely consumer demand, then it is possible to retain its status as a profession and not be seen as just another hawker of marketplace goods. When understood merely as a purveyor of goods in the marketplace, medicine loses its soul, and it will not save its soul if suffering is trivialized and serves only to mask the avaricious pursuit of profit. I believe Freidson is correct when he suggests that any theory that espouses that the primary purpose of work is to maximize personal gain "should be viewed as a frontal assault on professionalism."[44] The commoditization of suffering is just such a frontal assault. When infertility doctors sponsor contests for "free" cycles of IVF, when they show up on the doorsteps of the winners like Publishers Clearing House to videotape the reactions of the winners, they undermine professional practice and undercut any grounds for refusing procedures any "patient" happens to demand.

I believe Freidson is right to claim that only a robust commitment to professional ideals can withstand the corrosive effects of consumerist ideology. He writes:

> The functional value of a body of specialized knowledge and skill is less central to the professional ideology than its attachment to a transcendent value that gives it meaning and justifies its independence. By virtue of that independence members of the profession claim the right to judge the demands of employers or patrons and the laws of the state, and to criticize or refuse to obey them. That refusal is based not on personal grounds of individual conscience or desire but on the *professional* grounds that the basic value or purpose of a discipline is being perverted.[45]

Alas, the world of ART is too frequently one in which the profession of medicine is perverted. Physicians who practice in this world must not use suffering as an excuse to meet a patient's request for any procedure he may desire. Neither should a commitment to alleviate the suffering of the infertile be a vehicle for personal enrichment. Only if the dangers of the commoditization and trivialization of suffering are fully acknowledged and addressed can ART emerge from suffering's shadow.

Notes

1. Joseph A. Amato, *Victims and Values: A History and a Theory of Suffering* (New York: Greenwood, 1990), Kindle edition, location 2789.
2. Daniel Callahan, *What Price Better Health?* (Berkeley: University of California Press, 2003), 2.
3. Amato, supra note 1, 2802.
4. Ibid., 2819.
5. Ibid., 1767, 3537.
6. Callahan, supra note 2, 2.
7. Congregation for the Doctrine of the Faith, *Instruction on Respect for Human Life in Its Origin and the Dignity of Procreation* (Washington, DC: United States Catholic Conference, 1987) Publication No.156-3, 34.
8. American Society of Reproductive Medicine, "Patient Fact Sheet: Varicocele," accessed March 16, 2014, http://www.asrm.org/uploadedFiles/ASRM_Content/Resources/Patient_Resources/Fact_Sheets_and_Info_Booklets/Varicocele.pdf.
9. Ibid.
10. A varicocele may, however, lower testosterone levels and thus be associated with health, but this appears to be one of the few real health-related issues associated with the condition.
11. Franklin Miller, Howard Brody, and Kevin Chung, "Cosmetic Surgery and the Internal Morality of Medicine," *Cambridge Quarterly of Healthcare Ethics* 9/3 (2000): 353–364.
12. Ibid., 354.
13. Ibid., 356.
14. Ibid., 357.

15. For a discussion of cosmetic surgery that considers the possibility of feminist arguments in favor of the practice, see Kathy Davis, *Reshaping the Female Body* (New York: Routledge, 1995).

16. Canice Crerand, Martin Franklin, and David Sarwer, "Body Dysmorphic Disorder and Cosmetic Surgery," *Plastic and Reconstructive Surgery* 118/7 (2006): 167–180.

17. Amato, supra note 1, 1762–1765.

18. Ibid., 1768_1772.

19. Joseph E. Davis, "Medicalization, Social Control, and the Relief of Suffering," in *The New Blackwell Companion to Medical Sociology*, ed. William C. Cockerham (Malden, MA: Wiley-Blackwell, 2010): 211–243.

20. Miller, Brody, and Chung, supra note 11, 353–354.

21. Derek Bok, *Universities in the Marketplace: The Commercialization of Higher Education* (Princeton: Princeton University Press, 2003).

22. Justin Oakley and Dean Cocking, *Virtue Ethics and Professional Roles* (Cambridge, UK: Cambridge University Press, 2004), 87.

23. Miller, Brody, and Chung, supra note 11, 355.

24. Ibid., 355.

25. Douglas Quenqua, "Clinic Raffles Could Make You a Winner, and Maybe a Mother," *New York Times*, October 20, 2012. If the cost of the "free" cycle of IVF seems low, the fine print from the contest rules may explain why. The relevant section of the rules explains, in bold: "The Free Micro-IVF cycle is valued at $3,900.00 and is the basic Micro-IVF cycle offered by LIIVF. It covers the monitoring services of the LIIVF physicians and nurses for the duration of the cycle. It does NOT include the anesthesiologist, if needed, donor gametes, if needed, medications, cryopreservation, if applicable, required lab and screening tests, or other procedures, including but not limited to discretionary embryology services such as ICSI, assisted hatching, embryo glue, co-culture or other surgical or diagnostic procedures beyond the scope of the basic Micro-IVF program, if needed. The winner expressly understands and that these uncovered fees are payable prior to the commencement of treatment. It does not include any travel, lodging, food, or other such expenses."

26. Contest rules and entries in the essay portion of the contest can be found at: http://blog.longislandivf.com/2012/win-a-free-basic-micro-ivf-cycle-in-long-island-ivfs-extreme-family-building-makeover-contest/. Accessed March 16, 2014.

27. Ibid., n.p.

28. Ibid.

29. Marc Ereshefsky, "Defining 'Health' and Disease,'" *Studies in History and Philosophy of Biological and Biomedical Sciences* 40 (2009): 221–227. What Ereshefsky calls "naturalism" and "normativism" are sometimes referred to as objectivism and constructivism. See Dominic Murphy, "Health and Disease," in *A Companion to the Philosophy of Biology*, ed. Sahotra Sarkar and Anya Plutynski (Malden, MA: Blackwell, 2008).

30. As quoted by Ereshefsky, supra note 29, 223.

31. Ibid., 224.

32. Ereshefsky discusses "hybrid" accounts that combine aspects of both naturalism and normativism, but he argues that they are also inadequate. Murphy discusses a "two-stage" approach that involves both a scientific judgment that an abnormal bodily state has occurred and a normative judgment about the impact of such a state. I take Murphy's approach to be promising.

33. "Contest Rules and Entries." See supra note 26.

34. Ibid.

35. The YouTube video can be seen at: http://www.youtube.com/ecfertility. Accessed March 16, 2014.

36. M. Cathleen Kaveny, "Commodifying the Polyvalent Good of Health Care," *Journal of Medicine and Philosophy* 24/3 (1999): 207–223.

37. Practice Committee of the American Society for Reproductive Medicine, "Multiple Gestation associated with Infertility Therapy: An American Society for Reproductive Medicine Practice Opinion," *Fertility and Sterility* 97/4 (April 2012): 825–834.

38. Ibid., 826.

39. B. C. Fauser, P. Devroey, and N. S. Macklon, "Multiple Births Resulting from Ovarian Stimulation for Subfertility Treatment," *Lancet* 365 (2005) 1807–1816, 1813.

40. Steven Brint, *In an Age of Experts: The Changing Role of Professionals in Politics and Public Life* (Princeton, NJ: Princeton University Press, 1994), 7.

41. Ibid., 8.

42. Ibid., 17.

43. On this point, see Eliot Freidson, *Profession of Medicine: A Study of the Sociology of Applied Knowledge* (New York: Dodd, Mead, 1970): 91–92.

44. Eliot Freidson, *Professionalism: The Third Logic* (Chicago: University of Chicago Press, 2001), 218.

45. Ibid., 220–221.

19

Genomic Information and Suffering in the Genomic Era

Roberta M. Berry

Widespread access to a rapidly expanding array of genomic information has generated numerous ethical and policy controversies, some of them already addressed in legislation and court decisions. The quick march from controversy to policy response—for example, federal legislation restricting insurer and employer access to genetic test results and court decisions addressing the patentability of genes—may be taken as evidence of our capacity to understand and manage these controversies and the ethical puzzles they generate.

If we reconsider these controversies—and many more in prospect—from the perspective of their implications for human suffering, however, the puzzles appear more challenging and our capacity less certain. If the generation of genomic information is the halfway house to the generation of cures and consequent relief of suffering, surely there can be little doubt of the ethical imperative to generate that information as quickly and efficiently as possible. Yet, we know that the pursuit of our purposes is sometimes confounded despite—or due to—our exertions.

The first part of this chapter examines the complex operation of the genomic enterprise in pursuit of cures and the implications for human suffering. The second part examines questions posed by choices to undergo or forgo genetic testing while we reside in the halfway house, suspended between ignorance and capacity to cure. If the generation of genomic information is necessary to the pursuit of cures, it is also sufficient to serve the very different purposes of third parties. The third part addresses the consequences of harnessing the revelatory power of genomic information for third-party purposes that drive divisions among us, in the case of use by insurers and employers, and divisions within us, in the case of use by the criminal justice system. And the fourth part of this chapter considers the procreational choices opened up by the advance of the genomic enterprise. Parents equipped with genomic information must navigate the implications of their choices for the suffering of their potential children, themselves, and procreational partners they enlist in their efforts. The fifth part concludes with reflection on a deeper puzzle that awaits our progress through this collection of challenges, a puzzle requiring examination of our assumptions about the nature and meaning of suffering and our obligation to relieve it

The Genomic Enterprise and Human Suffering

On the cusp of modernity and the vast advances in science and technology that were to follow, Francis Bacon famously urged the pursuit of scientific knowledge for two purposes: "the glory of the Creator and the relief of man's estate."[1] Now, half a millennium later, the ascendancy of the science and technology enterprise—both in its awe-inspiring revelatory power and in its capacity to relieve the suffering associated with our embodiment—is arguably the central story of modernity.

THE SIMPLE TELLING: GOD'S GLORY AND THE RELIEF OF SUFFERING

In the simple telling, the genomic era is an unfolding chapter in that story, exemplifying the ascent of the science and technology enterprise and evincing Bacon's wisdom and prescience. An early highlight is Watson and Crick's discovery of the structure of DNA at mid-twentieth century, evidence of the transcendent unity of truth and beauty.[2] Following celebration of the glory comes the practical pursuit. At the close of the twentieth century, the federally funded Human Genome Project (HGP) marshals enormous effort to decipher the code written in our DNA with the expectation that this knowledge, coupled with ongoing dedication of both public and private resources and effort, would propel the advance to cures for a wide range of devastating and deadly diseases.[3] Genomic information begins to flow from the HGP and the research program grown up around it and following in its wake.[4] By the early twenty-first century, the flow turns to a torrent, carrying with it new understanding of disease processes, new diagnostics, new opportunities for personalized medicine, and glimmers of new cures.[5]

In this simple account, the actors in the story—the genomic scientists and technologists who engage in discovery and innovation, the public agencies that support their efforts, the commercial entities that translate their efforts into deliverables, the health care providers who deliver relief, and the policymakers who guide the enterprise—are allied in the pursuit of knowledge of our genomic being and application of that knowledge for the relief of human suffering. This simple telling dominates the public rhetoric surrounding the emergence and flourishing of the genomic enterprise.

There is essential truth to this simple version, as evidenced by the many achievements of the enterprise, including diagnostic and predictive tests, treatments, and cures—and the promise of more to come.[6] A more complete telling does not erase the simple one, but elaborates on it, to include a fuller account of the multiple actors and motivations that constitute the enterprise, the suffering it aims to relieve, and the implications for suffering of its operation.

THE GENOMIC ENTERPRISE: OF MULTIPLE ACTORS AND MIXED MOTIVES

On closer examination, the twin purposes recommended by Bacon and incorporated in the simple telling—the glory of the transcendent and the relief of suffering—do not encompass the full motivational set on display across the many actors constituting the genomic enterprise. Bacon, an acute observer of human motivation, admonished against a range of motivations displayed in his day—curiosity, enjoyment, reputation, repartee, profit, and professional advancement—and readily recognizable to the contemporary reader:

> But the greatest error of all the rest is the mistaking or misplacing of the last or furthest end of knowledge. For men have entered into a desire of learning and knowledge, sometimes upon a natural curiosity and inquisitive appetite; sometimes to entertain their minds with variety and delight; sometimes for ornament and reputation; and sometimes to enable them to victory of wit and contradiction; and most times for lucre and profession; and seldom sincerely to give a true account of their gift of reason to the benefit and use of men: as if there were sought in knowledge a couch whereupon to rest a searching and restless spirit; or a terrace for a wandering and variable mind to walk up and down with a fair prospect; or a tower of state, for a proud mind to raise itself upon; or a fort or commanding ground, for strife and contention; or a shop, for profit or sale; and not a rich storehouse for the glory of the Creator and the relief of man's estate.[7]

This motivational reckoning of sixteenth-century scientists resonates with the frank self-report, for example, of Watson, co-discoverer of the structure of DNA, about the many purposes motivating his effort—including reputation and professional advancement—and the effort of others engaged in the quest.[8] The race to map and sequence the human genome proceeded at breakneck speed in part because of competition between the HGP and a private competitor seeking the rewards of first completion.[9]

Other actors engaged in the enterprise reveal a similar mix of motivations. Along with the torrent of genomic information and the promise of eventual cures has come a torrent of patent filings securing rights to exclusive commercial exploitation by the entities that translate effort into deliverables.[10] The gene patents claimed in connection with the development of genetic tests for heightened risk of breast and ovarian cancer prompted one of the most prominent ethical and legal controversies associated with the genomic enterprise, concluding in the 2013 U.S. Supreme Court decision in the *Myriad* case that human genes were not patentable.[11]

Health care providers acting as investigators at the cutting edge of translation of the discoveries of the scientific endeavor into cures often hold financial stakes in the outcomes of their experimental efforts to discover and then deliver relief.[12] Concern about motivations—to financial gain and to reputational recognition—were cited in a prominent controversy associated with an early human subjects experiment in gene therapy gone wrong, resulting in the death of a human subject, Jesse Gelsinger.[13]

Policymakers who guide the enterprise have embraced incentives for research that recognize these motivations, justified by their instrumental efficacy in advancing the pursuit of cures. These include the grant of broad patent rights and of permission for academic researchers to commercialize the fruits of their publicly funded research.[14] In its decision in the *Myriad* case, the U.S. Supreme Court accepted this instrumental purpose; the Court's reasoning was guided by consideration of the net instrumental effect of gene patents on research and innovation.[15] Ongoing calls for reform of the 1980 Bayh-Dole Act authorizing the commercialization of publicly funded research also accept that Act's premise—incentives accelerate research toward cures—but seek refined instrumental design to maximize the efficacy of these incentives while minimizing collateral suffering imposed by the race to commercialization.[16]

If this recognition and instrumental use of the mix of motivations on display by actors engaged in the enterprise can succeed in generating cures, this suggests cause for celebration rather than admonishment: that from this crooked timber an enterprise can be built whose operation achieves the Baconian purpose of relieving human suffering. But a fuller account requires closer examination of suffering and its relief.

SUFFERING AND ITS RELIEF: CURING AND CARING

In the simple account, the genomic enterprise relieves suffering by discovering, innovating, translating, and delivering cures. We expect cures to relieve suffering by putting an end to the interwoven collection of experiences associated with serious illness, including pain, disability, and disfigurement, anticipatory fear of these, and fear of their continuation without relief; dependency and loss of control; isolation and increasing alienation from those who are not ill and who carry on the characteristic activities of those who are well; and dread of the ultimate personal dissolution foretold by these experiences.

Curing is the paradigm case of accomplishing relief, and treatment that falls short of curing is its very welcome close cousin to the extent it diminishes the magnitude or duration of these experiences. Like victory in a war of liberation curing is exhilarating in its vanquishment of the oppressor and stunning in its consequences for the patient set free. This story of curing we know to be an ideal, as rarely attained as final victory in a war and, even when attained, only interim for all of us. But, in the simple telling, we hold out curing as the aspirational ideal that galvanizes our hope and effort, and we savor each victory together with its inescapable hint of bittersweet.

A fuller account of suffering and our efforts to relieve it by curing complicates the story, even if its central truth remains. Curing is not a theoretical art, its victories are not won without battlefield costs, and the battlefield is the embodied patient. Curing can add to the measure of suffering when it fails and when it succeeds. For example, there has been and will be suffering imposed on first-generation patients by unintended failures of curing and treatment in emerging fields of practice, such as gene therapy, where knowledge is limited and technique uncertain, and the result may impose additional suffering without net gain in suffering relieved.[17] And the first-generation beneficiaries of the success of genetic testing for breast cancer risk combined with follow-on options for curing or preventing—watchful waiting and prophylactic mastectomies—know the high price in suffering endured to forestall worse.[18]

Instances of "iatrogenic suffering" imposed by failed and successful efforts at curing are common across domains of health care. They deserve reflection and study not just as occasions for ensuring informed consent and patient choice and guarding against researcher conflict of interest and error but also as occasions for improving our response to patients' suffering. We know, for example, that the mode of curing may add to the measure of suffering when health care providers fail to recognize, acknowledge responsibility for, and address suffering imposed both by the illness and the cure, as recounted by physician Eric Cassell in his story of a cancer patient and the treatments she endured—entailing pain, disability, disfigurement, and more—without evident concern by her physician for the suffering imposed.[19]

Relief of suffering requires empathic understanding and sympathetic response to experiences imposed both by illness and by the mode of curing or treatment. Caring responses to pain, disability, disfigurement, fear, dependency, alienation, and dread of death may include comforting, enabling, affirming, reassuring, empowering, embracing, and expressing solidarity in the face of death—the age-old repertoire of family, friends, and health care providers. A caring response, for example, may address pain and fear by reassuring explanation of the need to impose pain to accomplish a cure, or may modify a plan of treatment to limit the disability imposed.

Thus, as the simple story accurately tells, the genomic enterprise holds great promise, some of it already realized, to relieve suffering by the development and delivery of cures. As the more complete telling acknowledges, this is the result of coordinated efforts of multiple actors acting from a mix of motivations. And as the more complete telling also acknowledges, the risk of imposing iatrogenic suffering pervades the frontlines where cures are delivered. Another risk accompanies the operation of the enterprise as a system designed, like a machine, to generate results—the risk of imposing "systimagenic suffering."

SUFFERING IN THE GENOMIC ERA: THE OPERATION OF THE ENTERPRISE

The advent of modern technological medicine, with its machines that separate patients from the traditional ministrations of health care providers, has brought new opportunities to relieve and to impose suffering. Physician Lewis Thomas writes of the discomforts introduced by late-twentieth-century technological medicine, even as patients enjoyed better prospects for curing:

> In my father's time, talking with the patient was the biggest part of medicine, for it was almost all there was to do. The doctor-patient relationship was, for better or worse, a long conversation in which the patient was at the epicenter of concern and knew it.... [With] the advance of medicine's various and complicated new technologies... there is less time for talking.... The hospitalized patient feels, for a time, like a working part of an immense, automated apparatus.... The difference can be strange and vaguely dismaying for patients. But there is another difference, worth emphasis. Many patients go home speedily, in good health, cured of their diseases.[20]

Lifesaving technologies may cause more than discomfort even as they send patients home cured of the illnesses that prompted their use. A Johns Hopkins University School of Medicine study of patients treated in intensive care units (ICUs) concludes that a significant proportion developed post-traumatic stress disorder (PTSD) caused by the mode of operation of the ICUs. The results of the study, published in 2013, found:

> One in three people who survived stays in an... [ICU] and required use of a mechanical ventilator showed substantial... [PTSD] symptoms that lasted for up to two years....
>
> "We usually think of PTSD as something you develop if you go to war, are sexually assaulted or suffer a similar emotional trauma," says Dale Needham, M.D., Ph.D., a critical care specialist... and senior author of the study published online in *Psychological Medicine*. "Instead, it may be as common, or more common, in ICU patients as in soldiers, but it's something many doctors—including psychiatrists—don't fully appreciate."[21]

We are vulnerable to suffering imposed by lifesaving machines just as we are to iatrogenic suffering imposed by insufficient caring. These machines seize hold of us in a manner akin to the grip of the illnesses they are intended to vanquish. Patients may be immobilized, dependent, and powerless. They may experience pain and fear, isolation and alienation, and dread of their demise. The need to study and reflect on the operation of these machines and to develop and apply protocols that preserve their lifesaving power while limiting their collateral imposition of suffering is evident.

But could the operation of another kind of system aimed at curing—the genomic enterprise—also impose a similar "systimagenic suffering"? Consider, for example, the genetic tests for heightened risk of breast and ovarian cancer that prompted the controversy concluding in the *Myriad* case. The development of these tests and their use in combination with follow-on options for prevention and cure has rescued may women from the threat of serious illness or death and, accordingly, should count among the highlights in the story of the genomic era.

In fact, the operation of the genomic enterprise in this case generated a firestorm of legal and policy controversy.[22] The development and commercialization of the tests by Myriad Genetics was motivated, in part, by incentives crafted and implemented by policymakers in the U.S. Patent Act. Myriad obtained patents on *BRCA1* and *BRCA2* genes, and these patent rights anchored its exclusive right to develop and market its tests. Myriad refused to license these tests to others and enforced its patent rights to prevent others from offering alternative tests. In consequence, women were unable to obtain second-opinion testing, and they or their insurance pools were charged significant fees for Myriad's tests—although Myriad offered help for women unable to pay or obtain insurance coverage for its tests. In addition, researchers claimed a chilling effect on the pursuit of research that might lead to the development of cures because of the prospect of patent enforcement action by Myriad—a prospect that Myriad denied.

These operational effects generated a legal challenge that concluded in the U.S. Supreme Court decision in the *Myriad* case. The Court determined that isolated, naturally occurring human genes did not constitute patentable subject matter under the U.S. Patent Act, 35 U.S.C. §101. The Supreme Court's resolution of this interpretive question of the patentability of genes was informed by the underlying policy purpose of the U.S. Patent Act—to promote innovation for the benefit of society—and by consideration of the trade-offs between innovation incentivized and foreclosed by the grant of patent rights in human genes.[23]

Whether, in fact, the patenting of human genes generated net gains or losses in beneficial innovation is a complex question for which conclusive determination is impossible.[24] Empirical studies have found evidence of net losses from gene patenting with respect to the development of diagnostic testing, and many commentators have argued that the patents enforced by Myriad Genetics stifled innovation with respect to both the development of alternative diagnostic tests and the pursuit of therapeutic research.[25] Myriad and others made the case for net benefits: the patent system worked as intended, incentivizing research and generating lifesaving benefits that otherwise would not have been realized. Myriad's very large investment in developing its genetic tests could only be commercially justified by the promise of exclusive rights to market its tests for the limited period of time granted by patent law.[26]

Regardless of whether gene patenting generally or in the case of Myriad Genetics yielded net gains or losses, a fuller account of the genomic era recognizes the implications for suffering of the operation of the genomic enterprise in pursuit of net gains. As with the operation of the technological machines of modern medicine, the spinning of the gears of patent law, its incentives and its enforcement, in the commercialization of lifesaving innovation exacts a price from its beneficiaries. Women suffering in anticipatory fear of breast cancer—and their advocates—expressed dismay and outrage at their powerlessness to direct the impersonal operation of the enterprise to respond to their present and threatened future suffering—to expand options, reduce prices, and galvanize research effort to develop more and better tests and cures.[27]

Suffering is personal, as are the sympathetic responses that address its constitutive experiences, but the operation of the genomic enterprise is unavoidably and evidently impersonal, and the impact on its intended beneficiaries may include both relief from suffering because of the lifesaving cures it generates and discomfort or worse accompanying its operation. If we accept, on the more complete telling of the story, that the system is constituted of actors with mixed motivations, that incentives help turn its gears to lifesaving effect, and that its impersonal operation also exacts a price measured in suffering, then we can study and reflect on ways to reduce that price while preserving its lifesaving capacity. The end of gene patenting came in reactive response to complaint. Proactive policymaking efforts might consider ways to design or modify incentives to dampen or diffuse the impact of the operation of the enterprise, especially on its first-generation beneficiaries.[28]

We now turn to the implications for human suffering of rapidly expanding patient access to genomic information generated by the enterprise in the pursuit of cures. Here, too, study and reflection offer opportunities to manage the implications for suffering.

Genetic Testing: Knowing, Not Knowing, and in Between

Consider the potential impact of new genomic information offered up by an expanding array of genetic tests, including both tests that yield definitive news about present or future illness and tests that instead deliver news of susceptibility—probabilistic predictive risk information. The rapidly expanding technological capacity for inexpensive sequencing and advancing efforts to discern associations between genetic sequences and risk for disease will particularly press our capacity to understand and respond to the implications for suffering.

DIAGNOSTIC AND PREDICTIVE TESTING: CERTAINTY AND SUFFERING

As an adjunct to diagnosis, genetic testing is relatively new, but the relationship between definitive diagnosis—however accomplished—and suffering is familiar to every patient, her family and friends, and her health care providers. When the news is of a readily treatable condition—as with hemochromatosis, a condition that can be managed by means including therapeutic phlebotomy—diagnosis is the beginning of relief and restoration to a life interrupted by symptoms and the accompanying fear of the worst. When the news is of a dread disease—as with familial amyotrophic lateral sclerosis, in which a genetic test may aid diagnosis—vulnerability and fear penetrate to the core, and a new life, shaped by the suffering foretold, begins. Until the day that the genomic enterprise delivers new cures that move bad news to good, the impact on suffering of diagnostic genetic testing will consist primarily in its capacity to deliver definitive news quickly, cutting short the fearful anticipation of the symptomatic, delivering some to the old life and some to the new.

Rarely, genetic testing can yield definitive predictive results, as in the case of Huntington's disease (HD). A positive test result foretells a devastating degenerative decline typically beginning in middle age and concluding in premature death. The choice situation for most who might consider taking the test is unusual. Although asymptomatic, they know of their significant risk—fifty–fifty if a biological parent is afflicted. Initial expectations were that many or most at risk would choose to be tested. Attitudinal surveys of those at risk suggested this would be the case as well. The test results would put an end to the suffering associated with knowledge of significant risk but ignorance as to one's actual fate. Those tested would either be released from fear or released from uncertainty, with time to adjust to and plan for what would follow. In actual experience, however, relatively few choose to take the test, evidence of the challenge of understanding the experience of suffering by others, and the challenge of anticipating one's own experience until confronted with choices.[29]

For those who choose to undergo HD testing, studies indicate that the experience of suffering that follows bad news is most closely associated with the antecedent psychological state. Those who suffer from depression or hopelessness at the time of testing suffer more from bad news. Those in relatively less psychological distress at the time of testing suffer increased short-term distress at bad news but, in the long term, adjust well, at least as detected and measured by the psychological assessments employed and under conditions in which counseling support is available. There is also evidence of selection to undergo HD testing by those who are in less antecedent distress—those who, in fact, will experience less distress in consequence of bad news.[30] This suggests that, when confronted with the choice to risk receipt of definitive bad news, those at risk of HD anticipate with some accuracy the consequences for their own experience of suffering and choose to know or not know accordingly.

Past and future study and reflection may well yield understanding that can guide action for those concerned to reduce or limit the suffering of those at risk of HD. Counselors who provide information about the availability of HD testing can be attentive to the symptoms of suffering, including depression and hopelessness, that may be significant to the patient's choice.[31] There is also suggestive evidence of the implications for future suffering of learning of one's risk of HD—in this case, owing to revelation of family history—at a vulnerable developmental stage:

> Compared with test recipients, people who declined testing were significantly more depressed and pessimistic. They were more likely to expect to be carriers and anticipated more negative effects from a positive result. Interestingly, people who declined were more likely to have learned about their being at risk for Huntington's disease during adolescence rather than adulthood. [footnotes omitted][32]

Although there is no imminent hope that the genomic enterprise will yield relief from the suffering associated with HD—the decades-long dread followed by the reality of personal disintegration and the associated depression and hopelessness—there is hope to avoid doing additional harm through study of and reflection on the testing choices and experience of those at risk.

For the immediate future, definitive diagnostic and predictive testing will generate new occasions for the experience of suffering and for study and reflection to address them, but with the hope that one day the landscape of suffering will be radically revised as testing becomes routine preface to the administration of cures. More puzzling, for the near and long term, is the suffering occasioned by the second category of genomic information—predictive risk information—and the appropriate response to it. With the advent of ever better, quicker, and cheaper sequencing technologies, the current torrent of genomic information is rapidly turning to flood, much of it consisting of in-between knowledge of correlations with risk.

PREDICTIVE RISK TESTING: UNCERTAINTY AND SUFFERING

There will be challenges for individuals, in consultation with health care providers[33] or, increasingly, after information and consultation provided by direct-to-consumer genetic testing companies,[34] in deciding whether to undergo predictive risk testing. In response to a test revealing increased risk for Alzheimer's disease (AD), lifestyle changes might delay onset or reduce symptoms, and prudent life planning decisions might be undertaken, but there is no immediate hope of effective therapeutic intervention.[35] In contrast, the genetic test offered by Myriad Genetics for significantly increased risk of breast and ovarian cancer provides information of potentially lifesaving value, as summarized in one of the court decisions in the long-running dispute surrounding Myriad's patent rights:

> Certain mutations in the *BRCA* genes correlate with an increased risk of breast and ovarian cancer. The average woman in the United States has around a twelve to thirteen percent risk of developing breast cancer in her lifetime. Women with *BRCA* mutations, in contrast, face a cumulative risk of between fifty to eighty percent of developing breast cancer and a cumulative risk of ovarian cancer of between twenty to fifty percent. Diagnostic genetic testing for the existence of *BRCA* mutations is therefore an important consideration in the provision of clinical care for breast or ovarian cancer. This testing provides a patient with information on her risk for hereditary breast and ovarian cancers, and thus aids in the difficult decision regarding whether to undertake preventive options, including prophylactic surgery. Diagnostic results can also be an important factor in structuring an appropriate course of cancer treatment, since certain forms of therapy are more effective in treating cancers related to *BRCA* mutations.[36]

Positive test results in both cases carry a price in suffering, notably the heightened fear of disease and premature mortality, but other fears as well, including loss of insurance coverage and the additional threat this poses to control over one's future. On the simplest reckoning, this potential price would be weighed against the potential for relief if good news and against the availability of effective interventions if bad. Hence, the calculus might weigh in favor of testing for susceptibility to breast and ovarian cancer but against testing for predictive risk of AD.

The implications for suffering are more complex than this simple calculus, however, for several reasons. Most of us do not interpret risk information in the same way as those trained in the science of probability. We may well underestimate or overestimate the risk of disease in response to results, with confounding implications for suffering in the near term, and potentially the long term—if we respond inappropriately to test results in ways that increase the likelihood of disease.[37]

As with those who choose to undergo testing for HD, those who choose to undergo probabilistic testing for breast or ovarian cancer or AD are likely those who have reason to believe, because of family history, that they might be at high risk. Unlike HD testing, the news they receive will be probabilistic rather than definitive, moving them from the condition of knowing that they might be at high risk to knowing that they are at high risk—the position from which those who undergo HD testing begin. In the case of AD, as with HD, there is evidence that the suffering of those who receive bad news about their heightened risk is correlated to their antecedent psychological state.[38] But bad news from tests for heightened risk, even for a dread disease such as AD with no current hope for cure, allows room for the hope foreclosed by bad news from an HD test, with significantly different implications for the experience of suffering.

PREDICTIVE RISK TESTING: THE DIRECT-TO-CONSUMER INTERFACE AND SUFFERING

Other features of genetic risk testing introduce additional complexity to the assessment of the implications of predictive risk information. Direct-to-consumer (DTC) genetic testing companies using newer sequencing technologies have become significant conduits through which the flood of genomic information now flows, including risk information about a wide and growing range of conditions.[39] These sequencing technologies are rapidly increasing in power and decreasing in cost, with burgeoning potential to yield new knowledge about associations between DNA sequences and traits and conditions owing to information that their customers agree to contribute to company databases.[40] Some DTC companies market but do not sell their genetic testing services directly to consumers; instead, health care providers order and interpret the results for their patients. The DTC companies under consideration here, however, both market and sell their testing services directly to consumers with no required mediation by health care providers.[41]

The practices of some DTC companies have prompted controversy, centered on investigative findings of misleading information and the marketing of supplements with unproven value. Other concerns, extending to a broad array of genetic tests including DTC tests, include ensuring the analytical and clinical validity of the tests, that is, that the tests are accurate and reliable and that they in fact detect or predict a condition. There appears to be an emerging consensus among DTC companies and regulators that a more comprehensive and effective system of regulatory oversight to address these issues can and should be developed.[42]

More controversial and resistant to consensus resolution is disagreement about the implications of the DTC interface with customers. Consumers order and pay for their genetic tests online, receive DNA kits from the company and return DNA samples to the company, and then access test results on a secure company website, with additional written information about associations to conditions or traits provided on company webpages and through links to other resources and with telephone counseling available. DTC companies advise consumers to consult their health care providers for interpretation of results and guidance in determining any responsive course of action, but no involvement by health care providers is required to order tests or receive the results and information about the potential significance of the results.[43]

As genetic testing services have rapidly expanded in the early twenty-first century, federal regulatory agencies have paid increasing attention to a range of issues, including concerns about the direct DTC interface with consumers.[44] Some states have banned direct sales within their states, requiring that genetic tests be offered only on the order of a health care provider.[45] Several health care provider organizations and commentators have expressed opposition to the DTC model.[46] Other commentators, as well as DTC companies and consumers, have expressed support for the model.[47]

The debate is framed largely in terms of consumers' right to information about their own genomes versus protection against harm to consumers from access to genomic information unmediated by the expertise and support of health care professionals. Embedded in the debate are two contested issues with implications for human suffering: consumer capacity to understand and act on health-relevant information in ways that, at a minimum, do no harm; and potential infliction of suffering if bad news is delivered directly rather than mediated by delivery and counseling support from health care providers.

We might engage in study and reflection, as with traditional genetic testing, to guide future policy making. For example, a preliminary study of psychological harm from receipt of DTC AD risk information found no significant short-term risks.[48] A long-term study is underway to examine a wider array of potential impacts from DTC testing.[49]

Although these studies may well inform the current policy debate, the disruptive nature of the new technologies employed by DTC companies is likely to require us to recast our approach eventually. Efforts to regulate DTC testing may soon appear, in the rearview mirror, like the efforts of some jurisdictions to regulate the Internet and its interface with individuals around the globe: infeasible for technical reasons and ultimately infeasible because of the human appetite for knowledge. The technical infeasibility of restricting access to genomic information is a result of the ease of access to the source—one's own DNA—and the eventual diffusion of testing technologies around the globe. If there is sufficient demand for genomic information from new testing technologies, it will be relatively easy to supply.

And there is reason to believe there will be sufficient demand, even if, for some, the result will be an added measure of suffering. The desire for knowledge despite the implications for human suffering has long been observed. Pandora's insatiable curiosity released miseries that encircle the globe inflicting suffering on mortals for eternity, Eve could not resist the apple, and Faust sold his soul for knowledge. Friedrich Nietzche, in his *Beyond Good and Evil*, postulated a "will to knowledge" that ultimately derives from the will to power, knowledge constituting one of the instrumentalities for fulfillment of this bedrock desire. If Nietzsche is right, one reason we struggle with the implications of genomic information is its ambivalent allure: its promise of empowerment through knowledge and its threat to reveal the source of our ultimate disempowerment.

If efforts to restrict access to genomic information will eventually prove futile, then future study and reflection might helpfully turn to the implications of this for suffering and responses available to reduce them. It may be that we will observe selection to undergo testing by those who will suffer less from bad news, as observed among those choosing to undergo testing for HD. More broadly, perhaps the cultural template that influences our experience of suffering will shift, pushed by the widespread availability of genomic information about risk. Our cultural template once forbade open discussion of a diagnosis of cancer, inflicting early on the experience of isolation foretold by the diagnosis. Perhaps widespread knowledge and sharing of one's genomic risk profile will reduce isolation and contribute to empowerment through participation in efforts to expand knowledge and find cures and the opportunity to find support with "virtual friends" in addition to family, friends, and health care providers. And perhaps the widespread availability of genomic information will encourage wider and deeper training in genomics and counseling among health care providers, drawing patients to them for guidance and support.

As we anticipate the flood and engage in study and reflection on the opportunities for effective response, our efforts will be complicated by a set of unintended consequences generated by the advance of genetic testing. There will also be increasing demand for genomic information from third parties whose motivations fall outside the Baconian template.

Third-Party Uses of Genomic Information: Secrets and "Scarlet" Genetic Letters

While the shared purpose of relieving suffering, in concert with a range of other motivations, drives the genomic enterprise, there are by-products of the enterprise that serve unrelated purposes and that carry additional implications for human suffering. The genetic letters inscribed in our genomes, in combination with other influences, yield our phenotypes and associated risk profiles. With the exception of genetic twins, our genomes uniquely identify us. Third parties with reason to care about our phenotypes and risk profiles or about our identities may be motivated to apply testing technologies to serve their purposes, potentially contributing to the impact on suffering attributable to the genomic enterprise.

THIRD-PARTY BUSINESS USE OF GENOMIC HEALTH INFORMATION: THE POLICY DEBATE

As the genomic enterprise accelerated in the wake of the HGP, and an expanding array of genetic tests was developed, a serious concern emerged among actors in the genomic enterprise and those at risk of genetic conditions. The implications for suffering for those at risk extended well beyond the problems associated with genetic testing in the absence of cures. There were third parties—insurers and employers—whose business required them to assess the health risks of their potential insureds and employees.[50]

Insurance companies might require applicants to reveal the results of genetic tests so that they could use this information in setting rates for health, life, or disability insurance. If the results were dire, they might use the information to deny coverage altogether. Employers also might require applicants to reveal the results of genetic tests, and they might use this information to deny employment to otherwise qualified applicants because of projected costs for the employers' share of insurance costs or because the applicants might be especially vulnerable to potential risks in the workplace.[51]

The effect of these uses of genomic information by third parties would be to exclude those not yet ill, and who may never turn ill, from participation in the benefits of insurance and employment. The threat of exclusion might also dissuade individuals from obtaining genetic tests of potential value in preserving their own health and from obtaining genetic tests in conjunction with human subjects research to advance the development of cures. The proposed policy response was to impose limits on the ability of insurers and employers to access the results of genetic tests.[52]

Others engaged in the policy debate argued against this response as an inappropriate exercise in "genetic exceptionalism." Insurers routinely use risk information gathered from medical records, including family histories and the results of other medical tests, in setting rates or denying coverage. Their business requires that they do so because they must take in premiums at least sufficient to cover projected claims. Furthermore, it is only fair to charge higher premiums to those who are more likely to file claims or to file claims for larger amounts. For those who pose very high or unpredictable risks, it is only fair to exclude them from coverage to protect the viability of the insurance pool. Similarly, employers often require acceptable results of physical examinations as a condition of employment. They should not be denied access to relevant information for use in choosing among applicants for employment on the basis of projected costs to the business owing to risk of ill health.[53]

Those who favored restricting insurer and employer access to genomic information eventually prevailed. Several states enacted restrictions with some variation in their details. And, in 2005, Congress enacted the Genetic Information Nondiscrimination Act (GINA), which imposed nationwide restrictions applicable to the private health insurance market—although not to disability or life insurance—and to employers with fifteen or more employees.[54]

FIRST-GENERATION POLICY RESPONSE: GENOMIC HEALTH INFORMATION AND SUFFERING

The outcome of the debate points to the distinctive implications for suffering in third-party use of genomic information as opposed to other kinds of health care information. Those charged higher premiums or denied insurance coverage or employment on the basis of any kind of health care information endure suffering associated with loss of control and the power to provide for themselves and their loved ones, with the magnitude of the suffering dependent on the magnitude of the existential threat. There is also the experience of exclusion from the communities of the insured and employed following on a judgment that portends one's increasing isolation and ultimate exclusion from the human community.

There are distinctive implications for suffering associated with the use of genomic information, however. We come to know and come to terms with our family histories over time. We also are accustomed to receiving nongenetic test results, for better or worse, and to their changeability over time in response to changes in our habits or medical interventions. Genetic tests, on the other hand, entail sudden excavation of secrets previously hidden from view; some would prefer not to know these secrets about themselves, most would prefer not to share them with others. There is the peculiar indelibility of the information revealed; unlike most of our health indicators, genetic letters are written in permanent ink, inscribed in all but the red blood cells in our body, immutable to change or revision. There is the excavation of these indelible and inescapable secrets into the plain view of others who may use them to our detriment, including to exclude us from communities we hope will embrace us and offer us some measure of insulation against our fear of pain and disability, dependency and loss of control, isolation and alienation from others, and ultimate personal dissolution. From the perspective of risk assessment by third parties, genetic test results look like other risk data and should be used if they yield more accurate assessments; from the perspective of those whose results might be sought, the data are resonant with foreboding of suffering and should not be used.

This perspectival divide is relatively clear in the challenges it poses to policymakers: to identify the values at stake on both sides of the divide and craft policies that preserve them to the extent possible and sacrifice one for the other only after considered reflection. Although there is room for disagreement about the current balance struck in federal law, GINA reflects the choice to honor the threat of suffering for those who might be denied health insurance because of bad news from genetic test results and to honor the threat to the viability of life and disability insurance and to the fair allocation of costs to the insurance pools if individuals who receive bad news from genetic tests may use their private knowledge to obtain insurance significantly underpriced in light of their risk. The policy-making task will evolve, as will the assessment of threats to the values on both sides of the divide, as the implications of genetic test results are transformed by progress to cures.

CRIMINAL JUSTICE SYSTEM USE OF FORENSIC DNA IDENTIFICATION: THE POLICY DEBATE

The forensic use of DNA identification by the criminal justice system holds different and more confounding implications for human suffering. As the impetus to expansion of these databases continues, potentially extending to the creation of a universal database containing DNA profiles of everyone in the United States, we will face stark policy alternatives. The values at stake will not sort neatly across a perspectival divide, nor will they begin to dissolve as the genomic enterprise advances our knowledge and know-how—the choices in fact will be sharpened as techniques for identification improve in accuracy and affordability.

Current forensic DNA identification proceeds in two steps: first, establish and maintain DNA databases with DNA profiles of known individuals consisting of thirteen short tandem repeat (STR) core loci prepared from biological samples from the individuals; second, collect biological samples at crime scenes and compare the thirteen STR loci in the DNA from these samples against the DNA profiles in the databases in search of a match or "hit." A hit is probabilistic but not definitive evidence that the biological sample collected at the crime scene belongs to the known individual in the forensic DNA database. Assuming that the identification is correct, the likelihood that the individual in fact committed the crime is limited by many factors, including, for example, whether the individual's DNA was deposited at the crime scene before or after but not at the time of commission of the crime.[55]

The federal government maintains a Combined DNA Index System (CODIS), funded by the Federal Bureau of Investigation (FBI), which combines federal and state forensic DNA databases. All fifty states maintain databases, although they vary in their inclusion criteria; for example, some states include DNA profiles only for those individuals convicted of serious crimes, others include them for individuals convicted of lesser crimes as well, and some states include DNA profiles for individuals who are arrested but not convicted. Tens of thousands of investigations have been aided by the use of forensic DNA databases, which may help identify those who commit crimes and exclude others from suspicion.[56] In addition, hundreds of individuals convicted of crimes before the advent of modern genetic testing technologies or in the absence of opportunity to apply these technologies have subsequently been exonerated, in some cases after decades of imprisonment for crimes they did not commit.[57]

Genetic testing technology when applied to exclude individuals from suspicion or exonerate the innocent does not provoke controversy. The only concerns are technical: that the testing is accurate and that, under all the facts and circumstances, an accurate test result truly excludes or exonerates the individual.

The application of DNA profiling to help identify the potentially guilty, however, arouses considerable controversy. A "hit" could support a mistaken conclusion about identity for any of a wide variety of reasons, including unintentional contamination of a biological sample, intentional "planting" of evidence, deteriorated DNA at a crime scene that yields a partial match to a DNA profile, and juror confusion about the possibility that DNA from a crime scene belongs to a different individual despite a match or partial match with a DNA profile in the database. A mistaken conclusion about identity introduces the horrifying prospect of placing an innocent person under suspicion of a crime or even wrongfully convicting an innocent despite the very high burden of proof required for a criminal conviction.[58] A universal DNA database introduces a prospect far worse for most people: that wrongful suspicion or conviction might extend not only to those once convicted or arrested but also to all of us.

Those who favor a universal forensic DNA database point to the potential for solving more crimes, with benefits measured in justice for victims and prevention of future crimes by those caught and convicted. And the more efficient the criminal justice system, the more likely that potential future criminals will be deterred from their plans, with more benefits in crimes prevented.[59]

Opponents argue that those who have been convicted of crimes have surrendered some expectation of privacy even after completing their sentences, but others resident in the United States have not. And these privacy interests should preclude governmental intrusion to collect our biological samples and store our DNA profiles. In addition, a universal database would violate the spirit if not the letter of the presumption of innocence articulated in court decisions interpreting the U.S. Constitution, placing all of us at risk of wrongful suspicion and, potentially, wrongful conviction.[60]

FIRST-GENERATION POLICY RESPONSE: FORENSIC DNA IDENTIFICATION AND SUFFERING

In its 2013 decision in *Maryland v. King*, by a five to four decision and over a vigorous dissent, the U.S. Supreme Court approved the current practice of collecting DNA samples from arrestees, without consent or a warrant, and checking the arrestees' DNA profiles against profiles in the CODIS database.[61] The Supreme Court upheld the practice pursuant to the Maryland DNA Collection Act against a Fourth Amendment challenge in a case in which the practice yielded a "hit" and the conviction of an arrestee for a different crime than the crime for which he had been arrested. The policy and constitutional debates continue as policy makers and commentators contemplate expanded collection and use of forensic DNA, potentially including creation of a universal DNA database.[62]

These debates are framed in terms of justice, privacy, and security but include recognition of elements of suffering as well. In convictions, past victims of crimes receive some measure of relief for the past experiences and continuing threats imposed by intentional human infliction of pain, loss of control, and threat of dissolution. Potential future victims are spared the experience. All of us are potential victims and recognize the relief that more efficient identification and conviction of the guilty provides.

However, as we press toward efficiency in the criminal justice system and its promise of relief with more expansive forensic DNA databases, we introduce the prospect that any of us could be wrongfully suspected or convicted of crimes. This introduces a new measure of potential suffering detectable in debates surrounding other techniques deployed or proposed to guard against criminal, terrorist, or military threats, including video surveillance, Internet surveillance, monitoring of other communications, and universal identification cards. The prospect of a universal forensic DNA database evokes elements of "Orwellian suffering," in which governmental surveillance and control are a constant and sometimes extend to expunging all traces of the existence of those judged undesirable, the ultimate in alienation, disempowerment, and dissolution. There are also elements of "Kafkaesque suffering," the sense of fear, foreboding, and powerlessness at the threat of judgment and sentencing by criteria unintelligible to the accused, the letters of our DNA, applied by distant and inaccessible authorities.

As the advance of the genomic enterprise generates ever more accurate and inexpensive genomic information, it is likely to aggravate rather than relieve these stark tradeoffs and their implications for suffering. Study and reflection can assist at least in clarifying our choices.

These unintended consequences of the genomic era, involving applications of genomic information by third parties in realms that extend well beyond health care, pose significant challenges to our capacity to manage the implications for suffering. Even greater challenges will be posed in the last context of choice considered here, applications by potential parents.

Procreative Testing: The Ambiguous Future of Genomics and Suffering

In the genetic testing contexts discussed previously, our expectations of progress and of its effects are similar. We expect eventual progress to cures and, when curing is achieved, we expect that the experience of suffering associated with genetic testing will be radically revised. We expect the same trajectory of progress in the broader context of modern biomedical science. We once added to the measure of suffering by spreading infection among those gathered in hospitals, then advanced in our knowledge, discovered and applied cures, suffered setbacks from unintended consequences of our practices in administering the cures, revised our practices and regained some lost ground, and now seek new scientific breakthroughs and technologies that might replace old cures with better ones. In the same way, we expect progress from utter incapacity to address the suffering caused by genetic conditions, to a halfway house awash in genomic information with a mix of unintended consequences, to the beginnings of cures for some illnesses and, eventually, many more. In this respect, the implications for suffering ushered in by the genomic era—however distinctive in their details, regrettable in their impact, and deserving of our attention and efforts to do better—pose no challenge to the dominant Baconian template, a template whose replication across other fields of biomedical science contributes to the ascendancy of the science and technology enterprise in modernity.

But procreational testing, now in its infancy, challenges this familiar Baconian template. The trajectory to more and better testing and vastly expanded access to genomic information may well be prelude to more and better cures, but the implications for suffering are complicated and ambiguous, pressing against our assumptions about its nature and meaning. To see why this is so, consider, first, the choice contexts and motivations to make use of currently available and anticipated procreative genetic tests.

PROCREATIONAL TESTING: CHALLENGING CONTEXTS FOR CHOICES TO RELIEVE SUFFERING

One context for choice is that of potential future parents who undergo genetic testing to determine their carrier status and, hence, whether their biological offspring would be at risk of a heritable genetic condition. Typically, carrier testing is undertaken to avoid giving birth to biological offspring who will suffer a serious genetic condition such as infantile Tay-Sachs, a disease of the nervous system that results in progressive muscle weakness, loss of vision and hearing, paralysis, and death in early childhood.[63] The use of carrier testing to avoid the "vertical" transmission of a serious disease such as Tay-Sachs might be analogized to the use of inoculation to avoid "horizontal" transmission of serious infectious diseases to children-in-being. In both cases, parents are motivated to prevent suffering in their children and, because of the intense sympathetic connection between parent and child, their own associated suffering as well.

In the event that carrier testing indicates that biological offspring would be at risk, potential parents might proceed to any of a range of follow-on choices.[64] They might avoid biological procreation and instead adopt a child or obtain donated gametes and engage in vitro fertilization (IVF). They might engage in IVF using one potential parent's gametes plus donated gametes. They might engage in IVF using both potential parents' gametes and then use preimplantation genetic diagnosis (PGD)—genetic testing applied to the IVF embryos—to identify unaffected embryos for transfer to the womb. They might proceed with biological procreation and then engage in prenatal testing to determine whether the fetus is affected and, if so, terminate the pregnancy.

Carrier testing, combined with one of these follow-on choices, to avoid giving birth to a child with a serious genetic condition undoubtedly prevents grievous suffering in children and their parents and, in this respect, follows the familiar template of Baconian progress from testing to cure or, in this case, prevention. Some of the follow-on choices to accomplish prevention after carrier testing, however, introduce complications and ambiguities with their own implications for suffering and its relief and for the vindication of other values.

Regarding other values at stake, current IVF practices entail the eventual destruction of unused IVF embryos. For those who believe that life begins at conception and that the value of respect for persons supersedes the value of prevention of suffering in future children and parents, the use of IVF thus would be ethically unacceptable unless all IVF embryos, including those affected by the heritable genetic condition, were transferred to the womb of potential gestational mothers. The use of prenatal testing and possible termination of the pregnancy likewise would be unacceptable.

For those willing to consider options that entail the destruction of embryos or fetuses, the follow-on choices introduce the possibility of unintended consequences with potential implications for suffering. Some of these consequences might be diminished with advances in reproductive science and technology or by changes in policy guidelines; if so, new unintended consequences predictably would be introduced.

For those who proceed with biological procreation and prenatal testing, there are risks of unintended miscarriage associated with most current prenatal testing procedures and the attendant suffering experienced by those who lose wanted pregnancies.[65] For those willing to engage in IVF, the use of donated gametes introduces risks to egg donors as well as the children born of the IVF procedure. Known risks to egg donors include ovarian hyperstimulation syndrome (OHSS) caused by administration of fertility drugs to stimulate the release of eggs from the donor's ovaries. OHSS usually involves only mild discomfort but may lead to serious complications and the suffering that attends serious illness.[66] There is also some evidence of increased risk of cancer associated with administration of fertility drugs.[67] Another risk to egg donors suspected by some but as yet unproved is infertility, the loss of a highly valued human capacity that, for some, offers significant comfort and meaning in the encounter with one's ultimate dissolution.[68]

The risks to children born of IVF procedures include risks attendant on the greater frequency of multiple births and may include elevated risks of some birth defects.[69] Risks may also include psychological risks that derive from the current general practice in the United States of preserving the anonymity of gamete donors.[70] Some IVF children who learn of a biological parent who is unknown to them strongly desire to learn the identity and have contact with the biological parent; the denial of this knowledge is experienced as intense lifelong suffering, an irremediable absence in one's sense of personal integrity and identity, and a sense of isolation and alienation from the embrace of one's closest kin. Revision of policy guidelines to eliminate the practice of anonymity, on the other hand, might reduce the supply of donated gametes, with implications for suffering for those seeking to avoid the transmission of heritable genetic conditions as well as for the larger cohort of those who suffer from infertility.[71]

While this catalogue of implications for suffering and other values is perhaps no more challenging than that encountered by individuals faced with current choices to engage in nonprocreational genetic testing in the absence of cures, the catalogue is provocative in two respects. First, it reveals the complex implications of choices posed in the simplest procreational testing context, in which the unambiguous purpose is prevention of significant suffering associated with serious heritable genetic conditions. In this context, competing values will limit choices for some, and for those who proceed, all options include risks of adding to the measure of suffering for parents, children, or donors. Second, it invites reflection on the greater challenges posed in more complex procreational testing contexts.

PROCREATIONAL CHOICE: SUFFERING AND ITS RELIEF

The advance of the genomic enterprise is rapidly expanding our knowledge of associations between genetic sequences and a wide array of genetically influenced traits and conditions, and techniques for testing are growing more powerful and less costly. Use of assisted reproductive technologies, including IVF, is also growing rapidly. Procreational testing options may enable choices that are not motivated by the prevention of suffering attendant on serious genetic conditions, challenging our understanding of the nature and meaning of suffering and serving as prelude to the next frontier in the genomic era: the prospect of genetic engineering of future children.

The Baconian template assumes that we understand the nature and meaning of suffering and our obligation to relieve it, and that its relief is a good to which the scientific and technological enterprise should be dedicated. As procreational testing choices expand to address a wider array of traits and conditions, we will face questions that challenge our understanding. Do those who are dyslexic, near-sighted, short in stature, or shy suffer? Are we obligated to prevent the births of those who would manifest these traits or conditions to relieve their suffering?

If we conclude that these traits and conditions are different ways of experiencing embodiment rather than manifestations of suffering, then we might be obligated to accommodate or treat these children but not to prevent their birth. In fact, we might further conclude that the risk of some procreational choices to prevent their birth, including the unintended imposition of suffering on parents, children, or egg donors as noted previously, are not justified. This analysis would be somewhat different from that often invoked in policy debates involving distinctions between (acceptable) "therapeutic" choices and (unacceptable) "enhancement" choices, a distinction difficult to sustain in the absence of an anchor in a deeper assessment of the goods at stake.

But might we instead reach a different conclusion? As the genomic enterprise advances and cure or prevention increasingly relieves the suffering associated with serious illness to which we have long been vulnerable, our understanding of the nature and meaning of suffering and our obligation to relieve it will be tested. Perhaps the elimination of deviations from the mean will motivate us with the same thick imperative resonance that curing serious illness has inspired in the past. We might view these as all of a piece: imperfections associated with our embodiment that generate an imperative to marshal our resources and ingenuity to accomplish relief.

Concluding Reflection on the Nature and Meaning of Suffering and Our Obligation to Relieve It

In this chapter, we have seen how our exertions in pursuit of Bacon's call issued at the cusp of modernity have succeeded, in part, and hold promise for achieving far more. These exertions sometimes add to the measure of suffering, inviting study and reflection aimed at revising our course: delivering curing with caring, minimizing the implications of the genomic enterprise as system, tailoring our policies and protocols to track and address the impact of testing in the halfway house to cures, identifying and navigating the values at stake in third-party uses of genetic information. But the rapidly expanding options for procreative testing and follow-on choices noted previously invite further examination of the nature and meaning of suffering and our obligation to relieve it.

SUFFERING AND ITS RELIEF IN MODERNITY

We know that suffering associated with our embodiment is universal, as is the desire for relief from its grip. These facts anchor the continuing force, a half a millennium on, of Bacon's call.

Despite disagreement about the theoretical and practical terms of conversion of this universal desire into individual and social obligations, the call has largely united us, across worldviews and personal circumstances, in responsive action. Although the genomic era has been punctuated by controversies—about policies that govern the operation of the enterprise, the practice of genetic testing, and the uses of genetic information by third parties—from a step removed, these controversies appear relatively modest in scope, the range of contested resolutions tightly centered around broad agreement.

Tested by the advent of new procreative options, however, we may find that our broad consensus pulls apart. Our beliefs about the nature and meaning of suffering and our obligation to relieve it may overlap but not coincide, with significantly divergent implications for the future direction of the genomic enterprise.

SUFFERING AND ITS RELIEF IN POSTMODERNITY

In his later work, Bacon wrote of a religious conception of a perfected human estate, which he hoped might be realized by the advancement of science. In this work, his twin recommendations for the pursuit of knowledge—the glory of the Creator and the relief of suffering—are ultimately seen as one and the same:

> Men must realize...how great a difference there is between the idols of the human mind and the ideas of the divine mind.... [T]he latter are the Creator's true stamp upon created things, printed and defined on matter by true and precise lines. In this respect, therefore, truth and utility are the very things themselves, so works themselves are of greater value as pledges of truth than as comforts of life.[72]

And the advancement of science, although fraught with the dangers of corruption that characterize all earthly things, offered hope for the ultimate restoration of humankind's dominion over Nature, a return to a perfected embodiment free from the consequences of the Fall:

> [I]f objection is made to the corruption of the sciences and arts to evil purposes or to luxury and the like, not much notice should be taken of that, for as much could be said of all earthly goods.... Let the human race only recover its God-given right over Nature, and be given the necessary power; then right reason and sound religion will govern the exercise of it.[73]

In the voices of advocates of future procreational choices such as human genetic engineering, there is a similar longing to wield the power of science and technology to free humankind from the vulnerabilities and imperfections that accompany our embodiment, motivated now by a secularized vision of what could be if not what once was.[74] This longing encompasses relief from the experiences of pain, disability, and disfigurement, fear, dependency, and dread of death, but it aspires to something more and different: relief from man's humbled estate in virtue of our embodiment and ascent to a more perfected state in which we enjoy far greater control of our fate.

Suffering on this expansive vision includes the experiences associated both with serious illness and with other deviations from the mean of human functioning. Both signify our subjugation to nature and the denial of our aspiration to a more perfected state. Our obligation, on this view of the nature and meaning of suffering, extends beyond sympathetic responses to the experiences associated with serious illness. We are obligated to perfect ourselves: this is the form of human flourishing to which we can and should aspire by marshaling the power of the genomic enterprise. When genetic engineering is feasible, an extensive array of interventions may fall within the scope of this obligation.

An alternative conception instead aspires to perfect our response to suffering, a feature of our embodiment that signifies the terms of our participation in nature as embodied and, hence, vulnerable, mortal, and in need of curing and caring. Our obligation is to respond to the experiences associated with serious illness in ways that enable flourishing under these terms. This entails efforts to marshal our capacities for curing and for caring as effectively as we can while limiting our additions to the measure of suffering. On this view of the nature and meaning of suffering, traits and conditions that deviate from the mean call for accommodation and treatment to enable flourishing in the same way that serious illness calls for curing and caring to enable flourishing. When genetic engineering is feasible, only a narrow range of interventions will fall within the scope of our obligation to relieve suffering.

We now stand awash in genomic information let in after decades-long exertions to swing wide the sea gates. This vast sea will empower discoveries and inventions well beyond our achievements to date. The dominant rallying call throughout these exertions has been the imperative to relieve suffering associated with our embodiment. Our responses revealed in the collection of puzzles in this chapter are consistent with both visions above—and more. We will soon be pressed to choose among them.

Acknowledgments

I wish to thank Hillary Alberta for her excellent research assistance. I also wish to thank the Ivan Allen College of Liberal Arts, Georgia Institute of Technology, for the support provided by a Special Research Award, which enabled preparation of this essay. And I am grateful for the insightful comments of the editors of this volume, Ronald M. Green and Nathan Palpant, which were of great help to me in preparing this essay.

Notes

1. Francis Bacon, *The Advancement of Learning*, bk. 1, sec. 11 (1605).

2. James D. Watson, *The Double Helix: A Personal Account of the Discovery of the Structure of DNA* (New York: Atheneum, 1968); Leslie Roberts et al., "A History of the Human Genome Project," *Science* 291, no. 5507 (2001): 1195.

3. Ron Cowen et al., "Federal Budget 1996: R & D Would Fall," *Science News* 147, no. 86 (1995); Robert M. Cook-Deegan, "Mapping the Human Genome," *Southern California Law Review* 65 (1991): 579; Philip Kitcher, *The Lives to Come: The Genetic Revolution and Human Possibilities* (New York: Simon & Schuster, 1996), 87–126.

4. Human Genome Program, U.S. Department of Energy, "Evolution of a Vision: Genome Project Origins, Present and Future Challenges, and Far-Reaching Benefits," *Human Genome News* 7, no. 3 (1995), pt. 1, accessed March 17, 2014, http://www.ornl.gov/sci/techresources/Human_Genome/publicat/hgn/v7n3/02smithr.shtml, and pt. 2, accessed March 17, 2014, http://www.ornl.gov/sci/techresources/Human_Genome/

publicat/hgn/v7n3/03collin.shtml; U.S. Department of Energy, Office of Energy Research and Office of Biological and Environmental Research, *Human Genome Project Report*, Part I, Overview and Progress, Preface, page v, accessed March 29, 2014, http://web.ornl.gov/sci/techresources/Human_Genome/publicat/97pr/1997ProgramReport.pdf.

5. Human Genome Program, U.S. Department of Energy, "Genomes: 15 Years Later," *Human Genome News* 11, no. 3–4 (2001), accessed March 17, 2014, http://www.ornl.gov/sci/techresources/Human_Genome/publicat/hgn/v11n3/05delisi.shtml; Allen D. Roses, "The Genome Era Begins. . .," *Nature Genetics Supplement* 33 (2003): 217.

6. Anne Eisenberg, "Variations on a Gene, and Tools to Find Them," *New York Times*, April 27, 2013, accessed March 17, 2014, http://www.nytimes.com/2013/04/28/business/in-cancer-treatment-new-dna-tools.html?_r=0; Anemona Hartocollis, "Cancer Centers Racing to Map Patients' Genes," *New York Times*, April 21, 2013, accessed March 17, 2014, http://www.nytimes.com/2013/04/22/health/patients-genes-seen-as-future-of-cancer-care.html?pagewanted=all&_r=0; "Gene Therapy Is a 'Disruptive Science' Ready for Commercial Development, Experts Say," *Science Daily*, January 24, 2012, accessed March 17, 2014, http://www.sciencedaily.com/releases/2012/01/120124113203.htm.

7. Bacon, *The Advancement of Learning*, bk. 1, sec. 11.

8. Watson, *Double Helix*.

9. Leslie Roberts, "Controversial from the Start," *Science* 291, no. 5507 (2001): 1182–1188, accessed March 17, 2014, http://www.sciencemag.org/content/291/5507/1182.1.full.

10. Sabrina Safrin, "Hyperownership in a Time of Biotechnological Promise: The International Conflict to Control the Building Blocks of Life," *American Journal of International Law* 98 (2004): 641–685; Rebecca S. Eisenberg, "Re-Examining the Role of Patents in Appropriating the Value of DNA Sequences," *Emory Law Journal* 49 (2000): 783–800.

11. *Association for Molecular Pathology et al. v. Myriad Genetics, Inc. et al.*, No. 12-398, Slip Opinion, 569 U.S. ____ (2013); Law firm of Robinson, Bradshaw, & Hinson, "Myriad Gene Patent Litigation," *Genomics Law Report*, accessed March 17, 2014, http://www.genomicslawreport.com/index.php/category/badges/myriad-gene-patent-litigation/.

12. Kevin W. Williams, "Managing Physician Financial Conflicts of Interest in Clinical Trials Conducted in the Private Practice Setting," *Food and Drug Law Journal* 59 (2004): 45.

13. Robin Fretwell Wilson, "The Death of Jesse Gelsinger: New Evidence of the Influence of Money and Prestige in Human Research," *American Journal of Law and Medicine* 36 (2010): 295–325.

14. Legal Information Institute, "Patent," August 19, 2010, accessed March 17, 2014, http://www.law.cornell.edu/wex/patent; Wendy H. Schacht, "The Bayh-Dole Act: Selected Issues in Patent Policy and the Commercialization of Technology," Congressional Research Service, December 3, 2012.

15. *Association for Molecular Pathology et al. v. Myriad Genetics, Inc. et al.*, No. 12-398, Slip Opinion, p. 11, 569 U.S. ____ (2013).

16. Sara Boettiger and Alan B. Bennett, "Bayh-Dole: If We Knew Then What We Know Now," *Nature Biotechnology* 24 (2006): 320–323; Robert Gatter, "Human Subjects Research and Conflicts of Interest: Walking the Talk of Trust in Human Subjects Research: The Challenge of Regulating Financial Conflicts of Interest," *Emory Law Journal* 52 (2003): 327.

17. Doris Teichler Zallen, "US Gene Therapy in Crisis," *Genetics & Society 16*, no. 6 (June 2000): 272–275; Julian Savulescu, "Harm, Ethics Committees and the Gene Therapy

Death," *Journal of Medical Ethics* 27 (2001):148–150; "The Trials of Gene Therapy," *Nature* 420, no. 6912 (November 14, 2002): 107; Vicki Brower, "Cancer Gene Therapy Steadily Advances," *Journal of the National Cancer Institute News* 100, no. 18 (September 17, 2008): 1276–1278; "Gene Therapy Is a 'Disruptive Science,'" supra note 6.

18. Angelina Jolie, "My Medical Choice," *New York Times* (May 14, 2013), accessed March 17, 2014, http://www.nytimes.com/2013/05/14/opinion/my-medical-choice.html?_r=0 Page.

19. Eric J. Cassell, *The Nature of Suffering and the Goals of Medicine*, 2nd ed. (Oxford: Oxford University Press, 2004), 29–32.

20. Lewis Thomas, *The Youngest Science: Notes of a Medicine-Watcher* (New York: Penguin Books, 1995), 59.

21. Johns Hopkins Medicine, "PTSD Symptoms Common among ICU Survivors," news release, February 26, 2013, accessed March 17, 2014, http://www.hopkinsmedicine.org/news/media/releases/ptsd_symptoms_common_among_icu_survivors.

22. John Schwartz, "Cancer Patients Challenge the Patenting of a Gene," *New York Times*, May 12, 2009, accessed March 17, 2014, http://www.nytimes.com/2009/05/13/health/13patent.html?_r=1; E. Richard Gold and Julia Carbone, "Myriad Genetics: In the Eye of the Policy Storm," *Genetics in Medicine* 12, no. 4 Suppl. (2010): S39–S70; Mildred K. Cho et al., "Effects of Patents and Licenses on the Provision of Clinical Genetic Testing Services," *Journal of Molecular Diagnostics* 5, no. 1 (February 2003): 3–8; Timothy Caulfield et al., "Evidence and Anecdotes: An Analysis of Human Gene Patenting Controversies," *Nature Biotechnology* 24, no. 9 (September 2006): 1091–1094.

23. *Association for Molecular Pathology et al. v. Myriad Genetics, Inc. et al.*, No. 12-398, Slip Opinion, 569 U.S. ____ (2013); John Conley, "Some Thoughts on Myriad after the Supreme Court Argument," *Genomics Law Report*, May 1, 2013, accessed March 17, 2014, http://www.genomicslawreport.com/index.php/2013/05/01/some-thoughts-on-myriad-after-the-supreme-court-argument/#more-12729.

24. Caulfield et al., "Evidence and Anecdotes," supra note 22.

25. Jess Bravin and Brent Kendall, "Justices Strike Down Gene Patents," *Wall Street Journal*, June 13, 2013, accessed March 17, 2014, http://online.wsj.com/article/SB10001424127887324049504578543250466974398.html.

26. Kevin Noonan, "An Antidote to the Politics of the Human Gene Patenting Debate," Scotusblog, February 6, 2013, accessed March 17, 2014, http://www.scotusblog.com/2013/02/an-antidote-to-the-politics-of-the-human-gene-patenting-debate/.

27. "Outlaw Human Gene Patents," *Breast Cancer Action*, July 30, 2103, accessed March 17, 2014, http://www.bcaction.org/take-action/outlaw-human-gene-patents/; Anita Little, "People Over Profit: What the BRCA Ruling Means for Patients' Rights," *Ms. Magazine,* June 19, 2013, accessed March 17, 2014, http://msmagazine.com/blog/2013/06/19/people-over-profit-what-the-bcra-ruling-means-for-patients-rights/; David B. Agus, "The Outrageous Cost of a Gene Test," *International Herald Tribune*, May 20, 2013, accessed March 17, 2014, http://www.nytimes.com/2013/05/21/opinion/the-outrageous-cost-of-a-gene-test.html?_r=2&; Karuna Jaggar, "The Breast Cancer Gene and Control of Women's Bodies," *Ms. Magazine*, April 13, 2013, accessed March 17, 2014 http://msmagazine.com/blog/2013/04/13/the-breast-cancer-gene-and-the-control-of-womens-bodies/.

28. Jorge A. Goldstein et al., "Patent Pools as a Solution to the Licensing Problems of Diagnostic Genetics: United States and European Perspectives," *Drug Discovery World* (Spring 2005): 86–90; Tina Rosenberg, "Prizes with an Eye toward the Future," *New York*

Times, February 29, 2012, accessed March 17, 2014, http://opinionator.blogs.nytimes.com/2012/02/29/prizes-with-an-eye-toward-the-future/; Catherine Rampell, "Invent a Drug, Win $1 Million," *Slate*, January 23, 2008, accessed March 17, 2014, http://www.slate.com/articles/health_and_science/science/2008/01/invent_a_drug_win_1_million.single.html.

29. Bettina Meiser and Stewart Dunn, "Psychological Effect of Genetic Testing for Huntington's Disease," *Western Journal of Medicine* 174, no. 5 (2001): 336–340, accessed March 17, 2014 http://www.ncbi.nlm.nih.gov/pmc/articles/PMC1071392/;J. Scott Roberts and Sarah M. Tersegno, "Estimating and Disclosing the Risk of Developing Alzheimer's Disease: Challenges, Controversies, and Future Directions," *Future Neurology* 5, no. 4 (2010): 501–517, accessed March 17, 2014,http://www.ncbi.nlm.nih.gov/pmc/articles/PMC2941213/; Charlotte Raven, "Should I Take My Own Life?," *Guardian*, January 15, 2010, accessed March 17, 2014,http://www.guardian.co.uk/society/2010/jan/16/charlotte-raven-should-i-take-my-own-life.

30. Meiser and Dunn, "Psychological Effect of Genetic Testing," ibid.

31. T.-B. Robins Wahlin, "To Know or Not to Know: A Review of Behaviour and Suicidal Ideation in Preclinical Huntington's Disease," *Patient Education and Counseling* 65, no. 3 (2007): 279–287, accessed March 17, 2014, http://www.ncbi.nlm.nih.gov/pubmed/17000074.

32. Meiser and Dunn, "Psychological Effect of Genetic Testing," supra note 29.

33. J. C. Knight, "Genetics and the General Physician: Insights, Applications, and Future Challenges," *Quarterly Journal of Medicine* 102 (2009): 757–772; Richard L. Haspel et al., "Training Pathology Residents in Genomics and Personalized Medicine," *American Journal of Clinical Pathology* 133 (2010): 832–834.

34. Cinnamon S. Bloss et al., "Direct-to-Consumer Personalized Genomic Testing," *Human Molecular Genetics* 20, review issue 2 (2011): R132–R141; Karen Norrgard, "DTC Genetic Testing for Diabetes, Breast Cancer, Heart Disease, and Paternity," *Nature Education* 1, no. 1 (2008), accessed March 17, 2014, http://www.nature.com/scitable/topicpage/dtc-genetic-testing-for-diabetes-breast-cancer-698.

35. Roberts and Tersegno, "Estimating and Disclosing the Risk," supra note 29.

36. *Association for Molecular Pathology v. U.S. Patent and Trademark Office*, 689 F.3d 1303, 1314 (Fed. Cir. 2012).

37. Roberts and Tersegno, "Estimating and Disclosing the Risk," supra note 29.

38. Roberts and Tersegno, "Estimating and Disclosing the Risk," supra note 29.

39. Pascal Borry, Martina C. Cornel, and Heidi C. Howard, "Where Are You Going, Where Have You Been: A Recent History of the Direct-to-Consumer Genetic Testing Market," *Journal of Community Genetics* 1, no. 3 (2010): 101–106, accessed March 17, 2014, http://www.ncbi.nlm.nih.gov/pmc/articles/PMC3063844/; Roberta M. Berry et al., "Recent Developments in Health Care Law: Culture and Controversy," *HealthCare Ethics Committee Forum* 25, no. 1 (2013): 1–24.

40. Ricki Lewis, "Direct-to-Consumer Genetic Testing: A New View," *Plos Blogs*, November 8, 2012, accessed March 17, 2014,http://blogs.plos.org/dnascience/2012/11/08/direct-to-consumer-genetic-testing-a-new-view/;Timothy Caulfield et al., "Direct-to-Consumer Genetic Testing: Good, Bad or Benign?," *Clinical Genetics* 77 (2010): 101–105;Stuart Hogarth, Gail Javitt, and David Melzer, "The Current Landscape for Direct-to-Consumer Genetic Testing: Legal, Ethical, and Policy Issues," *Annual Review of Genomics and Human Genetics* 9 (2008): 161–182;Leslie Pray, "DTC Genetic Testing:

23andMe, DNA Direct, and Genelex," *Nature Education* 1, no. 1 (2008); 23andMe website, accessed March 17, 2014,http://www.23andme.com.

41. Borry et al., "Where Are You Going," supra note 39.

42. Daniel MacArthur, "My Submission to the FDA on the Regulation of Personal Genomics," *Wired.com*, May 3, 2011,http://www.wired.com/wiredscience/2011/05/my-submission-to-the-fda-on-the-regulation-of-personal-genomics/; Dan Vorhaus, "The FDA and DTC Genetic Testing: Setting the Record Straight," *Genomics Law Report*, March 11, 2011,http://www.genomicslawreport.com/index.php/2011/03/11/the-fda-and-dtc-genetic-testing-setting-the-record-straight/; J. K. Wagner, "Understanding FDA Regulation of DTC Genetic Tests within the Context of Administrative Law," *American Journal of Human Genetics* 87 (2010): 451–456; Dan Vorhaus, "The Past, Present, and Future of DTC Genetic Testing Regulation," Genomics Law Report, August 5, 2010,http://www.genomicslawreport.com/index.php/2010/08/05/the-past-present-and-future-of-dtc-genetic-testing-regulation/.

43. 23andMe website, accessed March 17, 2014, http://www.23andme.com.

44. Berry et al., ""Recent Developments in Health Care Law: Culture and Controversy," supra note 39.

45. Pray, "DTC Genetic Testing," supra note 40.

46. American Society of Human Genetics, "ASHG Statement on Direct-to-Consumer Genetic Testing in the United States," *American Journal of Human Genetics* 81 (2007): 635–637; American College of Medical Genetics, "ACMG Statement on Direct-to-Consumer Genetic Testing," April 7, 2008, accessed March 17, 2014, http://www.acmg.net/StaticContent/StaticPages/DTC_Statement.pdf; American Medical Association, "Comments to the Molecular and Clinical Genetics Panel," February 23, 2011, accessed March 17, 2014, http://www.ama-assn.org/ama1/pub/upload/mm/399/consumer-genetic-testing-letter.pdf.

47. Lewis, "Direct-to-Consumer Genetic Testing," supra note 40; Vorhaus, "The Past, Present, and Future," supra note 42; MacArthur, "My Submission to the FDA," supra note 42; Dan Vorhaus, Daniel MacArthur, and Luke Jostins, "DTC Genetic Testing and the FDA: Is There an End in Sight to the Regulatory Uncertainty?" *Genomics Law Report*, June 16, 2011, accessed March 17, 2014, http://www.genomicslawreport.com/index.php/2011/06/16/dtc-genetic-testing-and-the-fda-is-there-an-end-in-sight-to-the-regulatory-uncertainty/.

48. Dan Vorhaus, "Breaking: FDA Moves to Broadly Regulate LDTs," *Genomics Law Report*, June 16, 2010, http://www.genomicslawreport.com/index.php/2010/06/16/breaking-fda-moves-to-broadly-regulate-ldts/.

49. Brigham and Women's Hospital, "New Study Launched Investigating the Impacts of Personal Genomic Testing," press release, March 5, 2012, accessed March 17, 2014, http://www.brighamandwomens.org/about_bwh/publicaffairs/news/pressreleases/PressRelease.aspx?sub=0&PageID=1083.

50. Roberta M. Berry, "The Human Genome Project and the End of Insurance," *University of Florida Journal of Law & Public Policy* 7 (1996): 205–256.

51. Ibid.

52. Ibid.

53. Ibid.

54. U.S. Department of Health and Human Services, "GINA: The Genetic Information Nondiscrimination Act of 2008. Information for Researchers and Health Care Professionals," April 6, 2009, accessed March 17, 2014,http://www.genome.gov/pages/policyethics/geneticdiscrimination/ginainfodoc.pdf;Roberta M. Berry et al., "Recent

Developments in Health Care Law: Partners in Innovation," *HealthCare Ethics Committee Forum* 22, no. 2 (2010): 85–116.

55. Karen Norrgard, "Forensics, DNA Fingerprinting, and CODIS," *Nature Education* 1, no. 1 (2008), accessed March 17, 2014, http://www.nature.com/scitable/topicpage/forensics-dna-fingerprinting-and-codis-736.

56. Ibid.

57. Innocence Project, "Unreliable or Improper Forensic Science," accessed March 17, 2014, http://www.innocenceproject.org/understand/Unreliable-Limited-Science.php.

58. Andrea Roth, "Safety in Numbers? Deciding When DNA Alone Is Enough to Convict," *New York University Law Review* 85 (2010): 1130; Jenny Wise, "Providing the CSI Treatment: Criminal Justice Practitioners and the CSI Effect," *Current Issues In Criminal Justice* 21, no. 3 (2009–10): 383–399; Tania Simoncelli, "Dangerous Excursions: The Case Against Expanding Forensic DNA Databases To Innocent Persons," *Journal of Law, Medicine and Ethics* 34 (2006): 390.

59. Michael Seringhaus, "To Stop Crime, Share Your Genes," *New York Times*, March 14, 2010, accessed March 17, 2014, http://www.nytimes.com/2010/03/15/opinion/15seringhaus.html?_r=1&pagewanted=all; Paul M. Monteleoni, "DNA Databases, Universality, and the Fourth Amendment," *New York University Law Review* 82 (2007): 247.

60. Simoncelli, "Dangerous Excursions," supra note 58.

61. *Maryland v. King*, No. 12-207, Slip Opinion, 569 U.S. ___(2013).

62. Richard Lempert, "Maryland v. King: An Unfortunate Supreme Court Decision on the Collection of DNA Samples," *Brookings UpFront*. June 6, 2013, accessed March 17, 2014, http://www.brookings.edu/blogs/up-front/posts/2013/06/06-maryland-king-supreme-court-dna-samples-lempert.

63. American Congress of Obstetricians and Gynecologists, Committee on Genetics, "Screening for Tay-Sachs Disease," October 2005, accessed March 17, 2014, http://www.acog.org/Resources%20And%20Publications/Committee%20Opinions/Committee%20on%20Genetics/Screening%20for%20Tay%20-%20Sachs%20Disease.aspx.

64. Pascal Borry et al., "Preconceptional Genetic Carrier Testing and the Commercial Offer Directly-to-Consumers," *Human Reproduction* 26, no. 5 (2011): 972–977.

65. Susan Young, "A Brave New World of Prenatal DNA Sequencing," *MIT Technology Review*, January 30, 2013, accessed March 17, 2014, http://www.technologyreview.com/news/510181/a-brave-new-world-of-prenatal-dna-sequencing/; Jane E. Brody, "35 and Pregnant? Assessing Risk Becomes Easier," *New York Times*, December 27, 2005, accessed March 17, 2014, http://www.nytimes.com/2005/12/27/health/27brod.html?pagewanted=all.

66. American Society for Reproductive Medicine, "Repetitive Oocyte Donation," *Fertility and Sterility* 90 (2008): S194–S195; D. Bodri et al., "Complications Related to Ovarian Stimulation and Oocyte Retrieval in 4052 Oocyte Donor Cycles," *Reproductive Biomedicine Online* 17 (2008): 237–243; K. Jayaprakasan et al., "Estimating the Risks of Ovarian Hyperstimulation Syndrome (OHSS): Implications for Egg Donation for Research," *Human Fertility* 10 (2007): 183–187; Institute of Medicine and National Research Council, "Assessing the Medical Risks of Human Oocyte Donation for Stem Cell Research: Workshop Report," Washington, DC, 2007.

67. M. D. Althuis et al., "Uterine Cancer after Use of Clomiphene Citrate to Induce Ovulation," *American Journal of Epidemiology* 161 (2005): 607–615; Institute of Medicine and National Research Council, "Assessing the Medical Risks of Human Oocyte Donation," ibid.;J. Schneider, "Fatal Colon Cancer in a Young Egg Donor: A Physician Mother's Call

for Follow-Up and Research on the Long-Term Risks of Ovarian Stimulation," *Fertility and Sterility* 90 (2008): 2016.e1–2016.e5.

68. W. Kramer, J. Schneider, and N. Schultz, "US Oocyte Donors: A Retrospective Study of Medical and Psychosocial Issues," *Human Reproduction* 24 (2009): 3144–3149; D. Stoop et al., "Effect of Ovarian Stimulation and Oocyte Retrieval on Reproductive Outcome in Oocyte Donors," *Fertility and Sterility* 97 (2012): 1328–1330.

69. President's Council on Bioethics, "Reproduction and Responsibility: The Regulation of New Biotechnologies," chap. 2, "Assisted Reproduction," Washington, DC, March 2004, accessed March 17, 2014, http://bioethics.georgetown.edu/pcbe/reports/reproductionandresponsibility/chapter2.html.

70. G. Hewitt, "Missing Links: Identity Issues of Donor-Conceived People," *Journal of Fertility Counseling* 9, no. 3 (2002): 14–20, accessed March 17, 2014, https://www.infertilitynetwork.org/files/MissingLinks.pdf; Françoise Baylis, "The Forgotten Rights of Donor Offspring," *The Mark*, October 6, 2010, http://pioneers.themarknews.com/articles/2652-the-forgotten-rights-of-donor-offspring/#.UzZdFlzfazA.

71. Ian Craft et al., "Will Removal of Anonymity Influence the Recruitment of Egg Donors? A Survey of Past Donors and Recipients," *Reproductive BioMedicine Online* 10, no. 3 (2005): 325–329, March 17, 2014, http://download.journals.elsevierhealth.com/pdfs/journals/1472-6483/PIIS1472648310617919.pdf.

72. Francis Bacon, *Novum Organum*, trans. and ed. Peter Urbach and John Gibson (Chicago and La Salle, IL: Open Court, 1994), aph. 124, p. 126.

73. Bacon, *Novum Organum*, ibid., 131; Markku Peltonen, ed., *The Cambridge Companion to Bacon* (Cambridge, UK: Cambridge University Press, 1996), 176–177.

74. Roberta M. Berry, *The Ethics of Genetic Engineering* (New York: Routledge, 2007).

20

Preimplantation Genetic Diagnosis and the Prevention of Suffering

Mary Anderlik Majumder

> My story of living with OI [osteogenesis imperfecta], raising a beloved child with OI, and making reproductive decisions in light of OI really encompasses several stories. In one story, OI is a basic brokenness in need of fixing. In another, OI is just one of many human limitations in need of acceptance.... In reality, I believe each of these stories at different times, and sometimes several at once.
>
> Ellen Painter Dollar, *No Easy Choice*[1]

Preimplantation genetic diagnosis (PGD), like euthanasia, is cited by some as problematic because it prevents suffering by eliminating the potential sufferer. PGD also raises complex questions about family relationships and parental obligations in light of the possibility of suffering. I will begin with a brief explanation of PGD and will then explore three matters: the kinds of suffering that PGD may either prevent or create, the use of the rhetoric of suffering in discussions of PGD, and the policy questions raised by PGD that implicate views about suffering. Finally, I will offer some thoughts about the resolution of several policy questions in light of my own evaluation of these matters.

About Preimplantation Genetic Diagnosis

Preimplantation genetic testing, the process of removing one or more nuclei from an oocyte or embryo to test for mutations in gene sequence or aneuploidy (missing or extra chromosomes), may be used for either diagnostic or screening purposes. The term *preimplantation genetic diagnosis* is often used to refer to all genetic testing before implantation, but it is useful to review its precise definition. It refers to a scenario in which "one or both genetic parents carry a gene mutation or a balanced chromosomal rearrangement and testing is performed to determine whether that specific mutation or an unbalanced chromosomal complement has been transmitted to the oocyte or embryo."[2] With *preimplantation genetic screening*, in contrast, the genetic parents are known or presumed to be normal in genetic terms, and there is no specific target of the testing. In practice, however, the boundaries between PGD and genetic screening have been blurred by the advent of microarrays and whole genome sequencing because the platform used for diagnostic testing may allow for screening for other abnormalities.

What might be labeled *classic* PGD has a relatively straightforward moral justification: it permits couples to pursue the option of having genetically related children who are unaffected by a serious genetic condition. Without it, couples would have to rely solely on prenatal testing with the attendant possibility of pregnancy termination as the means to achieve this end.

Yet, even in the simplest cases of PGD, there are complexities. The process is arduous—it necessarily involves in vitro fertilization (IVF). It is also expensive, especially if the IVF and testing are not covered by insurance. Further, the odds of achieving an unaffected pregnancy may be small because success is dependent on the number and quality of the oocytes and embryos produced. Moreover, detection by means of PGD is imperfect, so prenatal testing is still recommended. There are also continuing concerns about risks, although no clear evidence of harm to children conceived using PGD has emerged to date. Finally, the process may conflict with various ethical viewpoints about suffering or disability or the status of preimplantation embryos. It may arouse concerns about human interference with nature or God's plan, or appear to have some kinship with past eugenic abuses. PGD is condemned by the Roman Catholic Church, and until very recently, it was illegal in Germany.

The advent of PGD has also given rise to a range of more particular controversies. Both public and academic spheres have debated its use in order to select for disability (e.g., deafness). More subtle dilemmas relate to the transfer of embryos with genetic abnormalities identified through testing, for example, when couples learn that none or few of the surviving embryos are normal and conclude that their desire for a child is stronger than their desire to avoid the birth of an affected child. The use of PGD for HLA matching—the creation of so-called savior siblings—has also generated concern. Other controversial practices include the use of PGD to detect disease susceptibilities, adult-onset conditions, and non-health-related traits. Recently, some have advocated for a legal duty on the part of prospective parents to use PGD to prevent the birth of a child with a serious genetic condition. Although much of the discussion that follows will be relevant to multiple issues, I will give specific attention to the first and last of these areas of controversy.

Finally, it is worth noting that there is a degree of commonality between PGD and prenatal testing. As with PGD, prenatal testing may be described as a means to avoid suffering by preventing individuals who might experience or cause suffering from coming into existence. Many observers anticipate a dramatic expansion in prenatal testing as more conditions become detectable and as more women choose such testing, especially if noninvasive testing early in pregnancy becomes widespread. Hopefully, reflection on PGD will have value in relation to this larger world of reproductive testing.

About Suffering

In *The Nature of Suffering and the Goals of Medicine*, Eric Cassell defines suffering as "a state of severe distress" associated with developments that "threaten the intactness" of a person.[3] Cassell draws attention to subjective and contextual aspects of suffering. For example, he points out that lives are lived and interpreted within a cultural and social matrix, including norms regulating whether the ill are embraced or isolated. Facial abnormalities and anomalies of the genitourinary system may cause great suffering because of such norms, even if they have little or no effect on physical or cognitive functioning.

Cassell also links suffering and narrative. While his focus is on personal narratives, this move, in conjunction with his recognition of cultural and social influences, suggests an important role for metanarratives addressing the place of suffering in human existence. Ronald Green points out that religious traditions are an important source of such metanarratives, having evolved distinctive ways of explaining and evaluating suffering.[4] Finally, Cassell offers a nuanced treatment of the notion of "meaningful suffering." Suffering *may* offer an opportunity for growth. However, such growth is neither uniform in its degree nor universal. Persons have also been destroyed by suffering.[5]

Cassell's work provides a valuable foundation for understanding the nature of suffering as, in part, a subjective and socially bound phenomenon. However, it has limits for an exploration of suffering in relation to PGD. When claims about young children or other individuals with certain genetic conditions are involved, it may matter how broadly suffering is understood. Is it enduring some experience generally regarded as negative? Or is it, as Cassell suggests, a more specific phenomenon requiring consciousness plus some cognitive ability to perceive what one is enduring in a particular way, for example, as a threat to intactness? In the absence of conscious awareness and any prospect for its emergence, it does seem confusing to describe what the person or entity experiences as suffering rather than injury or harm. Given some conscious awareness, though, perceptions of pain or discomfort, coupled with a lack of comprehension of any connection between what one is enduring and the satisfaction of one's needs, would bear a close family resemblance to Cassell's conception of suffering. Moreover, describing this experience as suffering is consistent with common use.

Undoubtedly, many individuals with a variety of genetic conditions will experience some associated suffering. Studies of suffering per se in connection with such conditions are uncommon, but there is a growing literature assessing quality of life. Although the concepts are obviously different, quality of life, like suffering, has subjective components, takes account of social relationships, and incorporates value judgments that are social, medical, and personal.[6] If there is a surprise in this literature, it may be the resilience on display across a range of challenges. In general, as children grow, physical and biomedical factors diminish in importance in shaping self-perceived well-being relative to psychosocial factors. It should be no surprise that material conditions matter; the prospects of children with impairments are strongly influenced by socioeconomic factors. But there is also evidence that that parents' ability to find meaning in their experience has the potential to improve their children's outcomes.[7]

When the focus shifts to parents or to persons contemplating parenthood, suffering certainly has an existential aspect. An affected child may threaten parents' life plans, expectations, and hopes. Parents may also suffer or anticipate suffering in a variety of concrete ways: trips to doctors and hospitals, battles with insurers, sleep deprivation, job losses, marital conflict, neglect of other children, or issues related to institutionalization. And most parents will suffer on behalf of the child, sympathetically experiencing what the child is enduring or might endure. Andrew Solomon notes that a widely cited article from the 1960s contained a disheartening conclusion that most parents who have a mentally disabled child "suffer chronic sorrow throughout their lives regardless of whether the child is kept at home or 'put away.'"[8]

Recent work presents a more complex and more positive portrait of life with children with physical and mental impairments. In one study, 94 percent of parents of children with mental impairments said they were getting along as well as most other families.[9] Solomon notes that other studies have indicated benefits in the following areas: greater intimacy, better priorities, increased empathy or compassion for others, and personal growth. Findings from studies of special needs children and divorce are contradictory. Drawing on the literature and his own interviews with three hundred families with children who fall into ten categories of difference (not all involving impairments), Solomon offers this summary:

> Constant high levels of stress may age parents of profoundly disabled children, making them crankier and more vulnerable, yet some cultivate a deep and abiding resilience. It turns out they have grown more skilled at handling other life stresses. Even as the downside wears you thin, the upside keeps on giving.[10]

Having a child who is different can also be the path into an identity and a social network that provides support, opportunities to form abiding friendships, and experiences of elevation and joy. An aware child may experience similar benefits.[11]

While the experiences of affected children and parents will be central to any consideration of suffering in the context of PGD, commentators have also noted the potential for collateral damage. The use of PGD may *cause* already existing affected siblings to suffer if they become aware of and perceive the choice as a rejection of them. People with disabilities generally may be vulnerable to a similar kind of damage, depending on their interpretation of what endorsements of prevention-of-existence express, over and above common and relatively uncontroversial endorsements of prevention-of-impairment. Societal investment in PGD and prenatal testing may also come at the expense of efforts to cure conditions or provide non-cure-directed care and social services for affected individuals and families.[12] Indeed, the availability of the technology may lead to more negative judgments about social support for parents who "chose" to have an affected child.[13] Finally, there is speculation about the consequences of the elimination of genetic conditions for the character of children or parents or societies. For example, what will become of unconditional love and acceptance?[14]

As broad generalizations about suffering become increasingly questionable, we may be motivated to redouble our efforts to draw distinctions. So, for example, we might try to distinguish "normal" suffering that should be accepted as a part of life from "excessive" suffering that should be prevented. Scholarly debates about PGD center in part on whether ethics and policy should be structured in terms of something similar to this distinction. Some articulate a standard that creates a single line of demarcation for suffering—hence the label *zero-line* for this position—such as whether or not a child will have a "life worth living." The assumption is that most people with an average amount of disappointment and disability lead lives that will satisfy the standard. The leading alternative is the maximizing or "perfectionist" position. Here, the standard may be something like create or select the "most advantaged" child, all other things being equal. Even the kinds and levels of suffering that most people experience will be viewed as proper targets for elimination through technology.[15]

Another possible distinction is between "serious" and "trivial" suffering. Should suffering count, or count as much, if it is generated as a result of an individual's or couple's own morally suspect value system (e.g., the prospective parent who will be terribly disappointed if her child doesn't get into Harvard or excel in sports)? Even if the parent's suffering is trivial, or in some sense morally condemnable, what about the suffering of the child who is poorly equipped to satisfy such a parent's aspirations? There are related questions about how to address the suffering created by social values and pressures to conform or suffer ostracism or bullying. While many respond that the proper remedy is to reorder societal values, some, such as Laura Purdy, believe it is legitimate to give weight to such suffering, even as we work for change.[16] Similar issues arise in relation to the suffering experienced by children and adults with special needs and their families when societies fail to provide services such as respite care.

Yet another approach, especially relevant to PGD, is to distinguish among genetic conditions according to severity. Tay-Sachs disease and Lesch-Nyhan syndrome are often mentioned as anchoring the severe end of the spectrum, but there is disagreement concerning the appropriate classification of many other conditions. A survey of North American and European geneticists found that 46 percent of conditions listed as "serious" by some respondents were listed as "not serious" by others.[17] Beyond the complexities introduced by ranges of underlying mutations and incomplete penetrance and variable expressivity, which complicate predictions about how a condition will manifest in a particular individual, efforts to create hierarchies of conditions are confounded by the kinds of social and other contextual factors already described.[18]

Consider two questions: Is higher functioning always better? Is extended survival always better? The first query, related to functioning, could be called the "Charlie" concern after the character in the story *Flowers for Algernon.* Charlie is happy in his initial state (mistaking teasing for friendship) but begins to suffer as he develops awareness of his limitations and his ill-treatment by others. Emily Kingsley, author of "Welcome to Holland," says of her son Jason, a leading example of achievement by a child with Down syndrome: "His intelligence has enriched our relationship so much and I would never want to give that up, but I'll admit that lower-functioning Down kids are happier, less obsessed with how unfair it is."[19] The second question is prompted by attention to the duration of suffering and by parents' reports of worries about their child's welfare after their own death as a major source of suffering. For parents, a child's early death may be devastating, but there is also the possibility of accepting the short life of a child with a lethal disorder as a precious gift to be embraced joyfully, as in the viral video "99 Balloons."[20]

Jeffrey Botkin hopes to escape from contestable value judgments by drawing lines based on the prevalence of a condition, rather than its severity, and the characteristics of the test for a condition, such as cost and predictive value. To the extent we are required to make value judgments about severity, our focus should be on the potential impact on the family, the parents, and existing or possible siblings, versus the child or society. The use of *impact* versus *burden* signals that some conditions are especially likely to move the family away from the typical family pattern, without implying that being part of such an atypical family is a negative experience overall. Botkin concludes that there should be no obligation to offer or provide testing for conditions that have only a mild potential impact on most families, or that only manifest phenotypically later in life when family impact is more attenuated.[21]

Suffering in Discussions of Preimplantation Genetic Diagnosis

PUBLIC PERSPECTIVES

The sociologist John Evans set out to study the relationship between attitudes about new reproductive technologies such as PGD and attitudes about suffering in the United States through qualitative interviews with 182 individuals. He included Roman Catholics, conservative Protestants, mainline and liberal Protestants, Jews, and "seculars." Evans found that, in general, almost everyone wanted to eliminate genetic disease—with caveats for the conservatives about harm to embryos—and to do so in order to avoid suffering. About 12 percent were flabbergasted that anyone would ask about *reasons* for stopping people from getting genetic diseases. They made statements along the lines of "if the technology exists, of course we should use it."

About half struggled with further questions about use of reproductive technologies and suffering. The majority of this group eventually settled on the idea of a threshold dividing suffering that might have some benefit from "too much" suffering. Concerns were most pronounced among religious conservatives and were concentrated in three areas: (1) opposition to ending suffering by ending or preventing the life of the sufferer; (2) the view that eliminating an entire group of people whom we have defined by their suffering appears antithetical to a commitment to acceptance of all people; and (3) the possibility of meaning or purpose in suffering, in the form of pedagogical value for the sufferer or the rest of society, the possibility of personal growth, or fostering empathy and caring.[22]

POTENTIAL AND ACTUAL PREIMPLANTATION GENETIC DIAGNOSIS USER PERSPECTIVES

A survey of patients with Marfan syndrome and their family members in France revealed a divergence between beliefs about the acceptability of testing to select against disability (70 percent) and personal willingness to use it (20 percent). Comments were about equally divided between those favoring and those concerned about testing. The favorable comments typically made some reference to suffering, for example: "Science has allowed us to get rid of suffering as a fact of life, and we should all be grateful." "In its suffering, the child could hold it against his parents for not doing something to avoid the syndrome." "As I am not a carrier, I was ready to accept the risk. . ., but I chose to follow the view of my affected husband, who, looking back at the suffering he had been through, didn't want to take this risk for his children." The concerned comments emphasized the preciousness of life "with all its flaws," the value of affected individuals to those in their circle and society, the presumptuousness in taking upon oneself the task of deciding that a life is not worth living, the unacceptability of "getting rid of those with the disease" as a response to the problems linked to a disease, and skepticism about the connection between normality and happiness.[23]

In an interview study, asymptomatic carriers of the Huntington mutation and their partners who had used PGD recounted the suffering associated with PGD, but also the greater suffering associated with prenatal diagnosis and pregnancy termination. Since Huntington's disease is an adult-onset condition, individuals and couples also wondered whether preventive steps were warranted given the prospect of a healthy life into early middle age. But many feared the burden of guilt and regret if they failed to use the available technology: "[W]e have the possibility to prevent the birth of a child at risk. So, we can't say anymore that we didn't know or that we couldn't do anything."[24]

Women participating in an online PGD bulletin board in the United States also expressed a sense of responsibility to avoid harm if possible. They distinguished their efforts to avoid the birth of a child (often a second child) with a serious genetic disorder from more frivolous uses of the technology and the idea of "designer babies."[25]

An ethnographic study in the United Kingdom highlighted the tension between the reproductive (best odds of taking home a baby) and genetic (best odds of avoiding birth of an affected baby) sides of IVF coupled with PGD. That study also revealed some mixed emotions. Knowing that a baby is going to die and in fact losing that baby after only a few months or years was consistently identified as a source of great suffering, and couples described their dread of repeating the experience. But at least one couple also judged their first, affected child's life "beautiful" in retrospect.[26]

Ellen Painter Dollar has written a memoir about her experience with PGD that addresses some of these themes in more depth. Painter Dollar has osteogenesis imperfecta (OI), a brittle bone disease. It is an incurable, lifelong condition, but fractures often lessen after puberty. Most cases have an autosomal dominant pattern of inheritance, meaning that, absent intervention, there is a 50 percent chance that a child of a parent with OI will be affected. Painter Dollar's position on the technology is complex and rooted in her Christian faith. She reports wrestling with how to understand suffering in light of that faith and writes:

> I view suffering as a characteristic of life in a fallen world: illness, disability, and disease are, quite simply, the result of life in a world that does not work as God intended. I believe they are bad things and that we are allowed to name them as bad things. This does not mean, however, that we have license to try to fix what is wrong at all costs or that we can't learn valuable lessons, find meaning, and come to know God and ourselves better as a result of suffering.[27]

She is especially struck by a friend's email that rejects the inherent value or goodness of suffering while also rejecting the view that suffering is an "ultimate disaster." She notes: "Again and again I have returned to this idea that avoidance of suffering, even for our children, is not our highest moral duty."[28]

Despite the importance of this idea, Painter Dollar works hard to acknowledge the toll taken by OI on her first child, Leah. It should be no surprise that in many of these descriptions, the suffering of child and parent intertwines, although as Painter Dollar points out, barriers exist to open acknowledgement of parents' mixed experience and emotions:

> There are reasons why parents wish and hope and pray for healthy babies, and those reasons go beyond cultural biases toward achievement and health. Quite simply, it is hard to care for a fragile child, a child for whom the most routine activities—walking in socks on a bare floor, speeding up to keep up with her class in the school hallway—are dangerous. And it is likewise hard to be that child.[29]
>
> We have never regretted our decision to have Leah in spite of the even odds that she would have OI. But we have certainly wished that she didn't have it. That is a difficult sentiment to admit: honest acknowledgement of the grief, envy, rage, and even regret that raising a child with a disability can bring is rare

> among parents. We don't want people to misunderstand. Of course we love our children fiercely, of course it's not all drudgery and pain, of course we have learned more than we could have imagined about acceptance and gratitude for unexpected gifts. But it is still heartbreaking and exhausting to raise a child who is in pain, who can't do what other children do easily, who looks or acts different enough that a trip to the grocery store or a dinner out can quickly become tiresome, even ugly, when strangers ask probing questions or make assumptions.[30]

These descriptions help explain why when they first heard about PGD, Painter Dollar and her husband felt as though they had encountered an opening in a door that seemed "locked tight."

These descriptions also help to explain Painter Dollar's distance from the view that conditions, or at least conditions like OI with their mix of physical and social suffering, are to be embraced as essential for good character or identity. On the first point, she writes:

> Whatever wisdom, gratitude, or kindness I have in me, and that Leah has in herself, have certainly been shaped by our experience with OI. But there are many wise, grateful, kind people who have never broken a bone in their lives, who have moved through life while experiencing plenty of disappointments and setbacks, but no major grief, ailment, or catastrophe.[31]

On the second point, Painter Dollar concludes that the disability-identity connection "*in and of itself* does not provide an adequate argument against seeking out new medical technologies and treatments for genetic disorders.... 'I want to be accepted as I am, but I'll take a cure too.'"[32]

Painter Dollar and her husband wanted more children to protect against random events that could render them childless, to provide companionship for Leah, and also to match the images they shared of an ideal family. However, the opening that PGD provided to the realization of this desire proved, upon investigation, no panacea. Painter Dollar's husband had the option of purchasing an insurance rider that would cover 80 percent of the costs of IVF itself, but this was limited to infertile couples, which technically they were not. Even if they were able to secure insurance coverage, they would still have to pay out-of-pocket for genetic testing plus 20 percent of the IVF costs. Painter Dollar had to consider the physical and psychological toll of the procedure and the possibility that a multiple pregnancy would be particularly dangerous given her condition. She also continued to wrestle with ethical questions. Her discomfort was made more acute by her realization that the clinic environment was ruled (with some reason) by the assumption that prospective parents would do *anything* to conceive a baby.

Despite qualms, Painter Dollar and her husband went forward with IVF and PGD. Only four of sixteen fertilized eggs developed, and only one embryo tested negative for OI. This embryo was transferred. No pregnancy resulted. This experience intensified doubt for Painter Dollar. The financial issues, the realization that she was slipping into a "consumer" mindset, and the feeling that all her agonizing was a matter of indifference to the clinic staff all crystallized in a question:

> I finally asked myself how I would feel if a second PGD cycle failed, after all of this. I realized that if it failed, I would want to try to conceive a baby on our own. I asked myself which scenario would grieve me more: never having another baby... or having two children with OI. The answer was suddenly clear: I wanted another baby no matter what his or her bones were like.... I could handle a second fragile baby, as hard as it would be. I did not want to handle the prospect of never having another baby at all because we feared OI too much.[33]

At this point, she and her husband decided not to pursue a second cycle of IVF and PGD. Painter Dollar subsequently gave birth to two more children, both of whom turned out to be unaffected by OI.

The moral Painter Dollar draws from this experience is not that the original decision to try PGD was mistaken, or that the later decision to proceed without it was unproblematic. Rather, she concludes that all options in this area are problematic:

> It's hard to cope with infertility or the harsh realities of genetic disease. It's hard to go through emotionally, physically, financially, and morally strenuous procedures such as IVF and PGD. It's hard to forego those procedures and the control (or illusion of control) over our procreation that they offer. It's hard to have a baby, and it's hard not to have a baby. It's hard to finally understand that no matter how we become parents... we can never clear the pain of life out of our children's paths.[34]

Since Painter Dollar's narrative is shaped by the Christian metanarrative, it is perhaps unsurprising that, for her, love is the solace in the face of these hard choices and unwelcome truths. On a more practical note, Painter Dollar offers recommendations that she believes would lessen the suffering of those weighing these choices. These include having clinics affirm that patients may have emotional, spiritual, and ethical questions and encourage access to professionals to help address these questions, and increasing awareness of the cultural context for personal choices.

Painter Dollar's own effort to carry out this project of consciousness raising has included writing an article titled "Rolling the Dice of a Genetic Legacy" for the *New York Times* Motherlode blog. The comments illustrate the diversity of experience and opinion. For example, a woman with scoliosis, inherited from her mother, acknowledges her aches and pains but affirms her mother's decision to have her because "otherwise I wouldn't be here." She also raises concerns about eugenics. Another author, while waiting for prenatal test results for autosomal recessive polycystic kidney disease (ARPKD), tried to imagine what "message" her existing, affected son would hear if he were to learn that she chose to terminate the pregnancy based on a positive result for ARPKD. Another cannot comprehend a decision to risk passing along a "serious genetic disorder." Yet another, affected by OI herself, "made sure" her own children did not have the condition but also counsels against judging others' choices.[35]

PHILOSOPHICAL PERSPECTIVES

Laura Purdy addresses these matters from a consequentialist perspective shaped by feminism. She argues that the difficulty we may experience in drawing lines between conditions suggests that more conditions should be considered potential or likely sources of significant suffering and therefore suitable targets for prevention, rather than the absence of distinctions. Regarding the possibility of personal growth through challenges associated with serious illness or disability, she remarks: "Since wise and compassionate folk exist who have not had such difficulties, it would surely be good to reduce the number who do to a minimum; the experiences of those who suffer from health catastrophes after birth will surely suffice."[36]

Purdy asserts that no logical or psychological link exists between our attempts to avoid foreseeable problems and our ability to cope with unexpected problems, or between contemporary prevention-of-suffering–oriented uses of reproductive technologies and past eugenic abuses. She believes the desire to lessen suffering that motivates efforts to secure future people against preventable suffering should strengthen efforts to alleviate the difficulties of existing people. Finally, she maintains that we should be wary of suggestions that there is something wrong with control over reproduction, especially because most of the sacrifice associated with reproduction is borne by women.

The work of other philosophers centers on harm, well-being, or life prospects, rather than suffering. The concepts are related, although suffering is subjective, while the other concepts may be discussed in more objective and abstract terms. Some philosophers treat suffering as a subset of harm, which can encompass, as well, limitations of opportunity and losses that may not even be recognized by the individuals affected. Julian Savulescu is one of the best-known proponents of a maximizing standard for reproductive decision making. The latest version of his "Principle of Procreative Beneficence," articulated in an article coauthored with Guy Kahane, provides: "If couples (or single reproducers) have decided to have a child, and selection is possible, then they have a significant moral reason to select the child, of the possible children they could have, whose life can be expected, in light of the relevant available information, to go best or at least not worse than any of the others."[37]

Savulescu and Kahane do not distinguish between disease and other characteristics that may affect well-being. They provide little specification of which characteristics subject to selection make lives go well or badly—although "chronic pain" is a candidate on the negative side and "joy" on the positive. They maintain that "aiming at the best is compatible with thinking that the concept of the most advantaged life is plural and open-ended."[38] For example, parents might determine that any disadvantages associated with manic depression or deafness are outweighed by its advantages.

John Harris, another prominent proponent of a duty to maximize well-being, asserts that choosing to implant an embryo with a genetic characteristic associated with illness is equivalent to inflicting the injury.[39] Along the same lines, Jeff McMahan argues that if there is no harm or misfortune associated with disability, then there is no basis for objecting to the infliction of prenatal injury that leads to disability. Further, McMahan argues that efforts to prevent disability through PGD are no more susceptible to the charge of devaluing persons with disabilities than efforts to prevent prenatal injury.[40] Both McMahan and Dan Brock question the ethics of the "ennobling others" argument for declining to prevent the birth of children with genetic disorders.[41] Brock offers this standard: "Individuals are morally required (or have a moral reason) not to let any child or other dependent person for whose welfare they are responsible experience serious and inadequately compensated harm or loss of benefit, if they can act so that, without affecting the number of persons who will exist and without imposing substantial burdens or costs or loss of benefits on themselves or others, no child or other dependent person for whose welfare they are responsible will experience serious and inadequately compensated harm or loss of benefit."[42]

Brock's reference to holding the number of persons constant, which may seem peculiar, is traceable to the "nonidentity problem" that plagues philosophers working in this area. Originally explored in the work of Derek Parfit, the problem arises in connection with policies or choices (e.g., choices about the timing of conception) that affect future generations. Parfit set out to show through hypotheticals that, in relation to such policies or choices, morality cannot be about what we owe particular people—cannot be wholly personal or person-affecting—because individuals cannot claim to be harmed or wronged by policies that are the very condition for their existence, as long as they consider their lives overall worth living.

There have been a number of responses to the nonidentity problem. A common one in the reproductive context is that there is a *relationally* rather than *genetically* defined future child who can be wronged by a parental choice not to pursue PGD or take other steps to minimize suffering. Another is the possibility of adopting a "wide person-affecting" view that permits a comparison of the relative suffering or well-being of two or more possible future children. Yet another is an impersonal view that considers the overall level of suffering or well-being in the world. On this view, the duty is to work for a world with less suffering rather than to prevent the suffering of anyone in particular. Some of these responses only make sense (or whatever sense they make) if the possible child with a genetic condition whose birth is prevented is "replaced" by a child with better prospects, hence Brock's concern about number.

Cynthia Cohen takes a different approach to the nonidentity problem within a zero-line framework. She notes that the claim "that you have done no harm to the child because you now have a child who lives a worthwhile life" is "odd because it justifies your act *after the fact*, that is, when you have a living child," but "the point of decision... comes *before the fact* of conception and birth." The possibility of wrong to the child at this point in time should be judged in relation to the alternative of *preconception nonexistence* rather than death: "Since preconception nonexistence is not as bad as death, a life that will be worse than preconception nonexistence will not have to be as bad as a life worse than death."[43] Her argument is predicated on the view that possible children have welfare interests that give rise to duties in advance of conception. The nonidentity problem does not arise because the possible child who was wronged by a decision (or careless conduct) that violates the prospective parents' duty is the same as the child who is conceived and born. Cohen cautions that we should avoid assuming that those who are not "normal" will inevitably experience suffering. She also suggests that any standard should factor in the degree to which prospective parents and society are able and willing to assume responsibility for addressing health problems.

In general, those who take issue with advocates for a duty to maximize well-being, inclusive of a duty to minimize suffering, are likely to emphasize the features of our lives that make line-drawing challenging. This appreciation, pace Purdy, is taken to support restraint rather than a more expansive prevention agenda.[44] For example, Michael Parker writes that "while it may be possible to delineate some conditions conducive to good lives, it is not going to be possible to relate the testable features of embryos in any useful or determinative sense to concepts as rich and complex as that of the 'good life,' thereby enabling the ranking of possible lives as better or worse."[45]

Adrienne Asch and David Wasserman emphasize the virtues of parents and families. A family is distinguished from a club precisely by its lack of selectivity and an ideal of unconditional devotion. Asch and Wasserman believe that the question that guides any line-drawing exercise should be: Does the presence of this impairment "preclude the enjoyment of goods central to parents and families"? In relation to prenatal testing, they assert that this amounts to asking whether an impairment would necessarily render the life of the child overall not worth living. They conclude that "perhaps no more than one or two" genetic conditions meet that standard.[46]

Wasserman undergirds these arguments with a discussion of role morality. In particular, he contrasts the role morality of parents, which is personal and entails acceptance of children with all their challenges, with the role morality of public officials, which is rightly impersonal and focused on maximizing the well-being of a population. Standards that are understood as deriving from an impersonal moral commitment to maximizing well-being would seem to fit better with the role morality of bureaucrats than that of parents. Wasserman is skeptical that human psychology will allow for a clear separation of and smooth transition between a "bureaucratic" morality for reproduction and a parental morality for actual child rearing. Finally, he asserts that prospective parents who choose not to use technologies of selection are not necessarily unconcerned with the welfare of the future child; they may have principled objections to the technology.[47]

McMahan's work in this area is distinguished by his attention to the psychological dynamics of parent–child relationships. He writes that we have evidence that individuals and couples do go through a successful psychological transition linked to a change in values in many cases. When contemplating parenthood, many will hope (or take active steps) to avoid having a child with disabilities. Yet, most will end up being grateful for the child they have, even if that child has disabilities. McMahan argues that this embrace of what they sought to avoid reflects their new parental values, as well as the completion of a process of adaptation, and a rational preference for one's actual life over some better but hypothetical alternative. He concludes: "Of course, programs for preconception screening cater to those who accept the prospective evaluation, not the retrospective evaluation. But rather than respond to this by seeking to discourage or prohibit screening for disabilities, perhaps we could seek to offset any expressive effect that screening programs might have by publicly acknowledging or giving social expression to the retrospective evaluation and to the values that support it."[48]

Approaches to Policy

McMahan mentions the possibility of prohibiting preconception screening, thereby moving the discussion into the realm of public policy. Proposals for flat prohibitions on PGD have not gained traction with policy makers outside of a few jurisdictions with special historical or cultural circumstances, such as Germany.[49] However, prohibitions on using PGD to select *for* disability are no longer unusual in jurisdictions that have comprehensive regulatory structures for PGD or assisted reproduction generally. For example, in the United Kingdom, PGD is regulated by the Human Fertilisation and Embryology Authority (HFEA) pursuant to the Human Fertilisation and Embryology Act. Clinics are only permitted to test for genetic conditions that HFEA has designated as sufficiently serious to warrant testing.[50] In 2008, the Act was amended to prohibit selection for disability. Embryos known to be at significant risk of developing "a serious physical or mental disability," "a serious illness," or "any other serious medical condition," "must not be preferred to those that are not known to have such an abnormality."[51]

The United States has no comparable body of regulation.[52] A survey published in 2008 found that 3 percent of clinics performing PGD reported having provided PGD to select for a disability.[53] That is a modest number, and most reports in the press concern prospective parents seeking gamete donors who will make conception of an affected child more likely rather than seeking out PGD solely for selection of disability.[54] Further, all such reports relate to two conditions, deafness and dwarfism, which are linked to strong social networks and, in the case of deafness, a complex history and culture.[55]

Positions on policy are related, but in complicated ways, to ethical stances. Dena Davis is one of the strongest critics of selection for disability, on the grounds that confining a child to a narrow group of people and a limited choice of careers violates the child's asserted "right to an open future." She aims to offer clinicians backing for their refusals of assistance, framing the issue in terms of the professional norm of respect for autonomy.[56] Savulescu opposes legal prohibitions on what he terms "designer disability," citing the principle of procreative liberty. While he supports dialogue and attempts at persuasion, he argues that individuals must have the ultimate freedom to act on their judgments of what will give their children the best prospects, at least as long as the "life worth living" standard is satisfied.[57] Asch and Wasserman, while asserting that almost every genetic condition is compatible with a worthwhile life for child and parents, nonetheless oppose selection for disability because it is contrary to the ideal of unconditional devotion.[58]

More recently, the policy debate has shifted to whether it is permissible to choose *not* to select *against* disability. This question comes up in a variety of contexts. For example, imagine a couple using IVF because of infertility but also known to be at risk of passing on a "serious" genetic disorder. The couple is offered PGD and refuses this intervention. Janet Malek and Judith Daar have argued that, in these circumstances, parents are violating an ethical duty that should be translated into a legal duty analogous to the legal duty to secure necessary medical care for an existing child.[59]

It is challenging to come up with a story that explains why such a couple, already using IVF, would have an objection to PGD. Perhaps the view that it is wrong to eliminate suffering by eliminating the sufferer, free of other convictions that would make IVF illicit, would suffice. In any event, application to couples that refuse IVF and PGD has the potential to generate more cases to test intuitions. One can construct many refusal narratives in which prospective parents neither display indifference to child welfare nor express religious or cultural beliefs about health and medical treatment at odds with modern science, distinguishing such cases from standard cases of medical neglect. For example, in Painter Dollar' s story, knowledgeable parents decided to forgo a second round of IVF plus PGD and instead engage in natural reproduction, with a 50 percent chance of having a child with OI. Although their course of action is influenced by religious convictions, their specific reasons would be endorsed by a significant number of people. These include a desire for additional biological children, a belief that avoidance of suffering is not the ultimate moral duty, and the high costs of assisted reproduction in financial, ethical, emotional, and physical terms.

Policy is not solely the province of governments. Professional guidelines or norms may also constrain options. Salvulescu and Kahane's Principle of Procreative Beneficence served as touchstone for conveners of two expert panels to address implications of the clinical introduction of comprehensive embryo testing in Europe. Among these sets of experts from the fields of assisted reproduction and genetics, there was almost unanimous agreement against transfer of embryos known to be affected by Down syndrome. However, there was apparent comfort with proceeding with transfer in the absence of (attainable) information about this genetic disorder.[60] The European Society of Human Reproduction and Embryology Task Force on Ethics and Law, in its statement on "The Welfare of the Child in Medically Assisted Reproduction," endorsed the last of three standards considered: (1) maximal welfare (no physician assistance if life conditions of future child will be less than optimal); (2) minimum threshold (physician assistance acceptable unless life conditions will be so poor that nonexistence would have been preferable); and (3) reasonable welfare (physician assistance acceptable if future child will have abilities and opportunities that make a human life valuable).[61]

Finally, the policies of insurers and funders play an important role in determining who has access to PGD. Although some U.S. states mandate coverage of infertility treatment, no state laws currently require insurers to cover genetic testing of embryos.[62] Insurers vary in their policies concerning payment for embryo biopsy and testing.[63] Even in countries that have national health insurance, such as the United Kingdom, approaches to funding PGD may vary by region.[64]

Concluding Thoughts

The ideas and arguments reviewed in this chapter regarding social, ethical, and policy approaches to PGD and the prevention of suffering make clear that individuals, because of their life experiences and their religious, cultural, and other beliefs, differ in their views of PGD and its relationship to suffering. Sometimes, the differences are so deep that another's viewpoint and the narrative in which it is embedded defy comprehension. At the same time, it is clear that many viewpoints and narratives reflect a measure of ambivalence. Typically, those who share the "every choice is hard" viewpoint also express reluctance to judge others' choices. Narratives about the experience of conceiving (or not), giving birth to (or not), and raising (or not) a child with a genetic or other disorder also vary. Not every parent finds the suffering associated with raising a child with a genetic disorder or being that child "compensated" and thus freed of moral disvalue.

The challenge for the field of bioethics and for policy makers is that suffering is a subjective phenomenon and each instance is unique, but often choices must be made. It seems this necessarily involves privileging some narratives over others. If we sometimes find ourselves, as Painter Dollar says, believing "several stories at once," is there a way to carry those plural and overlapping narratives into our evaluations, and ultimately, into policy?

Both as a nod to pluralism and as a reflection of what I currently see as the truth of the matter, I offer a few concluding thoughts. From a regulatory perspective, I believe the scope of permissible practice in the area of PGD should be broad enough to accommodate the range of reasonable viewpoints and the differing capacities of prospective parents. At least in the United States, this approach is consistent with a commitment to reproductive autonomy that has ethical and legal force. This commitment can be supported with a variety of arguments, including the following:

1. We should allow prospective parents to make their own choices concerning reproduction in recognition of their status as ends in themselves (as long as children have lives worth living or better than nonexistence overall).
2. Individuals know best, or at least know better than others, what will be good for them and for their families.

3. They, and not we, will have to live with the consequences.
4. Humility is appropriate given the limits of our knowledge and the absence of agreement.

For all these reasons, we should be cautious about imposing our views on others through the coercive power of the state. This approach is also consistent with the viewpoint of many professionals practicing in the field and so supportive of professional integrity.[65]

With reference to the debate about designer disability, legal prohibitions on the use of PGD to select for embryos at risk of a genetic disorder have not, I think, been adequately justified. As noted, reproductive autonomy is an important value for a variety of reasons. The idea that a child has a right to an open future that would outweigh parental autonomy in a significant number of cases has not been established as the consensus position. Further, given the very small number of relevant cases likely to emerge (because of limits on both demand and supply), the primary function of such laws is expressive. And because demand, if it exists, will probably come from those in the deaf community, the message is likely to be received as a hostile one, in continuity with a still little known and hence all the more shocking history of social oppression of persons with hearing impairments.[66]

As for a legal duty to select against disability, the case for mandatory use of PGD seems too weak to support such a policy for at least four reasons (in addition to the tension with respect for reproductive autonomy). First, it is hard to make the case that any condition is necessarily a source of severe suffering or harm to the child (given aggressive palliative care and adequate social support) or the family (with the same caveats). Second, even if severe suffering should occur in some instances, it may be meaningful in some circumstances. Here, it also important that any such suffering is more likely to fall on the parents, who had some say in the matter, rather than the children, who did not, because many of the most devastating conditions are incompatible with conscious awareness. Third, proponents of such a policy have yet to make a compelling case that preventing suffering by preventing the existence of a child is directly analogous to preventing suffering by treating the medical condition of a child. In other words, they have yet to make the case that refusing to select against a child likely to have a disability, especially in circumstances in which the child will have a life worth living, fits easily under the heading of medical neglect. Fourth and finally, the disagreement about the probable psychological effects of imposing a pro-selection policy on prospective parents has yet to be settled. McMahan's account seems realistic and reassuring, but others have argued that we have reason for concern. This is a matter that is hard to settle empirically in advance of implementation.

The case for mandating insurance coverage or providing public financial support for some uses of PGD strikes me as much stronger. Rather than endorsing selection, such a move removes a source of suffering for individuals and couples who do make an informed, autonomous decision to pursue PGD. Botkin suggests a promising approach to any necessary line drawing in this policy context, focusing attention on the clinical utility of particular tests and using a graded notion of family impact in evaluating condition significance.

The reasons for regulatory minimalism are not reasons for making PGD, and other forms of preconception and prenatal testing, an ethics-free zone. Given concerns about questionable social norms and inadequate social support, these are matters of public as well as private concern. At a minimum, we all have an obligation to support efforts to inform and to correct misinformation.[67] We should also do more to investigate what might be called the "hidden curriculum" of reproductive medicine—the "shoulds" and "should nots" embedded in offers of technology even when or perhaps especially when the surface commitment is to nondirectiveness. This is not to say that professionals involved in reproduction should abandon efforts to craft standards, including standards that may restrict the options of prospective parents. Rather, I wish to support critical reflection on practice, careful and compassionate listening to individuals and couples who make nonstandard requests, and humility. Finally, as Painter Dollar suggests, clinics might be encouraged to more readily recognize and offer resources to address patients' full range of possible concerns regarding PGD.

We also have a collective responsibility to destigmatize ambivalence. We should give parents the freedom to speak about the negative side of their experience in having a child with special needs. Solomon concludes that there is toll on parents from always having to wear a smile, and that this toll is unnecessary: "There is no contradiction between loving someone and feeling burdened by that person; indeed, love tends to magnify the burden.... For those who love, there should be no shame in being exhausted—even in imagining another life."[68] Painter Dollar contributes to this project by openly airing her ambivalence. Our companion responsibility is to recognize that often the smiles *are* authentic—to credit the positive side of parenting a child with a genetic disorder or other characteristic that moves the family out of the mainstream. If that positive side is widely understood, parents need not be fearful that their honesty about their ambivalence will fuel the "tragic" view of their experience or weaken social supports for their children and their choices.[69]

Solomon suggests that the counterpoint to suffering is joy. Just as suffering is deeper and more complex than pain, joy is deeper and complex than pleasure. In a piece entitled "Joy" that is also a meditation on parenthood, the writer Zadie Smith quotes a statement of fellow writer Julian Barnes about mourning: " 'It hurts just as much as it is worth.' " She adds: "It hurts just as much as it is worth. What an arrangement. Why would anyone accept such a crazy deal? Surely if we were sane and reasonable we would every time choose a pleasure over a joy, as animals themselves sensibly do."[70] But the question is rhetorical, and we do often choose the joy over the pleasure. To lessen suffering where and when we can at acceptable cost to ourselves and others does seem to be some kind of moral imperative—reflection leads away from the view that the suffering is valuable in and of itself. And surely our obligations are enhanced when we ourselves make decisions or take actions that bring others into being. Still, if we seek to establish relationships of worth, vulnerable to loss, it also seems we must pay the price in terms of continued vulnerability to suffering, both for ourselves and for others.

Acknowledgments

I thank Cynthia Cohen for her comprehensive review and many helpful suggestions throughout the manuscript. It is rare and wonderful to find a reader who is at once so kind and so exacting. Thanks, too, to my colleague Maggie Curnutte, for some terrific advice and for her gentle insistence that I not ignore the nonidentity problem. Any errors in grammar or judgment are entirely my own.

Notes

1. Ellen Painter Dollar, *No Easy Choice: A Story of Disability, Parenthood, and Faith in an Age of Advanced Reproduction* (Louisville: Westminster, 2012), 158.

2. Practice Committee of the Society for Assisted Reproductive Technologies and Practice Committee of the American Society for Reproductive Medicine, "Preimplantation Genetic Testing: A Practice Committee Opinion," *Fertility and Sterility* 90 (2008): S136–S143.

3. Eric J. Cassell. *The Nature of Suffering and the Goals of Medicine*, 2nd ed. (New York: Oxford University Press, 2004), 32.

4. Ronald M. Green, "Religions' 'Bioethical Sensibility': A Research Agenda," in *Notes from a Narrow Ridge: Religion and Bioethics*, ed. Dena S. Davis and Laurie Zoloth (Hagerstown: University Publishing Group, 1999), 165–181.

5. Cassell, supra note 3, 42–44.

6. Antoine Payot and Keith J. Barrington, "The Quality of Life of Young Children and Infants with Chronic Medical Problems: Review of the Literature," *Current Problems in Pediatric and Adolescent Health Care* 41 (2011): 91–101.

7. Andrew Solomon, *Far From the Tree: Parents, Children, and the Search for Identity* (New York: Scribner, 2012), 43(citingGlenn Affleck and Howard Tennen, "Cognitive Adaptation to Adversity: Insights from Parents of Medically Fragile Infants," in *Infants in Crisis: How Parents Cope with Newborn Intensive Care and Its Aftermath*, ed. Ann P. Turnbull, Joan M. Patterson, an Shirley K. Behr [New York: Springer-Verlag, 1991] 138). In general, the higher than expected quality-of-life ratings reported by people with disabilities (with a particular focus on those who transition from a normal to an impaired state) are often explained as a function of three processes: adaptation, coping, and accommodation. See, e.g.,Dan W. Brock, "Preventing Genetically Transmitted Disabilities while Respecting Persons with Disabilities," in *Quality of Life and Human Difference: Genetic Testing, Health Care, and Disability*, ed. David Wasserman, Jerome Bickenbach, and Robert Wachbroit (New York: Cambridge University Press, 2005), 73–74.

8. Solomon, supra note 7, 23 (quoting Simon Olshansky, "Chronic Sorrow: A Response to Having a Mentally Defective Child," *Social Casework* 43, no. 4 [1962]: 190–193, 190).

9. Douglas A. Abbott and William H. Meredith, "Strengths of Parents with Retarded Children," *Family Relations* 35, no. 3 [1986]: 371–375. For a recent review of the literature

concerning the effects on parental well-being of rearing neonates requiring long-term care (which would include some infants with serious genetic conditions but also premature infants and those with birth-related injuries), see Frank X. Placencia and Laurence B. McCullough, "Biopsychosocial Risks of Parental Care for High-Risk Neonates: Implications for Evidence-Based Parental Counseling," *Journal of Perinatology* 32 (2012): 381–386.

10. Solomon, supra note 7, 42. The evidence concerning the effects on siblings is also mixed. As a result of their experiences, groups studied have judged themselves more compassionate, responsible, tolerant, able to see the good in others, and flexible, but they are also at elevated risk of social ostracism and emotional and psychological problems (although not diagnosable psychiatric problems). Solomon synthesizes this literature on p. 204.

11. "Many of the worlds I visited were animated by such a fierce sense of community that I experienced pangs of jealousy. I would not wish to trivialize the difficulty of these identities, but I knew about that going in. The revelation was all the joy." Ibid., 41.

12. Roughly 25 years ago, Betsy Goodwin, whose daughter has Down syndrome, went to meet with officials at the National Institutes of Health (NIH). She recalls them telling her that with amniocentesis, Down syndrome would soon be a thing of the past. Ibid., 187. Although it is doubtful that today's officials would be so bald in their assessment, it is remarkable that total NIH funding for Down syndrome research is currently only about $20 million annually. See "National Down Syndrome Congress, National Down Syndrome Society, and Global Down Syndrome Foundation Express Disappointment in Federal Funding Decrease for People with Down Syndrome," Global Down Syndrome Foundation, accessed March 17, 2014, http://www.globaldownsyndrome.org/news-community/press-releases-2/2012-press-releases/down-syndrome-organizations-express-disappointment-in-federal-funding-decrease-for-people-with-down-syndrome.

13. Karen L. Lawson, "Perceptions of Deservedness of Social Aid as a Function of Prenatal Diagnostic Testing," *Journal of Applied Social Psychology* 33, no. 1 (2003): 76–90.

14. Interestingly, a recent study suggests that policies affecting reproduction can have significant unintended consequences for character. Specifically, compared with individuals born before implementation of China's One-Child Policy, individuals born after were significantly less trusting, less trustworthy, more risk averse, less competitive, more pessimistic, and less conscientious as measured by performance in standard economic experiments and responses to personality inventories. Lisa Cameron, Nisvan Erkal, Lata Gangadharan, and Xin Meng, "Little Emperors: Behavioral Impacts of China's One-Child Policy," *Science* 339, no. 6122, 953–957.

15. See notes 36–49 and accompanying text.

16. Laura M. Purdy, "Loving Future People," in *Reproduction, Ethics and the Law*, ed. Joan Callahan (Bloomington: Indiana University Press, 1995), 304.

17. Dorothy C. Wertz and Bartha Maria Knoppers, "Serious Genetic Disorders: Can or Should They Be Defined?" *American Journal of Medical Genetics* 108 (2002): 29–35. Schizophrenia is not a classic genetic disorder and does not figure on any respondent's list. However, recent research is finding associated genomic characteristics, and it is notable that schizophrenia is the one condition Solomon finds lacking in *any* upside for parents or affected individuals.

18. Some suffering is relatively context independent. The Groningen protocol contains the term "unbearable suffering." When I asked one of the authors about this at a presentation of the American Society for Bioethics and Humanities, he said they had not developed a more precise definition. However, all the recent cases of active euthanasia had involved

infants affected by the most severe form of epidermolysis bullosa (EB), a disease of the skin characterized by painful blistering. In one study, children with EB (along a spectrum but not including the most severe, and lethal, subtype) identified their most difficult problems as: (1) having an itchy skin, (2) being in pain, (3) having difficulties with participation, (4) lack of understanding of others, and (5) the feeling of being different. The parent list consisted of: (1) the child being different, (2) the child suffering pain, (3) feelings of uncertainty, (4) restrictions on employment and leisure time, (5) difficulties in organization of care, (6) never being off-duty, (7) family problems, (8) ignorance and lack of skills of care providers, and (9) resistance to difficult care. Note that even here there are major social components, and the researchers found variation across respondents not entirely explained by disease severity. See Corrine van Scheppingen et al., "Main Problems Experienced by Children with Epidermolysis Bullosa," *Acta Dermato-Venereologica* 88 (2008): 143–150; Corrine van Scheppingen et al., "The Main Problems of Parents of a Child with Epidermolysis Bullosa," *Qualitative Health Research* 18 (2008): 545–556.

19. Quoted in Solomon, supra note 7, 178. Solomon also notes that "[t]he worst disabilities seem to be associated with the best sibling adjustment" in part because the affected child's differences are obvious and do not require extensive explanation. Ibid., 380.

20. Wertz and Knoppers cite this issue as a possible explanation for the variability in geneticists' responses: "Early death, as in Tay-Sachs, may be regarded as a cause of suffering and parental grief and as a failure of medicine (serious). On the other hand, because the child's life is short and the parents may have time to bear other children without the condition, some might consider it as causing less grief than conditions requiring 10 or 20 years of care (not serious)." Wertz and Knoppers, supra note 17, 34.

21. Jeffrey R. Botkin, "Line-Drawing: Developing Professional Standards for Prenatal Diagnostic Services," in *Prenatal Testing and Disability Rights*, ed. Eric Parens and Adrienne Asch (Washington, DC: Georgetown University Press, 2000), 288–307.

22. John H. Evans, "Religious Beliefs, Perceptions of Human Suffering and Support for Reproductive Genetic Technology," *Journal of Health Politics, Policy and Law* 31, no. 6 (2006): 1047–1074; John H. Evans, *Contested Reproduction: Genetic Technologies, Religion and Public Debate* (Chicago: University of Chicago Press, 2010). Also, some respondents focused on individual suffering due to pain, while others focused on familial and other social suffering due to financial and emotional burdens. The "social burdens" group favored more extensive use of PGD, for example, to avoid deafness and adult-onset conditions. Assessing all the data, Evans concludes that views on suffering have about as much influence on opinions about reproductive technologies as views on embryonic life.

23. Fanny Caron et al., "What Do French Patients and Geneticists Think about Prenatal and Preimplantation Diagnoses in Marfan Syndrome," *Prenatal Diagnosis* 32 (2012): 1318–1323, 1321. Marfan syndrome is an autosomal dominant connective tissue disorder primarily involving the skeletal, ocular, and cardiovascular systems with significant phenotypic variability.

24. Marleen Decruyenaere, et al. "The Complexity of Reproductive Decision-Making in Asymptomatic Carriers of the Huntington Mutation," *European Journal of Human Genetics* 15 (2007): 453–462, 458. The authors note that available reports suggest that in general uptake of both PGD and prenatal testing in HD families is low.

25. Michelle McGowan, "Constructions of Good Motherhood in an Online Forum for Users of Preimplantation Genetic Diagnosis," in *Motherhood Online*, ed. Michelle Moravec (Newcastle upon Tyne, UK: Cambridge Scholars, 2011), 180–199.

26. Sarah Franklin and Celia Roberts, *Born and Made: An Ethnography of Preimplantation Genetic Diagnosis* (Princeton, NJ: Princeton University Press, 2006), 157.

27. Painter Dollar, supra note 1, 25.

28. Ibid., 65. For a lengthier exploration of similar themes, see Gerald P. McKenny, *To Relieve the Human Condition: Bioethics, Technology, and the Body* (Albany, NY: State University of New York Press, 1997).

29. Painter Dollar, supra note 1, 34.

30. Ibid., 33.

31. Ibid., 35.

32. Ibid., 27.

33. Ibid., 108.

34. Ibid., 143–144.

35. Ellen Painter Dollar, "Rolling the Dice of a Genetic Legacy," *New York Times*, July 20, 2012, accessed March 17, 2014, http://parenting.blogs.nytimes.com/2012/07/20/rolling-the-dice-of-a-genetic-legacy.

36. Purdy, supra note 16, 311.

37. Julian Savulescu and Guy Kahane, "The Moral Obligation to Create Children with the Best Chance of the Best Life," *Bioethics* 23, no. 3 (2009): 274–290, 274.

38. Ibid., 279

39. John Harris, "One Principle and Three Fallacies of Disability Studies," *Journal of Medical Ethics* 27 (2001): 383–387, 385

40. Jeff McMahan, "Causing Disabled People to Exist and Causing People to Be Disabled," *Ethics* 116 (2005): 77–99, 98.

41. Ibid., 84, 92–93; Brock, supra note 7, 88.

42. Ibid., 84. An earlier version in *From Chance to Choice* refers to "serious suffering or limited opportunity or serious loss of happiness or good." Allen Buchanan, Dan W. Brock, Norman Daniels, and Daniel Wikler, *From Chance to Choice: Genetics and Justice* (Cambridge, UK: Cambridge University Press, 2000), 249.

43. Cynthia B. Cohen, "The Morality of Knowingly Conceiving Children with Serious Conditions: An Expanded 'Wrongful Life' Standard," in *Contingent Future Persons: On the Ethics of Deciding Who Will Live, Or Not, in the Future*, ed. Nick Fotion and Jan C. Heller (Boston: Kluwer Academic, 1997), 27–40, 31, 35.

44. E.g., "In reality the 'zero line' is often hidden somewhere inside a huge grey area, where only a monster of self-confidence would come up with an easy judgement—or a judgement at all—about someone's life being above or below the line." Jonathan Glover, *Choosing Children: Genes, Disability, and Design* (New York: Oxford University Press, 2008), 58.

45. Michael Parker, "The Best Possible Child," *Journal of Medical Ethics* 33 (2007): 279–283, 281.

46. Adrienne Asch and David Wasserman, "Where Is the Sin in Synecdoche? Prenatal Testing and the Parent-Child Relationship," in *Quality of Life and Human Difference: Genetic Testing, Health Care, and Disability*, supra note 7, pp. 172–216, 204–205.

47. David Wasserman, "The Nonidentity Problem, Disability, and the Role Morality of Prospective Parents," *Ethics* 116 (2005): 132–152.

48. McMahan, supra note 40, 165–166.

49. A bill that passed the German Parliament in 2011 allows for testing when a parent has a high likelihood of passing on a genetic defect or experiencing a miscarriage or stillbirth. All other uses of PGD are still prohibited as contrary to a state policy of embryo protection. According to *Der Spiegel*, the bill passed by a wide margin, suggesting a lack of social polarization on this issue. The viewpoint of Labor Minister Ursula von der Leyen is presented as typical: "I am firmly convinced that we should not choose to close our eyes to how we

can use modern medicine appropriately to support and help these long-suffering families." However, some opponents argued that the stakes were high because the change provided an opening to a future of "designer babies" or human control of matters properly belonging to God (certain members of the conservative Christian Democratic Union Party and religious leaders), or decreasing diversity (members of the Green Party). "Controversial Genetic Tests: German Parliament Allows Some Embryo Screening," accessed March 17, 2014, http://www.spiegel.de/international/germany/controversial-genetic-tests-german-parliament-allows-some-embryo-screening-a-773054.html.

50. The list can be found at: http://www.hfea.gov.uk/cps/hfea/gen/pgd-screening.htm, accessed March 17, 2014. Most of the disorders manifest early, such as Tay-Sachs and OI, but the list has been expanded to include susceptibility to breast cancer.

51. Human Fertilisation and Embryology Act, sect. 14(4). Similarly, guidelines that bind clinics operating in Australia specify that PGD must not be used for "selection in favour of a genetic defect or disability in the person to be born," as well as non-medical gender selection and prevention of "conditions that do not seriously harm the person to be born." National Health and Medical Research Council, *Ethical Guidelines on the Use of Assisted Reproductive Technology in Clinical Practice and Research* (2007), sect. 12.2. However, greater ambivalence is on display here than in the United Kingdom, because these prohibitions are preceded by the proviso "[p]ending further community discussion," and another section notes that "what counts as a serious genetic condition is controversial" and "there are different perceptions of disability." Ibid., sect. 12.1.

52. For a review of the limited forms of regulation that exist in the United States, see President's Council on Bioethics, *Reproduction and Responsibility: The Regulation of New Biotechnologies*, March 2004, 99–103; Susannah Baruch, Gail Javitt, Joan Scott, and Kathy L. Hudson, Genetics and Public Policy Center, *Preimplantation Genetic Diagnosis: A Discussion of Challenges, Concerns, and Preliminary Policy Options Related to the Genetic Testing of Human Embryos*, January 2004, 7–10.

53. Susannah Baruch, David Kaufman, and Kathy L. Hudson, "Genetic Testing of Embryos: Practices and Perspectives of U.S. IVF Clinics," *Fertility and Sterility* 89 (2008): 1053–1058.

54. Darshak M. Sanghavi, "Wanting Babies Like Themselves, Some Parents Choose Genetic Defects," *New York Times*, December 5, 2006.

55. See, e.g., Solomon, supra note 7, 49–167.

56. Dena S. Davis, "Genetic Dilemmas and the Child's Right to an Open Future," *Hastings Center Report* 27, no. 2 (1997): 7–15, 14.

57. Julian Savulescu, "Deaf Lesbians, 'Designer Disability,' and the Future of Medicine," *British Medical Journal* 325 (2002): 771–773.

58. Asch and Wasserman, supra note 46.

59. Janet Malek and Judith Daar, "The Case for a Parental Duty to Use Preimplantation Genetic Diagnosis for Medical Benefit," *American Journal of Bioethics* 12, no. 4 (2012): 3–11.

60. Kristien Hens, Wybo Dondorp, and Guido de Wert, "Embryos without Secrets: An Expert Panel Study on Comprehensive Embryo Testing, and the Responsibility of the Clinician," *European Journal of Medical Genetics* 56, no. 2 (2013): 67–71. At least one couple with achondroplasia who sought PGD solely for the purpose of avoiding the lethal, double dominant form of the condition were repeatedly informed that clinics would not implant embryos affected by the milder form. Solomon, supra note 7, 156. Mitochondrial DNA

disorders have also provided an occasion for consideration of professional norms for transfer of potentially affected embryos because, in this context, the results of PGD can be difficult to interpret, and there may be few or no clearly unaffected embryos. See Annelien Bredenoord et al., "Preimplantation Genetic Diagnosis for Mitochondrial DNA Disorders: Ethical Guidance for Clinical Practice," *European Journal of Human Genetics* 17 (2009): 1550–1559.

61. ESHRE Task Force on Ethics and Law, "The Welfare of the Child in Medically Assisted Reproduction," *Human Reproduction* 22, no. 10 (2007): 2585–2588, 2586.

62. Baruch, Javitt, Scott, and Hudson, supra note 52, 9.

63. Painter Dollar reports that the insurance rider in her case covered only IVF and did not extend to genetic testing. Reports of such limitations are common among participants in chat groups and other online communities. At least one insurer does cover some instances of PGD. Specifically, Cigna covers PGD *as an alternative* to amniocentesis or chorionic villus sampling if a number of additional conditions are met: (1) testing is for a genetic disorder associated with "severe disability" and "limited treatment options," and (2) both partners are known carriers of a single gene autosomal recessive disorder, or one partner is a known carrier of a single gene autosomal dominant or a single X-linked disorder, or one partner has a balanced or unbalanced translocation. Cigna does not cover other uses, e.g., for screening, HLA typing, or detection of adult-onset disorders such as breast cancer. *Cigna Medical Coverage Policy on Preimplantation Genetic Diagnosis*, Policy No. 0108, eff. October 15, 2012.

64. Human Genetics Commission, Paper HGC 09/P18: Survey of Pre-implantation Genetic Diagnosis Funding [no date].

65. In the survey described supra note 17, the majority of respondents certified by either the American Board of Medical Genetics or the American Board of Genetic Counseling opposed using a seriousness standard to limit PGD. Other respondents were more receptive to limits, perhaps because they practiced within publicly financed health care systems. Reflecting on the survey results and arguments from representatives of the disability community, Wertz and Knoppers concluded: "Policy makers cannot realistically expect to develop a universally respected definition of serious genetic disorders. The term—if used—must be qualified to include the judgment of the patient and physician, with the patient making the final, and one hopes, informed, decision." Wertz and Knoppers, supra note 17, 35.

66. Solomon, supra note 7, 49–114.

67. The Prenatally and Postnatally Diagnosed Conditions Awareness Act authorizes funding and coordination of supportive services such as a telephone hotline, information clearinghouse, registry of families willing to adopt affected children, and awareness and education programs for providers. However, with no specific appropriation, these projects may have difficulty competing with other initiatives. Prenatally and Postnatally Diagnosed Conditions Awareness Act, compare S. 1810, July 18, 2007, and Public Law 110–374, 122 Stat. 4051, October 8, 2008.

68. Solomon, supra note 7, 21.

69. " 'I was determined not to be around folks who saw us as tragic,' one exasperated mother wrote. 'Unfortunately, that included my family, most professionals, and just about everyone else I knew.' " Ibid., 25.

70. Zadie Smith, "Joy," *New York Review of Books*, January 10, 2013.

PART SIX

Concluding Thoughts

21

Suffering and Ethics in an Age of Empowerment

Nathan J. Palpant

> There is all the difference in the world between the doctor performing an autopsy and the cadaver that is its victim. Modern man examines man the corpse and learns deadly things. There is a place for autopsies, namely, learning which things are deadly to life; however, an autopsy is a woefully bad way to learn about how to live. A more wholesome desire is to contemplate human *life* and the final causes that make it worth living.
>
> Lawrence Smith[1]

There is a natural desire for humans to avoid suffering. We are most often ushered into suffering by forces beyond our control. Suffering is a constant reminder of our vulnerability. Regardless of its etiology or manifestation, we speak of our concern about it in very particular ways: a fear of this rather than of that. Young couples can suffer, for example, in circumstances in which they have difficulty conceiving a child and face the need for assisted reproductive technologies. In these contexts, there is a particular fear of not being able to have a biological child. It is a fear that affects a couple's individual and relational senses of dignity and vitality. "There are times when adults hunger for children," writes ethicist Thomas Murray. "When we speak of the suffering of people who want to have children but cannot, 'suffering' is neither metaphor nor hyperbole: people who crave children to raise and love but cannot have them suffer because, for many of us, our children are a vital part of our own flourishing."[2] We know why we suffer or why we *might* suffer. We can foresee pain and death while keenly desiring bodily integrity and permanence. As such, threats to personal dignity are often understood as "suffering" and prompt a search for alternative outcomes and contingency plans. To counter vulnerability and suffering, contemporary Western philosophies, sociopolitical systems, and consumerist markets root us in self-determination, driving home the notion that we are entitled—entitled to alleviate or at least insure ourselves against vulnerability and suffering. Indeed, the rhetoric of suffering, which helps us orient ourselves in the human experience, is shaped by history, culture, and social expectations. In his seminal work on a history and theory of suffering, Joseph Amato writes in *Victims and Values:* "as the benefits of modernity permeate greater and greater sectors of society, it is increasingly assumed by larger and larger numbers of people that it is wrong not to be happy. As suffering becomes less and less expected in one's personal life, paradoxically it plays a greater and greater role in shaping the moral rhetoric of the public order."[3]

A misunderstanding of suffering has given rise to an inability to evaluate its moral purpose and significance, and Amato is suggesting that technological innovations providing a means to health and happiness may simultaneously contribute to our growing concern for suffering in our contemporary world. Current efforts in biomedicine have brought about a realization of the age-old maxims in which the goals of science, at a minimum, aim to ameliorate our mortality. As Mark J. Cherry points out in chapter 17 of this volume, "secular bioethics routinely sanctions access to nearly any means to satisfy individual lifestyle and death-style choices so as to avoid emotional, mental, or physical suffering, as at least morally permissible, if not obligatory." This has certainly become the normative expectation of science and medicine in our time. In an age of liberal individualized rights, "personalized medicine" and individual empowerment are the ethos of contemporary therapy.

In this essay, I aim to analyze suffering in light of two core principles that I believe significantly influence our ethics about how we make decisions about human suffering. In the first place, we cannot know how to alleviate suffering unless we know the good we seek in its remediation. Second, the good we seek is integrally tied to the powers we choose to employ. It is the relationship between the goods we prioritize and the powers we use that markedly influences our ethical priorities about how to approach human suffering. When it comes to protecting our ethical principles, I argue that there are many contexts when some moral good overrides our obligations to alleviate suffering, and that protecting those goods is integral to protecting the meaning of the human experience in the face of suffering. Lastly, I address our proclivity to evaluate suffering in light of powers we are capable of, which puts at risk our sensitivity to the meaning of suffering in the human experience. Instead of using power to define the goods we seek, desire, or are capable of achieving, it is the goods we value that ought to define the powers we employ.

In this approach, I am asserting that we have a moral obligation to discern and respect the boundaries to our responsibility to alleviate human suffering. To some, it may, for this reason, appear as though I am taking suffering too lightly in the way I emphasize the principles that I believe determine these boundaries. For one thing, I do not believe there is anything intrinsically good about suffering. I fully concur with Ronald Green's assertion that "suffering is evil." Second and on the flip side of this, I would argue that it is the *misunderstanding of the limits* to our obligation to alleviate suffering that opens us to callousness toward human suffering and undermines our sensitivity to discern those manifestations of suffering that absolutely and morally demand our intervention. Amato goes on to say in

Victims and Values that despite our increased sensitivity to suffering, we simultaneously "do not know what our suffering is; whether we should suffer at all; to which communities of suffering we belong; for what suffering we are responsible; in what sacrifices we are indebted; and what sacrifices should command our politics. With such elemental questions unanswered, we cannot set the moral boundaries of our world—and politics remain profoundly confused."[4] By clarifying these boundaries, we can make progress toward renewing the meaning of suffering as it informs our ethical priorities.

Setting the Stage

By nature of human vulnerability, we encounter suffering when our life experiences, the circumstances that define our social, psychological, and physical space, fail to align with our expectations of what we desire, hope for, or imagine. Schopenhauer gives a related interpretation that "all suffering actually emerges from the discrepancy between what we demand and expect and what happens to us"[5]. Although we do not always suffer *because* of a separation from "the discrepancy between what we demand and expect and what happens to us," I would assert that our suffering depends a great deal on whether our reality impinges on things like personal dignity, health, relationships, or other concepts that frame the meaning we seek in the human experience. I emphasize this definition because I believe it frames the most ethically problematic aspects of our moral decision making about suffering in the human experience.

As Bacon articulated centuries ago, the goals of biomedicine are built on the notion that human suffering requires remediation. This connection of suffering *in* disease has become infused into our language. We might say, "He is a sufferer of Parkinson's disease" or "I suffered from a heart attack." Suffering and disease are psychologically and linguistically coexistent—they are very often rhetorically inextricable. With our natural aversion to suffering and in fulfillment of Bacon's maxim, we advocate on behalf of science and medicine as a direct means of alleviating human suffering. To this end, in the past fifty years, we have seen the development of a wide range of pharmacological and technical applications in medicine including in vitro fertilization and other assisted reproductive technologies, psychotropic drugs, stem cell therapies, gene therapies, various life-sustaining therapies, and the like. With the increasing power of science and medicine, vulnerability for the modern individual is inexorably and progressively redefined.

With accounts accruing, evidence shows that our consumption of medical interventions is ever growing. Genetic knowledge using high-throughput gene sequencing technology is available for screening of DNA from in utero fetuses to adults seeking information about anything from diagnosis of genetic disorders to mapping genealogies. With prices sharply dropping for gene sequencing, scientists say that "a 'thousand-dollar genome' could become an important tool to realize personalized medicine."[6] To speak of changes in clinical neuropsychology, antidepressants are now the most highly prescribed drug according to the U.S. Centers for Disease Control and Prevention,[7] reaching an estimated 10 percent of the U.S. population. Some pharmaceutical companies are marketing "lifestyle drugs" aimed at improving quality of life regardless of any disease etiology. "Cosmetic neurology" is a new phrase in bioethics, a field where drugs are used for performance enhancement, to boost educational outcomes, or enable social recalibration. The list goes on: cosmetic surgery, stem cell therapy, antiaging therapies, gene therapy.

Our hunger for medicating the human experience supports the tacit assumption that human desire contributes to the confusion we feel about our moral priorities.[8] Facing these growing possibilities, there is a practical tension between the notion of a "cultural moral right to a basic minimum of accessible health care"[9] and patients' rights–based expectations of their health management. How does one measure "responsible" and "appropriate" care? With the subjective nature of values, the line between what merits a biomedical intervention as a prima facie moral obligation on the one end to morally impermissible (if not illegal) on the other end is defined by and large by how we conceive of, value, and measure human suffering.

As such, the capacity for us to shape the human experience through biomedicine, particularly as a result of advances developed since World War II, have given rise to outcomes that make us as a society concerned about the liberal stance we are taking toward the alleviation of human suffering. The statistics and rhetoric just described may seem sensationalistic, but let us all take pause now and consider that we are all part of a larger script of actors shaping the outcome of our society and the values that influence our priorities. I think we are all aware of these grave issues to some extent, and we may ask ourselves, "How did we get here"? What choices have driven the development of our positions toward medicine and suffering and our expectations for what medicine ought to do for our suffering?

To say "what medicine *ought* to do" makes the issue a moral matter, requiring an exercise of autonomy, evaluation of implications and responsibilities appropriately weighed, influences and coercions identified, a cost/benefit analysis of values gained or lost, a sensitivity to the moral risks associated with said decision. Like much of the human experience that functions at the level of hunches, inclinations, emotions, and moral ambiguities, I believe we have found ourselves in this place because of, first, our collective insensitivity to the meaning of suffering in the human experience and, second, the combined influences of technological advances, market pressures, and pure human desire converging to inform and shape our moral decisions. This combination is problematic among beings that are both morally responsible and morally ambivalent because our sensitivities to suffering and the power it holds in influencing our decision making far outweigh our sensitivities to the good we need to uphold the integrity of our character. We are inexorably trying to measure the powers we are capable of against the value of the goods we desire to uphold in an effort to position ourselves appropriately in the face of the vulnerabilities of the human experience.

In his seminal book, *Suffering and Moral Responsibility*, Jamie Mayerfeld presents an argument illustrating the point that the alleviation of human suffering is not always the highest moral good.[10] Mayerfeld writes, "there could be situations in which one could relieve suffering by killing someone painlessly. (Imagine that the rest of the person's life would have been miserable and that killing the person wouldn't be attended by any of the usual pain or inconvenience to others or yourself.) Nevertheless, in many of these situations, it would still be wrong to kill the person. This is because, in these situations, the prima facie duty not to kill outweighs or defeats the prima facie duty to relieve suffering." If killing people who are suffering is morally impermissible, then we must assert that this limit to our power affirms the need to understand what defines the rightness or wrongness of this way of dealing with human suffering and what other goods are valued higher than our obligations to alleviate that suffering.

History provides evidence of this repeated emergence of moral concern for advances in science and medicine aimed at alleviating suffering. The invention of surgical anesthesia by ether inhalation was decried by the president of the American Dental Association: "I am against these satanic agencies which prevent men from going through what God intended them to go through."[11] The antivivisectionists of the mid-1800s declared that no amount of human happiness, however merited, warranted suffering by animals. The development of in vitro fertilization techniques has long been criticized by the Catholic Church. Across the millennia, the debate is ongoing: what and who define the hierarchies and equivalencies of suffering?

There Are Limits to Our Obligation to Alleviate Human Suffering

Where does suffering situate in the context of our expectations of the goals of science and medicine? Posthumanist ethics touted by Nick Bostrom and David Pearce, among others, is one way to approach the issue. Posthumanism advocates for the movement to a society in which the enhancement of the human body and mind is achieved by any and all possible means.[12] However, in the face of every instinctual desire to eliminate suffering, in contemporary dialogue, we hear echoes of hesitancy, not to mention voices in outright opposition, running as a parallel discourse and raising the specter that such goals and ideals are merely primal as much as they are untenable.

The inconsistency in our public debate is emblematic of our moral confusion about suffering. There are, in fact, limits, practical and metaphysical, that impose a hierarchy of moral goods in the way we deal with human vulnerability and suffering. Instinctual desires to alleviate suffering clearly come into conflict with practical and metaphysical limits that shape our moral priorities. Jamie Mayerfeld has written, "too zealous a protection against suffering can deprive a person of non-hedonistic goods that would be worth their price in suffering."[13] Acknowledging the existence of limits and asserting that there are morally inadmissible means of contending with human vulnerability are affirmations of a moral hierarchy in which the alleviation of suffering is necessarily situated at a lower position than other moral goods.

In reacting to an advertisement in the *Harvard Crimson,* wherein a couple sought an egg donor five feet ten inches tall, athletic, without major family medical issues, and having combined SAT score of 1400 or higher for the price of $50,000, Michael Sandel wrote, "...something about the ad leaves a lingering moral qualm. Even if no harm is involved, isn't there something troubling about parents ordering up a child with certain genetic traits"?[14] Sandel refers to his moral hesitancy as "troubling." What is the meaning of this hesitancy when it comes to our ways of understanding our obligations toward human suffering?

William May referred to such moral qualms with his now famous phrase, "openness to the unbidden." What is it about the unbidden that we are so fearful of and concerned about? Is not the unbidden namely suffering and receptivity to our intrinsic vulnerability? May's phrase is a reaffirmation that there are real moral limits distinguished by identifiable principles that override our obligation to alleviate human suffering because there *is* meaning in the goods we uphold and the powers we seek in the face of suffering that define the values we prioritize in human life. "For it is in the choosing that enduring societies preserve or destroy those values that suffering and necessity expose. In this way societies are defined, for it is by the values that are foregone no less than by those that are preserved at tremendous cost that we know a society's character."[15]

Assertions of moral boundaries present a case that human suffering must exist and persist for the sake of protecting some more substantial human goods. Here we are faced with a complicated juxtaposition. On the one hand, we are all quite aware that suffering describes the worst experiences of human life, the one aspect of the human experience we are *most* driven to avoid, are deterred by, seek to suppress, are insured against, are angered by, and are strongly compelled to dispel relative to any other aspect of human existence. Any means to this end has been welcome in the history of moral beings: myth, magic, reason, faith, sacrifice, poetry, law, politics, commerce, medicine, suicide.[16] Yet we instinctively behave and make decisions as though the absence or elimination of suffering is not the greatest good. Why is this? If we accept the fact that there are morally inadmissible ways of intervening in human suffering, then we admit to the notion that there are limits to our moral obligation to alleviate human suffering. There is, in other words, some principle or set of principles that override, or have greater moral gravity, than the alleviation of human suffering.

Our Ethics toward Suffering Are Influenced by How We Define "Power for the Sake of Good"

How, then, do we determine the boundaries around which we have a moral obligation to alleviate suffering? To address this question, at least in part, I believe we must attempt to orient ourselves to those fundamental principles that define our relationship to suffering and how we negotiate with it in the human experience. What is it, specifically, that causes us to waver and shift about trying to identify the boundaries around our obligations to alleviate suffering? We don't want to suffer. By what means and to what ends ought we to address this want? What can we use as reference points to help interpret moral actions in the context of suffering? More so, what are the ethical principles most liable to influences and pressures that result in dulling of our moral sensitivity to the meaning of suffering in the human experience?

Although there are likely many ways to address these questions, I will focus on two closely intertwined factors. One is how we as individuals and as a society interpret the notion of good. That is, we can't know how to negotiate with suffering until we know the good we seek in its remediation, and therefore, I think our confusion about suffering is rooted inextricably in confusion about the "good" we value in the human experience. Different views of how we define "good" will markedly affect how we negotiate with suffering very generally and certainly within the context of bioethics, where we seek to understand how biomedicine ought to be used as a power for good as we negotiate with suffering in the human experience.

This brings me to my second factor influencing our negotiations with suffering, that is, how we interpret the notion of power.[17] More than most experiences in life, suffering (or the threat of it) tends to evoke in us the longing for power because suffering is so closely tied to feelings of vulnerability. In chapter 19 of this volume, Roberta Berry writes on genetic information as a source of power in our effort to negotiate with our intrinsic vulnerabilities, our "ultimate disempowerment": ". . .one reason we struggle with the implications of genomic information," writes Berry, "is its ambivalent allure: its promise of empowerment through knowledge and its threat to reveal the source of our ultimate disempowerment." Very often, our relationship to suffering is seen as an active trajectory into suffering or away from it, and power (like knowledge or technical savvy), more than anything else, is interpreted as our greatest means to manipulate our relationship to suffering. In bioethics, when we speak of using the power of medicine for the sake of good, what we mean by "power for good" can take varying forms, and it is our ethics that reveal the power we choose to employ and the good we seek to prioritize.

Although they are inextricably tied to each other's fate, goodness and power are often at odds with each other because they also, by nature, constrain each other. That is, choosing one power will automatically restrict the types of goods we are capable of achieving (and may even compromise other goods we value), and, on the other hand, defining the goods we seek compresses the available subset of powers capable of reaching those ends. Do we use the good we value to define the power best fit to protect that good, or do we use the power we have to acquire the goods we are capable of achieving?

I think that, in reality, to our detriment at times, it is typically the power at hand that defines the good we acquire and not the value of the good itself that retrospectively defines the powers we *ought* to invoke. As a consequence, I think that it is our inclination to seek power *over* suffering for the sake of achieving good instead of framing power in light of protecting the goods we value *in the face of* suffering that has, by and large, influenced the choices guiding contemporary ethics and the stance we now take toward suffering. As a consequence, external influences like market pressures and environmental pressures, as well as internal influences like desire, shape the nuances of our decisions in ways that cause us to evolve our moral decision making in line with the powers these influences provide. By nature of the relationship between desire and technology, these powers typically enable us to affirm goods that are valued hedonistically like longevity, happiness, and control.

In chapter 20, Mary Anderlik Majumder provides a prescient example of this when she cites a study finding that "[a]bout 12% were flabbergasted that anyone would ask about reasons for stopping people from getting genetic diseases. They made statements along the lines of 'if the technology exists, of course we should use it.'" and "'[s]cience has allowed us to get rid of suffering as a fact of life, and we should all be grateful.'" Much like these quotes portray, our ethics are influenced strongly by the powers we have that provide a means to the goods we seek in *overcoming* suffering.[18]

Power is our "present means to obtain some future apparent good" wrote Thomas Hobbes.[19] If power is meant to mean "*over* suffering" then *hedonistic* goods are elevated, and suffering indeed becomes an incontrovertible problem. With this ethical approach, vulnerability and suffering remain the greatest moral evils that we seek to control and against which we exert our greatest reasoned efforts. Unfortunately, when every instantiation of suffering demands the empowerment of our instrumental means, the moral value of suffering is trivialized and tends to give rise to victimization. This ethical approach interprets the notion of "power for good" in light of a commitment to individual rights, self-governance, and personal gain.

In contrast, using an ethical approach that reflects a commitment to citizenship, distributive justice, charity, and personal humility and that balances individual and social priorities, what I call a "principled ethic," the influence of suffering itself shifts away from its instrumental utility as a social or economic commodity. This helps protect the integrity of our sensitivity toward our moral obligations to suffering because, instead, suffering is interpreted as a part of our emotional and social rheostat that informs our relationship to personal and communal goods that merit our protection *in spite of* suffering.

As an example of this principled ethic, in chapter 20, Mary Anderlik Majumder writes of a family that struggled with the risks of passing on genetic diseases to their children but ultimately came to the conclusion that aversion to suffering cannot dictate the actions we take to bring meaning to the human experience.

> It's hard to cope with infertility or the harsh realities of genetic disease. It's hard to go through emotionally, physically, financially, and morally strenuous procedures such as IVF and PGD. It's hard to forego those procedures and the control (or illusion of control) over our procreation that they offer. It's hard to have a baby, and it's hard not to have a baby. It's hard to finally understand that no matter how we become parents... we can never clear the pain of life

> out of our children's paths.... Again and again I have returned to this idea that avoidance of suffering, even for our children, is not our highest moral duty.[20]

Instead of allowing the power of suffering to shape the goods we seek, in a principled ethic, the goods we value as citizens and individuals shape the powers we choose to employ.[21] Fear, in this case, functions to encourage humility and honesty by reminding us of our shared vulnerability, which acts as a substrate for solidarity as the fundamental moral act against suffering. Hobbes' definition of power interpreted in light of nonhedonistic goods confers energy to our ways of knowing the purpose of life over our means of manipulating the circumstances of life.

Notions of Power and Goodness Define Our Interpretation of Autonomy

As I stated at the outset of the previous section, power and goodness are values that by nature constrain and define each other. In this section, I will move to more specific concepts that reflect the conflicting relationship between power and goodness and the implications for bioethics. Specifically, freedom and security also, by nature, constrain each other and have significant implications for our definition of autonomy, a value that is directly put at risk in the context of suffering.[22] Since suffering is a manifestation of human vulnerability, it is often interpreted as a threat to our autonomy, where we define *autonomy* in a constrained fashion to mean the capacity for self-governance. I think it is acceptable, if not perfectly accurate, to state that vulnerabilities put at risk our ability to govern ourselves. However, for the modern individual, it is for this reason that security is simultaneously upheld as a means to protect autonomy because security gives us power over the vulnerabilities that put the capacity to govern our well-being at risk. The logic of this means that if we can secure the capabilities to govern our well-being, then the opportunity to exercise our rights is made available to us. This is an instinctively desirable position in which threats to suffering are controlled by securing our capacity to exercise our desires. Inasmuch as this is the inclination of our modern sensibilities, which we pursue indefatigably, it is fallacious. It is not the specific logic just outlined that is problematic but the definition of autonomy it employs, which misinterprets a proper relationship between the self, autonomy, and suffering.

The consequences of this reasoning end up leading us toward a place of absolute security completely defined by deterministic influences that undermine the very capacity for exercises of autonomy. To be blunt about the matter, with emotionally driven heuristics, we are instinctively functional egoists that use moral arguments to validate outcomes that affirm hedonistic self-interests, and these interests are often tied more to our pursuit of control and security, even at the cost of our freedom. Indeed, when hedonistic outcomes are the consequence of moral decisions, we become blinded to consequentialist deterministic influences, and the cost to our freedom is significant. At times, we may not actually be blinded to this at all, making it clear that we are very willing to forego freedom for the sake of gaining security.

To put this into context, let us quickly take up one example involving in vitro fertilization. Consider the situation in which a couple requires reproductive assistance by purchase of a gamete, and the genome of that gamete was fully known, with all of the variable attributes mapped out from risk factors for disease to hair color and likely IQ. For the sake of argument, let us consider that there was only one donor option to choose from, yet the donor was the perfect fit based on the desires of this couple. In a purely materialistic sense, this is an ideal situation.

In this case in which the couple is faced with such constraints, the hedonistic value of that gamete would actually not be perceived as limiting because the choice at hand affirmed every desire they wanted for a child that conformed to their interpretations of "valuable" characteristics. The singular option affirms fundamental inclinations toward well-being. So we can see that deterministic influences, in conjunction with limited possibilities that constrain freedom and autonomy, are instinctively acceptable if hedonistic outcomes are the consequence of such impositions. To the extent that technology and medicine provide sufficient options to curtail suffering and affirm mimesis (desire), even within *highly* limited possibilities, deterministic influences are in sync with instinctive notions of security, control, and self-governance that drive ethical decision making toward hedonistic ends. It doesn't so much matter whether the limits are seriously constraining as long as those options affirm the desire for well-being.

Examples like this reveal that deterministic influences are self-propagating, where the notion of "freedom" becomes increasingly constrained because the desire to transform the unknown exceeds the opportunity to accept the unknown. Furthermore, emphasizing this one side of autonomy, the desire to govern the self, however, undermines the other critical aspect of autonomy: to make an *uncoerced* choice. What do "freedom" and "autonomy" mean in the context of choices that affirm hedonistic desires, particularly in applications such as medicine that intrinsically affirm and act, at least in part, on behalf of the instrumental value of human life? For the functional egoist for whom hedonistic goods dictate moral decisions, what does it mean to make a choice?[23]

In this case, it is not medical or political paternalism that threatens autonomy as it did in historical eugenic practices, for example. The imposed deterministic and coerced constraint for eugenic purposes of old is, to the average modern individual, an obvious breach of moral integrity. But this sensitivity to the risk of coercive influences is all but stultified, if not fully eliminated, when it comes to the contemporary coordinated actions of market, environment, and desire, where self-governance retains the illusion of freedom. It is the desire for self-governance and the capacity to choose among the instrumental powers at hand for the sake of security that undermine the opposite side of the meaning of autonomy: that is, to have chosen without deference to persuasions, coercions, or the constraints of determinism. The loss of the latter means we are indeed fully self-governing but not autonomous.

In Sandel's critique of liberal eugenics, he argues that nonhedonistic goods such as liberty are only meaningful when our moral stance toward the world negotiates with that which we cannot control, or choose not to control. "Even if it does not harm the child or impair its autonomy," writes Sandel, "eugenic parenting is objectionable because it expresses and entrenches a certain stance toward the world—a stance of mastery and dominion that fails to appreciate the gifted character of human powers and achievements, and misses the part of freedom that consists in a persisting negotiation with the given."[24] This stance of mastery toward the world pervades our desire for genetic information and the free market capitalization of eugenic ideologies in embryo selection to the more general field of assisted reproductive medicine, psychotropic drugs, and the contemporary public ethos of personalized medicine.

Indeed, one might say we are "free" to navigate our way through the interventional storehouse, but this is the deceit of modernity. It is indeed a freedom to govern, but it is governance over a bounded subset of instrumental powers. Scott Veitch affirms the blinding deception bound within this mentality. "Busy with its choices," writes Veitch, "the modern Western individualized self does not, cannot, see conflict as genuinely incommensurable or tragic because there is nothing that will be beyond all measure, nothing that will not be able to be dealt with through the right form of social treatment: the right policy; the right product; the right therapy; the right price. On another view, of course, this is precisely the tragedy *of* the modern subject: that it cannot see this."[25] By restricting our view that the fundamental goal of medicine is the amelioration of vulnerability and suffering, we become, like all consumer-driven cultures, individuals swimming in strong current.

Biomedicine threatens liberty by usurping "our capacity to act freely, for ourselves, by our own efforts" writes Sandel, "and to consider ourselves responsible—worthy of praise or blame—for the things we do and for the way we are."[26] Consumerist inclinations and social treatments cloak determinism in the guise of autonomous decision making. With a failure to appreciate a proper moral orientation of our responsibility to suffering (we ought to prioritize the goods we value to identify the powers we choose to employ), we increasingly *have no choice* but to shape our ethical constitutions in a way that supports the moral obligation to alleviate suffering. A misunderstanding of our responsibility to suffering makes ethics in the public sphere tend toward a negative utilitarianist ethic.[27]

In the absence of said limits, consumerism and the fabrication of need undermine autonomy and liberty by binding us to deterministic ethics. Kant's autonomous moral subject has been reduced to a self defined as a "chooser between prescribed options," whose autonomy is fully manipulable and ersatz. This ethic mirrors aspects of a masochistic viewpoint that venerates one who is neither good (has aspects to his character that are intrinsically, nonhedonistically valuable) nor rational but only instrumentally powerful, who interprets suffering, if not as a problem to be overcome than as merely a matter to endure.

For the modern, writes Cherry, "[s]uffering is only appreciated as surd. Health care, as a result, is assessed primarily in terms of its ability to satisfy personal choice.

Physicians and other health care professionals have been reconceptualized as technicians, whose public role it is to help fulfill the autonomous lifestyle and death-style preferences of their patients" (see chapter 17). Progress and security for the sake of self-governance become the moral currency, and a sophisticated form of tribalism develops in which *instrumental* values shape ethics in the public square. We become kenotic victims sacrificed to the inexorably redefinable god of progress. "But let me tell Thee that now, to-day, people are more persuaded than ever that they have perfect freedom, yet they have brought their freedom to us and laid it humbly at our feet"—so says the Grand Inquisitor in Dostoyevsky's *The Brothers Karamazov*.[28]

So, what is the alternative? When we are faced with vulnerability and suffering, the meaning of autonomy can only be affirmed by a principled morality that respects the balancing work of protecting liberty in the activities of self-governance. I would define liberty in this context very simply as the freedom to choose among the *full* spectrum of goods in the human experience, not simply those that are hedonistically compelling. It ought to be, as I have said, the goods we value that define the powers we choose to employ for the sake of their protection. Since goods always restrict the powers we can employ, protecting liberty may in fact prohibit the use of instrumental powers that the governing self desires for the sake of pursuing well-being. But these constraints to power for the sake of liberty provide meaning to governance because it opens up the possibility to protect the full array of goods we value in the human experience, not simply those that are hedonistically desirable. Just as goodness and suffering give rise to the other's meaning, so is autonomy understood correctly when limits to the powers of self-governance are affirmed and respected by upholding principled morals that protect the good of liberty, the capacity to choose without coercion. Together, the exercise of self-governance, in balance with the requirements for liberty, frames the meaning and completeness of autonomy.

Quoting the contemporary philosopher Isaiah Berlin, Joseph Amato writes that "moral identities, truly diverse and differentiating and rooted in culture, religion, freedom, and aspirations, are formed around the values by which we live and for which we suffer and sacrifice. Morals cannot be empirically pieced away or compromised out of existence. They drive those who wish humans well to the assumption that 'the first public obligation is to avoid the extremes of suffering,' which include the destruction of values and freedom." In our pursuit of autonomy, exercising liberty protects those goods that comprise the meaning and mystery of the human experience and helps compensate for the arrogance we are prone to in self-governance.

Ethics and Suffering in Psychotropic Drug Prescriptions

To understand how this all fits together, let us undertake an analysis of a bioethical dilemma written about by Alan Schwartz in a *New York Times* article entitled, "Attention Disorder or Not, Pills to Help in School."[29] Schwartz describes a situation in which psychotropic drugs are prescribed for the purposes of "social justice," where parents are medicating their children with drugs typically used to treat attention-deficit/hyperactivity disorder (ADHD), but in this case are using them to "boost their academic performance."

For parents and physicians resorting to this strategy, it is clear that there is a discrepancy between the reality of their circumstances and the desire they have for better academic performance from their children, a frustration of desire. The desires to succeed, to be smart, to be socially adept are put at risk because of inept social systems. To deal with this, it is the power at hand (psychotropic modification of behavior) that defines the good we are capable of achieving (enhanced academic performance, increased socialization). Schwartz describes the work of one pediatrician, Dr. Anderson, who prescribes psychotropic drugs for learning enhancement to patients covered by Medicaid to help them compensate for underfunded public programs for education. The Rocaforts have four children under the care of Dr. Anderson, all of whom are on psychotropic drug regimens. The parents overtly admit that these prescriptions are not for ADHD but for academic purposes or, in the words of the father, "cosmetic" purposes: because Alexis was "a little blah." "If they're feeling positive, happy, socializing more," says the father, "and it's helping them, why wouldn't you? Why not?" Mr. Rocafort epitomizes the grip hedonistic influences have on shaping our moral decision making.

In this case, the evolution of market and environmental pressures, together with the pressure of personal desire, converge to identify a power (psychotropic drugs) that enables us to *overcome* suffering. For individuals involved in this case, there is insufficient sensitivity to the meaning of suffering in the human experience to alert them to "values in conflict" because the hedonistic desire for well-being far outweighs any awareness of subterfuge this ethic brings to other nonhedonistic goods put at risk by this approach.

In terms of autonomy, it is an affirmation of our inclinations for self-governance exercised for the sake of security at the cost of liberty, where the instrumental value of life is held above its intrinsic value and the alleviation of suffering becomes the highest moral prerogative. With complete disregard for honestly reporting the children's conditions to the doctor (an egregious breach of ethics designed to control the variables at hand and shape the circumstances to fit their desire), for the Rocaforts, it is the mere existence of suffering (frustration of desire) itself that provides the rationale for action.

"I don't have a whole lot of choice," said Dr. Anderson. "We've decided as a society that it's too expensive to modify the kid's environment So we have to modify the kid." Dr. Anderson sees this as a way of "evening the scales a little bit." Whether we are blinded to it or not, the coercive deterministic influences of the powers we are capable of that constrain freedom and autonomy are perfectly acceptable if hedonistic desires are the consequence of such impositions. Like individuals driven by strong current, deterministic pressures influence self-governance for the sake of mastery and security. Commenting on this case, Dr. Nancy Rappaport, a child psychiatrist in Cambridge, Massachusetts, said, "We are using a chemical straitjacket instead of doing things that are just as important to also do, sometimes more."

What Ought We to Do about Suffering?

Although the moral ambiguity we face regarding our obligation to suffering is likely not to get easier but rather to get more complicated given the trajectory of our social expectations, market pressures, technological advances, and so on, we must identify principles that remain a constant reference point. This reference point should aim to increase our sensitivity to the meaning of suffering in the human experience in order to determine and prioritize what interventions are morally appropriate, if not morally required, versus those that are morally questionable, if not morally impermissible. Principles that define these boundaries are difficult to come by, and I don't presume to be comprehensive as much as simply reflective about what may help in this regard. To this end, all of the principles outlined here revolve around what should be a more influential mantra of bioethics that the alleviation of suffering is not our highest moral obligation.

In the first place, we need to raise our awareness that the moral ambiguity around decisions made from the desire for circumstantial well-being present a great risk to our sensitivities to the role of suffering in the human experience. I believe that salubrity (promoting well-being) is one of the greatest threats to our moral sensitivities; it dulls our capacity to discern our moral priorities. Since we are inclined to measure characteristics of the salubrious life (such as happiness) as the opposite of suffering, interpreting issues of improving our "quality of life" entirely within a hedonistic framework disorients us to our moral obligations toward suffering. I would argue that when we use measures of salubrity to orient the trajectory of our decision making in response to desire, it is *more likely* in these situations that suffering *itself* is used as a justification for medical intervention. Suffering, not pathology, is the material currency. In these cases, the alleviation of suffering in exchange for improving the *instrumental* quality of life becomes the measure of what we value, our preimminent purpose, and the good we seek to prioritize.[30]

At least one way to counter this tendency is to increase our scrupulous analysis of decisions that are made on behalf of hedonistic ends and determine whether the mere existence of suffering defines the principal rationale for action. The greater the role of suffering alone (independent of malady or desire for species-normal functions, as described by Ronald Green in chapter 22) in defining the currency for our actions, the greater the moral burden to justify such interventions. This may sound obtuse, but I believe it comes across in this way only because people take personally matters that undermine individual rights, self-governance, and the pursuit of well-being.

The second principle refers to our relationship to the use of power in the context of suffering. Since hedonistic gains are so persuasive, the framework of goods defined by hedonism restricts the powers we are capable of employing toward those ends because such powers, particularly in reference to medicine, usually act on the instrumental value of the human experience. Medicine and biotechnology and the powers they employ fit by and large into this paradigm, and so limits to our power do not appear as restraining in this area simply because the opportunity to manipulate the circumstances of our life through medicine satisfy what is instinctively desirable for us. That is, medicine enables us to restore, maintain, if not notch up, our position on the hedonistic scale. In this context, medicine affirms our inclination to seek power *over* suffering for the sake of achieving good.

To recalibrate our orientation toward suffering, we must change how power is interpreted and used. Instead of using power to define the goods we seek, desire, or are capable of achieving, it is the goods we value that ought to define the powers we employ. This demands an evaluation and prioritization of the goods needed to make life meaningful and not simply circumstantially pleasant. These goods typically fall within the category of nonhedonistic goods in that they have intrinsic value and not simply market value; they are ontologically meaningful and not merely materialistically meaningful.[31]

Equally, if not more, pressing, it is a different set of powers that enable us to protect the goods we value despite the existence of suffering. In this case, suffering may very well persist simply because the goods we seek restrict the powers available to protect them, and these powers do not have the capacity to alter the circumstantial domain of the human experience like medicine and technology are designed to do. For example, in justifying her opposition to physician-assisted suicide in chapter 10, Margaret Somerville upholds the importance of moral values over the emotional desire to end life's suffering by this means. She writes,

> By arguing against physician-assisted suicide and euthanasia, I am proposing that there are and should be ethical and legal limits to our freedom to alleviate suffering and that these interventions are not legitimate means of doing so. Just as the axiom "freedom in fetters" tells us that we must restrict freedom to some extent, to protect and maintain the conditions that make freedom possible, so we must restrict what we do to relieve suffering to ensure that we protect and maintain the shared values that are necessary if we are not to risk creating a society in which no reasonable person would want to live.

Since suffering is integrally associated with the meaning of these nonhedonistic goods (such as charity or self-sacrifice), our moral caliper must rest first on the nonhedonistic goods we value and secondarily identify the powers required to protect (or even give meaning to) those goods in the face of suffering.

Conclusion

There is a tacit social agreement to treat suffering, vulnerability, and death with a "mutual pretense,"[32] an affectation designed to act as though life and health will persist despite the general knowledge that we exist in a world of suffering. Life is a constant practice in palliation. To complete Lawrence Smith's challenge, "to contemplate human *life* and the final causes that make it worth living" is to contemplate, at least in part, our suffering. The phrase "the problem of suffering," as we often think of it, reveals a serious misunderstanding of suffering. Although the sentiment describes matters that put everything from our desires, our well-being, and our very physical existence at risk, it would not be a "problem" except that alongside our encounters with a suffering world, we all have some conception that there is a good against which, like a map, we can discern the contours and nuances of its topography. Similarly, our greatest and most cherished goods are measured in light of the threat to suffering that we very willingly incur in order to acquire these goods.[33] The argument I have outlined here disposes of the *ultimate* importance of alleviating suffering as the highest moral good and claims, rather, that the protection of nonhedonistic goods holds greater moral gravity against which suffering ought to be measured and understood in the effort to guide decision making in medicine and science.

The premises outlined here build an ethic that supports the principle that the alleviation of suffering is not the greatest moral obligation. The alleviation of suffering is simply *a* goal among many that science and medicine can and must attend. I have set out here to argue for the presence of nonhedonistic principles that override our moral demand to alleviate human suffering, and we must approach bioethics primarily from the vantage point of our obligations to nonhedonistic goods, particularly the obligation to liberty and not simply the protection of self-governance. Suffering ought to inform our capacity to understand the meaning of life over our capacity to manipulate it. As such, we must learn to intentionally and proactively evaluate the consequences of actions as they pertain directly to the meaning of suffering in the human experience. In other words, despite the nature of suffering as unarguably and intrinsically bad, why must we leave suffering alone and let it be manifest in an individual or community?[34] How can we guide decision making now to allow this ethical framework to dictate our evaluation of scientific and medical advances and interventions? Therapeutic applications must jointly weigh our obligations to the healing imperative and the broader spectrum of goods we seek to protect, such as liberty, allowing us to carry forward our decisions in a morally principled manner.

Our interpretation of the relationship between power and goodness markedly shapes the priorities of our ethics. The purpose of this essay is to show that instead of using "power" to define the goods we seek, desire, or are capable of achieving, it is the goods we value that ought to define the powers we employ. This demands an evaluation and prioritization of the goods needed to make life meaningful and not simply circumstantially pleasant. The alleviation of suffering is not the greatest or highest moral good. In fact, there are limits to our obligation to remediate suffering, and the goals of science and medicine do not rest on the importance of attending to suffering *alone*. Suffering is not intrinsically good, but it is inextricable from the human experience. So our challenge is to come to terms with it, not in a reflexive manner, but rather through intentional examination of the nonhedonistic principles of the human experience that take constitutive or conditional precedence over the prima facie duty to alleviate suffering. Ultimately, these principles will provide prudent guidance for scientific and medical innovations or applications that aim to alleviate human suffering.

Acknowledgments

I would like to thank family, friends, and colleagues for valuable discussion and critical analysis of this manuscript during its various stages of development, including Darien, Sam, and Judy Palpant, as well as Stephen Dilley, Jeff Van Duzer, Thomas McCormick, Johnny Cox, Denise Dudzinski, Mary Anderlick Majumder, Barry Hoffmaster, Jeremiah Webster, and Ronald Green.

Notes

1. L C. Smith, "Distributist Perspectives: Introduction," in *Distributist Perspectives*, ed. T. Naylor (Norfolk, VA: IHS Press, 2004).

2. T. H. Murray, *The Worth of a Child* (Berkeley, Los Angeles, and London: University of California Press, 1996).

3. Joseph A. Amato, *Victims and Values: A History and a Theory of Suffering* (New York: Praeger, 1990), 170.

4. Ibid., 170.

5. I gleaned this from a translation from the German by Jens Schleiter in his essay on suffering in Buddhism in this volume. Arthur Schopenhauer, *Die Welt als Wille und Vorstellung, Bd. I* (Zürich: Haffmans, 1999 [1818]).

6. H. Wolinsky, 2007. "The Thousand-Dollar Genome," *EMBO Reports* 8 (2007): 900–903.

7. W. Cheshire, "Psychotropic Drugs and the Brain: A Neurological Perspective on Human Dignity," in *Human Dignity in Bioethics: From Worldviews to the Public Square*, ed. S. Dilley and N. Palpant (New York: Routledge, 2013), 300–323.

8. Mark J. Cherry affirms this in chapter 17 when he writes, "In short, contemporary medicine evokes a technological imperative; that is, a moral assumption that any health care technology that promises to satisfy human desire or to relieve suffering ought to be available for utilization at the patient's request. The very existence of such high-technology medical interventions for many demands its use. For many, any possibility to relieve human mental or physical suffering appears permissible, if not obligatory."

9. P. T. Menzel, "The Cultural Moral Right to a Basic Minimum of Accessible Health Care," *Kennedy Institute of Ethics Journal* 21 (2011): 79–119.

10. J. Mayerfeld, *Suffering and Moral Responsibility* (New York: Oxford University Press, 1999).

11. M. Thernstrom, *The Pain Chronicles: Cures, Myths, Mysteries, Prayers, Diaries, Brain Scans, Healing, and the Science of Suffering* (New York: Farrar, Straus, and Giroux, 2010).

12. Bostrom writes of the potential for "individuals to clip the wings of their own souls." This, he continues, "would be the result if we used emotional enhancers in ways that would cause us to become so 'well-adjusted' and psychologically adaptable that we lost

hold of our ideals, our loves and hates, or of our capacity to respond spontaneously with the full register of human emotions to the exigencies of life." N. Bostrom, "Dignity and Enhancement," in *Human Dignity and Bioethics*, ed. E. D. Pellegrino (Washington, DC: President's Council on Bioethics, 2009). While these images intrigue the moral imagination, they fail in the practical yet more difficult task of defining at what point such use would cross the threshold to a medicated existence null of meaning.

13. Ibid., 194. *Nonhedonistic* in this context simply refers very generally to those goods that do not have to do with notions of happiness or enjoyment. My use of the term also reflects this definition.

14. M. J. Sandel, *The Case Against Perfection* (Cambridge, MA: Harvard University Press, 2007), 3

15. I first encountered this insightful quote in Barry Hoffmaster's essay in this volume (see chapter 2). G. Calabresi and P. Bobbitt, *Tragic Choices* (New York: W. W. Norton, 1978), 17.

16. Margaret Somerville points out in her essay in this volume (see chapter 10) that one of the greatest influences for the legalization of euthanasia is our serious aversion to suffering, not necessarily the cultural desensitization of suffering within our culture. She writes, "I had suggested in my article that, among other causes of the move to legalize euthanasia, the vast exposure to death that we are subjected to in both current-affairs and entertainment programs might have overwhelmed our sensitivity to the awesomeness of death and, likewise, of inflicting it. But one of my students responded, 'If anything, I think many of our reactions come not from an overexposure to death, but from an aversion to suffering, and an unwillingness or hesitancy to prolong pain.'"

17. I use *power* here in the most fundamental definitional sense as the ability to produce an effect or possess control over something or someone.

18. As Mark J. Cherry points out in chapter 17, for the modern individual, the "focal point of the moral life is assumed to reside in autonomous self-determination, where liberty as the celebration of free individualistic choice is accented as integral to the good life for persons. . . . Moreover, because the focal point of the moral life is assumed to be autonomous self-determination, limits on the expression of one's autonomy are appreciated as unjust. Further accent is, therefore, given to health care services that are judged integral to the realization of important lifestyle projects so as to avoid the mental, emotional, or physical suffering resulting from their frustration." Cherry goes on to say that, "Each person is understood as possessing an equal liberty-based entitlement to realize his own understandings of the good life and the good death, unhampered by the choices of others or the constraints of nature."

19. Thomas Hobbes, *Leviathan* (New York: Oxford University Press, 2008).

20. Quoted in Mary Anderlik Majumder's essay in this volume (see chapter 20).

21. Karen Lebacqz provides a good example of this in chapter 13. She writes, "The unearned suffering that becomes redemptive is neither the 'natural' suffering of disease nor the unjust suffering of oppression; rather, it is the suffering voluntarily undertaken by those who struggle against oppression and injustice." Similarly, Margaret Somerville provides a good example, writing that "there is a radical difference between valuing only what we want in relation to our own life or also valuing the lives of generations to follow and deciding what we owe to them, and acting accordingly. Legalizing physician-assisted suicide or euthanasia in order to allow personal preferences concerning death to prevail . . . is an

example of the former. Rejecting physician-assisted suicide or euthanasia, because of the harm we believe it would do to individuals, our shared values, societal institutions, society, and future generations, is an example of the latter." In both these cases, these authors are making an argument on the basis that we ought to choose the powers we employ to first and foremost protect the goods we seek to protect.

22. This argument on the relationship between freedom and security has been shaped at least in part by the extensive works of polish sociologist Zygmunt Bauman and his writings on the "liquid modern culture."

23. On this point, Polish sociologist Zygmunt Bauman has written that, "when our dreams and hopes for a better life are concentrated entirely on our own egos, and are reduced to a tinkering with our bodies or souls, there are no limits to our ambitions and temptations, and so for the ego to grow, all limitations must go.... [T]he utopia of life revolving around the pursuit of constantly elusive fashion, does not give sense to life, whether authentic or fake. It merely helps to banish the question of life's meaning from our minds. Having turned life's journey into a never ending series of egotistical measures, making each episode experienced into an introduction to the next in the series, it does not offer an opportunity to consider its direction, or life's meaning as such." Z. Bauman, *Culture in a Liquid Modern World*, trans. Lydia Bauman (Polity Press, 2011), 26 and 30.

24. Ibid., 83.

25. S. Veitch, *Law and Irresponsibility: On the Legitimation of Human Suffering* (New York: Routledge-Cavendish, 2007).

26. Ibid., 25.

27. In chapter 8, Hinshaw, Jacobson, and Weisel bring up the point that this same type of rhetoric underlies our callousness toward human suffering. They write, "A more typical rationalization [for slavery] was the 1818 statement by the first congressman from the new state of Mississippi, George Poindexter, who said, 'It is not with us a matter of choice whether we will have slaves among us or not: we found them here, and we are obliged to maintain and employ them. It would be a blessing, could we get rid of them; but the wisest and best men among us have not been able to devise a plan for doing it.' Thus, the first rationalization for slavery was that 'we had no choice,' which was not essentially different than the Nazi defense that 'we were only following orders.'"

Similarly, Bobbit and Calabresi write, "The attitude consists of the avoidance of self-conscious choice: the method of choosing is not explicitly chosen and may not even be known by the mass of the people. The actual allocations evolve in the society without any explicit selection. The great advantage of this attitude is that as long as the belief in its society-intrinsic character holds, it seems to avoid the costs of fundamental values in conflict... and these incentives are rarely perceived as having been set up or chosen for such a purpose.... That the resulting allocation may or may not be desired or desirable is less important than the fact that no explicit choice of it was made.... Choice, however costly, is liberating and leads to progress; non-choice allows those already in power to hide the allocations they favor." Guido Calabresi and Philip Bobbitt, *Tragic Choices* (New York: W. W. Norton, 1978), 44–45.

So we can see that the issue of "having no choice" underlies a general misunderstanding of human suffering, where on the one side it can be used to justify terrible abuses of human rights and the perpetuation of suffering, while on the other side it can be used to alleviate suffering inappropriately by affirming the human desire to place the alleviation of suffering at the top of our moral priorities at the cost of protecting more substantial goods of the human experience. Protecting the nature of "choice," therefore, has significant implications for how we negotiate with human suffering, a topic that merits more discussion.28. F. Dostoevsky, *The Brothers Karamazov*, trans. Richard Pevear and Larissa Volokhonsky (New York: Farrar, Straus, and Giroux, 1990), 231.

29. A. Schwartz, "Attention Disorder or Not, Pills to Help in School," *The New York Times*, October 9, 2012.

30. Paul Lauritzen writes about this to a great extent in chapter 18 regarding the role suffering plays in decision making around assisted reproductive technologies. Lauritzen writes, "The further difficulty here is that when the market swallows up the personal and moral significance of individual pain and suffering, it becomes extremely difficult to evaluate and thus prioritize the sort of suffering that has a moral claim on us.... Here, we see one of the most serious threats that emerge from the medicalization of suffering. It obscures the consumerism in much of contemporary medicine."

31. In this section, I aim merely to assert that the goods we seek ought not simply to be defined by their capacity to enable us to *overcome* suffering and make life circumstantially pleasant in a hedonistic sense. The goods we prioritize ought to be protected because of the *meaning* they give to the human experience in spite of suffering. However, a more complete analysis of what these goods mean, how they are defined, what weight they ought to measure in influencing our ethical priorities, how worldviews influence these goods, and how defining these goods is undoubtedly different depending on the values one upholds. Such a discussion is merited yet beyond the scope of this essay. However, many of the essays in this volume, particularly those that address worldview perspectives on suffering, deal directly with this question. I also do not intend to portray hedonistic ends as inherently evil so much as I am seeking to emphasize the importance of nonhedonistic values in our ethical priorities because it is more so the latter than the former that are more often neglected in ethical decision making.

32. M. Bluebond-Langner, *The Private Worlds of Dying Children* (Princeton, NJ: Princeton University Press, 1978).

33. In her essay in chapter 20, Mary Anderlik Majumder provides an excellent reflection on this. She writes, "Just as suffering is deeper and more complex than pain, joy is deeper (or perhaps more exalted) and complex than pleasure. In a piece entitled 'Joy' that is also a meditation on parenthood, the writer Zadie Smith quotes a statement of fellow writer Julian Barnes about mourning: 'It hurts just as much as it is worth.' She adds: 'It hurts just as much as it is worth. What an arrangement. Why would anyone accept such a crazy deal? Surely if we were sane and reasonable we would every time choose a pleasure over a joy, as animals themselves sensibly do.' But the question is rhetorical, and we do often choose the joy over the pleasure. To lessen suffering where and when we can at acceptable cost to ourselves and others does seem to be some kind of moral imperative—reflection does seem to lead away from the view that the suffering is valuable in and of itself. And surely our obligations are enhanced when we ourselves make decisions or take actions that bring others into being. Still, if we seek to establish relationships of worth, vulnerable to loss, it also seems we must also pay the price in terms of continued vulnerability to suffering, both for ourselves and for others."

34. Joseph A. Amato reiterates this in chapter 4, where he writes, "As much as bioethics might wish to establish the most ambitious of programs of a curative and progressive humanism, it also must realistically recognize, lest it cut its tie with all of humanity's past, that humans will always suffer in some way."

22

The Evil of Suffering

Ronald M. Green

I begin with a forceful assertion: suffering is evil. However defined, whether "as the state of severe distress associated with events that threaten the intactness of person" (Cassell)[1] or "a highly unpleasant emotional experience associated with significant pain or distress" (DeGrazia),[2] suffering is something negative that all people strive to avoid. And not just people. As David DeGrazia argues, and as Buddhist teaching has long agreed, many animals, and certainly most vertebrates, can suffer. This has profound implications for biomedical research. Though not ruling out the use of animals in this context, it requires preventing or minimizing the forms of suffering they can experience.[3] Recent efforts to declare chimpanzees an endangered species and to thus significantly limit their use in biomedical research are steps in the right direction.[4]

All the authors in this book agree that suffering, as an aversive state, involves more than pain. There can be pain without suffering, as in normal childbirth, and there can be suffering without pain, as in the loss of a child or spouse. Nevertheless, pain, whether physical or psychological, is usually a central component of suffering, especially when it is allied with or produces emotional distress. As Cassell notes, "... people in pain frequently report suffering from pain when they feel out of control, when the pain is overwhelming, when the source of the pain is unknown, when the meaning of the pain is dire, or when the pain is apparently without end."[5] The lessons for medical care and biomedical research are clear. Although pain is often a necessary accompaniment of both illness and medical interventions, researchers and caregivers must strive to reduce it by palliation, by offering subjects and patients as much control over pain as possible, and by taking the time to carefully explain its onset and course. The neglect of attention to patients' pain and suffering in modern clinical care and medical education is a recurrent theme in this volume.

Our most basic moral obligations require us not to inflict suffering and to prevent or alleviate it when possible. This obligation does not derive from a particular religious or philosophical standpoint or a specific view of life's goods and evils. Here, I must disagree profoundly with Mark J. Cherry when he states in chapter 17 of this volume that "to make unequivocal moral judgments in response to suffering requires a canonical morality, a binding moral standpoint from which to know truly the nature of the right, the good, and the virtuous."[6] Cherry adds that "secular ethics, and thus secular bioethics, possesses no such definitive moral point of view." But the understanding that pain and suffering are evil does not depend on any specific moral view. This understanding is at the foundation of all moral views. Pain and suffering are states that all rational people ordinarily want to avoid. They can be regarded in Rawlsian terms as negative primary goods—as something that rational persons, regardless of their other values or life objectives, wish to minimize in their own lives.[7] Admittedly, from this basic understanding, there can arise different moral positions based on the rankings of these and many other goods and evils, but the wrongness of pain and suffering is universal and is an undeniable component of any moral view. In addition, the near universality and force of this aversion to pain and suffering places the prevention and elimination of both near the forefront of almost every moral perspective and every view of the good life. These insights ground the prestige of medicine as a profession. Sick monarchs, popes, presidents, and street people all willingly humble themselves before doctors and nurses.

Like many evil things, suffering can sometimes be accompanied by good things. Several of the essays in this volume develop the point that suffering can be enriching. Amato asserts, "Through love, pity, pardon, and mercy, suffering leads the self to associations, responsibilities, memories, and communal services and prayers."[8] Engelhardt observes that according to the teachings of the Christian Orthodox tradition, illness and suffering can provoke spiritual growth by breaking our habits of absorption in ourselves and by encouraging us to repent for sins.[9] Hoffmaster argues that suffering instructs us into the contingency of life and reveals "the finitude and fallibility" of our personal wills. And Majumder notes that, despite the many hardships faced by parents of children with severe genetic disorders, the "counterpoint" to this suffering sometimes is joy.

The Prima Facie Duty

There is a paradox here. While it may be true that suffering sometimes produces some of the highest of values and experiences, from moral integrity to joy, this in no way qualifies our basic moral obligation not to inflict suffering and to prevent or alleviate it when possible. Suffering has no intrinsic value, and, as DeGrazia observes, causing suffering remains "pro tanto wrong."[10] Or, as Jamie Mayerfeld puts it, "We have a prima facie duty to relieve suffering, because suffering is bad and ought not to occur."[11] Many considerations ground this duty. One is the sheer severity of suffering, which often destroys people as much or more than it builds them up. Another is the fact that suffering will always be with us. No matter how much we try to use biomedicine and other instrumentalities to achieve what Masahiro Morioka calls a "painless civilization," random events will always lead some persons to experience grievous suffering, and the ordinary vicissitudes of life will dole out a measure of suffering to each individual. There will always be ample opportunity for the development of character and experiences of triumph that suffering sometimes fosters.

Limits to This Duty

Our obligation to minimize suffering does not mean that we may never inflict suffering or refuse to alleviate it. As Mayerfeld observes, the demand to prevent or relieve suffering is only a prima facie obligation and can be overridden in specified circumstances. Mayerfeld himself offers four limits to the relief of suffering: consequentialist limits, deontological constraints, limits on obligatory sacrifice, and special obligations.[12] Consequentialist limits qualify our obligation to prevent or relieve suffering whenever inflicting or tolerating suffering is needed to reduce suffering overall. Deontological constraints refer to moral principles such as the duties not to kill, lie, cheat, or steal, respect for which may suspend our obligation to prevent or relieve suffering. The limits of obligatory sacrifice and special obligations both make room for people's legitimate personal concerns and other obligations and moderate the extent to which we must exert ourselves or sacrifice in the name of reducing suffering.

Understanding the links between these different moral constraints, especially between consequentialism and deontological principles, is the ongoing work of moral philosophy, which cannot be rehearsed here.[13] Nevertheless, without intending to present myself as purely a consequentialist or utilitarian, I can assert my conviction that the duty to prevent and relieve suffering underlies and explains all these limits. That is, the currency of such calculations is suffering itself. Sometimes, the link is direct and consequentialist, as when we actually impose suffering to relieve suffering. Painful cancer treatments are an example. Sometimes, the link is indirect and mediated by complex calculations of what will produce the most enduring and humane social policy—what will reduce suffering overall, if not in the instant case before us. Thus, many who argue against active euthanasia on deontological grounds also believe that policies permitting the direct killing of innocent human beings, even when motivated by the desire to relieve suffering, are likely to open the door to massive abuses of human life and incalculable new forms of suffering. Experience with the Nazi T-4 program, which traced a progression from involuntary euthanasia to genocide, still provides compelling evidence for these concerns. Whether euthanasia is likely to lead to mass killing today, under changed political, medical, and cultural conditions, remains one of the most urgent questions of bioethics. I'll return to this question momentarily. The point is that valid deontological constraints on the duty to prevent and relieve suffering can almost always be traced back to the concern to prevent or minimize suffering overall.

But we must be careful here. Not every deontological prohibition put forth as justifying limits to the prevention or reduction of suffering counts as such because the alleged moral rule or principle may have no compelling link to the reduction of suffering. One example helps make this point clearer. As Lisa Sowle Cahill reveals in chapter 11, Roman Catholic teaching remains opposed to the use of in vitro fertilization (IVF) as a way of relieving the suffering associated with infertility. Part of this opposition resides in the Church's belief that it is morally impermissible to destroy early human embryos, which it regards as fully moral persons. This, of course, raises the much-debated question of whether human embryos are in the class of beings that must be protected against suffering and death.[14] But even when no embryos are destroyed, as in single embryo transfer procedures, the Church contends that such procedures involve a violation of the morally inseparable link between procreation and sexuality.

But this link, originally introduced to ground the prohibition against the use of artificial birth control, makes little sense. So long as IVF is shown to be safe, there is no obvious reason related to human suffering that each conception must result from an act of sexual intercourse. Some Catholics may accept this logic (although studies suggest that Catholic affiliation has little effect on the attitudes of couples using IVF[15]), but such poorly founded positions do not make a compelling case for limiting resort to proven medical interventions. This is certainly true in the religiously pluralistic settings in which most bioethical debates take place, and it may even apply within religious traditions, like Catholicism, which seek to ground their moral norms in human reason generally. In all contexts, it is the currency of suffering that must be invoked to justify refusals to alleviate suffering, and the bases of deontological limits to this duty must be reasonably compelling.

We see these considerations at work in our ongoing debates about end-of-life decision making and euthanasia. As Margaret Somerville in chapter 10 indicates, some of the most forceful arguments for active euthanasia rely on its value in the relief of suffering. Although appeals to autonomy may also be invoked, these do not work in the case of incompetent patients. The fact that many proponents of active euthanasia want to extend its use even to such cases shows that the relief of suffering often plays a determinative role in such arguments.

The goal of relieving suffering in the context of medical care and especially at the end of life cannot be sufficiently emphasized. This consideration underlies the criticisms voiced throughout this volume against medical professionals who in the clinical context ignore the suffering of patients or who retreat into batteries of tests and standard procedures while ignoring the emotional needs of the patient before them. It also underlies the repeated observations of the importance of pain relief and palliation for dying patients, including resort to extreme or "terminal" sedation that may hasten death.

But the relief of suffering must always be approached through a broader analysis that takes into account the implications of policies in terms of that same value: the relief of suffering. Somerville, again, makes this clear when she rejects Canadian Judge Smith's "no difference" argument with respect to euthanasia. There is no difference, the judge asserts, between allowing a suffering terminal patient to die by withholding aggressive treatment and by actively ending that patient's life by administering a lethal drug. (Indeed, in terms of alleviating suffering, administering the drug may even be more efficient.) But there are, in fact, significant differences between these two policies. As Somerville makes clear, a policy of active euthanasia empowers medical practitioners to kill. It opens up a world in which venality, malevolence, or even medical error (e.g., a mislabeled syringe) can inflict anxiety and death on many patients, some of whom may not even be terminal or suffering. In contrast, withholding or withdrawing life-saving treatment risks only the very small subclass of apparently moribund patients who could recover if more aggressive treatment were not withheld. Here, we have a reasonable basis for drawing a line that prohibits medical professionals from ever becoming agents of death. The currency of this calculation, once again, is suffering in all its forms.

This does not mean that we must conclude that all forms of euthanasia are morally unacceptable. I personally believe that physician-assisted suicide (PAS) can pass muster as a morally permissible option in certain circumstances. Part of my calculus here reaches out to the patient suffering from amyotrophic lateral sclerosis who is forced to experience the torture of progressive loss of physical self-control and dignity. Part of it is the minimal role played in PAS by the physician, who only authorizes the patient's or family's access to the needed drugs. (Somerville stresses the physician's and state's involvement in PAS,[16] but one can reasonably construe the state's and physician's role here as merely unblocking obstacles that the state has erected to the patient's access to lethal drugs.) Nevertheless, I acknowledge a line of reasoning that begins with providing such access and then moves on to active physician involvement in cases in which patients are physically unable to end their own life. This could bring us back to crossing a line—the line that prohibits physicians from being agents of death—that I believe should not be crossed.

The point here is not to resolve this issue. Rather, it is to illustrate how our thinking in such instances must be governed not just by the impulse to prevent or relieve suffering but also by requirement that we take that impulse through the complex maze of social policy considerations, always with the ultimate purpose of preventing or relieving suffering. As Hinshaw, Jacobson, and Weisel make clear in chapter 8, it was the tendency of some researchers, as in the Tuskegee syphilis study, to impose unwarranted suffering in the name of relieving suffering that contributed to the rise of our elaborate structure of research regulations. Though frequently onerous from the researcher or institution's point of view, such regulations are meant to limit and control the suffering created by scientists' possibly overzealous pursuit of research results when they believe that the gain from such experiments may significantly reduce overall suffering.

Religion and Suffering

Understanding that preventing and alleviating suffering is the currency of medicine (and bioethics) provides guidance as we think about the role of religion in relation to healing. Here, we meet a problem that has significantly affected the field of bioethics: religious traditions sometimes have not just tolerated suffering but also seemingly lauded it in ways that invalidate medical efforts against suffering.

Part of the problem stems from the fact that the great world religions that continue to inform global culture antedate modern medicine. This often led them to tolerate suffering as an ineradicable fact of life. In some cases, as in the Buddhist tradition, this led to an emphasis, not on medical care, but on mental disciplines aimed at reducing suffering at the highest conceptual levels. Buddhists did not generally found hospitals, but rather sought to develop the monastic institutions where the religious and philosophic teachings that addressed and relieved suffering could be preserved and imparted.

In the case of the biblically derived traditions, medical care and medical institutions, with a few exceptions, were valued, with Christianity and Islam both notable for their development of hospitals, and Judaism for its veneration of the rabbi-physician.[17] But all these traditions also wrestled with the problem of theodicy: How can suffering be understood or justified in a world presumably created and ruled by a loving, all-powerful God? One answer to this question was to see suffering as the just result of human sin (a theodicy also mirrored in the Hindu-Buddhist idea of karma). Another answer, already suggested in the Hebrew prophetic tradition but brought to the center in Christian teaching, is that suffering is a form of fellowship with God, who himself suffers with us and on our behalf. While morally and spiritually salutary in many ways, these answers also had the effect of justifying suffering and making it an intrinsic good that might be actively pursued. In the words of Karen Lebacqz in chapter 13, suffering came to be seen not as something to be shunned but "as a discipline that can purify the soul and ennoble the person."[18] Various forms of ascetical self-abuse arose on this terrain. In some cases, these ideas fostered opposition to medical interventions, as when eighteenth-century Christians opposed vaccinations because they were seen as attempts to evade the penalty due for sin.[19] Thus, by means of profound religious reflection, and in a context in which medical science was still undeveloped, traditions sometimes represented suffering, not as an evil to be fought, but as something that was itself spiritually and morally desirable.

This kind of thinking is not wholly behind us, and it continues to have some resonance in contemporary bioethics. Catholic bioethics provides several examples. One appears in connection with the Church's formal teaching regarding homosexuality. In his October 1, 1986 letter to the bishops of the Catholic Church, "On the Pastoral Care of Homosexual Persons," Cardinal Joseph Ratzinger, leader of the Congregation for the Doctrine of the Faith (and subsequently Pope Benedict XVI), described homosexuality as an "intrinsically disordered" condition that could never be licitly expressed. The letter went on to ask, "What, then, are homosexual persons to do who seek to follow the Lord?" It answers:

> Fundamentally, they are called to enact the will of God in their life by joining whatever sufferings and difficulties they experience in virtue of their condition

> to the sacrifice of the Lord's Cross. That Cross, for the believer, is a fruitful sacrifice since from that death come life and redemption.

A few months later, on February 22, 1987, Cardinal Ratzinger applied a similar line of reasoning to infertility. Ruling out on various grounds resort to the newly available medical interventions to alleviate this problem, the cardinal concluded with this advice to couples facing infertility:

> The community of believers is called to shed light upon and support the suffering of those who are unable to fulfill their legitimate aspiration to motherhood and fatherhood. Spouses who find themselves in this sad situation are called to find in it an opportunity for sharing in a particular way in the Lord's Cross, the source of spiritual fruitfulness.

I will not rehearse here what I believe are the many problems in the cardinal's moral arguments against both homosexuality and IVF. My point is to illustrate how an argument for the moral and spiritual advantages of suffering (in this case, the way in which they offer an opportunity to participate in Christ's suffering) is introduced to undermine attention to biomedical information as well as resort to biomedical advances as a means of relieving suffering. Here, the experience of suffering becomes a valued *alternative* to biomedicine.

Catholicism is not alone in this recourse to the salvific and redemptive nature of suffering as a basis for counsels of nonaction in the face of new biomedical and bioethical possibilities. At some moments, too, Protestant bioethicists have urged a response to these questions that simply retreats into passivity before suffering. Consider the following remark by the progressive Protestant bioethicist Ronald Cole-Turner[20]:

> Increased use of prenatal genetic testing seems to fit within a larger popular tendency to avoid pain at all costs.... Is prenatal genetic testing just another way to shrink from the pain of others, in this case by preventing them from living with us? If that is all that prenatal testing is, then it should be resisted as incompatible with the meaning of Christian life in the community of the cross. The aim of the Christian life is not the avoidance of pain but the faithful following of One who enters into the pain of those who suffer.

As the essays in this volume by Roberta Berry and Mary Anderlik Majumder reveal, there are enormously complex issues raised by developing technologies of prenatal testing. For whom do we relieve suffering when the object of our interventions is not yet born or even conceived? To what extent does the use of genetic selection remove, not suffering, but the sufferer, and when, if ever, is this morally permissible? And what other new and unimagined forms of suffering might we unleash if we seek by genetic means to eliminate human imperfection? We have already witnessed the terrible dangers of abused and ill-informed eugenic thinking. I certainly do not want to argue here that genetic medicine should go forward without intensive bioethical reflection.

But I would say categorically that it is ethically mistaken to short-circuit the complex normative discussion that must accompany every decision in the genetic realm by passively accepting or tolerating the reality of suffering and disability. There may be many good reasons for allowing or not interfering with the birth of children suffering from serious genetic disorders, but the goodness of their suffering is not among them. Suffering is always an evil that should be prevented or reduced whenever possible and whenever efforts to do so do not bring greater evils in their train. Put religiously, the cross, and any similar validation of suffering, must be the last, not the first, resort in thinking about these problems.

An important contribution of several of the essays in this volume dealing with religion and suffering is that they offer new theological interpretations of the tradition that counter the positive valuation of suffering that sometimes marked religion in the premodern age. For example, H. Tristram Engelhardt emphasizes the fact that Orthodox Christianity, while valuing the spiritual learning that may accompany illness, refuses to see suffering itself as good. Afflictions may play an instrumental role in our spiritual self-discipline, says Engelhardt in chapter 12 of this volume, but they "are not in themselves valuable." It follows that although we are to accept with humility whatever God sends us, "the medical treatment of pain and even difficulty in sleeping is endorsed."[21] Apart from moral constraints, such as the prohibition on killing, resort to medical care and medical treatments is limited only by the consideration that it not interfere with the pursuit of salvation. This signals the belief that while suffering is an evil to be prevented or reduced, it does not always trump other goods cherished by individuals, including positive spiritual insights and experiences.

Lisa Sowle Cahill acknowledges in chapter 11 those motifs within traditional Catholic teaching that have stressed the redemptive nature of suffering. Foremost among these is the idea that suffering could serve as a "precondition of forgiveness of sins and reconciliation of humanity and God,..." Although still present in some authoritative Catholic documents and used as a warrant for the refusal of pain relief as a form of spiritual discipline, Cahill shows that this teaching is undergoing revision. In recent documents, she observes, suffering is presented as justified or meaningful when it serves a higher end or cause. In the context of illness, when no such cause is served, "the cross becomes rather a symbol of divine solidarity with human suffering, and in no way an encouragement to take on suffering that is pointless or unnecessary."[22]

Approaching the same issue from a Protestant perspective, and drawing on the writings of William Stringfellow, Karen Lebacqz argues in chapter 13 that to believe that enduring pain brings redemption is "a form of 'justification by works,' wherein bearing pain substitutes for doing good deeds."[23] The implications Lebacqz draws from this idea for the theological estimation of illness and suffering are striking: "The unearned suffering that becomes redemptive is neither the 'natural' suffering of disease nor the unjust suffering of oppression; rather, it is the suffering voluntarily undertaken by those who struggle against oppression and injustice." The cross is thus "a political symbol," pointing to the historical injustices under which Jesus suffered and died. Quoting theologian Sharon Thornton, Lebacqz states, "The political cross illumines the social contours of suffering."[24]

This returns suffering in a medical context to a wholly negative phenomenon that must be fought and reduced by every ethically permissible means. As Lebacqz puts it, "First, because suffering from disease is not redemptive, there is no reason to value such suffering. In general, therefore, we have a mandate to remove or reduce that suffering to the extent possible. . . ." In addition, "When suffering cannot be removed, it is the task of Christians to 'suffer with'—to have compassion, and to attempt to help the sufferers to find meaning in their illness."[25]

Lebacqz also identifies one other way that suffering figures importantly in biomedicine. Invoking the image of Christ as healer, she adds, "Christians who, out of compassion, risk their lives by exposing themselves to contagion in an effort to heal others could be said to be modeling Christ's compassion."[26] Here, it seems, we have a religious and spiritual reading of suffering with powerful implications for biomedicine. Sacred meaning is to be found, not in suffering, but in the frequently risky and sacrificial struggle against illness and disease and the suffering they bring, whether this takes place in the clinical or research setting of a developed society or in the more primitive confines of a third-world refugee camp.

Medicalization

I have argued that the medical prevention and relief of suffering is a moral obligation. This means that it is primarily limited by opposing moral obligations that either directly or through social policy arise from the same duty to prevent or relieve suffering. It is also true that only dedicated medical professionals possess full positive duties to actively reach out and prevent or relieve suffering in specified cases. The limits to self-sacrifice and the validity of conflicting personal obligations mean that lay people are not required to make active efforts to alleviate the distress of others who suffer from illness or disease, although, where appropriate, they can act on supererogatory obligations of this sort. Hospital and nursing home volunteers are good examples.

This raises a further question. Are medical professionals permitted or even required to reach out to prevent or alleviate suffering caused by nonmedical factors? This, in part, is the question of medicalization, defined as "the extension of the conceptual and normative domain of medicine to problems, states, or processes not previously within the medical sphere, leading to medical management and treatment of them."[27] As Paul Lauritzen shows in chapter 18, some contend that it is morally wrong for medical professionals, especially doctors, to treat nondisease conditions or those primarily caused by social or psychological factors. In this class falls nonreparative cosmetic surgery, some conditions whose meaning is contested such as body dysmorphic disorder, and, at least according to Lauritzen, some therapies that address infertility or childlessness.

There are two further questions here. One is what we mean by a disease or illness. For even if it is correct that physicians should not get involved in the treatment of nondisease conditions, in order to understand the meaning of this limit, we must first identify what counts as a disease. Second, there is the question of whether it is true that medical professionals should in fact confine their professional exertions to the treatment of illness and disease.

In thinking about the first of these questions, I have been much influenced by the definition of a *malady* (a synthetic term used to refer to illnesses, injuries, traumas, and disease conditions) offered by Bernard Gert, Charles Culver, and K. Danner Clouser. According to this definition, a person has a malady

> if and only if he has a condition [within the integument of his body], other than his rational beliefs or desires, such that he is suffering, or is at a significantly increased risk of suffering, a non-trivial harm or evil (death, pain, disability, loss of freedom, or loss of pleasure) in the absence of a distinct sustaining cause.[28]

Although it would require an additional chapter to fully explicate this definition, its most salient—and relevant—points can be quickly noted. First, using Lauritzen's terminology, this definition combines both naturalist and normative elements. The latter are contained in the evils, death, pain, disability, loss of freedom, or loss of pleasure, which all rational persons want to avoid, and which together might be summarized as suffering. Thus, maladies cause the evil of suffering, which all rational persons ordinarily want to avoid, and are rightly addressed by medicine for that moral reason. The naturalist component stems from the definitional requirement that a malady must involve an "increased risk" of suffering these evils. According to Gert, Culver, and Clouser, the baseline measurement of such risk is species normality. To have a malady, the bodily vulnerabilities exposing me to these evils must be significantly above or below that of the species. I do not have a malady if I am likely to die in an atmosphere saturated with carbon monoxide because all human beings perish in this environment. But if ordinary pollen or dust causes me to experience an asthmatic episode, I have a malady because my vulnerability to suffering in this environment is much greater than that of most other persons.

Three other features of this definition directly address the question of medicalization. First is the requirement that a malady be a condition residing within a person's body. A broken tendon causing pain and disability and a poorly functioning pancreas causing diabetes are both maladies, but living within proximity to the devastated Fukushima nuclear power plant is not a malady because, as a cause of increased risk of suffering, it is not a condition of the body (although it will likely cause such conditions—maladies). Second is the qualification that the suffering that is being experienced not be a result of a person's rational beliefs and desires. I do not have a malady if I suffer emotionally when the stock market collapses and decimates my retirement funds because it is perfectly rational to not want such a thing to happen and to suffer when it does. Finally, there is the requirement that a malady not have a distinct sustaining cause, understood as a cause that, once removed, immediately relieves the pain or suffering associated with its presence. A wrestler in a painful hammerlock does not have a malady because the pain will cease the moment his adversary moves away (although, again, such an episode may leave in its wake a malady in terms of tissue damage and inflammation). Gert, Culver, and Clouser argue that some conditions that have been previously diagnosed as maladies are not such because the sufferings associated with them are the result of such distinct sustaining causes. Homosexuality is a leading example. While homosexuals have frequently reported forms of psychological suffering, these appear to result not from homosexuality per se but from the social persecution and marginalization to which homosexuals have so often been subjected.

What are the implications of this definition for our question of medicalization? First, it suggests to me that some of the contentions made by Lauritzen and others regarding infertility are mistaken. Infertility is almost always a disease condition, a malady. It is a disability caused by some malfunctioning bodily organ or system, with *malfunctioning* here making reference to what is species normal. Most males and females of reproductive age and with the appropriate partner are able to reproduce. Those who cannot, because they have blocked fallopian tubes, inadequate endocrinal functioning, or too high temperature in the scrotum caused by a varicocele, have a malady. They have a species-abnormal bodily condition that places them at increased risk of being unable to do what most other human beings can do. Lauritzen claims that a malfunctioning varicocele is not a disease condition because it manifests only to those who want to have a child, but in terms of the definition of a malady, this is irrelevant. An individual with a frayed and vulnerable tendon may not suffer if she chooses not to engage in strenuous sports. But that does not mean that she does not have a malady, and one worthy of medical treatment. The measure here is not what one wants to do with one's body but rather whether a species-abnormal condition increases one's risk of suffering evils. In most cases, infertility is such a condition, even when its immediate bodily cause may be unknown, and even when the treatment may involve unusual medical regimens, such as the use of donor gametes.

These last points are important. We have never required that medical treatments be based on a full knowledge of the etiology of the disease, nor have we limited treatments to repairing the patient's bodily malfunction alone. Venereal diseases were successfully treated with various medications long before the causes of these diseases were well understood. When polio could neither be prevented nor cured at the biological level, iron lungs were successfully used to keep patients alive. In all these cases, efficacy in relieving disease symptoms and in restoring some measure of functioning has been the justifying consideration for therapies. Against this background, it is hard to see why the use of donor gametes does not qualify as an ethically acceptable therapy for infertility that medical professionals may appropriately offer and provide.

There may be reproductive technologies and other practices not easily explained in terms of this definition of malady. The provision of sperm donation, IVF, and donor gametes to homosexual persons to help them have children is an example. It is not species-abnormal for same-sex persons to be unable have children, and their inability to procreate is not a malady. Nevertheless, medical professionals are usually the only ones able to administer desired treatments, and it is hard to see why they should be prevented from applying their skills in such cases. The same logic applies to the broad sphere of cosmetic surgery. Although doctors cannot ethically perform such procedures if they significantly threaten the health of patients, the fact that medical expertise is needed for such procedures and renders them safer is widely regarded as a justification for physicians' involvement. This suggests that patients' desires are one valid component in our moral decision making about the use of medical technologies. They are not the only consideration, however, and as even these cases suggest, there are limits. Doctors should never become the deliberate agents of disease or death.

Although the definition of a malady thus makes clear why some conditions should be ethically suitable for medical treatment, it does not in and of itself decide the question of how far medical professionals may go in preventing or alleviating suffering. Here, a series of further ethically relevant considerations must be invoked. One is whether the condition is best addressed with the skills of medical professionals. A positive answer to this may explain why doctors are involved in assistive reproductive technology treatments, such as helping two lesbians with artificial insemination or IVF. It may explain why some doctors perform male circumcisions that are requested primarily for religious reasons. So long as such procedures are not shown to unnecessarily inflict a malady (where male circumcision is concerned, there is ongoing debate about both sides of this issue[29]), this has been an allowable sphere of medical activity.

Is there no such thing, then, as inappropriate medicalization? Are there no limits to what doctors can do in the relief of suffering? The concept of malady provides a partial answer in its insistence that such conditions be of the patient's body and not the result of a distinct sustaining cause. In general, this excludes physicians' professional attention to what are primarily socially caused evils. Doctors should stick to their area of expertise because it is not helpful, and sometimes is even dangerous, when they extend their prestige and exertions to matters for which they are not trained. No one can dispute the fact that racism and poverty cause many evils in our society, some of them manifest as bodily conditions (such as severe obesity and diabetes). But while doctors and biomedical researchers should legitimately address these medical sequelae and draw attention to the problems, there is no reason for them to be at the forefront of efforts to effect needed social reforms. There are also reasons for concern when doctors apply medical technologies, such as antidepression or antianxiety drugs, to suppress or relieve the symptoms of people suffering from socially caused psychological conditions that ought to be socially addressed. The extreme case—and negative example—of this was Soviet psychiatrists' collusion with authorities in silencing dissent.[30]

Lauritzen is also right to add professional integrity to our list of moral considerations that limit the medical relief of suffering. As he says, "Physicians are not, or at least should not be, 'hired guns' that sell their expertise to the highest bidder or anyone prepared to pay for their services."[31] The respect and trust accorded medical professionals is a socially precious possession that must not be squandered in the quest for riches. Of course, it is not easy to determine when the line is crossed that separates the pursuit of legitimate financial gain from the medical equivalent of ambulance chasing. But as is true in the famous Supreme Court description of pornography, in the more flagrant cases, "we know it when we see it."

To summarize, *medicalization* is a complex concept. Used as a pejorative term to critique activities that go beyond the bounds of what medicine should do, it does not appeal to a single authoritative conception of the limits of medicine. Instead, it is the result of a multifactorial moral decision involving a variety of discrete considerations that work together to warrant a judgment of appropriate or inappropriate behavior. Normally, medicine will focus on the prevention or treatment of maladies, although it can sometimes respond to purely discretionary patient requests and even enhancements, so long as doing so does not violate other medical-ethical obligations and so long as the procedures are best addressed with a medical technology and by a medical professional. Medical treatments should not be used where the causative problems are social or where medical interventions actually sustain or foment the causative evils. And medical professionals should avoid activities, from unrelated financial enterprises to tasteless advertising, that jeopardize respect for their profession.

Conclusion

I have argued that the prevention and relief of suffering, especially the suffering that is occasioned by conditions of the body, provides the moral grounding for medicine, in both its clinical and research dimensions. This understanding is reflected and developed in most of the essays in this volume and applied to such diverse matters as medical education, clinical care, and end-of-life decision making. The essays dealing with religion have the salutary effect of summoning these traditions back to this foundational understanding and away from any tendency, however understandable in historical terms, to value suffering as an intrinsic good. The importance of relieving suffering has ramifications for current debates in bioethics, including the emergent clinical area of genetics and reprogenetics.

I have also argued that the prevention and relief of suffering provides the most formidable justification for limiting the extension of biomedical activities. This concern underlies the structure of research protections that have been elaborated since World War II and the Tuskegee and Willowbrook disclosures. It provides the underlying rationale for those reasonable deontological limits that have been proposed in end-of-life and palliative medicine (as well as the positive rationale for palliative efforts). Despite the importance of autonomy and the relief of suffering, both must be resisted when they reasonably threaten even greater evils for many people. The key word here is *reasonably*. It is not enough to advance deontological principles to limit the relief of suffering or to simply assert that violating such principles threatens grave harms. Such claims must be supported by sound arguments and solid evidence where it is available. This is especially true in the setting of a religiously pluralistic society in which appeals to metaphysical beliefs and values must be set aside and only undeniably shared values invoked when justifying moral policies.

Finally, I have argued that medicine and medical professionals per se do not have to address all the evils that underlie or cause suffering. There are limits, the exceeding of which is well described as *medicalization*. Nevertheless, there is no magical formula for determining where these limits should be set. Distinctions such as "treatment versus enhancement" or "physiologically indicated versus merely desired" will not do. What is involved, instead, is a multifactorial judgment about which policy best serves all of our interests and is most likely to reduce suffering.

Notes

1. Eric J. Cassell, *The Nature of Suffering and the Goals of Medicine*, 2nd ed. (New York: Oxford University Press, 1991), 32.

2. *Suffering and Bioethics*, Chapter 7, p. 138.

3. Schlieter observes that early Buddhist texts suggest that animals may actually suffer more than human beings (Chapter 16, p. 312). The question of whether animals subjected to confinement and painful experiments suffer more than human beings, who at least have the advantage of comprehension of why they are suffering, is an important one for the evaluation of the use of animals in biomedical research.

4. James Gorman, "Changing Perspectives Propel Chimp Protections," *New York Times*, June 15, 2013. But see also John L. Vandeberg, "Apes Need Vaccines, Too," *New York Times*, August 1, 2013.

5. Cassell, *The Nature of Suffering*, 35.

6. *Suffering and Bioethics,* p. 338. I will not here develop my disagreements with Cherry's essay, other than to say that his presentation of Rawls's position raises many critical questions. Among other things, the essay takes Rawls's earlier and later qualifications of the universality of his two principles of justice as a critique and relativization of Rawls's entire moral approach. But Rawls never suggests that his basic Kantian moral methodology, with its reliance on impartiality and primary goods, is culturally specific or subject to change.

7. John Rawls, *A Theory of Justice* (Cambridge, MA: Harvard University Press, 1971), 62, § 15, 90–95.

8. *Suffering and Bioethics,* Chapter 4, p. 82.

9. *Suffering and Bioethics,* Chapter 12, p. 251.

10. *Suffering and Bioethics,* Chapter 7, p. 150.

11. *Suffering and Moral Responsibility* (New York: Oxford University Press, 1999), 111.

12. Ibid., chap. 8.

13. For one discussion of these links, see Bernard Gert, K. Danner Clouser, and Ronald M. Green, "The Method of Public Morality versus the Method of Principlism," *Journal of Medicine and Philosophy 18* (1993): 477–489.

14. For a presentation of my own views on this matter, see Ronald M. Green, *The Human Embryo Research Debates* (New York: Oxford University Press, 2001), chap. 2.

15. Several studies indicate that Catholic self-description does not appear to influence couples' attitudes to the disposition of their embryos used in IVF. See C. Laruelle and Y. Englert, "The Psychological Study of In Vitro Fertilization–Embryo Transfer Participants," *Fertility and Sterility 63* (1995), 1047–1050; C. Laruelle and Y. Englert, "Devenir des Embryons Surnuméraires et Risque de Grossesse Multiple en Fécondation In Vitro: Qu'en Pensent les Couple Concernés," *Revue Médicale de Bruxelles 17* (1996), 115–119; V. Provoost et al., "Infertility Patients' Beliefs about Their Embryos and Their Disposition Preferences," *Human Reproduction 1/1* (2009): 1–10. The widespread lay Catholic acceptance of IVF is also suggested by relatively unimpeded development and growth of IVF services in Ireland, where other Catholic teachings about sexuality continue to play a considerable role in public policy. See Robert Harrison "The Development of IVF Practice in Ireland: A Personal View," *Human Fertility 15/1* (2012): 3–10.

16. *Suffering and Bioethics,* Chapter 10, p. 210.

17. See Ronald M. Green, "Health and Disease in Religions," *International Encyclopedia of Ethics*, published online, February 1, 2013, DOI: 10.1002/9781444367072.wbiee784.

18. *Suffering and Bioethics,* Chapter 13, p. 264.

19. Green, "Health and Disease in Religions," supra note 17.

20. Ronald Cole-Turner and Brent Waters, *Pastoral Genetics: Theology and Care at the Beginning of Life* (Cleveland: Pilgrim Press, 1996), p. 139.

21. *Suffering and Bioethics,* Chapter 12, p. 255.

22. *Suffering and Bioethics,* Chapter 11, p. 237.

23. *Suffering and Bioethics,* Chapter 13, p. 265.

24. *Suffering and Bioethics,* Chapter 13, p. 268.

25. *Suffering and Bioethics,* Chapter 13, p. 269.

26. *Suffering and Bioethics,* Chapter 13, p. 269.

27. Joseph E. Davis, "Medicalization, Social Control, and the Relief of Suffering." In *The New Blackwell Companion to Medical Sociology*, ed. William C. Cockerham (Malden, MA: Wiley-Blackwell, 2010), 211–241.

28. B. Gert, C. M. Culver, and K. D. Clouser, "Malady," in *Bioethics: A Return to Fundamentals* (New York: Oxford University Press, 1997), chap. 5. I have inserted in parentheses wording from the authors' further description of the meaning of "a condition."

29. For treatment of two sides to the recent debates over male circumcision, see Brian D. Earp, "The Ethics of Infant Male Circumcision," *Journal of Medical Ethics 39/7* (2013): 418–420; and Joseph Mazor, "The Child's Interests and the Case for the Permissibility of Male Infant Circumcision," *Journal of Medical Ethics 39/7* (2013): 421–428. Other views are also found in this special issue of the journal.

30. United States Congress, House Committee on Foreign Affairs, Subcommittee on Human Rights and International Organizations, *Abuse of Psychiatry in the Soviet Union: Hearing before the Subcommittee on Human Rights and International Organizations of the Committee on Foreign Affairs and the Commission on Security and Cooperation in Europe, House of Representatives, Ninety-eighth Congress, first session*, September 20, 1983 (Washington, DC: U.S. Government Printing Office, 1984).

31. *Suffering and Bioethics,* Chapter 18, p. 361f.

INDEX

Page numbers followed by "f" and "t" indicate figures and tables.